PROBIOTIC BEVERAGES

PROBIOTIC BEVERAGES

Edited by

SANDEEP K. PANDA
School of Biotechnology, KIIT University, Bhubaneswar, Odisha, India

JULIE KELLERSHOHN
Ted Rogers School of Hospitality and Tourism Management, Ryerson University, Toronto, Ontario, Canada

INGE RUSSELL
Heriot-Watt University, Edinburgh, Scotland, United Kingdom

ELSEVIER

ACADEMIC PRESS
An imprint of Elsevier

Academic Press is an imprint of Elsevier
125 London Wall, London EC2Y 5AS, United Kingdom
525 B Street, Suite 1650, San Diego, CA 92101, United States
50 Hampshire Street, 5th Floor, Cambridge, MA 02139, United States
The Boulevard, Langford Lane, Kidlington, Oxford OX5 1GB, United Kingdom

Library of Congress Cataloging-in-Publication Data
A catalog record for this book is available from the Library of Congress

British Library Cataloguing-in-Publication Data
A catalogue record for this book is available from the British Library

ISBN 978-0-12-818588-9

For information on all Academic Press publications
visit our website at https://www.elsevier.com/books-and-journals

Publisher: Charlotte Cockle
Acquisitions Editor: Patricia Osborn
Editorial Project Manager: Lena Sparks
Production Project Manager: Kumar Anbazhagan
Cover Designer: Victoria Pearson

Typeset by SPi Global, India

Contents

Contributors **xiii**

I

Editorial chapter—Introduction

1. Introduction and overview
Sandeep K. Panda, Julie Kellershohn, and Inge Russell

1.1 Introduction 3
References 6

II

Geography and probiotic beverages

2. Probiotic beverages in India: History and current developments
Swati S. Mishra, Urmimala Das, Ramakrishna Biswal, and Sudhanshu S. Behera

2.1 Introduction 9
2.2 Principles and origins of probiotic systems 10
2.3 The history of probiotic beverages in India 11
2.4 An Indian perspective of probiotic beverages 12
2.5 Ethnic probiotic beverages in India 21
2.6 Probiotic beverages in modern India 25
2.7 Probiotic beverages as food and health supplements 26
2.8 Indian market of probiotic beverages 27
2.9 Indian government regulations on probiotic beverages 27
2.10 Conclusions and future prospectives 28
References 28

3. Probiotic beverages in Japan (some history and current developments)
Hirosuke Sugahara and Tatsuhiko Hirota

3.1 Introduction 35
3.2 Market trends and category of probiotic beverages in Japan 37

3.3 Drinkable yogurts with probiotic strains 38
3.4 Drinks based on fermented milk with probiotic strains 40
3.5 Other types of beverages containing probiotic strains 41
3.6 Beverages with paraprobiotic strains 42
3.7 Conclusions 44
References 45

4. Probiotic beverages in China
Wei Chen

4.1 Probiotic milk beverages in China 49
4.2 Probiotic fruit and vegetable beverages in China 51
4.3 Probiotic cereal beverages in China 55
References 57

5. Fermented foods and probiotic beverages in Korea
Kwangsei Lim and Jongho Koh

5.1 Introduction 61
5.2 Fermented foods in Korea 62
5.3 Health functional foods 66
5.4 Probiotic beverages and fermented products in Korea 70
5.5 Market perspectives 77
References 77

6. Probiotic beverages in Thailand: Health attributes and future trends
Sudsai Trevanich

6.1 Introduction 81
6.2 Current and future trends in research development of probiotic beverages in Thailand 82
6.3 Commercial probiotic beverage market in Thailand and health benefits of these beverages 91
6.4 Future considerations 95
References 95
Further reading 97

7. Probiotic beverages: Health benefits and current trends in the Middle East
Neda Mollakhalili Meybodi, Sarah Sanaei Nasab, Nasim Khorshidian, and Amir M. Mortazavian

7.1 Introduction 99
7.2 Health benefits of probiotic beverages 101
7.3 Types of probiotic beverage 102
7.4 Conclusions 121
References 121

8. Current trends and opportunities of plant-based non-alcoholic probiotic beverages: A European and African perspective

Juliana Mandha, Habtu Shumoy, Athanasia O. Matemu, and Katleen Raes

8.1 Introduction 127
8.2 Plant-based non-alcoholic beverages in Europe 128
8.3 Plant-based non-alcoholic beverages in Africa 139
8.4 Conclusions 149
Acknowledgments 149
References 149

9. The Americas

Inge Russell

9.1 Introduction 159
9.2 The USA and probiotic beverages 160
9.3 Regulation of use in the USA 160
9.4 Canada 162
9.5 Canadian regulations governing claims on probiotics 163
9.6 Mexico 164
9.7 Latin America 167
9.8 Concluding thoughts 169
References 170

III

Health and genomics

10. Probiotics: Emerging functional ingredients for healthy aging and age-related diseases

Pei Lei Tan and Sae Hun Kim

10.1 Introduction 175
10.2 Hallmarks of aging as a potential target for probiotics intervention 177
10.3 Probiotics for healthy aging 179
10.4 Probiotics for age-related diseases 187
10.5 Conclusions 202
References 202

11. TRP channels in the gut: Effect of probiotics and phyto-nutraceuticals on gut-brain-immune axis

Sushama Mohanta and Chandan Goswami

11.1 Introduction to TRP ion channels 213
11.2 Expression of TRPs in the gut 215
11.3 TRPs in gut epithelia 215

11.4 TRPs as regulators of the gut-neuronal system 216
11.5 TRPs as regulators of the gut-immune system 217
11.6 Involvement of TRPs in gut inflammation, irritable bowel syndrome, and other gut-related disorders 219
11.7 Bacterial lipopolysaccharides and bacterial toxins and their effects on TRPs 221
11.8 TRPs as regulators of the gut-brain axis 223
11.9 Evolution of gut function and TRPs 225
11.10 Variability in TRPs in the human population and choice of food/beverage selections 225
11.11 Food supplements and their effects on TRPs 226
11.12 Different probiotic factors that can target TRPs in the gut 227
11.13 Prospects and conclusions 230
Acknowledgment 230
References 230

12. Application of genomics, transcriptomics, and proteomics in probiotic research
Susrita Sahoo, Soumya R. Mahapatra, Namrata Misra, and Mrutyunjay Suar

12.1 Overview 235
12.2 OMICS-approaches to study probiotics and beneficial effects on the host 236
12.3 Probiotic focused bioinformatics databases 247
12.4 Future application of omics in development of engineered probiotics strains 247
References 249

IV

Production and quality

13. Starter cultures for probiotic beverages: A comparative study of traditional and modern approaches
Nasim Khorshidian, Mojtaba Yousefi, Neda Mollakhalili Meybodi, and Amir M. Mortazavian

13.1 Introduction 259
13.2 Starter cultures 260
13.3 Bacteria as starter cultures in probiotic beverages 263
13.4 Yeasts as starter cultures in beverages 270
13.5 Coculture/mixed culture application in probiotic beverages 270
13.6 Bioactive compounds in beverages produced by starter cultures 272
13.7 Immobilization technology for starter cultures 275
13.8 Conclusions 276
References 277

V

Technologies and legalities

14. Kefir, kombucha, and sour beers

Lopamudra Sahu and Sandeep K. Panda

14.1 Introduction 287
14.2 Brief background of kefir, kombucha, and sour beer 288
14.3 Preparation technology 291
14.4 Microbial dynamics in kefir, kombucha, and sour beer during the course of fermentation 294
14.5 Health-promoting potentials of kefir, kombucha, and sour beer 298
14.6 Current market status, consumers' preference and future of kefir, kombucha, and sour beer 299
14.7 Blending of beverages and the market purview! 300
14.8 Advances in technology and future perspectives 301
14.9 Conclusions 302
References 303

15. Probiotic lactobacillus strains for enhanced health benefits (genetic engineering and microencapsulation)

Gargi Dey, Didier Montet, and Phillippe Thonart

15.1 Introduction 309
15.2 Current global probiotic products 310
15.3 Emerging techniques for future probiotics 310
15.4 Conclusions 329
References 329
Further reading 337

16. Packaging for probiotic beverages

Natalia Lumby and Jonghun (Jay) Park

16.1 Introduction 339
16.2 The package 339
16.3 The packaging process 346
16.4 Future trends in probiotic beverage packaging 350
16.5 Conclusion 360
References 360

17. Microbial safety issues related to probiotic beverages and the organisms used in their manufacture

Md Latiful Bari and Md Arafat Al Mamun

17.1 Introduction 365
17.2 Safety of probiotic bacteria 368

17.3 Quality control of probiotic beverages 377
17.4 Conclusions 382
References 382

18. Quality control of probiotic beverages and organisms
Martins Ajibade Adefisoye, Ezekiel Green, Patrick Berka Njobeh, Ajibola Bamikole Oyedeji, and Oluwafemi Ayodeji Adebo

18.1 Introduction 389
18.2 Criteria for quality control of probiotics 391
18.3 Conclusion and future perspectives 397
Acknowledgment 400
References 400
Further reading 402

19. Legalities, intellectual property, ethical concerns and regulatory aspects in probiotics
Sripathi Rao Kulkarni

19.1 Introduction 403
19.2 Probiotic markets 405
19.3 Health claims 407
19.4 Intellectual property and probiotics—Some examples of products 407
19.5 Summary of patents and patent applications for probiotics 409
19.6 Intellectual property related disputes 412
19.7 Regulations: The need for probiotic guidelines 413
19.8 Genetically modified microorganisms 420
19.9 Gaps in policies 422
19.10 Summary 423
Acknowledgment 423
References 423

VI
Marketing probiotic beverages

20. Marketing probiotic beverages
Julie Kellershohn

20.1 Introduction 427
20.2 Global market size 427
20.3 Consumer needs and wants 428
20.4 The market for probiotic beverages spans dayparts, occasions, and consumer preferences 429
20.5 Beyond probiotics 431
20.6 "Clean label" and "absence of" 432

20.7 Benefit stacking and health halos in new product development 432
20.8 New technologies 433
20.9 Developing market opportunities—The young, the old, and the athlete 434
20.10 The market message in 2020 435
20.11 Concluding thoughts 439
References 439
Organization links 439
Product website links 440

21. Thoughts on the future of probiotic beverages

Spiros Paramithiotis, Maria K. Syrokou, and Eleftherios H. Drosinos

21.1 Introduction 441
21.2 Isolation of strains and the in vitro characterization of probiotic potential 442
21.3 Advances in dairy probiotic beverages 447
21.4 Development of nondairy probiotic beverages 449
21.5 Next-generation probiotics 456
21.6 Conclusions 458
References 458

Index 467

Contributors

Oluwafemi Ayodeji Adebo Department of Biotechnology and Food Technology, Faculty of Science, University of Johannesburg, Gauteng, South Africa

Martins Ajibade Adefisoye Department of Biotechnology and Food Technology, Faculty of Science, University of Johannesburg, Gauteng, South Africa

Md Latiful Bari Centre for Advanced Research in Sciences, University of Dhaka, Dhaka, Bangladesh

Sudhanshu S. Behera Ayurinno Legacy (OPC) Private Limited, Foundation for Technology & Business Incubation, TIIR Building, National Institute of Technology, Rourkela; Fisheries and Animal Resources Development Department, Directorate of Fisheries, Government of Odisha, Cuttack, Odisha, India

Ramakrishna Biswal Department of Humanities and Social Sciences, National Institute of Technology, Rourkela, Odisha, India

Wei Chen Jiangnan University, Wuxi, Jiangsu Province, People's Republic of China

Urmimala Das Ayurinno Legacy (OPC) Private Limited, Foundation for Technology & Business Incubation, TIIR Building, National Institute of Technology, Rourkela, Odisha, India

Gargi Dey School of Biotechnology, KIIT University, Bhubaneswar, India

Eleftherios H. Drosinos Laboratory of Food Quality Control and Hygiene, Department of Food Science and Human Nutrition, Agricultural University of Athens, Athens, Greece

Chandan Goswami National Institute of Science Education and Research, School of Biological Sciences, Khurda, Odisha; Homi Bhabha National Institute, Mumbai, India

Ezekiel Green Department of Biotechnology and Food Technology, Faculty of Science, University of Johannesburg, Gauteng, South Africa

Tatsuhiko Hirota Core Technology Laboratories, Asahi Quality & Innovations, Ltd., Moriya-shi, Ibaraki, Japan

Julie Kellershohn Ted Rogers School of Hospitality and Tourism Management, Ryerson University, Toronto, ON, Canada

Nasim Khorshidian Food Safety Research Center (Salt), Semnan University of Medical Sciences, Semnan, Iran

Sae Hun Kim College of Life Science and Biotechnology, Korea University, Seoul, South Korea

Jongho Koh Department of Bio-food Analysis and Technology, Bio Campus, Korea Polytechnics College, Nonsan, South Korea

Sripathi Rao Kulkarni Business Development-Intellectual Property Unit, CSIR-Central Drug Research Institute, Lucknow, Uttar Pradesh, India

Kwangsei Lim Research & Innovation Center, Danone Pulmuone Co., Ltd., Seoul, South Korea

Natalia Lumby School of Graphic Communications Management, Ryerson University, Toronto, ON, Canada

Soumya R. Mahapatra School of Biotechnology, Kalinga Institute of Industrial Technology (KIIT), Deemed to be University, Bhubaneswar, India

Md Arafat Al Mamun Centre for Advanced Research in Sciences, University of Dhaka, Dhaka, Bangladesh

Juliana Mandha Ghent University Campus Kortrijk, Kortrijk, West Flanders, Belgium; Nelson Mandela African Institution of Science and Technology, Arusha, Tanzania

Athanasia O. Matemu Nelson Mandela African Institution of Science and Technology, Arusha, Tanzania

Swati S. Mishra Department of Biodiversity and Conservation of Natural Resources, Central University of Odisha, Koraput, Odisha, India

Namrata Misra School of Biotechnology; KIIT-Technology Business Incubator (KIIT-TBI), Kalinga Institute of Industrial Technology (KIIT), Deemed to be University, Bhubaneswar, India

Sushama Mohanta National Institute of Science Education and Research, School of Biological Sciences, Khurda, Odisha; Homi Bhabha National Institute, Mumbai, India

Neda Mollakhalili Meybodi Department of Food Sciences and Technology, School of Public Health; Research Centre for Food Hygiene and Safety, Shahid Sadoughi University of Medical Sciences, Yazd, Iran

Didier Montet UMR95 QualiSud Cirad Université of Montpellier, Montpellier, France

Amir M. Mortazavian Department of Food Science and Technology, National Nutrition and Food Technology Research Institute, Faculty of Nutrition Sciences, Food Science and Technology, Shahid Beheshti University of Medical Sciences, Tehran, Iran

Sarah Sanaei Nasab Department of Food Sciences and Technology, School of Public Health, Shahid Sadoughi University of Medical Sciences, Yazd, Iran

Patrick Berka Njobeh Department of Biotechnology and Food Technology, Faculty of Science, University of Johannesburg, Gauteng, South Africa

Ajibola Bamikole Oyedeji Department of Biotechnology and Food Technology, Faculty of Science, University of Johannesburg, Gauteng, South Africa

Sandeep K. Panda School of Biotechnology, KIIT University, Bhubaneswar, India

Spiros Paramithiotis Laboratory of Food Quality Control and Hygiene, Department of Food Science and Human Nutrition, Agricultural University of Athens, Athens, Greece

Jonghun (Jay) Park School of Graphic Communications Management, Ryerson University, Toronto, ON, Canada

Katleen Raes Ghent University Campus Kortrijk, Kortrijk, West Flanders, Belgium

Inge Russell ICBD, Heriot Watt University, Edinburgh, United Kingdom

Susrita Sahoo School of Biotechnology, Kalinga Institute of Industrial Technology (KIIT), Deemed to be University, Bhubaneswar, India

Lopamudra Sahu Department of Botany, Utkal University, Bhubaneswar, India

Habtu Shumoy Ghent University Campus Kortrijk, Kortrijk, West Flanders, Belgium

Mrutyunjay Suar School of Biotechnology; KIIT-Technology Business Incubator (KIIT-TBI), Kalinga Institute of Industrial Technology (KIIT), Deemed to be University, Bhubaneswar, India

Hirosuke Sugahara Core Technology Laboratories, Asahi Quality & Innovations, Ltd., Moriya-shi, Ibaraki, Japan

Maria K. Syrokou Laboratory of Food Quality Control and Hygiene, Department of Food Science and Human Nutrition, Agricultural University of Athens, Athens, Greece

Pei Lei Tan College of Life Science and Biotechnology, Korea University, Seoul, South Korea

Phillippe Thonart Walloon Center for Industrial Biology, Microbial Technology Unit, University of Liège, Gembloux, Belgium

Sudsai Trevanich Department of Food Science and Technology, Faculty of Agro-Industry, Kasetsart University, Bangkok, Thailand

Mojtaba Yousefi Food Safety Research Center (Salt), Semnan University of Medical Sciences, Semnan, Iran

PART I

Editorial chapter—Introduction

CHAPTER

1

Introduction and overview

Sandeep K. Panda[a], *Julie Kellershohn*[b], *and Inge Russell*[c]

[a]School of Biotechnology, KIIT University, Bhubaneswar, India
[b]Ted Rogers School of Hospitality and Tourism Management, Ryerson University, Toronto, ON, Canada
[c]ICBD, Heriot Watt University, Edinburgh, United Kingdom

1.1 Introduction

Probiotic beverages have been around for thousands of years, so why have they recently become one of the trendiest and best-selling health drink products on the market?

The Romans drank fermented milk to treat intestinal problems over 1000 years ago, yet we only now are starting to understand how the probiotic bacteria in these drinks provide health benefits. In the 1800s, scientist Ilya Mechnikov identified that it was the bacteria in the milk products that were providing health benefits; yet 200 years later, why is there still controversy over which probiotic bacteria provide which benefits? This confusion among consumers about microorganisms and the health-promoting potential of probiotic beverages has persisted for decades. Questions are still not wholly resolved regarding which organisms provide the most benefit and which benefits have been scientifically proven to the satisfaction of the general consumer.

If we look at purchase survey results, then we see that consumers clearly believe that they are experiencing benefits from probiotic beverages, otherwise there would not be the global consumer market for these drinks, even though the specific health concerns that the beverages are marketed to address varies in the different countries. The large proportion of consumers that take some type of probiotic product for their health is demonstrated by consumer demand and interest by geography. In Germany, 54% of the population claim to take probiotic products to boost

Probiotic Beverages
https://doi.org/10.1016/B978-0-12-818588-9.00020-6

the immune system (FMCG Gurus—Probiotic Survey Germany, 2018), in China, 62% take probiotics to aid the digestive system (FMCG Gurus—Probiotic Survey China, 2018), in the USA 67% take probiotics to promote a healthy gut (Mintel, 2020), and in Argentina 85% take probiotics to aid in digestion (FMCG Gurus—Probiotic Survey Argentina, 2019).

In the midst of a global health pandemic, there is even greater interest in foods that support immune health and consumers want more access to information. There is a hunger for clarity in 2020 and 4 out of 10 surveyed consumers describe wanting to know more about the effectiveness of probiotics in terms of ingredients and efficacy (GlobalData Coronavirus (COVID-19), 2020).

Both producers and consumers struggle with what is the best format for a probiotic drink? Which bacterial strains have been proven to provide a health benefit and to which consumers? What other ingredients in the product offer health benefits? How tasty and appealing is the drink? Modern consumers are aware of the functional attributes of different food products and there is a growing research field focused on the health-promoting potential of probiotic drinks. The millennial consumer is particularly interested in novelty and variety and they look for more than classical flavors and formats. Probiotic beverages containing prebiotics, probiotics and postbiotics are emerging as a "smart beverage" appropriate for the times.

How can one evaluate the drink's safety? What regulations are in place in different countries to ensure that the labelling is truthful about the effectiveness of the drink's contents? Every day we hear more in the popular press about the microbiome and how it is now viewed as a new organ system in the body. How does drinking a probiotic beverage align with having a healthy microbiome?

When a consumer is trying to select the best probiotic drink for their needs, the choices are abundant. How can they decipher the accuracy of product claims, which are often based on marketing material or on information from social media?

What are the local country regulations for a probiotic drink? Local regulations may be nonexistent where any claim can be made regardless of scientific truth or they may be very strong and well monitored for adherence. Today's consumer values honesty and demands transparency. Are the probiotic organisms in the drink appropriate for the benefit being sought and are the organisms alive and active? At what level are they present in the drink? Are the company's claims about sustainability and social responsibility factual? In 2020, consumers are embracing the buyer philosophy of "good for me and good for we."

Probiotic beverages vary by geographical location, depending on the local cultural practice. This book extensively covers the probiotic beverages of different continents and countries. Kombucha's move from an ancient Chinese beverage to a mainstream global commercial product in the North American market is one such example. Other drink success stories include similar mainstream moves for kefirs and sour beers.

In separate chapters, Africa, China, Europe, Japan, India, Korea, The Americas, The Middle East, and Thailand are geographies where their local probiotic drinks are explored and their history and their current production methods provide the reader with a better understanding of how some of these local beverages, combined traditional local wisdoms with broader market opportunities, to create global drinks.

The importance of probiotics in human health is one of the most debated areas. Three chapters in the book are dedicated to critically explaining and illustrating the potential of probiotics in age-related disease, impacts on the gut-brain axis, and the application of microengineering to enhance the efficacy of probiotics. The application of genomics is an important facet of the latest research trends, and one chapter exclusively covers the advances in genomics, transcriptomics, and proteomic studies with probiotic organisms and what these advances may mean for the future.

A chapter of the book is dedicated to the very important issue of starter cultures as well as chapters on quality control and microbial safety. A separate chapter is dedicated to packaging and how can the producer maintain quality and safety in product packaging. Although regulations are important as a consumer protection tool, legalities, intellectual property, and ethical concerns can pose barriers to innovation and new product development.

Last, the book examines the marketing of some new probiotic drinks on the market. How has the marketing focus changed for these new drinks and why are social media tools and influencers so important? What will consumers be looking for in 2021 and how do the current products on the market address consumer articulated and unarticulated needs?

The editors of this book come from three very different backgrounds—research on probiotic organisms, the challenges of biotechnology, especially in the area of fermentation science, new product development, and marketing. By reaching out to their global colleagues, the editors were able to ask experts to summarize for the reader highlights in the various areas of interest, from local history to global production, to packaging, and marketing.

COVID-19 has greatly disrupted the entire probiotic market. However, it has also generated more interest in probiotic beverages in a short period of time than in what would normally have been much slower market growth. Consumers are looking for ways to increase their health and immunity status. The beverage route is appealing as it fits easily into their lifestyle and is preferred by many to ingesting probiotics in pill form. This book was never meant to provide recipes for producing probiotic drinks at home—there are many other books in the marketplace that provide that information. Rather, this book provides the reader with a depth of knowledge that spans more than just one product or one promise of a health benefit. Without understanding the wider view of probiotic beverages globally, one cannot process the deluge of information available today—some being found in high-quality research (in trusted scientific journals), some that is interesting speculation and food for thought, and some that is blatant misinformation.

This book provides a concise and up to date collection of information that is valuable, and indeed critical, to anyone working in the area of probiotic beverages, whether that be production, marketing, or as a consumer who wishes to be well informed. It is a must-read textbook on what you need to know about probiotic beverages in today's marketplace.

References

FMCG Gurus—Probiotic Survey Argentina (2019).
FMCG Gurus—Probiotic Survey China (2018).
FMCG Gurus—Probiotic Survey Germany (2018).
GlobalData Coronavirus (COVID-19) (2020). *Consumer survey consolidated results, week 1-6.*
Mintel (2020). *The future of nutrition, health and wellness.*

PART II

Geography and probiotic beverages

CHAPTER

2

Probiotic beverages in India: History and current developments

Swati S. Mishra[a], *Urmimala Das*[b], *Ramakrishna Biswal*[c], *and Sudhanshu S. Behera*[b,d]

[a]Department of Biodiversity and Conservation of Natural Resources, Central University of Odisha, Koraput, Odisha, India[b]Ayurinno Legacy (OPC) Private Limited, Foundation for Technology & Business Incubation, TIIR Building, National Institute of Technology, Rourkela, Odisha, India[c]Department of Humanities and Social Sciences, National Institute of Technology, Rourkela, Odisha, India[d]Fisheries and Animal Resources Development Department, Directorate of Fisheries, Government of Odisha, Cuttack, Odisha, India

2.1 Introduction

Beneficial bacteria, called 'probiotics," have been used for the fermentation of foods/drinks for over 6000 years, mainly in cultures developed in Babylon, Egypt, and the Indus Valley (Beniwal, Semwal, & Navani, 2019). In various rural areas of India, people have relied on fermentation to develop different flavor characteristics of foods prepared by various traditional processing techniques from available raw materials as per their sociocultural ethics, religion and ethnic preferences (Mishra, Ray, & Rosell, 2017; Sharma, Attri, & Goel, 2019).

The achievement/probability of a probiotic drink depends on the effectiveness of probiotics in providing/nurturing cells capable of effectively modifying the host's effective microbiota (Angmo, Kumari, & Bhalla, 2016). However, traditional functional foods/fermented foods/probiotic

Probiotic Beverages
https://doi.org/10.1016/B978-0-12-818588-9.00010-3

drinks have been made in many parts of India for centuries. These juices/drinks are made by tribal people using indigenous knowledge and local raw materials. Depending on the raw material used, two essential groups of probiotic drinks (dairy and non-dairy) are produced by natural/spontaneous fermentation or probiotic addition. The addition of active bacterial cultures can be considered by the consumer as an added value and a high-quality marker (Saranraj, Behera, & Ray, 2019). Due to the rise in dynamic lifestyles and culture of fast food/junk food, people all over the world are facing challenges and this has led to the preference for alternative foods and many probiotic health products (Lakshmy, Devi, & Ramesh, 2018; Mishra, Ray, Panda, & Montet, 2017). The presence of probiotics is behind the enhanced sensory and medical properties of many fermented beverages. Adoption of probiotics in commercial fermented food/beverages, in a country such as India, to prevent various diseases rather than seeking them through the production of probiotic beverages at the household level was inevitable (Lakshmy et al., 2018). In recent years, the biggest market segment of probiotics is in the form of liquid products. Fluid probiotics were readily accepted for infants and consumers that face difficulty in consuming pills. Novel products are accessible in the marketplace, such as yogurt-based drinks and probiotic-infused juices, which give consumers new choices of probiotic sources and are regarded as offering a functional improvement in consumer health (Garcia, Guerin, Souidi, & Remize, 2020).

The use of probiotics in dairy and non-dairy beverages has been extensively investigated worldwide, while other metrics, particularly India's interest, is less documented (Behera, Bal, Das, Panda, & Mohanty, 2018). This chapter includes literature on indigenous probiotic drinks, new trends related to traditional probiotic drinks, lactic acid bacteria (LAB) diversity, the effect of processing steps, and perceived nutritional and health benefits in the Indian context.

2.2 Principles and origins of probiotic systems

The concept of 'probiotic' has been precisely defined as "living microorganisms," which when consumed in certain numbers have far more health benefits than general nutrition (Prado, Parada, Pandey, & Soccol, 2008). In general, beneficial microorganisms can thrive and be present in high numbers in the gastrointestinal (GI) tract, when consumed in oral doses (about $>10^9$ cells per day) (Behera, Ray, Das, Panda, & Saranraj, 2019; Vasudha & Mishra, 2013). These probiotic microorganisms/beneficial microorganisms are already present in the GI tract and hence are "generally regarded as safe" (GRAS) (Angmo et al., 2016). Lactic acid bacteria (LAB) strains have been the most evaluated probiotics in the previous decades. They are known to perform some fundamental tasks such as nourishment safeguarding, improve nourishment stockpiling, and limiting food-borne microorganisms or pathogens through the generation of biochemicals such as lactic acid (LA), acetic acid, hydrogen peroxide, bacteriocin, diacetyl and carbon dioxide (Angmo et al., 2016). The most common probiotics are members of the genera *Lactobacillus* and *Bifidobacterium*. They are established in a variety of environmental niches, including dairy beverages and unfermented probiotic drinks made from dairy products (Angmo et al., 2016; Beniwal et al., 2019).

2.3 The history of probiotic beverages in India

The methods for the preparation of the probiotic beverage/alcoholic drink '*soma runs*' might have developed in the Vedic period (2500–200 BCE) of Indian history, around the Indus River (Tamang, Thapa, Tamang, Rai, & Chettri, 2015). Alcohol is widely consumed in India (from the Vedic East) and special mention of this consumption among tribes is referred in the Ramayana (during 300–75 BCE) and is well established in Asia, and still continues today (Tamang, Thapa, & Bhalla, 2016).

Both wine fermentation and malting processes, are thought of as one of the oldest food processing practices in food history but are rarely used in traditional fermentation processes in India. As an alternative, an amylolytic mixed starter is commonly used, which is obtained from cultivated strains of LAB and/or yeast and/or mold on cooked or raw cereals/legumes - cereals/vegetables/fruits (Tamang, 2010; Behera & Panda, 2020). Historical records give some data on the fermented alcohol beverages in India. For instance, *Kodo Koh Jaan*, a blended beverage of developed finger millet from the Himalayas region, is referred to all through the Nepal in the Kirat Dynasty (625 BCE–100 CE) (Adhikari & Ghimirey, 2000; Tamang et al., 2015).

2.4 An Indian perspective of probiotic beverages

Probiotic drinks have traditionally been made by the local population and have preserved a unique microflora over the centuries. Ethnic fermented/probiotic drinks are a study focus for developing new probiotic microorganisms and novel biologically active compounds (Beniwal et al., 2019; Mishra, Behera, Kar, & Ray, 2018; Sahu & Panda, 2018).

2.4.1 Dairy-based probiotic beverages

Traditional fermented probiotic beverages, such as yogurts and fermented kinds of milk, are marketed in India. The fermented milk products are different from yogurts as they use starters of mixed cultures (i.e., mesophilic *Lactococci)* (Routray & Mishra, 2012). Naturally/spontaneously fermented and processed milk foods, such as *dahi, chhu, chhurpi, lassi* and *mohi* (from cow/buffalo/yak milk) are rich sources of nutrition and are found in many societies (Kemgang, Kapila, Shanmugam, & Kapila, 2014). *Dahi*/curd/Indian yogurt is a famous and frequently consumed conventional Indian fermented milk product. It is prepared by the maturation/fermentation of milk utilizing the mesophilic *Lactococcus*, to which *Leuconostoc* is sometimes included as a partner organism (Routray & Mishra, 2012). Lactobacillus strains are the most predominant microorganisms in different Indian fermented milk products (but are not limited to *Streptococcus* and *Lactococcus* species) (Routray & Mishra, 2012). *Dahi* is the main spontaneous/natural fermented milk product for the consumption in Darjeeling Hills, Sikkim, and is a part of the diet of the Himalayan tribal people as well (Beniwal et al., 2019). Beniwal et al. (2019) reported that the LAB strains from *dahi* were identified as *Enterococcus faecalis, E. faecium* and *Lc. lactis* based on 16S rRNA gene sequencing analysis. Kemgang et al. (2014) reported that *Lb. rhamnosus* S1K3 in *dahi* produces antimicrobial compounds that resist foodborne pathogens. Naturally fermented milk (NFM) products from cow and/or yak milk are common in Sikkim and Arunachal Pradesh, India; *chhurpi* (a protein-rich supplement) and *gheu/mar* (a fat-rich food additive) contribute significantly to the livelihood of the local community (Shangpliang, Rai, Keisam, Jeyaram, & Tamang, 2018). *Gheu/mar* (a crude butter) is a product that is rich in fat and obtained by churning milk. *Chhurpi/Churapi* (a cottage cheese–like product) is a casein-rich soft variety of a popular NFM ethnic product. Predominant LAB strains (*Lb. fermentum, Lc. lactis* and *Lb. helveticus*) and major acetic acid bacteria (*Acetobacter* spp., and *Gluconobacter* spp.) are present in *Chhurpi/Churapi* (Shangpliang et al., 2018). Dan et al. (2019) reported that strains such as *Lb. plantarum* can be used together with *S. thermophilus* as a mixed starter to enhance the flavor and consistency of fermented dairy beverage products.

Lassi is mentioned in ancient Indian scriptures along with the precursor *dahi*. Since ancient times, it has been used either with sugar or with black salt and cumin seeds. There is a high consumption of *lassi* in India. The texture and composition of *lassi* changes essentially relying upon the kind of milk utilized, the strategies for preparation, and the effectiveness of fat removal. *Lassi* is low in fat and contains a large consortium of beneficial bacteria. It is viewed as beneficial to the stomach, nutritive and supportive in alleviating gastrointestinal sicknesses, for the most part, due to the

TABLE 2.1 Traditional dairy-based probiotic beverages/drinks associated molecular techniques of identification.

Dairy-based probiotic beverages	Probiotics involved	Molecular technique for identification	References
Dahi	*Enterococcus faecalis, E. faecium, Lactococcus lactis, Lb. rhamnosus*	16S rRNA gene sequencing analysis	Beniwal et al. (2019)
Chhurpi/Churapi	*Lc. lactis, Lb. fermentum, Lb. helveticus, Acetobacter* spp., *Gluconobacter* spp.	(%) content of G+C of DNA, phenotypic	Shangpliang et al. (2018)
Gheu	*Lc. lactis, Lb. helveticus, Acetobacter* spp., *Gluconobacter* spp.	(%) content of G+C of DNA, phenotypic	Shangpliang et al. (2018)
Mar	*Lc. lactis, Lb. helveticus, Acetobacter* spp., *Gluconobacter* spp.	(%) content of G+C of DNA, phenotypic	Shangpliang et al. (2018)

bioactive mixes present in the local milk and balanced by the effect of the LAB strains (*Lactobacillus* and *Lactococcus*) (Ghosh, Mondal, & Mondal, 2020; Padghan, Mann, Sharma, & Kumar, 2015).

Mohi is buttermilk, made by the churning of yogurt and taken as a refreshing drink, mainly in Nepal. (Dewan & Tamang, 2007; Ghosh et al., 2020). Dairy-based refreshments (Table 2.1) are a wellspring of probiotics, have a good taste and are useful for lactose intolerant individuals (Behera, Ray, & Zdolec, 2018; Routray & Mishra, 2012).

2.4.2 Non-dairy probiotic beverages

Interest in non-dairy probiotic beverages rather than dairy-based probiotic products is due to consumers' health concerns regarding the cholesterol in dairy-related products (Behera & Panda, 2020; Panghal et al., 2018). This has led to the development of diverse non-dairy probiotic beverages made from grains, legumes, fruits and vegetables. (Table 2.2). These alternative sources of non-dairy probiotic drinks are low in cost, high in phytochemical/biotic compounds, can decrease cholesterol concerns and are of interest to lactose intolerant individuals (Panghal et al., 2018). The grains, organic produce and vegetable juices (Fig. 2.1) contain minerals, nutrients, dietary fiber and cancer prevention agents, making them appropriate for healthy food category. Additionally, juices contain oxygen scavenging additives (e.g., ascorbic acid) and high sugar content,

TABLE 2.2 Traditional non-dairy-based probiotic beverages/drinks/juices of India.

Name of beverage	Probiotics involved	Fermentation conditions	References
Cereal and legume based probiotic beverages			
Probiotic drink (barley, finger millet, and moth bean)	*Lb. acidophilus*	6 h at 37°C, 10^4 CFU mL^{-1}	Chavan, Gat, Harmalkar, and Waghmare (2018)
Yogurt-like germinated brown rice	FD-DVS YC-180 Yo-Flex® (diverse LAB strains)	2×10^7 CFU mL^{-1}, 42 °C, pH 4.2	Cáceres, Peñas, Martínez-Villaluenga, García-Mora, and Frías (2019)
Rice-based fermented beverage/ bhaati jaanr	*Lb. plantarum* L7	35 °C for 48 h, 10^6 CFU mL^{-1}	Giri, Sen, Saha, Sukumaran, and Park (2018)
Fermented wheat flour dough/roti/ bobroo	*Lb. plantarum* K90, *Lb. fermentum* K75, and *Lb. fermentum* K78	37°C for 48 h	Sharma et al. (2019)
Chhang	*Lb. plantarum, Lb. casei, Enterococcus faecium, Pediococcus pentosaceus* and yeasts such as *Saccharomyces cerevisiae, S. fibuligera, Pichia kudriavzevii* and *Candida tropicalis*	3.5×10^4 CFU mL^{-1}, 30 °C for 24–48 h	Thakur, Saris, and Bhalla (2015)
Vegetable based probiotic beverages			
Tomato juice	*Lb. acidophilus* LA39, *Lb. plantarum* C3, *Lb. casei* A4, and *Lb. delbrueckii* D7	30 °C for 24 h, 10^6 to 10^8 CFU mL^{-1}	Yoon, Woodams, and Hang (2004)
Beetroot drink	*Lb. rhamnosus, Lb. plantarum, Lb. delbrueckii*	pH 6.5, 37°C	Panghal et al. (2017)
Cabbage juice	*Lb. brevis, Lb. rhamnosus, Lb. plantarum* C3, *Lb. casei* A4 and *Lb. delbrueckii* D7	8 log CFU mL^{-1}, 24 h, 37°C	Jaiswal and Abu-Ghannam (2013)
Probiotic drink/ vegetable juice	Lb. *acidophilus* NCDC 11, *Lb. plantarum* NCDC 414, *Pediococcus pentosaceus* MTCC 2819	30°C for 72 h; 8 log CFU mL^{-1}, pH ›3.5	Sharma and Mishra (2013)

TABLE 2.2 Traditional non-dairy-based probiotic beverages/drinks/juices of India—cont'd

Name of beverage	Probiotics involved	Fermentation conditions	References
Soymilk	*Lb. acidophilus* La-5, *Bifidobacterium animalis* Bb-12 and *Streptococcus thermophilus*	10^8 CFU mL^{-1}, 3.2h, pH4.8	Battistini et al. (2018)
Kale juice	*Lb. acidophilus* IFO 3025, *Lb. casei* KCTC 12452, *Lb. brevis* FSB-1 and *Lb. plantarum* KCTC 3104	10^9 CFU mL^{-1}, 48h	Kim (2017)
Probiotic drink (Sohiong juice)	*Lb. plantarum, Lb. rhamnosus, Lb. delbrueckii*	37°C for 72h, 10^6 CFU mL^{-1}	Vivek, Mishra, Pradhan, and Jayabalan (2019)
Probiotic beverage (Moringa leaves and beetroot)	*Lb. plantarum, Enterococcus hirae*	37°C for 48h, 10^3–10^7 CFU mL^{-1}	Vanajakshi, Vijayendra, Varadaraj, Venkateswaran, and Agrawal (2015)
Khalpi	*Leuconostoc fallax, Lb. brevis, Pediococcus pentosaceus, Lb. plantarum*	20–25°C for 3days	Tamang and Tamang (2010)
Fruits based probiotic beverages			
Mango juice	*Lb. acidophilus* MTCC 10307, *Lb. delbrueckii* MTCC 911, *Lb. plantarum* MTCC 9511 and *Lb. casei*	30°C for 72h, 10^7 CFU mL^{-1}	Reddy, Min, and Wee (2015)
Sohiong juice	*Lb. plantarum* MCC 2974	37°C for 72h; 6 log CFU mL^{-1}	Vivek et al. (2019)
Pomegranate juice	*Lb. plantarum, Lb. delbruekii, Lb. paracasei, Lb. acidophilus*	30°C for 72h	Mousavi, Mousavi, Razavi, Emam-Djomeh, and Kiani (2011)
Pineapple juice	*Lb. casei* NRRL B442	6.03 log CFU mL^{-1}, 31°C and pH5.8	Costa, Fonteles, de Jesus, and Rodrigues (2013)
Apple juice	*Lb. paracasei*	Anaerobic incubation at 37°C for 72h	Pimentel, Madrona, Garcia, and Prudencio (2015)

Continued

TABLE 2.2 Traditional non-dairy-based probiotic beverages/drinks/juices of India—cont'd

Name of beverage	Probiotics involved	Fermentation conditions	References
Cashew apple juice	*Lb. casei* NRRL B-442	30°C, 7.48 log CFU mL^{-1} and pH5.0	Pereira, Almeida, Lima, da Costa, and Rodrigues (2014)
Probioticated grape juices	*Pediococcus pentosaceus*	pH3.1–3.2, 6.2–6.5 log CFU mL^{-1} for 72h	Kumar, Umamahesh, and Reddy (2017)
Amla juice	*Lb. paracasei* HII01	pH4.3, 10^9 CFU mL^{-1}, 35–37°C for 12h	Peerajan et al. (2016)
Probiotic honey beverage	*Lb. acidophilus* MTCC 10307	9 log CFU mL^{-1}, 30°C for 3–9h	Nath, Ukkuru, and Kumari (2015)
Orange juice			
Mixed probiotic beverages			
Whey and pineapple juice	*Lb. acidophilus*	1% (v/v); 48h at 30°C ± 1°C	Shukla, Jha, and Admassu (2013)
Vegetable-fruit beverage	*Lb. plantarum* 115, *Lb. plantarum* Vege Start 60	20% (m/v) sugar solution, 35°C, 14 d	Yang et al. (2018)
Fruit juice (tomato, orange, and grape)	*Lb. plantarum* and *Lb. acidophilus*	48h, 37°C, 8.1–9.0 × 10^8 CFU mL^{-1}	Nagpal, Kumar, and Kumar (2012)
Probiotic mixed juice (watermelon and tomato)	*Lb. fermentum* and *Lb. casei*	48h, 30–37°C, ~10^6 CFU mL^{-1}	Sivudu, Umamahesh, and Reddy (2014)
Mixed juice (sugarcane and sweet lime)	*Lb. acidophilus*	24h, 37°C, 10^8 CFU mL^{-1}	Khatoon and Gupta (2015)
Vegetable fermented juice (carrot and orange)	*Lb. plantarum* CECT 220	24h, 37°C, 10^8 CFU mL^{-1}	Valero-Cases and Frutos (2017)
Fermented mixture juice (carrot, beet and apple)	*Lb. casei*	48h, 37°C, 10^6 CFU mL^{-1}	Zandi, Hashemiravan, and Berenjy (2016)

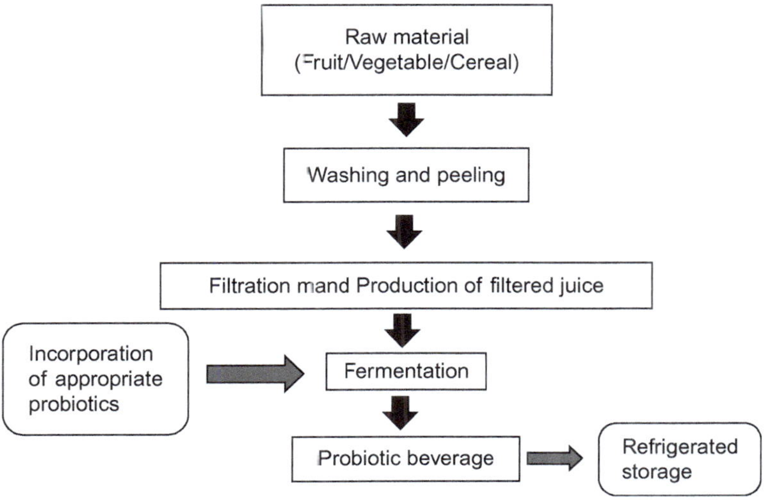

FIG. 2.1 Preparation of probiotic beverages.

which maintains anaerobic conditions and supports probiotic growth and viability (Roberts et al., 2018).

2.4.2.1 Cereal and legume-based probiotic beverages

Cereal and legume–based probiotic beverages can facilitate the development of an improved functional beverage with probiotic benefits (Das, Patra, Singdevsachan, Gouda, & Shin, 2016; Panda et al., 2018). *Chhang* is a traditional alcoholic brew produced by the ethnic people of Himachal Pradesh and the North-West Himalayas. This is a relative of beer and ingredients, such as barley, millet and rice grains, are used to brew this drink. Several LAB strains (e.g., *Lb. plantarum, Lb. casei, Enterococcus (E.) faecium* and *Pedicoccus (P.) pentosaceus*) and yeasts (e.g., *Saccharomyces (Sacch.) cerevisiae, Sacch. fibuligera, Pichia kudriavzevii* and *Candida tropicalis*) are implicated in the fermentation of *chhang* (Thakur et al., 2015). *Chhang* (prepared from rice) and *sura* (prepared from millet) are the most accepted traditional cereal-based fermented alcoholic drinks consumed by the tribal and rural residents of Himachal Pradesh using traditional inoculums of *"dhehli"* and *"phab"* (Thakur et al., 2015). Microbial examinations of *sura* uncovered that *Sacch. cerevisiae* is a prevailing microorganism in maturation along with species of *Candida, Leuconostoc* and *Lactobacillus* (Thakur & Bhalla, 2004).

More recently, Chavan et al. (2018) reported a probiotic beverage using seeds (germinated and non-germinated) of barley, finger millet and moth bean inoculated with *Lb. acidophilus*. Fermentation with this starter culture

(*Lb. acidophilus*) improved the functional properties (bacterial counts, 2,2-diphenyl-1-picrylhydrazyl- (DPPH) -assay and polyphenol content) and overall acceptability of the beverage.

Bhaati jaanr is an Indian Himalayan fermented beverage made from rice and used as a staple food. It has a gentle alcoholic, tangy taste. This high calorie drink is used for postpartum women and sick older people in the villages. Giri, Sen, et al. (2018) studied the use of *Lb. plantarum* L7 for this traditional rice-based fermented beverage *bhaati jaanr*.

In 2019, Sharma et al. (2019) identified potential LAB strains from conventionally fermented wheat flour dough known as "*babroo*." The phylogenetic analysis discovered that three probiotic strains (*Lb. fermentum* K78, *Lb. plantarum* K80 and *Lb. fermentum* K75) were involved in *babroo* fermentation. Cáceres et al. (2019) evaluated the suitability and consequence of fermentation on dietary and health benefits of germinated brown rice (supplemented with 7% sucrose, 5% glucose and 0.5% gelatin) for developing a yogurt-like product. Lactic acid (LA) fermentation was performed at 42°C using a commercial starter culture (FD-DVS YC-180 Yo-Flex® containing LAB strains). The fermented beverage showed a high phenolic (15.2 mg/100 g) and γ-aminobutyric acid (GABA) (1.9 mg/100 g) content, antioxidant activity (46.9 μg/100 g) and angiotensin I-converting enzyme (ACE)-inhibition (61.5%) properties.

Gupta and Bajaj (2017) studied a fermented oat flour beverage using probiotic strain Lb. *plantarum* M-13 and honey (a health enhancer). The optimized process variables (concentration of oat flour, 8.0%, *w/v*; honey, 3.0%, w/v, incubation time, 48 h) enhanced the probiotic viability (up to 4 weeks).

2.4.2.2 *Fruit-based probiotic beverages*

In recent years, consumers' interest in fruit-based probiotic beverages has increased. However, the use of probiotic cultures in fruit-based beverages and their environment remains a challenge. Juice/beverage manufacturers are interested in designing new/alternative products to expand the existing functional drink/drink category (Panda et al., 2017; Prado et al., 2008). Suitability of probiotic cultures as fruit juice supplements/additives for acid tolerance activity was studied by Sheehan, Ross, and Fitzgerald (2007). Some LAB strains (*Lb. rhamnosus* GG, *Lb. casei* DN-114001 and *Lb. paracasei* NFBC 43338) were found to have potential in fruit juices because of their tolerance to acid-like environments (Sheehan et al., 2007).

The production of probiotic pomegranate juice, through maturation/fermentation, by four strains of LAB (*Lb. plantarum, Lb. delbruekii, Lb. paracasei and Lb. acidophilus*) was studied by Mousavi et al. (2011). The fermentation process was performed at 30°C for 72 h under microaerophilic conditions. The probiotic LAB strains notably consumed citric acid and showed higher viability in pomegranate juice during the storage time (4 weeks).

Probiotic fruit (mango) drinks have inherent health benefits. Mango probiotic juice/beverages were fermented with probiotics (e.g., *Lb. acidophilus*, *Lb. delbrueckii*, *Lb. plantarum* and *Lb. casei*) at 30°C for 72 h under micro-aerophilic conditions, and the juice was rated good in sensory attributes (color, taste and flavor) (Reddy et al., 2015). Ranjitha, Oberoi, Upreti, and Redappa (2018) reported that a mango beverage is inoculated with *Lb. helveticus* MTCC 5463 had the potential for developing a probioticated mango beverage. The pH decreased to 3.2 in the process of fermentation.

Apple juice was found to be an appropriate medium for fermentation by the probiotic *Lb. plantarum* PCS 26, resulting in a functional drink with potentially increased shelf-life and good sensory acceptance (Dimitrovski, Velickova, Langerholc, & Winkelhausen, 2015). Roberts et al. (2018) evaluated the feasibility of *Lb. plantarum* NCIMB 8826 in a non-alcoholic-based fermented apple juice in a period of 15 days of storage at 4°C. The viability of the bacteria, in a simulated gastric and intestinal environment, remained above 10^7 colony forming units (CFU) mL^{-1} under storage conditions.

Sohiong (*Prunus nepalensis*) fruit is an under-utilized fruit of the Northeastern part of India. It is known to be an affluent resource of vitamins, minerals, polyphenols and anthocyanin and has been explored for the development of probiotic drinks (Vivek et al., 2019). Vivek et al. (2019) investigated the appropriateness of sohiong juice for the manufacturing of a probiotic drink (37°C for 72 h) using *Lb. plantarum*. The probiotic microorganism population was still elevated (6 log CFU mL^{-1}) even after 4 weeks of storage at 4 ± 1°C. The beverage met with consumer approval.

Peerajan et al. (2016) investigated the fermentation of the amla fruit (*Phyllanthus emblica*) by *Lb. paracasei* HII01 with reference to carbon sources, polyphenols and antioxidant properties (FRAP and ABTS assays). The study revealed that the amla juice product produced by *Lb. paracasei* HII01-mediated fermentation, resulted in a high quality nutritional drink for consumption, with significant polyphenolic content and antioxidant properties.

Kumar et al. (2017) studied the quality of fermented/probioticated grape (white and red) juices with the probiotic bacterium *P. pentosaceus*. Fermented red grape juice (pH 3.1 and viable bacteria (6.5 log CFU mL^{-1}) was compared to fermented white grape juice (pH 3.2 and 6.2 log CFU mL^{-1}) at 72 h of fermentation. Fermented red grape juice showed a titrate capacity of 0.34% compared to fermented white grape juice at 0.72%.

Hashemi, Haridy, and Qashqari (2018) studied the effect of leaf extract of *Moringa oleifera* (a fast-growing, drought-resistant tree native to the Indian subcontinent) and found that it increased the shelf-life and the quality of sweet orange juice.

2.4.2.3 Vegetable-based probiotic beverages

Vegetable-based (e.g., cabbage, carrot root, onion, ginger, peanuts, tomato) probiotic drinks/beverages are beneficial to health (Nychas, Panagou, Parker, Waldron, & Tassou, 2002; Wootton-Beard & Ryan, 2011) and are generally produced with a lactic acid fermentation using probiotic LAB strains. These drinks are an alternative beverage for consumers who cannot tolerate milk protein and serve as a health drink for vegetarians. (Nychas et al., 2002). Yoon et al. (2004) studied the appropriateness of tomato juice as a raw material for the manufacture of a probiotic juice product using four LAB strains (*Lb. acidophilus* LA39, *Lb. plantarum* C3, *Lb. casei* A4 and *Lb. delbrueckii* D7). This probiotic juice had a decreased pH (3.5) and increased acidity (1.67%) and reached a cell viability of 10^8 CFU mL^{-1} after a 30°C fermentation for 72 h.

Khalpi is a fermented cucumber-based probiotic beverage consumed in the North-Eastern (Sikkim and Darjeeling hills) states and the Himalaya region of India. In a *khalpi* fermentation, some heterofermentative LAB strains (e.g., Leu. *fallax*, *Lb. brevis* and *P. pentosaceus*) are used for initiating the fermentation, with a final finish by *Lb. plantarum* (Tamang & Tamang, 2010).

Jaiswal and Abu-Ghannam (2013) investigated the production of a probiotic cabbage juice drink utilizing numerous strains of LAB (*Lb. brevis, Lb. plantarum* and *Lb. rhamnosus*). Lactic acid (LA) was the most important end product of the fermented cabbage juice, and the juice retained more than 75% of the phytochemicals (total phenolic and total flavonoid content) and bioactivity.

Rafiq, Sharma, Nazir, Rashid, and Sofi (2016) concluded that carrot juice is a suitable raw material/media for the growth of probiotic organisms, such as *Lb. plantarum, Lb. casei* and *Bifidum longum*.

Vanajakshi et al. (2015) reported that the fermentation of a moringa leaf–based beetroot beverage (1:2) was suitable for a probiotic drink (*Lb. Plantarum* and *Enterococcus hirae*). This fermented moringa leaf–based beverage showed commercial potential as a refreshing healthy drink. Beetroot juice also shows good potential for the development of probiotic drinks. Beet juice is free of cholesterol and contains health-promoting ingredients (Panghal et al., 2017). Panghal et al. (2017) studied a probiotic drink using beetroot and fermented at optimum conditions (pH 6.5, 37°C, *Lb. rhamnosus, Lb. plantarum* and *Lb. delbrueckii*). They examined the probiotic potential of this beetroot juice based on the viability of the LAB. Probiotic beet juice showed a gradual decrease in pH and sugar over time, while the total amount of phenols, flavonoids and antioxidants in the probiotic beverage increased, compared to the fresh juice sample.

Vegetable juices, perceived as healthy and refreshing foods, have been proposed as an ideal carrier for functional health components such as minerals, vitamins, dietary fibre and bioactive compounds such as phenolic compounds, choline, carotenoids, phytoestrogens and glucosinolates (Kim, 2017). Kim (2017) studied fermented kale juice potential using four lactobacilli strains (*Lb. acidophilus* IFO 3025, *Lb. casei* KCTC 12452, *Lb. brevis* FSB-1 and *Lb. plantarum* KCTC 3104).

2.4.2.4 *Mixed probiotic juices*

Mixed fruit and/or vegetable juices have proven to be capable carriers or growth media for probiotics. Sharma and Mishra (2013) investigated alternative food matrices such as the suitability of a mixed vegetable juice composed of bitter gourd, bottle gourd and carrot as a raw material for the production of a probiotic drink (Lb. *acidophilus* NCDC 11, *Lb. plantarum* NCDC 414, and *Pediococcus pentosaceus* MTCC 2819). A maize vegetable juice was fermented at 30°C for 72 h and changes in the microbial population and pH were observed during the fermentation period. Vegetable juice has been proven to be a good base for fermented probiotic beverage preparation.

Sivudu et al. (2014) studied the appropriateness of watermelon and tomato juice as a raw material for the production of probiotic mixed juices using Lb. *fermentum* and *Lb. casei*. Zandi et al. (2016) reported on the production of fermented functional beverages based on mixtures of carrot, beet and apple juice using *Lb. casei*. Nagpal et al. (2012) investigated probiotic-fortified fruit juices (tomato, orange and grape) as functional beverages using two *Lactobacillus* isolates, Lb. *plantarum* and *Lb. acidophilus*, for the fermented juice.

Khatoon and Gupta (2015) reported on the suitability of sugarcane and sweet lime juices as sole sources for the growth of beneficial *Lb. acidophilus*. Juices were inoculated with a 24-h lactic acid bacteria (*Lb. acidophilus*) culture. The viable cell counts of *Lb. acidophilus* reached 10^8 CFU mL^{-1} after 24 h of fermentation at 37°C. *Lb. acidophilus* was capable of utilizing sugarcane and sweet lime juice for growth and lactic acid production, suggesting that these juices served as a good quality medium for the growth of probiotics.

Probiotic beverages from whey and pineapple juice were studied by Shukla et al. (2013) using *Lb. acidophilus* as the probiotic organism. The study revealed a satisfactory quality of probiotic beverage along with health beneficial properties. The whey and pineapple juice (65:35 blend) were inoculated with 1% (*v*/v) of *Lb. acidophilus* and the product had a shelf-life of 24 days at 5°C ± 1°C and 48 h at 30°C ± 1°C.

2.5 Ethnic probiotic beverages in India

Ethnic beverages are fermented naturally using a consortium of probiotics in the form of dry, cereal-based starters (Table 2.3). Various strains from the LAB species are used to create ethnic beverages with different sensory attributes (Tamang, 2015).

TABLE 2.3 Application of selected microorganisms in ethnic beverages in India.

Ethnic beverage	Microorganisms involved	Reference
Rice beer	*Lb. plantarum, Lb. acidophilus, S. cerevisiae, Lb. fermentum, Bifidobacterium sp.*	Kardong et al. (2012)
Xaj-pani (Rice-wine)	*Lb. plantarum, Lb. brevis, Leuco. lactis, Weissella cibaria, Lc. lactis, Weissella para mesenteroides,* and *Leuco. pseudomesenteroides*	Bora, Keot, Das, Sarma, and Barooah (2016)
Bas-tenga	*Lb. plantarum, Lb. acidophilus*	Das et al. (2016)
Kanji	*Lb. plantarum, Lb. acidophilus, Hansenula anomala, Candida guilliermondii, C. tropicalis, G. candidum, Lb. dextranicum, Lb. paraplantarum,* and *Lb. pentosus*	Tamang (2012) and Lamba, Goomer, and Saxena (2019)
Haria	*Bifidobacterium* sp., *Pediococcus* sp., and *Lactobacillus* sp.	Ray, Hor, Singh, and Mondal (2017)
Raabadi	*Lb. plantarum* RYPR1	Yadav, Puniya, and Shukla (2016)

2.5.1 Rice beer

Apong (rice beer) is a mild alcoholic refreshing/energizing beverage and an essential element of the social, cultural, and religious living of the *mising* (also known as *mishing*) community/tribes of North-East India (Arunachal Pradesh) (Das et al., 2016). This drink is well known to nearly all the tribes of the state. *Apong* is produced by fermenting cooked rice with herbal-based yeast starter cakes called "*aopo pitha*" (Tiwari & Mahanta, 2007). *Po:ro apong* (*saimod*) is very similar to *apong* and a socio-culturally important alcoholic rice beverage unique to the *missing* tribes of Assam in India. About 16 different plant species are used for the preparation of the yeast starter culture (*epop*) (Kardong et al., 2012). Rice beer (*Kiad lieh*) (a distilled, clear and alcoholic drink) is used by the natives of *Khasi* (Khasi Hills) (Tamang, 2010) and *Pnar* or *Synteng* (Jaintia Hills) in Meghalaya during various religious festivals and ceremonies (Sawian, Nongkynrih, Anand, & Charan, 2018). The dry and mixed starter prepared for *Kiad lieh* is "*Thiat*" (natural LAB, mold and yeast) in combination with dried and milled leaves of *Amomum aromaticum* (khaw-iang), milled local red rice, *Oryza sativa* (khaw saw) and spring water (umpohliew) to form a paste (Sawian et al., 2018). *Zutho* (rice beer) is a conventional alcoholic brew made from rice (*Oryza sativa* L.) and is a well-liked alcoholic drink in Nagaland (Jamir & Deb, 2014; Tamang et al., 2016). It has a fruity aroma and sour taste, and its unique aroma has characteristics similar to those of Japanese sake and sprouted rice sake (Tamang et al., 2016). Ghosh et al. (2015) prepared the rice-based fermented beverage using the probiotic strain *Lb. fermentum* KKL1. The fermented rice-based beverage liberated enzymes (amylase and phytase) and showed strong antioxidant activity.

2.5.2 Rice-wine

Rice wine (from glutinous rice) is a conventional alcoholic drink in North-Eastern India (Manipur and Assam). It is locally named *"xaj-pani"* especially by the *Ahoms* community of Assam. Rice wine is a significant beverage used in religious functions among the *Ahoms* (Saikia, Tag, & Das, 2007). The standard to prepare rice wine involves the process of saccharification of steamed rice starch. This is achieved by fungal enzymes under aerobic solid-state fermentation (SSF) conditions. Molds are mixed with water and allowed to undergo a submerged alcoholic fermentation (SmF) by various yeast cultures (*Pichia anomala, Saccharomyces cerevisiae* and *Trichosporon*) using traditional starter flat cakes (Jeyaram, Singh, Capece, & Romano, 2008). The starter culture used in rice wine is locally recognized as *xaj-pitha*, a combination of mixed culture of molds, yeasts and bacteria (LAB) that are maintained on substrates, such as rice powder and fortified with several herbs. Some of the most frequently appearing LAB strains are *Lb. plantarum, Lb. brevis, Leuco. lactis, Weissella cibaria, Lc. lactis, W. para mesenteroides, Leuco. pseudomesenteroides and Pediococcus pentosaceus* (Bora et al., 2016). The ethnic starter *'hamei'* (flat rice cake and wild herbs) is also used to make a rice beverage (rice wine) indigenously called *'atingba'*, from which a clear liquor can be distilled that is called *'yu'* in Manipur (Tamang, 2010). The drink is prepared under a non-sterile environment as a home-scale fermentation, using conventional solid flat rice cakes. The LAB strains of *"hamei"* do not create biogenic amines, useful knowledge for a starter culture (Tamang, 2010).

2.5.3 Bastanga

Ethnic people of the North-East States of India consume bamboo shoot–based fermented products as a traditional food (Jamir & Deb, 2014). People of Nagaland, typically by the *Lotha* Naga tribe, called *"Rhujuk"* in *Lotha* dialect, consume these bamboo shoots in a fermented form, called "sour bamboo" and locally known as *Bastanga/Bas-tenga* (Das et al., 2016).

2.5.4 Kanji

Kanji is an indigenous natural/spontaneous fermented gentle alcoholic drink mainly consumed by people in Northern India throughout the summer season. *Kanji* is prepared, using a traditional household method, with black carrot (*Daucus carota*)/beetroot (*Beta vulgaris*) and by additions of salt, crushed mustard, and/or red chili powder. In the process of preparation, carrots or beetroots are cleaned and washed, finely shredded and with additions (salt and mustard seeds), finally, the drink is placed into earthen pots. Here, it is left to ferment naturally at 26–34°C for 4–7 days (Tamang, 2012). The alcohol content of *kanji* is ~2.5% and the pH is ~4.0, resulting in a mild alcoholic product with an acidic taste (Tamang et al., 2016). Microorganisms, such as *Hansenula anomala, Candida guilliermondii, C. tropicalis, G. candidum, Lb. plantarum, Lb. dextranicum, Lb. paraplantarum* and *Lb. pentosus,* are involved in *kanji* fermentations. *Kanji* is a well-liked remedy for the treatment of many stomach ailments such as indigestion, loss of appetite and liver disorders (Lamba et al., 2019; Tamang, 2012).

2.5.5 Haria

Haria (or *Harhia*) is an alcoholic drink consumed by the tribal communities of West Bengal, Bihar and Jharkhand states of India. It is an energy loaded drink with ethnomedicinal importance. *Haria* is made using boiled scorched rice, mixed with a traditional starter named *'bakhar/dabai'* (1:100) and fermented in an earthen pot kept in a dark room for 3–5 days. This mixture is later thinned/diluted with water and sieved to produce *haria*. For generations, *haria* has been popular among the several tribes (East-Central India) for treatment of gastrointestinal ailments such as acidity, dysentery, diarrhea, amebiasis and vomiting. Also, a significant level of antioxidant activity has been noted (Ray, Ghosh, Singh, & Mondal, 2016). During a haria fermentation, there is an amassing of starch hydrolytic enzymes, along with different types of maltooligosaccharides (maltotetraose, maltotriose and maltose) (Ghosh et al., 2015). Several microbial species, such as *Sacch. cerevisiae, Sacch. boulardii, Zygosaccharomyces cidri, Candida tropicalis, C. musae, C. nitratophila, Issatchenkia* sp., *Pediococcus* sp., *Lactobacillus* sp. including LAB strains are involved in the *haria* fermentation process (Sha, Thakur, Tamang, & Tamang, 2012). The health beneficial/probiotic microbes present in *haria* belong to *Bifidobacterium* sp., *Pediococcus* sp., and *Lactobacillus* sp., and their presence was confirmed through PCR-Denaturing Gradient Gel Electrophoresis (PCR-DGGE) fingerprinting (Ghosh, Ray, Adak, Dey, et al., 2015; Ray et al., 2017).

2.5.6 Raabadi

'Raabadi' is the name of a much-loved local beverage in the Rajasthan and Haryana states of India. The primary ingredients to produce Raabadi are grain and pearl millet-flour, buttermilk, salt, dark pepper, cumin seed

powder and dry green coriander. It is an invigorating and a cooling drink, for the most part, consumed during the summer (Yadav et al., 2016). Yadav et al. (2016) isolated the probiotic bacteria from *raabadi*. An aggregate of five *raabadi* samples was gathered and 54 isolates were filtered utilizing a Man, Rogosa and Sharp (MRS) medium. The isolates were surveyed for resilience to low pH and bile salts. Isolate *Lb. plantarum* RYPR1 showed good probiotic potential. An anti-nutritional factor in the beverage called phytate prevents the bioabsorption of minerals (Fe^{2+}, Zn^{2+}, Ca^{2+} ions) in the gastrointestinal tract. Basu, Tomar, and Hati (2015) studied the isolation of phytate degrading *lactobacilli* from *raabadi* samples. Isolates such as *Lb. fermentum, Lb. rhamnosus* and *Lb. brevis* were found to have the potential to degrade phytate content in this cereal-based fermented product.

2.6 Probiotic beverages in modern India

In today's modern India, due to urbanization, the changes in dietary habits and lifestyle patterns have health-conscious consumers searching for alternative treatment regimens and so probiotics and probiotic-based food supplementations have drawn attention.

2.6.1 Application of modern techniques

Although spray drying procedures are used for probiotic dairy-based drinks, a few investigations have assessed the spray drying process for use with probiotic natural product juices. Pereira et al. (2014) assessed the lack of hydration by the spray drying of cashew squeezed apple containing Lb. *casei* NRRL B-442, and decided the practicality, stockpiling temperature and physical properties of the powder during 35 days of storage. Microbial endurance rates (Lb. *casei* NRRL B-442) were higher than 90% (at 4°C for 35 days).

Sonication (use of sound energy to shake particles) was used with pineapple juice, to produce an appropriate substrate for *Lb. casei* growth to produce a non-dairy probiotic refreshment by Costa et al. (2013) along with strain *Lb. casei* NRRL B442. The *Lb. casei* strain was viable under optimized conditions (31°C and pH 5.8). The pH was further reduced over time due to the production of lactic acid (post-acidification) and browning was not observed to be an issue.

2.6.2 Effect of prebiotics

Prebiotics (defined as non-digestible fiber compounds in this context) in the fruit and vegetable beverages support and induce the growth of probiotics in the gastrointestinal tract. Pimentel et al. (2015) assessed the consequence of the fortification (using oligofructose) of apple juice on the physicochemical juice properties and the probiotic's (*Lb. paracasei*) viability during refrigerated storage (4°C for 28 days). Squeezed apple juice was seen as a reasonable vehicle for Lb. *paracasei* as a probiotic. Further, the oligofructose utilized as a prebiotic prolonged the viability of the probiotic (*Lb. paracasei*) in the apple juice.

Nath et al. (2015) developed a honey beverage (30°C for 3–9 h) using *Lb. acidophilus* as the probiotic microorganism and ascertained its quality, viable count and shelf-life. The probiotic beverage produced high scores for overall acceptability and showed a viable count of more than 9 log CFU mL^{-1}, with a shelf-life of 15 days.

Valero-Cases and Frutos (2017) researched the prebiotic impact of various concentrations (0%, 1%, and 2%) of inulin on the development and endurance of *Lb. plantarum* CECT 220 in mixed carrot and squeezed orange juice after 24 h of aging. An expanded span time of usability was seen in the aged juices with inulin. At 30 days, the aged juices with 2% inulin (after in vitro absorption) showed a noteworthy survival of *Lb. plantarum.*

Bernal-Castro, Díaz-Moreno, and Gutiérrez-Cortés (2019) investigated the viability of commercial probiotics (*Lb. casei*) in the development of a functional tropical/red fruit beverage (20% strawberry, 10% blackberry and 5% papaya) enriched with prebiotics (inulin and fructooligosaccharides). The effect on the viability of *Lb. casei* inoculated into the fruit beverage was monitored using growth kinetics (37°C for 50 h). The findings indicated that fortification with 1% inulin had a protective effect on the stability of *Lb. casei* in the fruit beverage.

Giri, Venkatachalam, Sen, and Park (2018) fermented coconut (*Cocos nucifera* L.) water (35 °C for 48 h) using the probiotic *Lb. casei* L4, and found it could serve as a good functional beverage since it contained both electrolytes and probiotics.

2.6.3 Application of nanotechnology

Nanotechnology has the potential in improving sensorial, nourishing, and quality characteristics of drinks, and also nanoparticles can be utilized as conveyance frameworks for different bioactive compounds into functional beverages. ur Rahman, Sahar, Ishaq, and Khalil (2020) have recently reviewed the various opportunities and challenges regarding the use of nanotechnology in the beverage industry.

2.7 Probiotic beverages as food and health supplements

A number of probiotic refreshments that are popular around the whole north-eastern locale of India has various medical advantages, are wholesome and have nutraceutical potential. They provide expanded sustenance, for example, proteins, minerals, phytochemicals, phytosterols and dietary fibers (Behera, Bal, et al., 2018). Probiotic drinks can be rich in various bioactive mixes and maltooligosaccharides (e.g., maltotetraose, maltotriose and maltose), which can repress the development of intestinal pathogens and be nutritious for babies and seniors (Ghosh, Ray, Adak, Dey, et al., 2015). Panghal et al. (2018) suggest that the utilization of probiotic drinks results in lower serum cholesterol levels, invigorate calcium retention, improve protein absorbability and counteract the effects of foodborne pathogens (Panghal et al., 2018). Generally, log6-log7 of probiotic organisms per mL (or g) of drink has been suggested as the level for a presentation of a medical advantage (Angmo et al., 2016; Desobgo, Mishra, Behera, & Panda, 2017). Utilization of probiotic drinks has been demonstrated as useful in improving different clinical conditions such as puerile loose bowels, supplanting *Clostridium difficile* colitis, *Helicobacter pylori* contamination, incendiary entrail sicknesses and female urogenital diseases (Angmo et al., 2016). Other gainful impacts include improvement in lactose digestion, lowering serum cholesterol and effects as anti-toxins (Angmo et al., 2016).

2.8 Indian market of probiotic beverages

Probiotics are non-pathogenic microorganisms, which upon ingestion impart a positive medical advantage on the host (Das et al., 2016). Probiotics perform an extraordinary job as preventive medicine. The global probiotics market is projected to reach over USD 74.7 billion by 2025 and develop at a compound annual growth rate of over 7% in the next decade (Grand View Research, 2019; Kumar et al., 2020). In 2019, a Rakuten Insight survey (Rakuten.com) found that a majority of Indian respondents consumed functional beverages (functional meaning conveying a health benefit) several times a week, 15% consumed once daily and only 11% never consumed functional beverages. The functional or fortified food market in India in 2018 was USD 3.9 billion and is forecast to reach USD 6 billion by 2023.

2.9 Indian government regulations on probiotic beverages

Currently in India, there are no general expressed guidelines for probiotics. In Europe, guidelines are being kept up by the European Food Safety Authority (EFSA) under the 'guideline 178/2002/EC; order 2000/13/EU' act. In the United States, probiotics are being managed by 403 (a) (1) of the government Food, Drug, and Cosmetic Act; however, the focus is on the legitimacy of claims, rather than efficacy, safety and quality (de Simone, 2018).

A team has been established by the Indian Council of Medical Research (ICMR), consisting of specialists from different fields to create rules for the assessment and application of probiotics in India. This endeavor has been made by the ICMR and the Department of Biotechnology (DBT) to outline the rules to manage the utilization of probiotics in nourishment and to provide prerequisites to evaluate the safety and viability of the probiotic strains, well-being cases, and labeling of items with probiotics (Ganguly et al., 2011; Ramakrishna, 2014). Probiotics in India are described as useful nourishment and as of now are controlled by food laws that manage general food as opposed to pharmaceuticals or medications (Tingirikari, Sarathy, & Karthigarani, 2019). Regulatory bodies of India will need to ensure that probiotic beverages are regulated by lawful approval processes in a manner that will lead to maximal health benefits and minimal health risk for consumers (Arora, Arora, Bansal, & Baldi, 2019).

2.10 Conclusions and future prospectives

There is every reason to believe that probiotic beverages will be the next food category where the healthy bacteria (LAB) will make their mark. The acceptable commodities are cereal, vegetable, and fruit-based beverages for the development of such products. Producers should continue to improve and add advantageous probiotic microorganisms to beverages (Prado et al., 2008; Tingirikari et al., 2019). To better understand the useful properties of probiotic drinks, investigations on this topic will need to continue. The ongoing advancements in metabolomics and new techniques will help to further elucidate some of the fermentative pathways. Governments could provide facilities for cottage industries to help with the commercialization of novel products; this could generate revenue among the indigenous tribes dealing with particular beverages. Further, in vivo investigations should be carried out to establish the health promotional attributes and to allow for the establishment of new health claims for Indian probiotic beverages.

Conflict of interest

All authors declare that they do not have any conflict of interest in the publishing of this chapter.

References

Adhikari, R. R., & Ghimirey, H. (2000). *Nepalese society and culture*. Kathmandu (Nepali): Vidharthi Pushtak Bhandar.

Angmo, K., Kumari, A., & Bhalla, T. C. (2016). Probiotic characterization of lactic acid bacteria isolated from fermented foods and beverage of Ladakh. *LWT- Food Science and Technology*, *66*, 428–435.

Arora, M., Arora, M., Bansal, P., & Baldi, A. (2019). Need and recommendations for universal guidelines on regulatory status and quality control/safety of probiotic products. *Applied Clinical Research, Clinical Trials and Regulatory Affairs*, *6*(3), 231–249.

Basu, S., Tomar, S. K., & Hati, S. (2015). Isolation and identification of phytate-degrading lactobacilli from Indian cereal-based fermented milk product-"Raabadi" *International Journal of Fermented Foods*, *4*(1and2), 49–59.

Battistini, C., Gullón, B., Ichimura, E. S., Gomes, A. M. P., Ribeiro, E. P., Kunigk, L., & Jurkiewicz, C. (2018). Development and characterization of an innovative synbiotic fermented beverage based on vegetable soybean. *Brazilian Journal of Microbiology*, *49*(2), 303–309.

Behera, S. S., Bal, P., Das, S., Panda, S. H., & Mohanty, N. (2018). Advances in microbial fermentation and fermented food for health. In *Innovations in technologies for fermented food and beverage industries* (pp. 53–69). Cham: Springer.

Behera, S. S., & Panda, S. K. (2020). Ethnic and industrial probiotic foods and beverages: Efficacy and acceptance. *Current Opinion in Food Science*, *32*, 29–36.

Behera, S. S., Ray, R. C., Das. U., Panda, S. K., & Saranraj, P. (2019). Microorganisms in fermentation. In *Essentials in fermentation technology* (pp. 1–39). Cham: Springer.

Behera, S. S., Ray, R. C., & Zdolec, N. (2018). *Lactobacillus plantarum* with functional properties: an approach to increase safety and shelf-life of fermented foods. *BioMed Research International*,9361614 18 pages (2018). https://doi.org/10.1155/2018/9361614.

Beniwal, A., Semwal, A., & Navani, N. K. (2019). Mechanistic insights into probiotic properties of lactic acid bacteria associated with ethnic fermented dairy products. *Frontiers in Microbiology*. *10*, 502https://doi.org/10.3389/fmicb.2019.00502.

Bernal-Castro, C. A., Díaz-Moreno, C., & Gutiérrez-Cortés, C. (2019). Inclusion of prebiotics on the viability of a commercial *Lactobacillus casei subsp. rhamnosus* culture in a tropical fruit beverage. *Journal of Food Science and Technology*, *56*(2), 987–994.

Bora, S. S., Keot, J., Das, S., Sarma, K., & Barooah, M. (2016). Metagenomics analysis of microbial communities associated with a traditional rice wine starter culture (Xaj-pitha) of Assam, India. *3 Biotech*, *6*(2), 153. https://doi.org/10.1007/s13205-016-0471-1.

Cáceres, P. J., Peñas, E., Martínez-Villaluenga, C., García-Mora, P., & Frías, J. (2019). Development of a multifunctional yogurt-like product from germinated brown rice. *LWT*, *99*, 306–312.

Chavan, M., Gat, Y., Harmalkar, M., & Waghmare, R. (2018). Development of non-dairy fermented probiotic drink based on germinated and ungerminated cereals and legume. *LWT*, *91*, 339–344.

Costa, M. G. M., Fonteles, T. V., de Jesus, A. L. T., & Rodrigues, S. (2013). Sonicated pineapple juice as substrate for *L. casei* cultivation for probiotic beverage development: Process optimisation and product stability. *Food Chemistry*, *139*(1–4), 261–266.

Dan, T., Chen, H., Li, T., Tian, J., Ren, W., Zhang, H. , et al. (2019). Influence of *Lactobacillus plantarum* P-8 on fermented milk flavor and storage stability. *Frontiers in Microbiology*, *9*, 3133. https://doi.org/10.3389/fmicb.2018.03133.

Das, G., Patra, J. K., Singdevsachan, S. K., Gouda, S., & Shin, H. S. (2016). Diversity of traditional and fermented foods of the seven sister states of India and their nutritional and nutraceutical potential: A review. *Frontiers in Life Science*, *9*(4), 292–312.

de Simone, C. (2018). The unregulated probiotic market. *Clinical Gastroenterology and Hepatology*, *17*(5), 809–817. https://doi.org/10.1016/j.cgh.2018.01.018.

Desobgo, S. C., Mishra, S. S., Behera, S. K., & Panda, S. K. (2017). Scaling-up and modelling applications of solid-state fermentation and demonstration in microbial enzyme production related to food industries. In *Microbial enzyme technology in food applications* (pp. 452–468). Boca Raton, FL: CRC Press.

Dewan, S., & Tamang, J. P. (2007). Dominant lactic acid bacteria and their technological properties isolated from the Himalayan ethnic fermented milk products. *Antonie Van Leeuwenhoek*, *92*(3), 343–352.

Dimitrovski, D., Velickova, E., Langerholc, T., & Winkelhausen, E. (2015). Apple juice as a medium for fermentation by the probiotic *Lactobacillus plantarum* PCS 26 strain. *Annals of Microbiology, 65*(4), 2161–2170.

Ganguly, N. K., Bhattacharya, S. K., Sesikeran, B., Nair, G. B., Ramakrishna, B. S., Sachdev, H. P. S. , et al. (2011). ICMR-DBT guidelines for evaluation of probiotics in food. *The Indian Journal of Medical Research, 134*(1), 22. (2011). 21808130.

Garcia, C., Guerin, M., Souidi, K., & Remize, F. (2020). Lactic fermented fruit or vegetable juices: Past, present and future. *Beverages*, 6(1), 8. https://doi.org/10.3390/beverages6010008.

Ghosh, K., Mondal, S. P., & Mondal, K. C. (2020). Ethnic fermented foods and beverages of West Bengal and Odisha. In *Ethnic fermented foods and beverages of India: Science history and culture* (pp. 647–685). Singapore: Springer.

Ghosh, K., Ray, M., Adak, A., Dey, P., Halder, S. K., Das, A. , et al. (2015). Microbial, saccharifying and antioxidant properties of an Indian rice based fermented beverage. *Food Chemistry, 168*, 196–202.

Ghosh, K., Ray, M., Adak, A., Halder, S. K., Das, A., Jana, A. , et al. (2015). Role of probiotic *Lactobacillus fermentum* KKL1 in the preparation of a rice based fermented beverage. *Bioresource Technology, 188*, 161–168.

Giri, S. S., Sen, S. S., Saha, S., Sukumaran, V., & Park, S. C. (2018). Use of a potential probiotic, *Lactobacillus plantarum* L7, for the preparation of a rice-based fermented beverage. *Frontiers in Microbiology, 9*, 473. https://doi.org/10.3389/fmicb.2018.00473.

Giri, S. S., Venkatachalam, S., Sen, S. S., & Park, S. C. (2018). Use of a potential probiotic, *Lactobacillus casei* L4, in the preparation of fermented coconut water beverage. *Frontiers in Microbiology. 9*, https://doi.org/10.3389/fmicb.2018.00473.

Grand View Research (June 2019). *Press release. Probiotics market worth $77.09 billion By 2025 | CAGR: 6.9%. (June 2019). https://www.grandviewresearch.com/press-release/global-probiotics-market.*

Gupta, M., & Bajaj, B. K. (2017). Development of fermented oat flour beverage as a potential probiotic vehicle. *Food Bioscience, 20*, 104–109.

Hashemi, J. M., Haridy, L. A., & Qashqari, R. J. (2018). The effect of *Moringa oleifera* leaves extract on extending the shelf life and quality of freshly sweet orange juice. *Journal of Biochemical Technology, 9*(4), 63–76.

Jaiswal, A. K., & Abu-Ghannam, N. (2013). Kinetic studies for the preparation of probiotic cabbage juice: Impact on phytochemicals and bioactivity. *Industrial Crops and Products, 50*, 212–218.

Jamir, B., & Deb, C. R. (2014). Some fermented foods and beverages of Nagaland, India. *International Journal of Food and Fermentation Technology, 4*(2), 87–92.

Jeyaram, K., Singh, W. M., Capece, A., & Romano, P. (2008). Molecular identification of yeast species associated with 'Hamei'—A traditional starter used for rice wine production in Manipur, India. *International Journal of Food Microbiology, 124*(2), 115–125.

Kardong, D., Deori, K., Sood, K., Yadav, R. N. S., Bora, T. C., & Gogoi, B. K. (2012). Evaluation of nutritional and biochemical aspects of *Po:ro apong* (Saimod)—A home made alcoholic rice beverage of *Mising* tribe of Assam, India. *Indian Journal of Traditional Knowledge*,(2012). http://nopr.niscair.res.in/handle/123456789/14392.

Kemgang, T. S., Kapila, S., Shanmugam, V. P., & Kapila, R. (2014). Cross-talk between probiotic lactobacilli and host immune system. *Journal of Applied Microbiology, 117*(2), 303–319.

Khatoon, N., & Gupta, R. K. (2015). Probiotics beverages of sweet lime and sugarcane juices and its physiochemical, microbiological & shelf-life studies. *Journal of Pharmacognosy and Phytochemistry, 4*(3), 25–34.

Kim, S. Y. (2017). Production of fermented kale juices with lactobacillus strains and nutritional composition. *Preventive Nutrition and Food Science, 22*(3), 231–236.

Kumar, R., Sood, U., Gupta, V., Singh, M., Scaria, J., & Lal, R. (2020). Recent advancements in the development of modern probiotics for restoring human gut microbiome dysbiosis. *Indian Journal of Microbiology, 60*, 12–25. https://doi.org/10.1007/s12088-019-00808-y.

Kumar, B. V., Umamahesh, K., & Reddy, O. V. S. (2017). Isolation and identification of *Pediococcus pentosaceus* from cow's milk curd and its use in grape juices fermentation. *Journal of Advances in Biology & Biotechnology*, 1–11. https://doi.org/10.9734/JABB/2017/34440.

Lakshmy, G., Devi, B. S., & Ramesh, B. (2018). The blooming prospects of probiotic products in India. *International Journal of Recent Technology and Engineering*, *7*, 253–259.

Lamba, J., Goomer, S., & Saxena, S. K. (2019). Study the lactic acid bacteria content in traditional fermented Indian drink: Karji. *International Journal of Gastronomy and Food Science*. *16*, 100143https://doi.org/10.1016/j.ijgfs.2019.100143.

Mishra, S. S., Behera, P. K., Kar, B., & Ray, R. C. (2018). Advances in probiotics, prebiotics and nutraceuticals. In *Innovations in technologies for fermented food and beverage industries* (pp. 121–141). Cham: Springer.

Mishra, S. S., Ray, R. C., Panda, S. K., & Montet, D. (2017). Technological innovations in processing of fermented foods an overview. In *Fermented foods, part II* (pp. 21–45). Boca Raton, FL: CRC Press.

Mishra, S. S., Ray, R. C., & Rosell, C. M. (2017). Microbial enzymes in food applications: History of progress. In *Microbial enzyme technology in food applications* (pp. 17–32). Boca Raton, FL: CRC Press.

Mousavi, Z. E., Mousavi, S. M., Razavi, S. H., Emam-Djomeh, Z., & Kiani, H. (2011). Fermentation of pomegranate juice by probiotic lactic acid bacteria. *World Journal of Microbiology and Biotechnology*, *27*(1), 123–128.

Nagpal, R., Kumar, A., & Kumar, M. (2012). Fortification and fermentation of fruit juices with probiotic lactobacilli. *Annals of Microbiology*, *62*(4), 1573–1578.

Nath, A. H., Ukkuru, M., & Kumari, M. K. S. (2015). Development of a probiotic honey beverage. *Optimization*, *1*(9), 1–9.

Nychas, G. J. E., Panagou, E. Z., Parker, M. L., Waldron, K. W., & Tassou, C. C. (2002). Microbial colonization of naturally black olives during fermentation and associated biochemical activities in the cover brine. *Letters in Applied Microbiology*, *34*, 173–177.

Padghan, P. V., Mann, B., Sharma, R., & Kumar, A. (2015). Studies on bio-functional activity of traditional Lassi. *Indian Journal of Traditional Knowledge*, *1*, 124–131.

Panda, S. K., Behera, S. K., Qaku, X. W., Sekar, S., Ndinteh, D. T., Nanjundaswamy, H. M., et al. (2017). Quality enhancement of prickly pears (*Opuntia sp.*) juice through probiotic fermentation using *Lactobacillus fermentum*-ATCC 9338. *LWT*, *75*, 453–459.

Panda, S. H., Das, S., Bal, P., Panda, S. K., Goli, J. K., & Mohanty, N. (2018). Characterization of novel folate producing *Lactobacillus rhamnosus* and its appliance in fortification of ragi (*Eleusine coracana*) gruel. *Food Bioscience*, *21*, 100–106.

Panghal, A., Janghu, S., Virkar, K., Gat, Y., Kumar, V., & Chhikara, N. (2018). Potential non-dairy probiotic products–a healthy approach. *Food Bioscience*, *21*, 80–89.

Panghal, A., Virkar, K., Kumar, V., Dhull, S. B., Gat, Y., & Chhikara, N. (2017). Development of probiotic beetroot drink. *Current Research in Nutrition and Food Science Journal*. *5*(3) https://doi.org/10.12944/CRNFSJ.5.3.10.

Peerajan, S., Chaiyasut, C., Sirilun, S., Chaiyasut, K., Kesika, P., & Sivamaruthi, B. S. (2016). Enrichment of nutritional value of *Phyllanthus emblica* fruit juice using the probiotic bacterium, *Lactobacillus paracasei* HII01 mediated fermentation. *Food Science and Technology*, *36* (1), 116–123.

Pereira, A. L. F., Almeida, F. D. L., Lima, M. A., da Costa, J. M. C., & Rodrigues, S. (2014). Spray-drying of probiotic cashew apple juice. *Food and Bioprocess Technology*, *7*(9), 2492–2499.

Pimentel, T. C., Madrona, G. S., Garcia, S., & Prudencio, S. H. (2015). Probiotic viability, physicochemical characteristics and acceptability during refrigerated storage of clarified apple juice supplemented with *Lactobacillus paracasei ssp. paracasei* and oligofructose in different package type. *LWT- Food Science and Technology*, *63*(1), 415–422.

Prado, F. C., Parada, J. L., Pandey, A., & Soccol, C. R. (2008). Trends in non-dairy probiotic beverages. *Food Research International*, *41*(2), 111–123.

Rafiq, S., Sharma, V., Nazir, A., Rashid, R., & Sofi, S. A. (2016). Development of probiotic carrot juice. *Journal of Nutrition & Food Sciences*, *6*(534), 2. https://doi.org/10.4172/2155-9600.1000534.

Ramakrishna, B. S. (2014). *FAO/WHO guidelines to assess probiotic efficacy for human consumption–would they suffice? ECAB health impact of probiotics: Vision & opportunities-E-book*: (p. 105). .

Ranjitha, K., Oberoi, H. S., Upreti, K. K., & Redappa, K. (2018). Screening of probiotic strains for development of ready-to-serve probioticated mango beverage. *Journal of Horticultural Sciences*, *13*(2), 164–171.

Ray, M., Ghosh, K., Singh, S., & Mondal, K. C. (2016). Folk to functional: An explorative overview of rice-based fermented foods and beverages in India. *Journal of Ethnic Foods*, *3*(1), 5–18.

Ray, M., Hor, P. K., Singh, S. N., & Mondal, K. C. (2017). Screening of health beneficial microbes with potential probiotic characteristics from the traditional rice-based alcoholic beverage, haria. *Acta Biologica Szegediensis*, *61*(1), 51–58.

Reddy, L. V., Min, J. H., & Wee, Y. J. (2015). Production of probiotic mango juice by fermentation of lactic acid bacteria. *Microbiology and Biotechnology Letters*, *43*(2), 120–125.

Roberts, D., Reyes, V., Bonilla, F., Dzandu, B., Liu, C., Chouljenko, A., et al. (2018). Viability of *Lactobacillus plantarum* NCIMB 8826 in fermented apple juice under simulated gastric and intestinal conditions. *LWT*, *97*, 144–150.

Routray, W., & Mishra, H. N. (2012). Sensory evaluation of different drinks formulated from dahi (Indian yogurt) powder using fuzzy logic. *Journal of Food Processing and Preservation*, *36*(1), 1–10.

Sahu, L., & Panda, S. K. (2018). Innovative technologies and implications in fermented food and beverage industries: An overview. In *Innovations in technologies for fermented food and beverage industries* (pp. 1–23). Cham: Springer.

Saikia, B., Tag, H., & Das, A. K. (2007). Ethnobotany of foods and beverages among the rural farmers of Tai Ahom of North Lakhimpur district, Asom. *Indian Journal of Traditional Knowledge*, *6*(1)(2007). http://nopr.niscair.res.in/handle/123456789/843.

Saranraj, P., Behera, S. S., & Ray, R. C. (2019). Traditional foods from tropical root and tuber crops: Innovations and challenges. In *Innovations in traditional foods* (pp. 159–191). UK: Woodhead Publishing.

Sawian, P., Nongkynrih, K. J., Anand, U., & Charan, A. A. (2018). Biochemical tests performed for the identification of the isolates collected from local rice beer (Kiad). *Journal of Pharmacognosy and Phytochemistry*, *7*(1), 395–397.

Sha, S. P., Thakur, N., Tamang, B., & Tamang, J. P. (2012). Haria, a traditional rice fermented alcoholic beverage of West Bengal. *International Journal of Agriculture Food Science and Technology*, *3*(2), 157–160.

Shangpliang, H. N. J., Rai, R., Keisam, S., Jeyaram, K., & Tamang, J. P. (2018). Bacterial community in naturally fermented milk products of Arunachal Pradesh and Sikkim of India analysed by high-throughput amplicon sequencing. *Scientific Reports*, *8*(1), 1532. https://doi.org/10.1038/s41598-018-19524-6.

Sharma, K., Attri, S., & Goel, G. (2019). Selection and evaluation of probiotic and functional characteristics of autochthonous lactic acid bacteria isolated from fermented wheat flour dough babroo. *Probiotics and Antimicrobial Proteins*, *11*(3), 774–784.

Sharma, V., & Mishra, H. N. (2013). Fermentation of vegetable juice mixture by probiotic lactic acid bacteria. *Nutrafoods*, *12*(1), 17–22.

Sheehan, V. M., Ross, P., & Fitzgerald, G. F. (2007). Assessing the acid tolerance and the technological robustness of probiotic cultures for fortification in fruit juices. *Innovative Food Science & Emerging Technologies*, *8*(2), 279–284.

Shukla, M., Jha, Y. K., & Admassu, S. (2013). Development of probiotic beverage from whey and pineapple juice. *Journal of Food Processing and Technology*, *4*(206), 1–4.

Sivudu, S. N., Umamahesh, K., & Reddy, O. V. S. (2014). A comparative study on probiotication of mixed watermelon and tomato juice by using probiotic strains of lactobacilli. *International Journal of Current Microbiology and Applied Sciences*, *3*(11), 977–984.

Tamang, J. P. (2010). Diversity of fermented beverages and alcoholic drinks. In *Fermented foods and beverages of the world* (pp. 85–125). Boca Raton, FL: CRC Press.

Tamang, J. P. (2012). Plant-based fermented foods and beverages of Asia. In *Handbook of plant-based fermented food and beverage technology* (pp. 49–92). Boca Raton, FL: CRC Press.

Tamang, J. P. (2015). Naturally fermented ethnic soybean foods of India. *Journal of Ethnic Foods*, *2*(1), 8–17.

Tamang, B., & Tamang, J. P. (2010). In situ fermentation dynamics during production of gundruk and khalpi, ethnic fermented vegetable products of the Himalayas. *Indian Journal of Microbiology*, *50*(1), 93–98.

Tamang, J. P., Thapa, N., & Bhalla, T. C. (2016). Ethnic fermented foods and beverages of India. In *Ethnic fermented foods and alcoholic beverages of Asia* (pp. 17–72). New Delhi: Springer.

Tamang, J. P., Thapa, N., Tamang, B., Rai, A., & Chettri, R. (2015). Microorganisms in fermented foods and beverages. In *Health benefits of fermented foods and beverages* (pp. 1–110). Boca Raton, FL: CRC Press.

Thakur, N., & Bhalla, T. C. (2004). Characterization of some traditional fermented foods and beverages of Himachal Pradesh. *Indian Journal of Traditional Knowledge*, *3*, 325–335.

Thakur, N., Saris, P. E., & Bhalla, T. C. (2015). Microorganisms associated with amylolytic starters and traditional fermented alcoholic beverages of North Western Himalayas in India. *Food Bioscience*, *11*, 92–96.

Tingirikari, J. M. R., Sarathy, M. V., & Karthigarani, A. K. (2019). Impact of probiotics in human health and disease treatment. In *Nutraceutical and functional foods in disease prevention* (pp. 35–67). Hershey, PA: IGI Global.

Tiwari, S. C., & Mahanta, D. (2007). Ethnological observations on fermented food products of certain tribes of Arunachal Pradesh. *Indian Journal of Traditional Knowledge*, *6*(1)(2007). http://nopr.niscair.res.in/handle/123456789/839.

ur Rahman, U., Sahar, A., Ishaq, A., & Khalil, A. A. (2020). Design of nanoparticles for future beverage industry. In *Nanoengineering in the beverage industry* (pp. 105–136). UK: Woodhead Publishing.

Valero-Cases, E., & Frutos, M. J. (2017). Effect of inulin on the viability of *L. plantarum* during storage and in vitro digestion and on composition parameters of vegetable fermented juices. *Plant Foods for Human Nutrition*, *72*(2), 161–167.

Vanajakshi, V., Vijayendra, S. V. N., Varadaraj, M. C., Venkateswaran, G., & Agrawal, R. (2015). Optimization of a probiotic beverage based on Moringa leaves and beetroot. *LWT- Food Science and Technology*, *63*(2), 1268–1273.

Vasudha, S., & Mishra, H. N. (2013). Non dairy probiotic beverages. *International Food Research Journal*, *20*(1), 7–15.

Vivek, K., Mishra, S., Pradhan, R. C., & Jayabalan, R. (2019). Effect of probiotification with *Lactobacillus plantarum* MCC 2974 on quality of Sohiong juice. *LWT*, *108*, 55–60.

Wootton-Beard, P. C., & Ryan, L. (2011). Improving public health?: The role of antioxidant-rich fruit and vegetable beverages. *Food Research International*, *44*(10), 3135–3148.

Yadav, R., Puniya, A. K., & Shukla, P. (2016). Probiotic properties of *Lactobacillus plantarum* RYPR1 from an indigenous fermented beverage Raabadi. *Frontiers in Microbiology*, *7*, 1683. https://doi.org/10.3389/fmicb.2016.01683.

Yang, X., Zhou, J., Fan, L., Qin, Z., Chen, Q., & Zhao, L. (2018). Antioxidant properties of a vegetable–fruit beverage fermented with two Lactobacillus plantarum strains. *Food Science and Biotechnology*, *27*(6), 1719–1726.

Yoon, K. Y., Woodams, E. E., & Hang, Y. D. (2004). Probiotication of tomato juice by lactic acid bacteria. *The Journal of Microbiology*, *42*(4), 315–318.

Zandi, M. M., Hashemiravan, M., & Berenjy, S. (2016). Production of probiotic fermented mixture of carrot, beet and apple juices. *Archives of Advances in Biosciences (Journal of Paramedical Sciences)*, *7*(3), 17–23.

CHAPTER

3

Probiotic beverages in Japan (some history and current developments)

Hirosuke Sugahara and Tatsuhiko Hirota
Core Technology Laboratories, Asahi Quality & Innovations, Ltd., Moriya-shi, Ibaraki, Japan

3.1 Introduction

There are many traditional fermented foods in Japan such as miso, soy sauce, natto, sake, amazake and vinegar, but in terms of probiotic beverages in Japan, these are mostly fermented dairy products, products similar to those found in other countries. This chapter depicts Japanese history and market trends of various probiotic beverages. According to the Japanese literature, milk or dairy products used to be uncommon and were recognized as medicine in ancient Japan. These products were consumed by a limited number of people, such as nobility. There was little consumption of dairy products until the late 19th century. Since the 1950s, dairy products have been increasingly consumed. Although dairy products were not generally consumed in Japan at the beginning of the 20th century, two unique dairy products did emerge in Japan.

Kaiun Mishima, the founder of the CALPIS brand, visited Inner Mongolia on business and found people drinking cultured milk, which was milk fermented with lactobacilli. Mishima was surprised by the good flavor of the drink and found that the healthful properties of the drink improved his own health condition. He was convinced that the secret of the tastiness and the healthy function of the drink lay in the milk and the lactobacilli. After returning to Japan, he devoted his time to developing a tasty and healthy cultured milk product. As a result, this product, which was the first lactic acid drink in Japan, was launched in 1919

https://doi.org/10.1016/B978-0-12-818588-9.00005-X

(Fig. 3.1). The product was made from skim milk and other ingredients and fermented slowly by adding a starter culture that included *Lactobacillus helveticus* as the predominant microorganism (Ohsawa, Uchida, Ohki, Nakamura, & Yokogoshi, 2015).

Minoru Shirota was a Japanese microbiologist, who discovered that certain lactic acid bacteria survived passage through the gut after ingestion. He isolated and cultivated *Lactobacillus casei* strain Shirota in 1930. The *L. casei* strain Shirota is thought to be beneficial to maintain gut health. This strain has been cultivated in a mixture of skim milk or skimmed milk powder, sugar and glucose, and this cultivated mixture has been commercially marketed as the probiotic milk beverage Yakult since 1935 (Gogineni, Morrow, Gregory, & Malesker, 2013). The beverage contains a high concentration of sugar. This sugar-enriched milk is usually subjected to high heat treatment. Therefore, Maillard types of reactions are induced between sugar and amino acids, resulting in a light coffee brown beverage color (Turkmen, Akal, & Özer, 2019).

Nowadays, these two products are manufactured and marketed not only in Japan but in other countries as well. CALPIS and Yakult are long selling products that celebrated their 100th and 80th anniversary in 2019 and 2015, respectively. Today, the former product is marketed with line extensions containing various flavors and fruit juices by Asahi Soft Drinks Co. Ltd. Many papers have shown that the *L. casei* strain Shirota contained in the latter product has various functionalities for host health. Since the

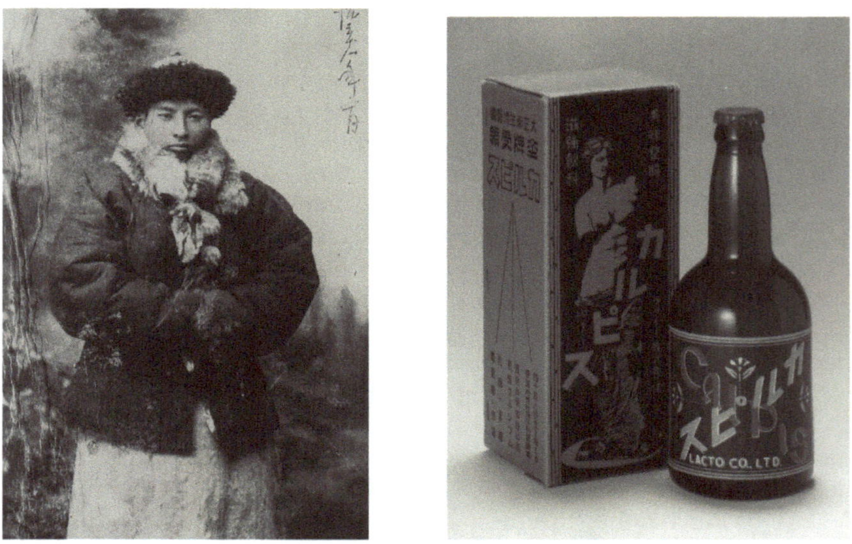

FIG. 3.1 Photograph of Kaiun Mishima in 1906 and photo of CALPIS bottle packaging for the product launch in 1919.

health benefits of lactic acid bacteria are now widely understood in Japan, many beverages containing lactic acid bacteria have been developed since the 1950s. However, there were few probiotic strains whose functionality was already as well elucidated in the 1950s. In 1991, there was the approval of the "*F*oods for *S*pecialized *H*ealth *U*se" (FOSHU), which permits labelling of health claims on foods that meet specific requirements for safety and efficacy and this had a major impact on the development of each company's own probiotic strains (Yamada, Sato-Mito, Nagata, & Umegaki, 2008). For the present-day Japanese consumer market, each company develops probiotic beverages using various probiotic strains based on their own research.

3.2 Market trends and category of probiotic beverages in Japan

Market research in 2019 indicated that the Japanese market size for probiotic beverages was around 2 billion USD and that market size has been stable or slightly increasing over the past few years. The Japanese market share of the probiotic beverage category is as follows: Meiji Co. Ltd. ~40% share, Yakult Honsha Co. Ltd. ~35%, Morinaga Milk Industry Co. Ltd. ~7% and Megmilk Snow Brand Co. Ltd. ~5%. The market share is highly concentrated in the above four companies, and it has been maintained in this manner over the past few years. In the probiotic beverage market, there are about 20 products with major sales. Other than the above mentioned companies, Nissin York Co. Ltd., Ezaki Glico Co. Ltd. and Kagome Co. Ltd. are companies that also produce major beverage products.

There are several categories of probiotic beverages in Japan, such as drinkable yogurt, drinks based on fermented milk, and other types of beverages. Drinkable yogurts are liquid types of yogurt in which stabilizers, sugars, flavors and other ingredients are mixed with plain yogurt and homogenized (Nagaoka, 2019). Drinkable yogurts, as probiotic beverages, contain strains of lactic acid bacteria or bifidobacteria with specific functionality. Most of the strains with these functionalities were originally developed for use in semi-solid yogurt. Since drinkable yogurt can be easily consumed anywhere, unlike semi-solid yogurt, tastes and flavors of drinkable yogurt containing certain probiotic strains are preferred by consumers.

Drinks based on fermented milk are composite milk products obtained by mixing fermented milk with potable water, with or without the addition of other ingredients, such as whey, other non-dairy ingredients and flavorings. Drinks based on fermented milk must contain a minimum of 40% fermented milk (CODEX STAN 243-2003). In this chapter, probiotic beverages containing certain probiotic strains and their health benefits, supported by clinical studies, will be elucidated.

3.3 Drinkable yogurts with probiotic strains

Each Japanese dairy company has marketed drinkable yogurt with their own probiotic strain. Meiji Co. Ltd. mainly uses three probiotic strains: *Lactobacillus gasseri* OLL2716, *Lactobacillus delbrueckii* subsp. *bulgaricus* OLL1073R-1 and *Lactobacillus gasseri* PA-3 for their product marketed as 'drinkable yogurt with probiotic strains'. In a human clinical study, *L. gasseri* OLL2716 containing yogurt reduced gastric mucosal inflammation related to *Helicobacter pylori* infection (Sakamoto et al., 2001) and it had beneficial effects on functional dyspepsia without *H. pylori* involvement (Ohtsu et al., 2017). *L. bulgaricus* OLL1073R-1 produces extracellular polysaccharides that induce natural killer cell activation in vivo (Makino et al., 2016) and intake of yogurt fermented with *L. bulgaricus* OLL1073R-1 was reported to reduce the risk of catching the common cold and to enhance natural killer cell activity in the elderly people (Makino et al., 2010). *L. gasseri* PA-3 showed high incorporation of purines (Yamada et al., 2016) and oral intake of yogurt containing *L. gasseri* PA-3 alleviated increases in serum uric acid levels of the subjects (Kurajoh et al., 2018). Even though these findings were elucidated using a semi-solid yogurt, these benefits are thought to derive from the specific lactic acid bacteria rather than from the nutrition of the yogurt. Therefore, drinkable yogurt containing *L. gasseri* OLL2716 has the potential to maintain the health of the upper digestive tract; drinkable yogurt containing *L. bulgaricus* OLL1073R-1 has the potential to reduce the risk of infection; while drinkable yogurt containing *L. gasseri* PA-3 is helpful for alleviating conditions with high serum uric acid levels.

Megmilk Snow Brand Co. Ltd. mainly uses two probiotic strains: *Lactobacillus gasseri* SBT2055 and *Bifidobacterium longum* SBT2928 for their "drinkable yogurt with probiotic strains." The fermented milk containing *L. gasseri* SBT2055 is reported to exhibit a lowering effect on abdominal adiposity in human (Kadooka et al., 2010, 2013), thus drinkable yogurt containing *L. gasseri* SBT2055 should be helpful for reducing visceral fat. In addition, the intake of the fermented milk is reported to promote the production of specific IgA, an acquired immune function, and also to promote the activation of NK cells, an innate immune function (Nishihira et al., 2016), thus suggesting that *L. gasseri* SBT2055 has potential in this area. Some studies have shown beneficial effects of *B. longum* SBT2928 (Nishihira et al., 2016), however, most of the studies used it as an admixture with *L. gasseri* SBT2055.

The functionality of *B. longum* SBT 2928 alone is still unclear. The genus *Bifidobacteria* is a natural resident bacterial group in the human gut microbiota (Bottacini, Ventura, Sinderen, & Motherway, 2014). Since *Bifidobacteria* are obligate anaerobes and dairy products contain certain concentrations of dissolved oxygen, the survival rate of *Bifidobacteria* in dairy products needs to be improved. It is thought that the capsules improve the survival rate of *B. longum* SBT 2928 by protecting the bacteria from the dissolved oxygen in the dairy product. For this reason, capsules enclosing the *B. longum* SBT 2928 are included in drinkable yogurt.

The Morinaga Milk Industry Co. Ltd. mainly uses *Bifidobacterium longum* subsp. *longum* BB536 for "drinkable yogurt with probiotic strains." Since 1971, *B. longum* BB536 has been used for "Bifidus Yogurt," which was the first dairy product in Japan containing a bifidobacterial strain. *B. longum* BB536 is reported to have several beneficial effects such as alleviation of gastrointestinal disorders, improvement of intestinal environment, immuno-modulation, anti-allergy and anti-infections. It is considered that the modulation of gut microbiota is the principal beneficial action of live *B. longum* BB536 cells in promoting human health (Wong, Odamaki, & Xiao, 2019) as the live cells act in concert with the gut microbiota to improve intestinal health. A human clinical study indicated that defecation frequency was significantly increased by the oral intake of yogurt containing live *B. longum* BB536 cells compared to the oral intake of yogurt without the probiotic strain (Ogata et al., 1997), inferring that yogurt with *B. longum* BB536 was more effective than yogurt without the probiotic strain. Since viability of *B. longum* BB536 cells in a dairy product is an important factor, a technique for the improvement of growth and viabilities in dairy products was developed using the *Lactococcus lactis* subsp. *lactis* MCC866, which has a cell wall–anchored proteinase and an active oxygen species reducer (genes coding for alkyl hydroperoxide reductase). The *L. lactis* MCC866-induced growth of *B. longum* BB536 by supplementation of nutrients derived from the degradation of protein and enhanced viability of *B. longum* BB536 by reducing active oxygen species contained in dairy product (Odamaki, Xiao, Yonezawa, Yaeshima, & Iwatsuki, 2011; Yonezawa et al., 2010).

Improvement of intestinal health is the most well-known beneficial function in probiotic strains and the company Chr. Hansen has commercially marketed many probiotic strains such as *Lactobacillus rhamnosus* GG and *Bifidobacterium animalis* subsp. *lactis* BB-12 that globally are the most documented probiotic *Lactobacillus* and *Bifidobacterium* strains (Jungersen et al., 2014; Segers & Lebeer, 2014).

In Japan, drinkable yogurt containing *L. rhamnosus* GG has till date only been marketed by Takanashi Milk Products Co. Ltd., while drinkable yogurt containing *B. animalis* BB-12 has been marketed by several companies such as Koiwai Dairy Products Co. Ltd. and Furuya Milk Products

Co. Ltd. Drinkable yogurts containing *B. animalis* GCL2505 (Ishizuka et al., 2012) and *B. animalis* LKM512 (Matsumoto, Aranami, Ishige, Watanabe, & Benno, 2007) have been marketed by Ezaki Glico Co. Ltd. and Kyodo Milk Industry Co. Ltd., respectively. Japanese companies have used *B. animalis* for drinkable yogurt as *B. animalis* has a higher tolerance for dissolved oxygen compared to other bifidobacterial strains (Meile et al., 1997).

Since 1970, the company Yakult Honsha Co. Ltd. has marketed a drinkable yogurt named 'Joie'. This product contains one of the most famous probiotic strains, the *L. casei* strain Shirota, which was originally first used for Yakult. The cell numbers of *L. casei* strain Shirota in the product number over 1.25 billion cells per bottle and this strain has also now been used in various fruit juices for further commercialization. Since 1978, Yakult Honsha Co. Ltd. also has marketed drinkable yogurt named "Mil-Mil," which contains *Bifidobacterium breve* strain Yakult. Administration of *B. breve* strain Yakult has been reported to show clinical benefits in immunocompromised patients by improving their intestinal environments (Wada et al., 2010). The beverage tastes more like milk rather than exhibiting the flavors of fermented milk. The product is packaged in a container consisting of five layers: three layers of polyethylene, one layer of paper and one layer of aluminum foil. Atmospheric oxygen is blocked by the container and it is thought that viability of the *B. breve* strain Yakult in the product is therefore improved.

3.4 Drinks based on fermented milk with probiotic strains

Drinks based on fermented milk were defined by CODEX (CODEX STAN 243-2003) in 2010, a relatively new definition for dairy products. In Japan, the most famous drink based on fermented milk with a probiotic strain is Yakult, marketed by Yakult Honsha Co. Ltd. As mentioned previously, this product contains the *L. casei* strain Shirota and many research articles have explored the health benefits of the *L. casei* strain Shirota on the host, including improving the intestinal environment, contributing to weight loss and contributing to higher perceived sleep satisfaction (Matsumoto et al., 2010; Nagata, Chiba, Wang, & Yamashiro, 2017; Takada et al., 2017). Research of new functionality in *L. casei* strain Shirota has continued and Yakult as a manufactured product has changed since 2013. The former Yakult contained 15 billion cells of *L. casei* strain Shirota per bottle, while the currently manufactured product contains 20 billion cells of *L. casei* strain Shirota per bottle. The product has been renamed "New Yakult." Already since 1999, there was a line extension of the product, containing 40 billion cells of *L. casei* strain Shirota per bottle, marketed as "Yakult 400."

As the other drinks based on fermented milk, Yakult Honsha Co. Ltd. also markets BF-1, which contains the probiotic strain named *Bifidobacterium bifidum* YIT10347. The product is also enclosed in the five-layer package. Drinks based on fermented milk containing *B. bifidum* YIT10347 are reported to exert beneficial effects on gastrointestinal discomfort and symptoms such as postprandial discomfort and epigastric pain in healthy adults (Gomi et al., 2018).

Nissin York Co. Ltd. has marketed a beverage based on fermented milk containing the probiotic strain named *Lactobacillus casei* NY1301. This product is reported to improve the intestinal environment (Azuma et al., 2001). The Morinaga Milk Industry Co. Ltd. markets "Caldus Milk," which contains more than 2 billion cells of *B. longum* BB536 per bottle. This beverage tastes like milk rather than fermented milk and has the benefits of intestinal environment improvement derived from *B. longum* BB536.

In the Japanese market, there are many drinks marketed that are based on fermented milk other than the manufactured products described above, however, the functionality of the strains used in most of these fermented milk drinks has not yet been elucidated.

3.5 Other types of beverages containing probiotic strains

The company Kagome Co. Ltd. markets a probiotic drink containing a low concentration of milk product named Labreα, which contains *Lactobacillus brevis* KB290. Research on the consumption of capsules containing *L. brevis* KB290 reported on the improvement of non-pathological diarrhea-predominant irritable bowel syndrome symptoms and inflammatory status in healthy volunteers (Fuke, Aizawa, Suganuma, Takagi, & Naito, 2017). Therefore, *L. brevis* KB290 addition to a probiotic beverage is thought to improve the intestinal environment.

Yakult Honsha Co. Ltd. markets soymilk fermented by the *L. casei* strain Shirota. Soymilk contains glycosides forms of isoflavones, which not only have estrogen-like effects but also can suppress the effects of excessive estrogen. Glycosidic activity in the *L. casei* strain Shirota produces aglycones forms of isoflavone from glycoside forms of isoflavones, thereby improving human intestinal absorption of isoflavones (Nagino et al., 2016). The improvement of isoflavone absorption has the potential in promoting health. The functionality of the product is mainly considered to be the result of improved absorption of the soy isoflavone rather than the health benefit of the *L. casei* strain Shirota. As well as drinks based on fermented milk, many beverages containing lactic acid bacteria are marketed in Japan, however, the functionality of the strains used in most of these beverages has not yet been elucidated.

3.6 Beverages with paraprobiotic strains

Almost all probiotic beverages in Japan are distributed as chilled beverages for a number of reasons. The viabilities of the cells affect the properties of the manufactured product by their fermentation. The temperature of the manufactured product requires regulation to improve the viability of the probiotic strain, as the health benefits of the probiotic strains are highly dependent on their cell number. On the other hand, most of the non-probiotic beverages distributed in the Japanese market are packed in plastic bottles. For usefulness in distribution, beverages packed in plastic bottles are usually favored since they can be stored at room temperature.

Taverniti and Guglielmetti (2011) reviewed the effect of non-viable lactic acid bacteria and proposed a new concept regarding the immunomodulatory properties of probiotic microorganisms beyond their viability (Taverniti & Guglielmetti, 2011). This new concept was defined as "paraprobiotics"; non-viable microbial cells (intact or broken) or crude cell extracts, which, when administered in adequate amounts, confer a benefit on the human or animal consumer. Several studies described in the review indicate that non-viable probiotic strains can have immunomodulatory effects. Paraprobiotics have certain advantages over probiotics in allowing for the development of safer, more stable, and more numerous different products (Adams, 2010). Piqué et al. (2019) reviewed paraprobiotic treatments and effects on the improvement of intestinal health (Piqué et al., 2019).

Asahi Soft Drinks Co. Ltd. has used three paraprobiotic strains for beverages: *Lactobacillus acidophilus* L-92, *Lactobacillus amylovorus* CP1563 and *Lactobacillus gasseri* CP2305. Research on the administration of tablets containing heat-killed *L. acidophilus* L-92 showed that it was effective for atopic dermatitis symptoms in adults (Inoue et al., 2014), and that tablets containing heat-killed *L. acidophilus* L-92 could reduce symptoms by suppressing type-2-helper-T-cell-dominant inflammation by activating regulatory T-cells and type 1 helper T-cells (Yamamoto et al., 2016). Paraprobiotic beverages containing *L. acidophilus* L-92 have the potential in reducing allergic symptoms such as atopic dermatitis. The strain *L. amylovorus* CP1563 firstly selected for it PPARα/γ activation ability contributes to ameliorating metabolic disorders. For the upregulation of PPARα/γ activation ability, the *L. amylovorus* CP1563 culture was heat-killed and fragmented. The fragmented *L. amylovorus* CP1563 induced decreased levels of low-density lipoprotein cholesterol and triglycerides in mouse plasma (Nakamura, Ishida, Sawada, et al., 2016). Since consumption of a beverage containing fragmented *L. amylovorus* CP1563 indicated a reduction in body fat and prevention of metabolic syndrome in a human clinical study, beverages containing fragmented *L. amylovorus* CP1563 are also thought to reduce body fat (Nakamura, Ishida, Aihara, et al., 2016). Sugawara et al. (2016) reported that the administration of beverages containing heat-killed *L. gasseri* CP2305 had a beneficial effect on the regulation of intestinal function (Sugawara et al., 2016). In addition, ingestion of beverages containing heat-killed *L. gasseri* CP2305 ameliorated chronic stress-associated behavior such as sleep quality (Nishida et al., 2017) and improved mental, physical, and sleep quality (Sawada et al., 2017). Based on these insights, a beverage containing heat-killed *L. gasseri* CP2305 is thought to improve intestinal health and stress-associated symptoms such as sleep quality.

Other paraprobiotic beverages containing *Lactobacillus paracasei* MCC1849, *Lactococcus lactis* JCM5805 and *Lactobacillus plantarum* L-137 have been marketed by Morinaga Milk Industry Co. Ltd., Kirin Beverage Company, Limited and House Wellness Foods Corporation, respectively. All paraprobiotic strains have shown the immunomodulatory effects in human clinical studies (Hirose, Murosaki, Yamamoto, Yoshikai, & Tsuru, 2006; Maruyama et al., 2016; Shibata et al., 2016). Table 3.1 summarizes the main probiotic beverages and probiotic/paraprobiotic strains on the Japanese market in 2019.

TABLE 3.1 Summary of the main Japanese companies and probiotic/paraprobiotic strains used for their beverages.

Main company	Beverage type	Probiotic strains	Paraprobiotic strains
Meiji Co. Ltd.	Drinkable yogurt	*Lactobacillus gasseri* OLL2716	–
		Lactobacillus delbrueckii subsp. *bulgaricus* OLL1073R-1	–
		Lactobacillus gasseri PA-3	–
Yakult Honsha Co. Ltd	Drinks based on fermented milk and Drinkable yogurt	*Lactobacillus casei* strain Shirota	–
	Drinkable yogurt	*Bifidobacterium breve* strain Yakult	–
	Drinks based on fermented milk	*Bifidobacterium bifidum* YIT10347	–

Continued

TABLE 3.1 Summary of the main Japanese companies and probiotic/paraprobiotic strains used for their beverages—cont'd

Main company	Beverage type	Probiotic strains	Paraprobiotic strains
Morinaga Milk Industry Co. Ltd	Drinkable yogurt and drinks based on fermented milk	*Bifidobacterium longum* subsp. *longum* BB536	–
	Drinkable yogurt and milk beverage	–	*Lactobacillus paracasei* MCC1849
Megmilk Snow Brand Co. Ltd.	Drinkable yogurt	*Lactobacillus gasseri* SBT2055	–
		Bifidobacterium longum SBT2928	–
Nissin York Co. Ltd.	Drinks based on fermented milk	*Lactobacillus casei* NY1301	–
Ezaki Glico Co. Ltd.	Drinkable yogurt	*Bifidobacterium animalis* GCL2505	–
Kagome Co. Ltd.	Lactic fermenting beverage	*Lactobacillus brevis* KB290	–
Asahi Soft Drinks Co. Ltd	Soft drink	–	*Lactobacillus acidophilus* L-92
		–	*Lactobacillus amylovorus* CP1563
		–	*Lactobacillus gasseri* CP2305
Kirin Beverage Company, Limited	Soft drink	–	*Lactococcus lactis* JCM5805
House Wellness Foods Corporation	Soft drink	–	*Lactobacillus plantarum* L-137

3.7 Conclusions

Along with the overall increase in the consumption of dairy products, many probiotic beverages have been developed. Two events have had a major impact on the development of probiotic beverages in Japan. The first event was health claims labelling regulations with "*F*oods for *S*pecialized *H*ealth *U*se" (FOSHU) described in the introduction leading to probiotic beverages being marketed and widely distributed that mainly focus on improving the intestinal environment. The second event was the launch of a new food labeling system known as "Food with Function Claims" (FFC) in 2015. Under this system, industry producers independently evaluate the scientific evidence on healthy foods such as food ingredients, and products containing the health foods are permitted to describe the functional properties that warrant health claims (Maeda-Yamamoto & Ohtani, 2018). Development of probiotic beverages with several new functionalities, such as alleviating increases of the serum uric acid levels and improving metabolic function was promoted by this system. Paraprobiotic beverages also now have the chance to be more widely marketed. Currently, probiotic beverages with new functionality are being developed under the "food with function claims," and innovative new probiotic beverages based on additional scientific knowledge are expected to continue to be developed for both the Japanese and global markets.

References

Adams, C. A. (2010). The probiotic paradox: Live and dead cells are biological response modifiers. *Nutrition Research Reviews*, *23*(1), 37–46.

Azuma, Y., Ito, K., Ohki, A., Inoue, A., Inoue, K., Sato, M., & Benno, Y. (2001). Effects of a milk drink fermented with *Lactobacillus gasseri* NY0509 and *Lactobacillus casei* NY1301 on fecal microflora in healthy volunteers. *Nippon Shokuhin Kagaku Kogaku Kaishi*, *48*(1), 35–43.

Bottacini, F., Ventura, M., Sinderen, D., & Motherway, M. (2014). Diversity, ecology and intestinal function of bifidobacteria. *Microbial Cell Factories*, *13*(Suppl 1), S4.

Fuke, N., Aizawa, K., Suganuma, H., Takagi, T., & Naito, Y. (2017). Effect of combined consumption of *Lactobacillus brevis* KB290 and β-carotene on minor diarrhoea-predominant irritable bowel syndrome-like symptoms in healthy subjects: A randomised, double-blind, placebo-controlled, parallel-group trial. *International Journal of Food Sciences and Nutrition*, *68*(8), 973–986.

Gogineni, V. K., Morrow, L. E., Gregory, P. J., & Malesker, M. A. (2013). Probiotics: History and evolution. *Journal of Ancient Diseases & Preventive Remedies*, *01*(02).

Gomi, A., Yamaji, K., Watanabe, O., Yoshioka, M., Miyazaki, K., Iwama, Y., & Urita, Y. (2018). *Bifidobacterium bifidum* YIT 10347 fermented milk exerts beneficial effects on gastrointestinal discomfort and symptoms in healthy adults: A double-blind, randomized, placebo-controlled study. *Journal of Dairy Science*, *101*(6), 4830–4841.

Hirose, Y., Murosaki, S., Yamamoto, Y., Yoshikai, Y., & Tsuru, T. (2006). Daily intake of heat-killed *Lactobacillus plantarum* L-137 augments acquired immunity in healthy adults. *The Journal of Nutrition*, *136*(12), 3069–3073.

Inoue, Y., Kambara, T., Murata, N., Komori-Yamaguchi, J., Matsukura, S., Takahashi, Y., … Aihara, M. (2014). Effects of oral administration of *Lactobacillus acidophilus* L-92 on the symptoms and serum cytokines of atopic dermatitis in Japanese adults: A double-blind, randomized, clinical trial. *International Archives of Allergy and Immunology*, *165*(4), 247–254.

Ishizuka, A., Tomizuka, K., Aoki, R., Nishijima, T., Saito, Y., Inoue, R., … Ikeda, T. (2012). Effects of administration of *Bifidobacterium animalis* subsp. *lactis* GCL2505 on defecation frequency and bifidobacterial microbiota composition in humans. *Journal of Bioscience and Bioengineering*, *113*(5), 587–591.

Jungersen, M., Wind, A., Johansen, E., Christensen, J. E., Stuer-Lauridsen, B., & Eskesen, D. (2014). The science behind the probiotic strain *Bifidobacterium animalis* subsp. *lactis* BB-12 (®). *Microorganisms*, *2*(2), 92–110.

Kadooka, Y., Sato, M., Imaizumi, K., Ogawa, A., Ikuyama, K., Akai, Y., … Tsuchida, T. (2010). Regulation of abdominal adiposity by probiotics (*Lactobacillus gasseri* SBT2055) in adults with obese tendencies in a randomized controlled trial. *European Journal of Clinical Nutrition*, *64*(6), 636–643.

Kadooka, Y., Sato, M., Ogawa, A., Miyoshi, M., Uenishi, H., Ogawa, H., … Tsuchida, T. (2013). Effect of *Lactobacillus gasseri* SBT2055 in fermented milk on abdominal adiposity in adults in a randomised controlled trial. *The British Journal of Nutrition*, *110*(9), 1696–1703.

Kurajoh, M., Moriwaki, Y., Koyama, H., Tsuboi, H., Matsuda, H., Yamada, N., … Yamamoto, T. (2018). Yogurt containing *Lactobacillus gasseri* PA-3 alleviates increases in serum uric acid concentration induced by purine ingestion: A randomized, double-blind, placebo-controlled study. *Gout and Nucleic Acid Metabolism*, *42*(1), 31–40.

Maeda-Yamamoto, M., & Ohtani, T. (2018). Development of functional agricultural products utilizing the new health claim labeling system in Japan. *Bioscience, Biotechnology, and Biochemistry*, *82*(4), 554–563.

Makino, S., Ikegami, S., Kume, A., Horiuchi, H., Sasaki, H., & Orii, N. (2010). Reducing the risk of infection in the elderly by dietary intake of yoghurt fermented with *Lactobacillus delbrueckii* ssp. *bulgaricus* OLL1073R-1. *The British Journal of Nutrition*, *104*(7), 998–1006.

Makino, S., Sato, A., Goto, A., Nakamura, M., Ogawa, M., Chiba, Y., … Asami, Y. (2016). Enhanced natural killer cell activation by exopolysaccharides derived from yogurt fermented with *Lactobacillus delbrueckii* ssp. *bulgaricus* OLL1073R-1. *Journal of Dairy Science*, *99*(2), 915–923.

Maruyama, M., Abe, R., Shimono, T., Iwabuchi, N., Abe, F., & Xiao, J. Z. (2016). The effects of non-viable *Lactobacillus* on immune function in the elderly: A randomised, double-blind, placebo-controlled study. *International Journal of Food Sciences and Nutrition*, *67*(1), 67–73.

Matsumoto, M., Aranami, A., Ishige, A., Watanabe, K., & Benno, Y. (2007). LKM512 yogurt consumption improves the intestinal environment and induces the T-helper type 1 cytokine in adult patients with intractable atopic dermatitis. *Clinical and Experimental Allergy : Journal of the British Society for Allergy and Clinical Immunology*, *37*(3), 358–370.

Matsumoto, K., Takada, T., Shimizu, K., Moriyama, K., Kawakami, K., Hirano, K., … Nomoto, K. (2010). Effects of a probiotic fermented milk beverage containing *Lactobacillus casei* strain Shirota on defecation frequency, intestinal microbiota, and the intestinal environment of healthy individuals with soft stools. *Journal of Bioscience and Bioengineering*, *110*(5), 547–552.

Meile, L., Ludwig, W., Rueger, U., Gut, C., Kaufmann, P., Dasen, G., … Teuber, M. (1997). *Bifidobacterium lactis* sp. nov., a moderately oxygen tolerant species isolated from fermented milk. *Systematic and Applied Microbiology*, *20*(1), 57–64.

Nagaoka, S. (2019). Yogurt production. In M. Kanauchi (Ed.), *Lactic acid bacteria. Methods in molecular biology, (Book 1887)* (pp. 45–54). Totoway, NJ: Humana Press.

Nagata, S., Chiba, Y., Wang, C., & Yamashiro, Y. (2017). The effects of the *Lactobacillus casei* strain on obesity in children: A pilot study. *Beneficial Microbes*, *8*(4), 535–543.

Nagino, T., Kano, M., Masuoka, N., Kaga, C., Anbe, M., Miyazaki, K., … Tanaka, A. (2016). Intake of a fermented soymilk beverage containing moderate levels of isoflavone aglycones enhances bioavailability of isoflavones in healthy premenopausal Japanese women: A double-blind, placebo-controlled, single-dose, crossover trial. *Bioscience of Microbiota, Food and Health*, *35*(1), 9–17.

Nakamura, F., Ishida, Y., Aihara, K., Sawada, D., Ashida, N., Sugawara, T., … Fujiwara, S. (2016). Effect of fragmented *Lactobacillus amylovorus* CP1563 on lipid metabolism in overweight and mildly obese individuals: A randomized controlled trial. *Microbial Ecology in Health and Disease*, *27*, 30312.

Nakamura, F., Ishida, Y., Sawada, D., Ashida, N., Sugawara, T., Sakai, M., ... Fujiwara, S. (2016). Fragmented lactic acid bacterial cells activate peroxisome proliferator-activated receptors and ameliorate dyslipidemia in obese mice. *Journal of Agricultural and Food Chemistry*, *64*(12), 2549–2559.

Nishida, K., Sawada, D., Kuwano, Y., Tanaka, H., Sugawara, T., Aoki, Y., ... Rokutan, K. (2017). Daily administration of paraprobiotic *Lactobacillus gasseri* CP2305 ameliorates chronic stress-associated symptoms in Japanese medical students. *Journal of Functional Foods*, *36*, 112–121.

Nishihira, J., Moriya, T., Sakai, F., Kabuki, T., Kawasaki, Y., & Nishimura, M. (2016). *Lactobacillus gasseri* SBT2055 stimulates immunoglobulin production and innate immunity after influenza vaccination in healthy adult volunteers: A randomized, double-blind, placebo-controlled, parallel-group study. *Functional Foods in Health and Disease*, *6*(9), 544–568.

Odamaki, T., Xiao, J. Z., Yonezawa, S., Yaeshima, T., & Iwatsuki, K. (2011). Improved viability of bifidobacteria in fermented milk by cocultivation with *Lactococcus lactis* subspecies *lactis*. *Journal of Dairy Science*, *94*(3), 1112–1121.

Ogata, T., Nakamura, T., Anjitsu, K., Yaeshima, T., Takahashi, S., Fukuwatari, Y., ... Iino, H. (1997). Effect of *Bifidobacterium longum* BB536 administration on the intestinal environment, defecation frequency and fecal characteristics of human volunteers. *Bioscience and Microflora*, *16*(2), 53–58.

Ohsawa, K., Uchida, N., Ohki, K., Nakamura, Y., & Yokogoshi, H. (2015). *Lactobacillus helveticus*—Fermented milk improves learning and memory in mice. *Nutritional Neuroscience*, *18*(5), 232–240.

Ohtsu, T., Takagi, A., Uemura, N., Inoue, K., Sekino, H., Kawashima, A., ... Koga, Y. (2017). The ameliorating effect of *Lactobacillus gasseri* OLL2716 on functional dyspepsia in *Helicobacter pylori*-uninfected individuals: A randomized controlled study. *Digestion*, *96*(2), 92–102.

Piqué, N., Berlanga, M., Miñana-Galbis, D., Piqué, N., Berlanga, M., & Miñana-Galbis, D. (2019). Health benefits of heat-killed (tyndallized) probiotics: An overview. *International Journal of Molecular Sciences*, *20*(10)E2534.

Sakamoto, I., Igarashi, M., Kimura, K., Takagi, A., Miwa, T., & Koga, Y. (2001). Suppressive effect of *Lactobacillus gasseri* OLL 2716 (LG21) on *Helicobacter pylori* infection in humans. *The Journal of Antimicrobial Chemotherapy*, *47*(5), 709–710.

Sawada, D., Kawai, T., Nishida, K., Kuwano, Y., Fujiwara, S., & Rokutan, K. (2017). Daily intake of *Lactobacillus gasseri* CP2305 improves mental, physical, and sleep quality among Japanese medical students enrolled in a cadaver dissection course. *Journal of Functional Foods*, *31*(April), 188–197.

Segers, M. E., & Lebeer, S. (2014). Towards a better understanding of *Lactobacillus rhamnosus* GG-host interactions. *Microbial Cell Factories*, *13*(Suppl 1), S7.

Shibata, T., Kanayama, M., Haida, M., Fujimoto, S., Oroguchi, T., Sata, K., ... Ishii, N. (2016). *Lactococcus lactis* JCM5805 activates anti-viral immunity and reduces symptoms of common cold and influenza in healthy adults in a randomized controlled trial. *Journal of Functional Foods*, *24*(June), 492–500.

Sugawara, T., Sawada, D., Ishida, Y., Aihara, K., Aoki, Y., Takehara, I., ... Fujiwara, S. (2016). Regulatory effect of paraprobiotic *Lactobacillus gasseri* CP2305 on gut environment and function. *Microbial Ecology in Health and Disease*, *27*, 30259.

Takada, M., Nishida, K., Gondo, Y., Kikuchi-Hayakawa, H., Ishikawa, H., Suda, K., ... Rokutan, K. (2017). Beneficial effects of *Lactobacillus casei* strain Shirota on academic stress-induced sleep disturbance in healthy adults: A double-blind, randomised, placebo-controlled trial. *Beneficial Microbes*, *8*(2), 153–162.

Taverniti, V., & Guglielmetti, S. (2011). The immunomodulatory properties of probiotic microorganisms beyond their viability (ghost probiotics: Proposal of paraprobiotic concept). *Genes & Nutrition*, *6*(3), 261–274.

Turkmen, N., Akal, C., & Özer, B. (2019). Probiotic dairy-based beverages: A review. *Journal of Functional Foods, 53*(February), 62–75.

Wada, M., Nagata, S., Saito, M., Shimizu, T., Yamashiro, Y., Matsuki, T., … Nomoto, K. (2010). Effects of the enteral administration of *Bifidobacterium breve* on patients undergoing chemotherapy for pediatric malignancies. *Supportive Care in Cancer: Official Journal of the Multinational Association of Supportive Care in Cancer, 18*(6), 751–759.

Wong, C. B., Odamaki, T., & Xiao, J. (2019). Beneficial effects of *Bifidobacterium longum* subsp. *longum* BB536 on human health: Modulation of gut microbiome as the principal action. *Journal of Functional Foods, 54*(March), 506–519.

Yamada, N., Iwamoto, C., Kano, H., Yamaoka, N., Fukuuchi, T., Kaneko, K., & Asami, Y. (2016). Evaluation of purine utilization by *Lactobacillus gasseri* strains with potential to decrease the absorption of food-derived purines in the human intestine. *Nucleosides, Nucleotides & Nucleic Acids, 35*(10 – 12), 670–676.

Yamada, K., Sato-Mito, N., Nagata, J., & Umegaki, K. (2008). Health claim evidence requirements in Japan. *The Journal of Nutrition, 138*(6), 1192S–1198S.

Yamamoto, K., Yokoyama, K., Matsukawa, T., Kato, S., Kato, S., Yamada, K., & Hirota, T. (2016). Efficacy of prolonged ingestion of *Lactobacillus acidophilus* L-92 in adult patients with atopic dermatitis. *Journal of Dairy Science, 99*(7), 5039–5046.

Yonezawa, S., Xiao, J. Z., Odamaki, T., Ishida, T., Miyaji, K., Yamada, A., … Iwatsuki, K. (2010). Improved growth of bifidobacteria by cocultivation with *Lactococcus lactis* subspecies *lactis*. *Journal of Dairy Science, 93*(5), 1815–1823.

CHAPTER

4

Probiotic beverages in China

Wei Chen

Jiangnan University, Wuxi, Jiangsu Province, People's Republic of China

The production of commercial probiotic beverages in China was rather late compared to Japan, although in certain regions of China people have a long history of consumption of traditionally fermented beverages. The health benefits of these naturally fermented beverages were documented in ancient scripts, which may be associated with the function of natural probiotics in these beverages. According to a recent survey, probiotic beverages have gained significant traction in China's beverage market. Probiotic products, including fermented foods and beverages, have ranked in China's top 10 food trends since 2016.

4.1 Probiotic milk beverages in China

The past decades have witnessed a steady growth in the sales of probiotic milk beverages in China. In 2018, the growth rate of dairy consumption in China was higher than in other food sectors such as snacks. Currently, the vast majority of probiotic beverages in China are dairy-based, with fermented milk as the product leader among the various probiotic beverages.

4.1.1 History of probiotic milk beverages in China

For a long time in Chinese history, fermented milk beverages were prepared and consumed mainly by the northern nomadic tribes, whereas the diet of people of the Central Plains generally did not contain dairy products. The first written documentary of koumiss, a fermented beverage prepared with mare's milk, may date back 2500 years, and it is believed that koumiss may possess health benefits for digestive and chronic diseases such as bronchitis and tuberculosis (Zhang, 1994). It was recorded that the Mongols collected mare's milk in leather containers and the milk

Probiotic Beverages
https://doi.org/10.1016/B978-0-12-818588-9.00003-6

was usually held for a few days until it turned sour before drinking. However, koumiss consumption is rather limited due to its high acidity and the weak coagulation properties of mare's milk, compared to fermented milk prepared from other mammalians, particularly bovine milk. The nomadic people in Northern China had clearly already mastered the production technique of fermented milk over 2000 years ago (Zhang, Chen, Dan, & Dong, 2014).

Besides koumiss, fermented yak milk is another traditional fermented milk beverage. It is estimated that over 90% of the yak population, in the world resides in China, particularly in the Himalaya region of Central Asia, the Tibetan Plateau. Naturally fermented yak milk and cheese products are known for their microbial biodiversity including *Lactobacillus, Bifidobacterium, Streptococcus, Lactococcus,* and *Leuconostoc* species, in addition to yeasts.

However, for quite a long period China's R&D capacity in probiotics and related fermented milk products lagged behind the rate of this fast-growing market and its global counterparts. To counter this problem, in the past few decades, the collection of traditional fermented products and fecal samples were conducted in different regions of China (Tibet, Inner Mongolia, Yunnan, Sichuan, etc.) for the isolation of lactic acid bacteria for screening and the application of probiotic strains. With the efforts of Chinese scientists and the food industry, many more probiotic strains, with independent intellectual rights, have been developed and applied for use in probiotic milk beverages.

4.1.2 Market overview

China's dairy production and dairy product import rates continue to grow, indicating a strong demand for dairy products. In the past 2 years, around 30% of new supermarkets, which specialize in the sale of fresh produce and specialized products, have included probiotic milk beverages in their offerings.

In 2002, Yakult (a fermented milk drink developed by Japanese scientists in the 1930s) first entered the Chinese market and the dairy firm Yakult currently owns five production plants in China. However, it is facing challenges with more new products entering the market from Chinese competitors. The market share of Yakult in China has been decreasing over the past few years. Chinese consumers are demanding probiotic milk beverages with a more diversified flavor profile and textural properties.

Increasing health concerns, along with rising demand for functional beverage products, continue to stimulate industry application of probiotics in dairy beverages. Throughout China, the Yili, the Mengniu, and the Bright Dairy & Food Co., Ltd. dominate over 50% of the dairy market share. The products of the Bright Dairy & Food Co., Ltd. have popularity in Shanghai and nearby regions. Within the category of the fermented milk beverages of the Bright Dairy & Food Co., Ltd., "Taojingaoshou," a newly launched probiotic fermented milk beverage is leading the sales growth rate.

Although currently the majority of the probiotic strains utilized in commercial probiotic milk beverages in China are still dominated by strains developed and manufactured by oversea companies such as Chr. Hansen and DuPont (Danisco), more domestic competing players are emerging with the fast growth of the Chinese market.

Lactobacillus plantarum ST-III, a probiotic strain isolated from Chinese kimchi, was developed and applied in fermented milk products by the Bright Dairy & Food Co., Ltd. since 2004, and a series of products named "Jianneng" have been developed based on *L. plantarum* ST-III with different nutritional and functional properties (Liu, Gu, Zhang, Zhao, & Chen, 2019; Yan et al., 2018). Another example is *L. plantarum* CCFM8661, which was applied in "Taojingaoshou," a fermented milk beverage commercialized in 2018. Besides the common functional benefits of probiotics, such as improving intestinal flora balance and boosting immune function, *L. plantarum* CCFM8661 possesses a strong ability to alleviate heavy metal toxicity (Zhai et al., 2017, 2018, 2019). It has been granted multiple international and domestic patents. *L. casei* Zhang, isolated from koumiss, is another probiotic strain that has been applied in fermented milk beverages since 2015 (Hor et al., 2018; Xu et al., 2019).

In summary, although new beverage categories are emerging in the Chinese beverage market, probiotic milk beverages are retaining their popularity, as most of the probiotic beverages in China's marketplace are still dairy-based. Moreover, with the advancement of biotechnology in China, the development of probiotic strains and innovation of products will continue to support this market growth.

4.2 Probiotic fruit and vegetable beverages in China

The most popular and well-known fermented beverage in the world is yogurt, however globally, approximately 2%–3% of people are allergic to lactoprotein. In addition, the high fat and high cholesterol content found in many dairy products is not conducive to the health of people with chronic diseases such as diabetes, hypertension, hyperlipidemia, etc. Therefore, the development and promotion of new fermented fruit and vegetable beverages have become a research "hotspot," as fruits and vegetables themselves are rich in vitamins, minerals, dietary fiber and other nutrients. In addition, after fermentation by probiotic organisms, the flavor of the fruits and vegetables is increased and their antioxidant ability and immune regulatory functions are enhanced (Kumar, Vijayendra, & Reddy, 2015), which better meets the dual pursuit of nutrition and flavor and, therefore, has broad market application prospects.

4.2.1 Development history of probiotic fermented fruit and vegetable beverages

The application of probiotics in fermented fruits and vegetables can be traced back to the 1960s. Pederson (1961) first applied pure-fermentation inoculation techniques in kimchi research in 1961. Subsequently, in 1998, Caldwell Bio Fermentation Canada Inc. Used patented technology for inoculating fermented vegetables with composite strains.

The development of probiotic-fermented drinks in China is roughly divided into three stages. The first stage is lactic acid bacteria (LAB) fermented beverages, which are relatively simple in terms of fermentation time and fermentation raw materials. Represented by-products such as Wahaha's vitamin A, D calcium-enriched milk and Robust's Health Express, these sold well in the late 1980s, and the rapid rise of LAB beverages in recent years is regarded as their continuation and upgrade. The second stage is represented by fruit vinegars and grain-fermented drinks. In the mid-to-late 1990s, various types of fruit vinegars, such as McKinley Apple Cider Vinegar, opened a new era in the development of acetic acid drinks, espousing a variety of health effects. While some grain and plant-fermented beverages had become popular, the concept of fermented beverages had not been widely adopted. With the evolvement of society and the improvement of people's consumption levels, the domestic beverage market was undergoing massive changes, and people's demands for beverages have gradually turned to natural, nutritious, and healthy directions. Probiotic fermented fruit and vegetable beverages are considered to be "natural, healthy and a return to nature," exactly meeting consumer's rising demands. In the third stage, the concept of fermented fruit and vegetable beverages has been officially put forward and has gradually matured since 2014 and is now widely regarded as the milestone stage for fruit and vegetable juice beverages (Wang, 2017).

4.2.2 Probiotic function and research advances in probiotic fermented fruit and vegetable beverages

Probiotic fermented fruit and vegetable juice products are complex and diverse. For example, Xia et al. (2007) used bayberry as the main raw material, mixed carrot and tomato juice, and added *Lactobacillus bulgaricus*, *Streptococcus thermophilus* and *Lactobacillus plantarum* for fermentation. Finally, the optimum fermentation process and juice-mixing method were determined. Zhou et al. inoculated the mixed bacterial powder of *Lactobacillus plantarum, 'Bulgarian bacillus' (currently named "Lactobacillus delbrueckii"* subsp. *bulgaricus)* and *Streptococcus thermophilus* at a ratio of 2:1:1 into a mixed fragrant pear-cucumber juice for fermentation (Zhou & Liu, 2017). Zhou and Han (2011) fermented an apple-carrot mixed juice with *Lactobacillus bulgaricus* and *Streptococcus thermophilus* at a ratio of 1:1, when studying the production technology of fermented beverages.

Different fruit and vegetable juices can be fermented using different probiotics, and their probiotic functions are also different, including regulating intestinal flora, regulating immunity, antioxidant properties, lowering cholesterol and alleviating heavy metal toxicity. Zhan et al. used carrot papaya juice fermented by *Lactobacillus plantarum* DMDL 9010 to produce a mixed fermented fruit and vegetable juice. This particular probiotic strain is reputed to reduce high cholesterol in serum and has bile salt hydrolase activity, with the resultant mixed fermented fruit and vegetable juice exhibiting a rich taste and flavor, as well as good antioxidant activity (Zhan, Li, Huang, Huang, & Liu, 2019). Lan et al. developed a new pomegranate beverage fermented by LAB including *Lactobacillus casei* and *Lactobacillus rhamnosus* (Lan et al., 2017). This pomegranate beverage, fermented by LAB, exhibited a higher polyphenol content and antioxidant ability. Guan et al. described an apple juice fermented by *Bifidobacterium*, which had an inhibitory effect on four harmful bacteria (*Salmonella typhimurium, Shigella, Salmonella paratyphoid B* and *Staphylococcus aureus)* (Guan, Zhang, & Xi, 2010). Lu et al. used fermented fruit and vegetable juice to inhibit the growth of tumor cells, and the inhibition rate of lymphosarcoma was 28%, whereas that of H22 hepatoma cells was 49.1% (Lu, Toshima, Wu, Zhang, & Cai, 2007). Fruit juice fermented by LAB has been reported to significantly reduce the cholesterol content in the blood of rats (Foo et al., 2003), the mechanism may be that the LAB culture produces some active substances in the fermentation process. Zhai et al. found that fruit and vegetable juice fermented by *Lactobacillus plantarum* CCFM8610 could reduce the content of the heavy metal in mouse tissues and alleviate oxidative stress in mice.

4.2.3 Industrial progress of probiotic fermented fruit and vegetable beverages

Zenith International, a well-known global food and beverage consultancy, recently released a market analysis report on fruit and vegetable juices, pointing out that in the next 5 years, global fruit and vegetable juice beverages will grow at an average annual growth rate of 5%. They predicted that by 2020, the global consumption of fruit and vegetable juice beverages will reach 105 billion liters. Countries such as Germany, Japan and South Korea have already conducted extensive research on fermented fruit and vegetable juices and have developed a variety of fruit and vegetable beverages fermented by probiotic organisms (Ares, Giménez, & Deliza, 2010; Coïsson, Travaglia, Piana, Capasso, & Arlorio, 2005; Li, Chen, Ruan, Zhu, & He, 2010; Marafon, Sumi, Alcantara, Tamime, & Oliveiraa, 2011; Oliveira, Perego, Oliveira, & Converti, 2011; Sandoval-Castilla, Lobato-Calleros, Aguirre-Mandujano, & Vernon-Carter, 2004; Xie, Xiong, & Guan, 2014). For example, the product "The vegetable warrior" is a fruit and vegetable juice fermented by *Lactobacillus plantarum*. It contains eight kinds of fruits and vegetables such as garlic, pumpkin, sweet potato, banana, etc. It is mixed with a certain proportion of milk and has a unique flavor and rich nutrition and is very popular in the marketplace.

The research on probiotic fermented fruit and vegetable beverages in China started relatively late, but with extensive research and development potential. According to the National Bureau of Statistics, the output of fruit and vegetables is 669 million tons, accounting for more than 40% of the world's total output, but the processing rate of fruits and vegetables is very low, including less than 10% of fruits and less than 1% of vegetables. The processing technology for fruits and vegetables in foreign countries is relatively mature, and their processing rates of fruits and vegetables is over 40%. The high yield and low processing rate make the loss rate of fresh fruits and vegetables in China exceed 30%, while that of fruits and vegetables in foreign countries is less than 7% (Chen et al., 2012). The rapid development of the fermentation industry, the changes in consumption trends, and the low deep processing rate of fresh fruits and vegetables, together have laid a solid foundation for the requirement of the development of fermented fruit and vegetable juice beverages in China.

In addition, the standardization of the fermented fruit and vegetable juice beverage industry in China is currently in the promotion stage. The authoritative standards are "General Principles of Beverage" of GB/T10789-2015, "Fruit and Vegetable Juice and its Beverage" of GB/T31121-2014, "Apple Cider Vinegar Beverage" of GB/T30884-2014 and other national standards. At present, many of these products on the market are mainly implemented according to corporate standards. With the continuous growth of the fermented fruit and vegetable juice beverage industry, the market is urgently in need of corporate champions in the industry to formulate relevant national standards and industry standards, leading to the healthy development of the industry.

The research focus of fermented fruit and vegetable juice beverage products is about technology and the craft of strain fermentations, which are concentrated in three aspects: the breeding of fermentation strains, optimization of fermentation technology and flavor modification. The Nanchang University of China and Jiangxi Jiangzhong Pharmaceutical (Group) Co., Ltd., jointly, completed the "key technology and industrial application of probiotic fermented fruits and vegetables," and they won the 2016 National Science and Technology Progress Award second prize. This project introduced probiotic fermentation technology into the field of deep processing of fruit and vegetable foods and created a key technology innovation system for the upper, middle and lower reaches of probiotic fermented fruits and vegetables. A new series of products have been popularized and applied in 71 enterprises in 19 provinces and cities in China, which has effectively enhanced the international competitiveness of fruit and vegetable foods in China and promoted the scientific and technological progress of the fruit and vegetable processing industry.

4.3 Probiotic cereal beverages in China

In China, cereals are the main components in the daily diet and the important role of cereals was addressed in Huangdi's Classic on Medicine 2000 years ago. According to the Dietary Guidelines for China, cereals are a staple food and a very important energy source that can also provide protein, dietary fiber, vitamin B and minerals to guarantee a balance of dietary nutrients. Cereal beverages can satisfy the requirements for nutrition supplements for the rapid pace of modern life, which focuses on natural and healthy properties and is the main trend for beverage developments. Probiotic fermentation can improve the nutritional value and provide special flavors of cereal beverages, with large market potential. In 2007, the Hui Erkang Corporation took the lead in promoting a series of cereal beverages called "Guli" and a variety of cereal beverages made of coarse grains were continually developed by COFCO Limited and the Yili Group.

4.3.1 Development of probiotic fermented cereal beverages

Unlike fermented milk and fruit beverages, researchers had already begun to study fermented cereal beverages in the 1990s. Mercier et al. studied the kinetics of lactic acid fermentation on corn by *Lactobacillus amylophilus* in 1992 (Mercier, Yerushalmi, Rouleau, & Dochain, 1992). In Japan, rice germ was fermented to produce beverages that could provide rich nutrition and benefit human health (Chen, 2004).

In 1994, Lu et al. from Anhui Agricultural University studied the transformation of wheat starch, which was fermented by lactic acid bacteria to produce lactic acid beverages (Lu & Xiong, 1994). This may be the first report on fermented cereal beverages in China. Sticky rice, corn juice and oats are also very good materials for probiotic fermentation and provide both nutrition and beneficial health effects (Luo, Lu, Yu, Wang, & Gao, 2011).

In 2010, the Ministry of Health P.R. China released a list of bacterial cultures permitted in foods, and only the bacterial cultures in this list were allowed to be used in food products. The list in 2010 included six *Bifidobacterium* species, 14 *Lactobacillus* species and *Streptococcus* thermophiles. Since then, new species of cultures have been added and the list has been updated yearly.

Probiotic organisms are beneficial to human health and are mainly *Bifidobacterium* and *Lactobacillus* species. *Lactobacillus* species are more commonly used in cereal beverage fermentation; whereas sometimes yeasts are applied for co-fermentation to form better and more mellow flavors (Gao et al., 2014; Luo, Kong, Guo, Jia-li, & Kong, 2015). The fermentation can be achieved by single or multi bacterial cultures (Chen et al., 2014; Jiang et al., 2018). Chen et al. fermented cargo rice with six different cultures (*Lactobacillus casei, L. acidophilus, L. delbrueckii, L. salivarius, Bifidobacterium* and *Saccharomyces cerevisiae)*, and showed advantages in high protein/fiber content and low fat/energy (Chen et al., 2014). In addition, the transformation of bioactive substances may occur during cereal beverage fermentations, such as an increase in organic acids and β-glucans. Probiotic fermentation can also improve the bioavailability of the iron and zinc present in cereals (Enujiugha, 2006). Arora et al. reported how probiotic fermentation can be a potential process to enhance the nutritional quality of mixed coarse cereals (Arora, Jood, & Khetarpaul, 2010).

4.3.2 Probiotic function and research advances in probiotic fermented cereal beverages

In recent years, as more attention has been paid to health and nutrition, fermented beverages have become more popular. There is a very long history of milk-based beverages in probiotic fermentation. However, the probiotic potential of cereal-based beverages is now attracting more attention. Cereals are rich in water-soluble fibers and oligosaccharides, which can act as substrates for probiotic organism fermentations and cereals are becoming one of the favored probiotic carriers (Enujiugha & Badejo, 2017; Lamsal & Faubion, 2009). For example, Charalampopoulos et al. found that malt, wheat and barley extracts exhibited protective effects on the viability of *L. plantarum, L. acidophilus* and *L. reuteri* in acidic conditions, which may be due to the sugars present in the cereal extracts (Charalampopoulos, Pandiella, & Webb, 2003). Angelov et al. developed an oat-based probiotic drink using *Lactobacillus plantarum* B28 as the starter and found that the β-glucan content in the drink remained unchanged during the fermentation (Angelov, Gotcheva, Kuncheva, & Hristozova, 2006). Beta-glucan is reported to have effects on glycemic, insulin and cholesterol responses to foods and is regarded as a functional food ingredient (Brennan & Cleary, 2005). Arora et al. found that germination and fermentation caused significant improvements in reducing the sugar, thiamine, niacin, lysine and soluble dietary fiber content of barley-based food mixtures, which enhanced the nutritional quality of these food mixtures (Arora et al., 2010).

In China, using health functional claims is another way to create added value for consumers. Nowadays, there are only 18 listed health claims that are allowed to be used on health foods, which decreased from the previous 27 claims. Probiotics can also be tested for their potential for these claims. It should be stated that any product aiming to offer health functions should apply for health food registration in advance.

4.3.3 Industrial progress of probiotic fermented cereal beverages

Probiotics are widely accepted in China and new probiotic products are continually developed and introduced to the market. Currently, the vast majority of probiotic beverages are dairy-based, and to date cereal-based beverages only have a very small market portion. However, many studies suggest that cereals have very important nutritive values. One type of fermented cereal beverage is made by mixing cereal pulp with fermented milk, which can either be a probiotic beverage with live strains or a non-viable bacteria beverage with a longer shelf life.

The second type of beverage uses cereal pulp as a substrate and then adds probiotic organisms to produce a fermented beverage, which can be preserved with the live probiotic strains under cold chain storage. The organic acids produced by the probiotic organisms can help to maintain a balanced digestive system and also moderate the beverage's flavor and taste. In addition, the cereal-based probiotic beverages can be alternatives for consumers who have limitations on their consumption of dairy products, in addition to providing exotic and unique tastes.

Probiotic products offer great potential in China's markets for their health benefits and the refined tastes. Research indicates that consumer awareness of probiotics has reached 70% in first-tier cities. For Chinese consumers, the taste is everything and today still outranks health benefits on people's purchasing decisions. Therefore, taste and health benefits should be combined together to develop cereal-based probiotics beverages. The development of new probiotic strains and various types of products to meet the needs of these ever increasing markets an exciting opportunity.

References

Angelov, A., Gotcheva, V., Kuncheva, R., & Hristozova, T. (2006). Development of a new oat-based probiotic drink. *International Journal of Food Microbiology, 112*, 75–80.

Ares, G., Giménez, A., & Deliza, R. (2010). Influence of three non-sensory factors on consumer choice of functional yogurts over regular ones. *Food Quality and Preference, 21*, 361–367.

Arora, S., Jood, S., & Khetarpaul, N. (2010). Effect of germination and probiotic fermentation on nutrient composition of barley based food mixtures. *Food Chemistry, 119*, 779–784.

Brennan, C. S., & Cleary, L. J. (2005). The potential use of cereal (1→3, 1→4)-β-D-glucans as functional food ingredients. *Journal of Cereal Science, 42*, 1–13.

Charalampopoulos, D., Pandiella, S., & Webb, C. (2003). Evaluation of the effect of malt, wheat and barley extracts on the viability of potentially probiotic lactic acid bacteria under acidic conditions. *International Journal of Food Microbiology, 82*, 133–141.

Chen, Z. (2004). The developmental trend of rice intensive utilization in 21st century. *Journal of Wuxi University of Light Industry, 23*(4), 104–110.

Chen, L. S., Ding, Q. B., Wu, W. L., Liu, J., Su, X. X., & Zhao, Y. (2012). Research progress in functional characteristics of fermented fruit and vegetable juices. *Science and Technology of Food Industry, 33*(11), 418–421.

Chen, H.-X., Zhao, L.-Q., Yun, T.-T., Liu, S., Li, Y.-R., Yang, Z.-Q., et al. (2014). Study on manufacturing process and nutritional value of brown rice beverage by probiotic fermentation. *Food and Fermentation Industries, 40*(11), 269–275.

Coïsson, J. D., Travaglia, F., Piana, G., Capasso, M., & Arlorio, M. (2005). *Euterpe oleracea* juice as a functional pigment for yogurt. *Food Research International, 38*, 893–897.

Enujiugha, V. N. (2006). Supplementation of ogi, a maize-based infant weaning food, with African oil bean seed (*Pentaclethra macrophylla* Benth). *International Journal of Postharvest Technology and Innovation, 1*, 202–211.

Enujiugha, V. N., & Badejo, A. A. (2017). Probiotic potentials of cereal-based beverages. *Critical Reviews in Food Science and Nutrition, 57*(4), 790–804.

Foo, H. L., Loh, T. C., Lim, Y. S., Shukriyah, M. H., Kufi, C. N., & Law, F. L. (2003). Effects of fermented fruits on growth performance, shedding of Enterobacteriaceae and lactic acid Bacteria and plasma cholesterol in rats. *Pakistan Journal of Nutrition, 2*(4), 228–233.

Gao, Y., Han, Y.-Q., Yu, M., Lu, M., Zhang, C. H., Li, C.-Y., et al. (2014). Optimization on the technology of fermented brown rice beverage. *Food Science and Technology, 39*(2), 121–124.

Guan, X. R., Zhang, D. C., & Xi, Q. (2010). Biological antagonism of *Bifidobacterium* fermented mixed fruit and vegetable juice *in vitro*. *Chinese Journal of Microecology, 22*(3), 202–204.

Hor, Y. Y., Lew, L. C., Lau, A. S. Y., Ong, J. S., Chuah, L. O., Lee, Y. Y., et al. (2018). Probiotic *Lactobacillus casei* Zhang (LCZ) alleviates respiratory, gastrointestinal and RBC abnormality via immuno-modulatory, anti-inflammatory and anti-oxidative actions. *Journal of Functional Foods, 44*, 235–245.

Jiang, Y.-X., Zhang, Y., Yu, A.-T., Wang, S.-Y., Zhou, Q., Zhang, T.-C., et al. (2018). Optimizing the preparation technics of *Lactobacillus plantarum*-fermented cereals beverage. *Food Science and Technology, 43*(11), 83–89.

Kumar, B. V., Vijayendra, S. V. N., & Reddy, O. V. S. (2015). Trends in dairy and non-dairy probiotic products—a review. *Journal of Food Science and Technology, 52*(10), 6112–6124.

Lamsal, B. P., & Faubion, J. M. (2009). The beneficial use of cereal components in probiotic foods. *Food Reviews International, 25*, 103–114.

Lan, Y., Wu, J., Wang, X., Sun, X., Hackman, R. M., Li, Z., et al. (2017). Evaluation of antioxidant capacity and flavor profile change of pomegranate wine during fermentation and aging process. *Food Chemistry, 232*, 777–787.

Li, Q. Q., Chen, Q. H., Ruan, H., Zhu, D. S., & He, G. Q. (2010). Isolation and characterisation of an oxygen, acid and bile resistant *Bifidobacterium animal* subsp. *lactis* Qq08. *Journal of the Science of Food and Agriculture, 90*, 1340–1346.

Liu, J., Gu, Z., Zhang, H., Zhao, J., & Chen, W. (2019). Preventive effects of *Lactobacillus plantarum* ST-III against Salmonella infection. *LWT- Food Science and Technology, 105*, 200–205.

Lu, M., Toshima, Y., Wu, X. L., Zhang, X., & Cai, Y. Q. (2007). Inhibitory effects of vegetable and fruit ferment liquid on tumor growth in Hepatoma-22 inoculation model. *Asia Pacific Journal of Clinical Nutrition*, *16*, 443–446.

Lu, Y., & Xiong, J. (1994). Functional cereal beverages fermented by lactic acid bacteria. *Technical Information from China and Foreign Countries*, *4*, 16–17.

Luo, Y.-Y., Kong, L.-L., Guo, J.-L., Jia-li, & Kong, J. (2015). Research of compound cereal fermented drink. *Food Research and Development*, *36*(14), 57–62.

Luo, C., Lu, Z., Yu, W., Wang, Q., & Cao, X. (2011). Study on production process of several cereal drinks fermented by probiotics. *Journal of Northeast Agricultural University*, *42*(5), 127–129.

Marafon, A. P., Sumi, A., Alcantara, M. R., Tamime, A. Y., & Oliveiraa, M. N. (2011). Optimization of the rheological properties of probiotic yoghurts supplemented with milk proteins. *LWT- Food Science and Technology*, *44*(2), 511–519.

Mercier, P., Yerushalmi, L., Rouleau, D., & Dochain, D. (1992). Kinetics of lactic acid fermentation on glucose and corn by *Lactobacillus amylophilus*. *Journal of Chemical Technology and Biotechnology*, *55*(2), 111–121.

Oliveira, R. P. D. S., Perego, P., Oliveira, M. N. D., & Converti, A. (2011). Growth and survival of mixed probiotics in nonfat fermented milk: The effect of inulin. *Chemical Engineering Transactions*, *24*, 457–462.

Pederson, C. S. (1961). The effect of pure-culture inoculation on fermentation of cucumbers. *Food Technology*, *15*, 351–354.

Sandoval-Castilla, O., Lobato-Calleros, C., Aguirre-Mandujano, E., & Vernon-Carter, E. J. (2004). Microstructure and texture of yogurt as influenced by fat replacers. *International Dairy Journal*, *14*, 151–159.

Wang, N. (2017). Analysis on development status and trend analysis of fermented fruit and vegetable juice beverage. *Agricultural Science and Technology and Equipment*, *5*, 75–76. (in Chinese).

Xia, Q. L., Xing, J. R., Chen, J. B., Yang, Y., Zhu, Z. J., Chen, G. F., et al. (2007). Research of blended fermented fruit and vegetable juice drink. *Storage and Process*, *7*(4), 46–48.

Xie, M. Y., Xiong, T., & Guan, Q. Q. (2014). Research progress on the key techniques of the fruit and vegetable products fermented by probiotics. *Journal of Chinese Institute of Food Science and Technology*, *14*(10), 1–8.

Xu, H., Huang, W., Hou, Q., Kwok, L. Y., Laga, W., Wang, Y., et al. (2019). Oral administration of compound probiotics improved canine feed intake, weight gain, immunity and intestinal microbiota. *Frontiers in Immunology*, *10*, 666. https://doi.org/10.3389/fimmu.2019.00666.

Yan, M., Chen, W., Li, N., Ren, J., Chen, C., You, C., et al. (2018). Impact of *Lactobacillus plantarum* ST-III on the composition of infant gut microbiota and its potential synergism with breast milk and infant formula as revealed by an in vitro study. *International Dairy Journal*, *85*, 66–72.

Zhai, Q., Liu, Y., Wang, C., Qu, D., Zhao, J., Zhang, H., et al. (2019). *Lactobacillus plantarum* CCFM8661 modulates bile acid enterohepatic circulation and increases lead excretion in mice. *Food & Function*, *10*(3), 1455–1464.

Zhai, Q., Wang, H., Tian, F., Zhao, J., Zhang, H., & Chen, W. (2017). Dietary *Lactobacillus plantarum* supplementation decreases tissue lead accumulation and alleviates lead toxicity in Nile tilapia (*Oreochromis niloticus*). *Aquaculture Research*, *48*(9), 5094–5103.

Zhai, Q., Yang, L., Zhao, J., Zhang, H., Tian, F., & Chen, W. (2018). Protective effects of dietary supplements containing probiotics, micronutrients, and plant extracts against lead toxicity in mice. *Frontiers in Microbiology*, *9*, 2134. https://doi.org/10.3389/fmicb.2018.02134.

Zhan, S., Li, Q. L., Huang, Y. Y., Huang, J., & Liu, D. M. (2019). Development and oxidation resistance of mixed fermented fruit-vegetable juice of carrot and papaya. *Food Science and Technology*, *44*(1), 146–153.

Zhang, H. (1994). Ancient Chinese dairy products. *China Dairy Industry*, *22*(4), 161–167 (in Chinese).

Zhang, H., Chen, X., Dan, T., & Dong, J. (2014). Traditional Chinese fermented dairy foods. In *Lactic acid bacteria* (pp. 493–535). Dordrecht: Springer.

Zhou, Y. H., & Han, Q. X. (2011). Studied on fruit and vegetable juice beverages fermented by lactic acid bacteria. *Food Research and Development*, *32*(3), 113–116.

Zhou, Q., & Liu, M. J. (2017). Technology optimization of bergamot pear-cucumber juice fermented by mixed *Lactobacillus*. *Food Industry*, *12*, 68–72.

CHAPTER

5

Fermented foods and probiotic beverages in Korea

Kwangsei Lim[a] *and Jongho Koh*[b]

[a]Research & Innovation Center, Danone Pulmuone Co., Ltd., Seoul, South Korea

[b]Department of Bio-food Analysis and Technology, Bio Campus, Korea Polytechnics College, Nonsan, South Korea

5.1 Introduction

There have been many changes in definition since the concept of probiotics was introduced, but one thing that has not changed is that it can help the health of the host when ingested. Currently, the definition of probiotics uses what was proposed by FAO/WHO (2001). As you can see from the definition "live microorganisms which, when administered in adequate amounts, confer a health benefit on the host" it is a very broad and general requirement (FAO/WHO, 2001). Probiotics have been naturally recognized and consumed as functional products by the beneficial actions of the probiotics themselves. Although some problems may arise with the recognition of lactic acid bacteria and probiotics as the same, foods containing probiotics have been able to achieve the same success as the current ones by inheriting consumer expectations for the safety of GRAS (Generally Regarded As Safe) status and effectiveness.

The Korean food and beverage cultures are showing many changes due to geographical characteristics, living environments, traditional lifestyles, religious rites, and the living standards of the times. Traditional beliefs show the religious and cultural features of Buddhism, Confucianism, and Christianity, which are entrenched deeply into life, according to the times based on history. Agriculture began around 3–4000 BCE in the Korean Peninsula and the farming life was settled from 500 BCE.

Despite a short history of consumption of less than 50 years in Korea, the belief in the beneficial effects of fermented milk itself or lactic acid

Probiotic Beverages
https://doi.org/10.1016/B978-0-12-818588-9.00016-4

bacteria has strongly developed thanks to the promotion and education of active business entities. It may be natural for Koreans, who have encountered a variety of fermented foods based on vegetables, grains, and even fish, other than fermented milk products, that the Western-style yogurt market has achieved remarkable growth in such a short time. This success, followed by probiotic products, especially functional foods that could claim functionalities, has resulted in explosive growth in a short period of about 10 years.

5.2 Fermented foods in Korea

The unique geographical location of Korea and its isolation from neighboring countries has contributed to the development of a distinct ethnic group with a unique culture. Through time, simplicity has become a basic notion of Korean philosophy, and this simplicity is also reflected in food habits. In Korea, where dairy farming is not developed, fermented foods using vegetables and grains rather than milk have evolved. Various types of traditional fermented foods, such as doenjang, chungkookjang, ganjang (soybean sauce), gochujang (fermented soybean paste made of red pepper powder), and kimchi are the essential elements of Korean cuisine and these are consumed by many people around the world as healthy foods. Everyone would agree that kimchi, which is fermented vegetables, is a typical traditional fermented food that represents Korea (Patra, Das, Paramithiotis, & Shin, 2016; Surh, Kim, & Kwon, 2008).

5.2.1 Kimchi

Kimchi, a representative Korean fermented vegetable, consisting of mixing salted napa cabbage and other ingredients, such as red pepper powder, garlic, ginger, scallions, and salted fish, is a side dish that is often served on tables. The term kimchi originated from Chimchae, which means soaking vegetables, and it is recorded in the ancient Korean book, Samkuksaki, published in 1145 CE (Cheigh & Park, 1994; Surh et al., 2008). The appearance of kimchi began to be similar to that of traditional kimchi of the late Joseon Dynasty (1392–1897). There are many kinds of kimchi, depending on ingredients, seasons, and regions. Kimchi is still mainly made and consumed by each household, and due to changes in the social environment and the demand of the younger generation for convenience, branded kimchi produced in commercial mass production systems is also growing (Cheigh & Park, 1994; Patra et al., 2016).

As kimchi is prepared from fresh vegetables, the fermentation processes occur via the microbial succession of various microorganisms naturally present in the raw materials in kimchi. The concentration of salt in kimchi is about 2%–3%, so only salt-resistant microorganisms can survive. In an air-blocked environment, lactic acid bacteria increase rapidly, and then, kimchi develops a unique taste and aroma with lactic acid, acetic acid, carbon dioxide, and alcohol. The lactic acid bacteria, such as *Leuconostoc citreum, L. mesenteroides, L. gasicomitatum, L. gelidum, L. carnosum, Weissella cibaria, W. koreensis, W. confusa, Lactobacillus sakei, Lb. brevis,* and *Lb. plantarum* are commonly present, and members of the genera *Lactococcus* and *Pediococcus* are present in lesser abundance (Chang, 2018; Chang & Chang, 2010; Jung, Lee, & Jeon, 2014; Lee et al., 2015). *Leuconostoc mesenteroides* is the primary bacterium that leads the fermentation until kimchi tastes delicious. In the early stages of fermentation, *Leuconostoc* species, such as *L. citreum, L. lactis,* and *L. mesenteroides* are dominant and predominantly produce carbon dioxide, acetic acid, ethanol, various ester compounds, mannitol, and dextran together with lactic acid (Cho et al., 2006; Kim & Chun, 2005; Lee, Kim, Cho, & Kim, 2008; Lim, Park, & Han, 1989). When the pH of kimchi drops due to the organic acid produced, the number of microorganisms with weak acid resistance decreases sharply. The acid-tolerant *Lactobacillus* spp. appear after the middle of fermentation, and *Lb. plantarum* and *Lb. brevis* dominate the flora. The number of lactic acid bacteria in kimchi is counted at an initial level of about 10^4–10^5 CFU/g, up to 10^8 CFU/g, when it is fully ripened (Chang, Choi, & Chang, 2011; Shin, Kim, Han, Lim, & Bak, 1996).

Recent studies have revealed that kimchi has nutritional and health-promoting properties, as it is rich in vitamins, minerals, dietary fibers, and other functional components, including lactic acid bacteria (Islam & Choi, 2009; Kim et al., 2011; Park, Jeong, Lee, & Daily, 2014). Several studies have found that kimchi, which was recognized as healthy oriental food, has excellent potential as a source of probiotics (Chang & Chang, 2011; Dharaneedharan & Heo, 2016; Park, Jeong, et al., 2014). Consumption of kimchi, as a part of the daily diet, exhibits a series of positive effects on a variety of factors associated with metabolic syndrome, including blood pressure, body fat, blood glucose, and total cholesterol (Park, Jeong, et al., 2014; Patra et al., 2016).

5.2.2 Fermented soy pastes

Soybeans are known to be native to China (Manchuria area) and Korea (in the Northeast Asia region), and their usage dates back to 4000 years ago. Soy-based products include cheonggukjang (quick fermented soybean paste), doenjang (soybean paste), ganjang (soy sauce), and gochujang (hot pepper-soybean paste) and these are prepared once in a year, stored in large clay pots and consumed throughout the year. These fermented soybean foods have become an essential part of the Korean diet, used as a seasoning and found in side dishes and soups that are consumed daily (Patra et al., 2016; Shin & Jeong, 2015).

To make doenjang, the beans are mashed to make a lump of soybean paste (meju, Korean-style soybean koji), fermented for growth of bacteria and fungi, and the fermented soybean paste is soaked in salty water for 40–60 days for maturation (further fermentation). After, the meju is taken out from a container (porcelain pot), the liquid is made with soy sauce (ganjang), and the remaining solids are placed into another container and salted, more cooked cereals and meju are added into it and it is matured for 3–6 months to make traditional doenjang. Doenjang varies depending upon the ingredients used, the ripening time, and the ripening method. The unique flavors and tastes are due to the decomposed products of soybean proteins, from the soybean seed, by the action of microorganisms during fermentation. *Bacillus subtilis* and *B. licheniformis* are the dominant microbes in doenjang, along with *Aspergillus*, *Mucor*, and *Rhizopus* species, all of which originate from airborne microorganisms or which exist naturally in raw soybean materials (Kang, Kim, Joo, Lee, & Yim, 2000; Nam, Won, Chung, Kwak, & Kwon, 2015; Patra et al., 2016; Shin & Jeong, 2015).

The history of cheonggukjang production dates back to BEC, but the oldest on record dates back to the period of the Three Kingdoms (683 CE) in the Korean Peninsula. Cheonggukjang is a fermented product that is manufactured with a short fermentation period (2–4 days) of boiled soybeans using the *B. subtilis* in the rice straw. During the short fermentation, with high temperatures (40–43°C), soybeans are converted into a viscous substance with a distinctive aroma. Koreans have been consuming cheonggukjang for hundreds of years, and significant amounts of data suggest that cheonggukjang contains bioactive potentials for human health (Anthony, Clarkson, & Williams, 1998; Barnes, Sfakianos, Coward, & Kirk, 1996; Choi, Chung, Jeong, & Oh, 2014; Kang, Lee, Yoo, & Seo, 1998; Kim, Song, Kwon, Kim, & Heo, 2008; Shin & Jeong, 2015).

Recent studies have revealed the health benefits of cheonggukjang. The key components are enzymes that function similarly to nattokinase and *Bacillus* species, such as *B. subtilis*, *B. licheniformis*, and *B. amyloliquefaciens* (Kim et al., 1996; Lee, Yang, Song, Chai, & Kim, 2006; Ryu et al., 2017). These strains have mainly been used in animal feed additives rather than in food, but recent studies have shown more attempts made to apply these spore-forming microbes to food, and one nattokinase powder has been approved as a health functional food (HFF) ingredient in Korea, with a health claim to help improve blood circulation.

5.2.3 Makgeolli: A Korean fermented grains alcoholic beverage

Makgeolli is a traditional alcoholic beverage prepared from rice, barley, wheat, or malt grains by fermentation using a natural starter called nuruk. The flavors and tastes of makgeolli depend mainly on the content of metabolic products, such as sugars, amino acids, organic acids, and aromatic compounds produced during the fermentation of rice by molds and yeasts. Compared with other alcoholic beverages, makgeolli contains high concentrations of nutrients, organic acids, and 6%–8% alcohol, as well as a significant amount of lactic acid bacteria and yeast (Jin, Kim, Jin, Eom, & Han, 2008; Kim & Han, 2006; Nile, 2015).

Nuruk is a traditional starter culture made from wheat, rice, or grits, which allows for the growth of various natural types of microorganisms, such as fungi, yeast, and lactic acid bacteria, which are useful for the parallel processes of saccharification of the rice starch and alcohol fermentation. In nuruk, *Rhizopus* species, *Aspergillus* species, *Lichethemia* species, and *Mucor* species are inhabitants, and *Saccharomyces* species *B. subtilis*, and lactic acid bacteria have been identified (Baek et al., 2010; Song et al., 2013; Park, Song, et al., 2014). It has been reported that 20 kinds of unpasteurized makgeolli in the market contain more than 10^8 CFU/mL of lactic acid bacteria. *Lactobacillus plantarum*, *L. casei*, and *L. paracasei* were dominant species, and *L. fermentum*, *L. harbinensis*, *L. ingluviei*, *L. curvatus*, *L. curstorum*, *L. rhamnosus* were also isolated (Lee, Seol, Jeong, & Kim, 2016).

Studies report that makgeolli has various biological properties, including anticancer properties, positive effects on blood circulation and lipids, antihypertensive, fibrinolytic and superoxide dismutase-like activity, and antibacterial and antioxidant properties (Kang, Kim, Ahn, & Lee, 2012; Kim, Lee, Choi, & Lee, 2002; Ryu et al., 2007).

5.2.4 Dairy fermented milk products

The birth of fermented milks, including cheese, originally began with the natural power of fermentation, when lactic acid bacteria accidentally contaminated stored milk. These serendipitous events did not occur early in Korea as the modernized breeding of milking cows only began in the early 1900s, and the production of pasteurized milk started at the Gyeongsung Milk Cooperative in 1937. A fermented milk (lactic fermented dairy drink) was first introduced to Korean consumers in 1976, as a technical partnership with Yakult Honsha. This product, packaged in a small plastic bottle, was very different in taste, flavor, color, and appearance from the traditional yogurts consumed in the Middle East or Europe. About 20 years later, a western-style spoonable yogurt was introduced to the domestic market, and over the next two decades, fermented dairy products of various formats and functions entered the local market. Global brands Yoplait (1983) and Danone (1989 and relaunched in 2009) also established their production plants in Korea and entered the market.

The local standards for fermented milks were divided into fermented milk (lactic fermented drink), thick fermented milk (yogurt), and a lactic

TABLE 5.1 Standards for fermented milks and lactic beverage in Korea.[a]

	Fermented milk (lactic fermented drink)	Thick fermented milk (yogurt)	Lactic beverage
Category	Dairy products	Dairy product	Beverage (general food)
MSNF[b] (%)	Not less than 3%	Not less 8%	Less than 3%
Lactic acid bacteria or yeast counts (CFU/mL)	More than 10^7 CFU/mL	More than 10^8 CFU/mL	More than 10^6 CFU/mL

[a] *Reference: Ministry of Food and Drug Safety (2019b).*
[b] *MSNF, milk solid non-fat.*

beverage based on MSNF (Milk Solid Non-Fat) and total counts of lactic acid bacteria (Table 5.1).

Yogurt can be divided into spoonable and drinkable forms depending on the physical properties, and most functional fermented milk products containing probiotics are drinkable yogurts. Unlike European countries where consumption of spoonable yogurt contributes significantly to the market, Korea has been leading the growth of the yogurt market with the liquid format, which accounts for a large portion of consumption. This majority is because a drinkable format product was first introduced to consumers, and it is a relatively familiar and suitable format for busy social venues. As a result, the perception that a functional yogurt is a form of drinkable beverage is firmly established by consumers to date, and even now, there are few spoonable yogurts in the market that have enhanced functionality. The Korean fermented milk market is 970 Billion Won (USD 907 Million) based on 2017 retail distribution point data (Korea Agro-Fisheries & Food Trade Corporation, 2017), and the total market is estimated to reach about 2 Trillion Won (USD 1.87 Billion) considering that about 40% of the total market is not included in the POS data because it is sales in the form of door-to-door sales. (Note – In 2017 1 US dollar = roughly 1070 Korean WON).

5.3 Health functional foods

5.3.1 Definition and regulations

HFF is a product manufactured, including processing, using functional ingredients that are nutritious and harbor beneficial functions for the body. All of the HFFs officially distributed in the Korean domestic market are ingredients that have passed the meticulous evaluation of the Ministry of Food and Drug Safety (formerly known as Korea Food and Drug Administration) for their safety and functionality, through a strict review system with human studies and animal testing and manufactured in GMP (Good Manufacturing Practice)-certified facilities.

For the distribution of HFF products in the market, each product is strictly controlled by the government with preliminary reviews against the advertising and health claims on the labels and also managed through the record tracking system to ensure product quality and to provide consumers with accurate information. Therefore, all of the HFF products approved by the government's system are required to have the proper health claims in order to be able to use the official "Health Functional Food" mark (Ministry of Food and Drug Safety, 2018).

There are two types of approved functional ingredients for HFFs in Korea as listed below:

(1) Notified in the codes of HFFs: a manufacturer can use publicly notified functional ingredient(s) for its HFF product(s) by the standards and specifications prescribed in this code.

(2) Individually recognized by the government: a business operator who wants to operate a HFF business can apply for individual recognition of functional ingredients or HFFs, and they apply for recognition to the Minister of Food and Drug Safety with the relevant data related to safety, functionality, and other requirements.

5.3.2 Probiotics as a health functional food

Sales of local HFFs have continued to grow steadily and were estimated to be 2.4 Trillion Won (USD 2.16 Billion) in 2018, and their 5-year CAGR (Compound Annual Growth Rate) was almost 9% from 2014 to 2018. Probiotics recorded the highest growth rate among HFF ingredients over the past 5 years, growing approximately 300 Billion won (USD 269 Million) in sales and moved up to third place in 2018 (Table 5.2).

While the term probiotic may seem somewhat unfamiliar to consumers, the growth of the functional drinkable yogurts that have led the domestic yogurt market since the mid-1990s, active promotion, and communication of manufacturers have made it easier than expected for consumers to understand the term probiotic. So, it is perhaps quite natural to achieve such success with probiotic products that can harbor health claims on the label. Health functional probiotic products are classified into two types of products as mentioned above, as one notified in the codes or individually recognized by the government. In the case of the notified probiotic cultures, these consist of 19 species of bifidobacteria and lactic acid

TABLE 5.2 Annual turnover and market share of health functional foods (HFF) and top five ingredients in Korea.[a]

		2014		2015		2016		2017		2018		
Rank[b]	**Ingredient**	**Sales[d]**	**MS (%)[e]**	**Sales**	**MS (%)**	**Sales**	**MS (%)**	**Sales**	**MS (%)**	**Sales**	**MS (%)**	**CAGR[c] (2014–2018) (%)**
1	Ginseng	633	38.8	694	38.1	990	46.6	1036	46.3	1110	44.0	11.88
2	Individuals[f]	318	19.5	320	17.5	236	11.1	245	11.0	323	12.8	0.29
3	Probiotic	139	8.5	158	8.7	190	9.0	217	9.7	299	11.9	16.62
4	Vitamins and minerals	142	8.7	208	11.4	184	8.7	226	10.1	248	9.8	11.91
5	Milk thistle	69	2.4	71	3.9	109	5.1	104	4.7	82	3.3	4.01
Total sales of health functional foods		1564		1733		2018		2130		2396		8.91

[a] *Source: Ministry of Food and Drug Safety (2019a).*
[b] *Rank in 2018.*
[c] *CAGR, compound annual growth rate.*
[d] *Annual turnover of local sales (Billion Korean Won).*
[e] *MS, market share.*
[f] *Individually approved ingredients as health functional foods.*

TABLE 5.3 List of probiotic cultures notified as ingredients for health functional foods in Korea.[a]

Genus	Species
Lactobacillus	*L. acidophilus, L. casei, L. gasseri, L. delbrueckii* subsp. *bulgaricus, L. helveticus, L. fermentum, L. paracasei, L. plantarum, L. reuteri, L. rhamnosus, L. salivarius*
Bifidobacterium	*B. bifidum, B. breve, B. longum, B. lactis (B. animalis* subsp. *lactis)*
Lactococcus	*L. lactis*
Streptococcus	*S. thermophiles*
Enterococcus	*E. faecium, E. faecalis*

[a] *Source: Ministry of Food and Drug Safety (2018).*

bacteria, as shown in Table 5.3. These probiotic cultures were peer-reviewed by experts in advance and health claims are only for intestinal health as below:

(1) Claims allowed: It can help to increase beneficial bacteria and suppress harmful bacteria and facilitate bowel movement.
(2) Product specifications: 10^8 to 10^{10} CFU/day.

Therefore, in order to roll out probiotic products as HFFs, it is only possible to use the specified 19 species listed or to use strains approved under the Individual Certification Approval Procedures established by the Ministry of Food and Drug Safety if a product wishes to claim functionality other than intestinal health. To date, functional claims of species/strains licensed under Individual Certification Approval Procedures are shown in Table 5.4, and only the claim statements allowed by law are available. Functional health claims added to individual certification include improving skin diseases through control of immune hypersensitivity, reduction of body fat, preventing skin damage from ultraviolet rays, and improving the vaginal health of women. Also, dead cells (postbiotic), which have been proven to be effective, have been added as individual certificated ingredients despite the WHO's definition of probiotic.

Probiotics as HFFs are mostly products packaged with sticks or sachet in powder form, and very few products have been launched into the market in a drinkable format. Powder-type products can be stored at room temperature. They are easy to carry in small quantities and can be consumed without water. Some probiotic products have been developed using micro-encapsulation techniques to increase their preservation at room temperature or to increase their survival in the digestive organs when ingested.

TABLE 5.4 List of individually approved probiotic cultures as health functional food ingredients.[a]

Microorganisms[b]	Health claims	Recommended dose (/day)
Lb. plantarum IM76 and *B. longum* IM55	Immune control (alleviation of hypersensitivity)	1×10^{10} CFU[c]
Lb. acidophilus GLA-14 and *Lb. rhamnosus* HN001	Vaginal health	5×10^{9} CFU
Lb. acidophilus YT1(HU038)	Women's health after menopause	1×10^{8} CFU
Lb. curvatus HY7601 and *Lb. plantarum* KY1032	Weight management (body fat)	1×10^{10} CFU
Lb. rhamnosus IDCC3201, heat-treated	Skin health	400 mg of powder (as 1×10^{10} CFU)
Lb. gasseri BNR17	Weight management (body fat)	1×10^{10} CFU
Lb. plantarum HY7714	Skin health	1×10^{10} CFU
Lb. rhamnosus GR-1 and *Lb. reuteri* RC-14	Vaginal health	1×10^{9} CFU
Lb. casei CBT-LC5, *Lb. rhamnosus* CBT-LR5, *Lb. plantarum CBT-LP3,* and *B. lactis* CBT-BL3	Skin health	2×10^{9} CFU
Lb. sakei Probio65	Skin health	1×10^{10}–1×10^{12} CFU
Lb. plantarum CJLP133	Skin health	1×10^{10}–1×10^{12} CFU
S. thermophilus DSM24731, *Lb. acidophilus* DS24735, *Lb. delbrueckii* subsp. *bulgaricus* DSM24734, *Lb. paracasei* DSM24733, *Lb. plantarum* DSM24730, *B. longum*	Digestive health	1×10^{8}–3×10^{12} CFU
E. faecalis FK-23, heat treated	Alleviation of allergy caused by pollen	1 g of powder

[a] *Reference: National Food Safety Information Service (2020).*
[b] B = Bifidobacterium, Lb = Lactobacillus, Lc = Lactococcus, S = Streptococcus, E = Enterococcus.
[c] *CFU, colony forming unit.*

5.4 Probiotic beverages and fermented products in Korea

5.4.1 Opportunities and restraints of the global probiotics market

The global probiotics market was estimated at USD 49.4 Billion in 2018 and projected to grow at a CAGR of 7.0%, to reach USD 69.3 Billion by 2023. The growth of the market is driven by factors such as promising health benefits of foods containing probiotics and increasing consumer awareness about healthy diets. Probiotics have proven substantial benefits related to health, more specifically to the human digestive system. Huge R&D investment has increased innovation in products and process tools for probiotics. Probiotics are found in supplement form or as components of foods and beverages. Their integration with inexpensive health foods, such as yogurt, fruit juices, and cultured dairy drinks has contributed to this significant market size. Based on the application, the food and beverage segment is estimated to account for the largest share in the probiotics market. The demand for liquid probiotics has increased as compared to dry probiotics, due to its application in yogurt, which is the most popular source of probiotics. Other products that use liquid probiotics include kefir water, probiotic juices, and yogurt-based drinks, which are healthy options for daily supplementation. The major restraints in the growth of the market are the lack of international quality standards, regulations for probiotic products, and the high R&D costs for developing new probiotic strains and scientific validations for their probiotic cultures. Due to the high cost of production, the price of the final product is also high. Marketing and distribution of these products also add to the product price, as they require different packaging and distribution channels as compared to more common products. Although consumers are aware of the health benefits of probiotics, the high prices are restraining them from buying these products, which is a challenge for manufacturers (Markets and Markets Research, 2019).

5.4.2 Probiotic drinkable yogurts

Most of the products containing probiotics in the Korean market consist of yogurts, lactic fermented milks, and powdered dietary supplements. A few probiotic juices, pasteurized milk with added probiotics, and probiotic chocolate are on the market. Among them, liquid-type products can be classified as probiotic beverages. The most popular probiotic beverages in the Korean market are definitely drinkable yogurts with probiotics. Korean consumers are very familiar with scientific or microbiological terms such as lactic acid bacteria and probiotics, as the introduction of fermented milk included communicating and focusing messages to consumers on the explanation and efficacy of lactic acid bacteria. This is why functional yogurt containing probiotics has grown so rapidly in Korea, which has a relatively short 50-year intake history compared to Europe.

Most functional fermented milk sold in Korea contains at least one probiotic strain, in addition to yogurt starters (*Lb. delbrueckii* subsp. *bulgaricus* and *S. thermophilus*), most of which are bifidobacteria and lactobacilli. Most of these starters and cultures are supplied by global culture companies (CHR. Hansen Holding A/S, Dupont-Danisco, or DSM Food

Specialties, etc.) and some strains are from dairy companies, universities, and research institutes with their own research capabilities. The origin of isolates is an essential part of the differentiation strategy for products. For example, a variety of claims can be found, such as isolates from famous longevity villages in Korea, isolates from the Caucasus region where traditional fermented milks came from, or strains certified by the Bulgarian government. Although the scientific background is weak, a wide variety of claims are utilized such as lactic acid bacteria isolated from breast milk, isolated from traditional fermented foods such as kimchi, and isolated from Korea where dietary habits were quite different from that of Western countries. However, it is not easy to validate the difference in effect attributable to the origin of the strain and to identify where it was actually isolated. Table 5.5 lists probiotic dairy products and the probiotic strains noted on the label and sold in Korea by 10 companies. Most are probiotic drinkable yogurts, claiming intestinal health with indirect expression, the primary role of lactic acid bacteria and probiotics on the host.

Since the mid-1990s, when functional yogurt was introduced, fermented dairy products that claimed various functionalities, such as lowering serum cholesterol or blood pressure control, have been developed and launched. Although there were side effects to the exaggerated advertising, as products with insufficient scientific evidence or small amounts of active ingredients appeared in the market, these drivers led to the overall growth of the yogurt market in Korea. Since 2002, functional claims have been banned in general foods and dairy products, but consumers are already aware of the beneficial effects of yogurts and probiotics even by direct or indirect expressions that are metaphorical. Nearly 30 years before the ban, consumers had already been educated through communications by manufacturers. This is why probiotic yogurts still maintain high sales performance through indirect claims without claiming specific functionality.

The controversial debate over the survivability of lactic acid bacteria in yogurt through the human digestive tract began a long time ago, but it has not been noticed in the market. However, in the various formats of probiotic products that are stored in ambient conditions, it is easy to find a product containing microencapsulated or multiple-layered probiotics.

5.4.3 Probiotic beverages as health functional foods

Apart from powdered probiotic supplements, liquid products similar to drinkable yogurt with physicochemical properties and appearance are also on the market. All products contained notified probiotics among 19 species for the intestinal health claim, and some of these emphasize additional functional claims, such as liver health, synbiotic functionality with prebiotics, or immune stimulation by adding approved ingredients as HFFs (Table 5.6).

TABLE 5.5 Korean market examples of probiotic dairy fermented milks and their microorganisms from ten companies.

Company	Product type[a]	Microorganisms on the label[b]
A	Yogurt	*B. animalis* subsp. *lactis*, *Lb. delbrueckii* subsp. *bulgaricus*, *Lc. lactis*, *S. thermophiles*
	Fermented milk	*Lb. delbrueckii* subsp. *bulgaricus*, *S. thermophilus*, *Lb. paracasei*
	Yogurt	*Lb. delbrueckii* subsp. *bulgaricus*, *Lb. rhamnosus*, *S. thermophilus*, *B. animalis* subsp. *lactis*, *Lb. helveticus*, *Lb. acidophilus*
	Fermented milk	*Lb. delbrueckii* subsp. *bulgaricus*, *Lb. rhamnosus*, *S. thermophilus*, *Lb. paracasei*
	Fermented milk	*Lb. delbrueckii* subsp. *bulgaricus*, *S. thermophilus*, *B. animalis* subsp. *lactis*, *Lb. helveticus*, *Lb. acidophilus*
	Fermented milk	*Lb. casei*
B	Yogurt	*S. thermophilus*, *Lb. acidophilus*, *B. animalis* subsp. *lactis*, *Lb. fermentum*, *Lb. plantarum*
	Yogurt	*S. thermophilus*, *Lb. acidophilus*, *B. animalis* subsp. *lactis*, *Lb. confusus*, *Lb. gasseri*, *Lb. plantarum*
	Yogurt	*B. animalis* subsp. *lactis*, *S. thermophilus*, *L. acidophilus*
	Fermented milk	*B. animalis* subsp. *lactis*, *S. thermophilus*, *Lb. delbrueckii* subsp. *bulgaricus*
C	Yogurt	*Lb. plantarum*, *S. thermophilus*, *Lb. delbrueckii* subsp. *bulgaricus*
	Fermented milk	*Lb. plantarum*, *Lb. casei*
D	Yogurt	*Lb. rhamnosus*, *B. animalis* subsp. *lactis*, *S. thermophilus*, *Lb. delbrueckii* subsp. *bulgaricus*
	Yogurt	*B. animalis* subsp. *lactis*, *Lb. acidophilus*, *S. thermophilus*
	Yogurt	*Lb. rhamnosus*, *B. animalis* subsp. *lactis*, *S. thermophilus*, *Lb. delbrueckii* subsp. *bulgaricus*, *Lc. lactis*
E	Yogurt	*Lb. acidophilus*, *Lb. casei*, *Lb. plantarum*, *Bifidobacterium* sp., *S. thermophilus*, *Lb. paracasei*
	Fermented milk	*Lb. casei*, *Bifidobacterium* sp., *Lb. plantarum*
	Fermented milk	*Lb. casei*
F	Yogurt	*Bifidobacterium* sp.(encapsulated)
G	Fermented milk	*B. animalis* subsp. *lactis*, *S. thermophilus*, *Lb. delbrueckii* subsp. *bulgaricus*
H	Fermented milk	*B. animalis* subsp. *lactis*, *S. thermophilus*, *Lb. delbrueckii* subsp. *bulgaricus*
I	Yogurt	*B. longum* (encapsulated)

[a] *Classified by milk solid non-fat content (%) of products as Food Code.*
[b] B = Bifidobacterium, Lb = Lactobacillus, Lc = Lactococcus, S = Streptococcus, E = Enterococcus.

TABLE 5.6 Probiotic beverages as health functional foods and their microorganisms and functionalities as claimed on the label.

Company	Microorganisms[a]	Health claims on the label and active ingredients[b]
A	*B. animalis* subsp. *lactis*, *Lb. delbrueckii* subsp. *bulgaricus*, *Lc. lactis*, *S. thermophilus*	Intestinal health by probiotics
B	*S. thermophilus*, *B. animalis* subsp. *lactis*, *Lb. acidophilus*, *L. casei*	1. Intestinal health by probiotics 2. Liver health by *Hovenia dulcis* berry extract and Milk thistle
C	*B. animalis* subsp. *lactis*, *Lb. casei*, *Lb. plantarum*, *S. thermophilus*	1. Intestinal health by probiotics 2. Intestinal health by prebiotics (lactulose)
D	*Lb. sakei*	1. Skin health and intestinal health by aloe gel 2. Skin health (alleviation of hypersensitivity) by a probiotic

[a] B = Bifidobacterium, Lb = Lactobacillus, Lc = Lactococcus, S = Streptococcus.
[b] *Some products can separate claims with different functional ingredients.*

5.4.4 Milk and vegetable beverages containing probiotics

Unlike the fermented probiotic yogurt, products that add probiotic strains directly into the pasteurized milk and package them have come to market again. Milk containing probiotic bacteria (*Bifidobacterium* sp., or *Lb. acidophilus*) had already debuted in the Korean market in the late 1990s, but there was a problem with cold chain distribution that caused a sour taste over time. Due to these quality problems, this product failed to prosper in the market; but recently, a milk product using *Lb. plantarum* strains has again been introduced into the market (Table 5.7). *Lb. plantarum* perhaps consumes less lactose than other lactic acid bacteria, and therefore acid production is more unlikely to develop during refrigeration or distribution.

Probiotic products based on vegetable or fruit juices are divided into fermented or non-fermented (added) products. For most of the fermented vegetable juices, some of the raw materials are fermented separately and mixed with other non-fermented ingredients instead of fermented as whole products such as yogurt. Raw materials used in fermentation are very diverse, such as fruit juices, vegetable juices, red ginseng, and black garlic. Non-fermented products, which are added probiotics after heat treatment, emphasize live bacteria, but most of the fermented products are pasteurized or sterilized to facilitate distribution conditions. Strains used in probiotic beverages are of so-called vegetable-plant origin lactic

TABLE 5.7 Milk and vegetable juices containing probiotic beverages and their microorganisms.

Company	Product type	Microorganisms[a]
A	Milk	*Lb. plantarum*
B	Milk	*B. animalis* subsp. *lactis*
C	Juice	*L. plantarum*
D	Juice	*Lb. sakei*
E	Juice	*Lb. acidophilus, S. thermophiles, B. animalis* subsp. *lactis, Lb. delbrueckii* subsp. *bulgaricus*
F	Juice	*E. faecalis*
G	Juice	*Lb. acidophilus, Lb. salivarius, Lb. brevis, Lb. casei, Lb. plantarum, Lb. sakei, Lb. rhamnosus, Lb. paracasei, Lb. reuteri, Lb. helveticus, Lb. gasseri, Lb. fermentum, L. delbrueckii* subsp. *bulgaricus, B. bifidum, B. breve, B. longum, Lc. lactis, Bacillus subtilis, Weissella koreensis, Leuconostoc mesenteroides*

[a] B = Bifidobacterium, Lb = Lactobacillus, Lc = Lactococcus, S = Streptococcus, E = Enterococcus.

acid bacteria, including *Lb. plantarum* and this claim was made using the healthy hallowed image of kimchi, the representative traditional fermented food in Korea. There is even a product containing multiple strains of probiotics, consisting of 20 different species of lactic acid bacteria, even though currently there is no positive evidence of multiple strain use versus single strain use advantage (Table 5.7).

5.4.5 Fermented herbal and plant-based products

5.4.5.1 Fermented red ginseng

Ginseng has been widely used as a food and for its medicinal value for thousands of years in the Orient. Ginsenoside, a saponin family, is known as a key ingredient that shows various effects, such as anti-cancer, anti-inflammatory activity, anti-stress, and antioxidant (Lee, Jung, Kim, Lee, & Chung, 2006; Park et al., 2005). Ginseng saponins (ginsenoside glycosides) are converted by microflora in the digestive tract and absorbed into the human body (Akao, Kanaoka, & Kobashi, 1998). Red ginseng, when steamed and dried, contains low-molecular ginsenosides such as ginsenosides Rg2, Rg3, Rh2, and compound K, which are not found in unsteamed ginseng. Its excellent physiological activities have attracted attention as a raw material for functional food and medicine (Kim, Choi, Kim, Suh, & Park, 2010).

Research studies on the bio-conversion of ginsenoside Rd to compound K by fermentation of lactic acid bacteria, isolated from kimchi a representative traditional fermented food, have been reported (Lee et al., 1993; Quan et al., 2008), and this process also has the advantage of supplying beneficial microbes and increasing the absorption rate by decomposing ginsenosides (Kim, Kim, & Cha, 2007). Research work on improving the absorption rate of ginsenosides and exploring useful physiological active substances has been actively conducted since around 2000 with red ginseng by fermentation or bio-conversion technology using lactic acid bacteria (Park, Moon, et al., 2014; Shin, 2010).

Despite the long intake experience of red ginseng and the benefits of increasing the bio-availability of its beneficial ingredients through the lactic fermentation, there are no beverage products yet in the market containing live probiotics that are mainly fermented red ginseng. Probably the reason for this limitation is caused by the distribution conditions of beverage products, where a long shelf life at ambient temperature is required.

5.4.5.2 Fermented plant-based products

With the trends of vegetarianism and dairy-free in the United States and Europe, a need for milk-alternative products, which can be drunk instead of milk, has emerged. To date, soy milk, almond milk, oat milk, and rice milk made from plant-based ingredients are good alternatives, and these have quickly eroded the milk market. With the healthy image of plant-based raw materials and the avoidance of animal resources, the development of new products using various plant-based ingredients has been attempted. However, in the case of yogurt, things are a little different. Yogurt produced using soy or almond has been attempted for quite a long time, but it has not been able to make its way to the market due to limitations in improving the off-notes and rough texture that appear after fermentation. However, recent increases in consumer demand, changes in perceptions, and advanced processing technology has raised the need for the development of yogurt using plant-based ingredients only or dairy-free. With companies specializing in plant-based products, such as Alpro and Silk, various plant-based yogurts are now increasing their market share in the traditional dairy yogurt market. To date, companies and products that claim the effectiveness or differentiation of plant-based yogurt containing probiotics are few.

In Korea, yogurt made from plant-based ingredients, including soy milk, has not yet settled in the market. The absence of soy yogurt may be challenging to explain, given the considerable amount of consumption that had already formed a large market for soy milk from a long time ago. Although attempts have been ongoing, many quality inferiorities have prevented plant-based yogurts from settling in the market. However, this market is expected to change gradually as more needs from vegetarians push demand.

5.5 Market perspectives

Despite the shorter history of probiotic products in Korea, the local probiotics market has been snowballing over the past 30 years and has reached 3 trillion Won (USD 2.6 Billion), including HFFs and probiotic drinkable yogurts. There are many products with various formats and functionalities on the shelves. Due to legal restrictions of functional or health claims on the label, probiotic yogurt sales had been slowing down, but probiotic products as functional foods have filled the market and continue to lead market growth. In the past 5 years, probiotic functional foods have grown more than 6% on a CAGR basis, recording sales of 300 Billion Won (USD 269 Million) in 2018 and third place of sales value. Although powdered supplement products still dominate in the local market, liquid-type products are being introduced to the market, and individually approved strains claiming various functionalities have been developed and commercialized beyond intestinal health claims. Attempts are being made steadily.

Currently, Korea is the fastest country to transition to an aging society. As baby boomers, who have led consumption over the last two decades, have started to retire, the number of consumers who want to age healthy and still have purchasing power has increased consumption of functional foods, including probiotics. As a result of this increasing interest in health and the active research on the human microbiome, the role and function of intestinal bacteria are being re-enlightened, and the consumption of various foods, especially probiotics, is expected to rise constantly. Also, through the ongoing steady research on Korean traditional fermented foods, such as kimchi and soy pastes, (doenjang and cheonggukjang) is the focus, also various functionalities have been confirmed and there are attempts to commercialize them. Apart from the traditional types of fermentations of milk, attempts have been made using various raw materials, such as plant-based (soy, almond, oat, or coconut) and fruits and vegetable juices. More probiotic products for animals are also expected to be on the market.

References

Akao, T., Kanaoka, M., & Kobashi, K. (1998). Appearance of compound K, a major metabolite of ginsenoside Rb1 by intestinal bacteria, in rat plasma after oral administration measurement of compound K by enzyme immunoassay. *Biological & Pharmaceutical Bulletin, 21*(3), 245–249.

Anthony, M. S., Clarkson, T. B., & Williams, J. K. (1998). Effects of soy isoflavones on atherosclerosis: Potential mechanisms. *American Journal of Clinical Nutrition, 68*(6), 1390S–1393S.

Baek, S. Y., Yun, H. J., Choi, H. S., Hong, S. B., Koo, B. S., & Yeo, S. H. (2010). Screening and characteristics of useful fungi for brewing from commercial nuruk in Chungcheong Province. *Korean Journal of Microbiology and Biotechnology, 38*(4), 373–378.

Barnes, S., Sfakianos, J., Coward, L., & Kirk, M. (1996). Soy isoflavonoids and cancer prevention. Underlying biochemical and pharmacological issues. *Advances in Experimental Medicine and Biology, 401*, 87–100.

Chang, H. C. (2018). Healthy and safe Korean traditional fermented foods; kimchi and chongkukjang. *Journal of Ethnic Foods, 5*(3), 161–166.

Chang, J. Y., & Chang, H. C. (2010). Improvements in the quality and shelf life of kimchi by fermentation with the induced bacteriocin-producing strain, *Leuconostoc citreum* GJ7 as a starter. *Journal of Food Science, 75*(2), 103–110.

Chang, J. Y., & Chang, H. C. (2011). Growth inhibition of foodborne pathogens by kimchi prepared with bacteriocin-producing starter culture. *Journal of Food Science, 76*(1), 72–78.

Chang, J. Y., Choi, Y. R., & Chang, H. C. (2011). Change in the microbial profiles of commercial kimchi during fermentation. *Korean Journal of Food Preservation, 18*(5), 786–794.

Cheigh, H. S., & Park, K. Y. (1994). Biochemical, microbiological, and nutritional aspects of kimchi (Korean fermented vegetable products). *Critical Reviews in Food Science and Nutrition, 34*, 175–203.

Cho, J. H., Lee, D. G., Yang, C. N., Jeon, J. I., Kim, J. H., & Han, H. U. (2006). Microbial population dynamics of kimchi, a fermented cabbage product. *FEMS Microbiology Letters, 247* (2), 262–267.

Choi, J. H., Chung, N. J., Jeong, D. Y., & Oh, D. H. (2014). Immunostimulatory activity of isoflavone-glycosides and ethanol extract from a fermented soybean product in human primary immune cells. *Journal of Medicinal Food, 17*(10), 1113–1121.

Dharaneedharan, S., & Heo, M. S. (2016). Korean traditional fermented foods—A potential resource of beneficial microorganisms and their applications. *Journal of Life Science, 26*(4), 496–502.

FAO/WHO (2001). *Evaluation of health and nutritional properties of powder milk with live lactic acid bacteria*: (pp. 1–4). Cordoba, Argentina: Report from FAO/WHO Expert Consultation.

Islam, M. S., & Choi, H. (2009). Antidiabetic effect of Korean traditional baechu (Chinese cabbage) kimchi in a type 2 diabetes model of rats. *Journal of Medicinal Food, 12*(2), 292–297.

Jin, J. B., Kim, S. Y., Jin, Q., Eom, H. J., & Han, N. S. (2008). Diversity analysis of lactic acid bacteria in Takju Korean rice wine. *Journal of Microbiology and Biotechnology, 18*(10), 1678–1682.

Jung, J. Y., Lee, S. H., & Jeon, C. O. (2014). Kimchi microflora: History, current status, and perspectives for industrial kimchi production. *Applied Microbiology and Biotechnology, 98* (6), 2385–2393.

Kang, M. G., Kim, J. H., Ahn, B. H., & Lee, J. S. (2012). Characterization of new antihypertensive angiotensin I-converting enzyme inhibitory peptides from Korean traditional wine. *Journal of Microbiology and Biotechnology, 22*(3), 339–342.

Kang, M. J., Kim, S. H., Joo, H. K., Lee, G. S., & Yim, M. H. (2000). Isolation and identification of microorganisms producing the soy protein-hydrolyzing enzyme from traditional mejus. *Journal of the Korean Society Agricultural Chemistry and Biotechnology, 43*(2), 86–94.

Kang, S. M., Lee, C. S., Yoo, C. K., & Seo, W. S. (1998). Purification and characterization of fibrinolytic enzyme excreted *by Bacillus subtilis* K-54 isolated from Chung Guk Jang. *Korean Journal of Applied Microbiology and Biotechnology, 26*(6), 507–515.

Kim, E. K., An, S. Y., Lee, M. S., Kim, T. H., Lee, H. K., Hwang, W. S., et al. (2011). Fermented kimchi reduces body weight and improves metabolic parameters in over-weight and obese patients. *Nutrition Research, 31*(6), 436–443.

Kim, W., Choi, K., Kim, Y., Park, H., Choi, J., Lee, Y., et al. (1996). Purification and characterization of a fibrinolytic enzyme produced from *Bacillus* sp., strain CK 11-4 screened from chungkook-jang. *Applied and Environmental Microbiology, 62*(7), 2482–2488.

Kim, B. G., Choi, S. Y., Kim, M. R., Suh, H. J., & Park, H. J. (2010). Changes of ginsenoside in Korea red ginseng (*Panax ginseng*) fermented by *Lactobacillus plantarum* M1. *Process Biochemistry, 45*(6), 1319–1324.

Kim, M. J., & Chun, J. S. (2005). Bacterial community structure in kimchi, a Korean fermented vegetable food, as revealed by 16S rRNA gene analysis. *International Journal of Food Microbiology, 103*(1), 91–96.

Kim, Y. J., & Han, Y. S. (2006). The use of Korean traditional liquors and plan for encouraging it. *Journal of the Korean Society of Food Culture, 21*(1), 31–41.

Kim, H. G., Kim, K. Y., & Cha, C. J. (2007). Screening for ginseng fermenting microorganisms capable of biotransforming ginsenosides. *Korean Journal of Microbiology, 43*(2), 142–146.

Kim, J. H., Lee, D. H., Choi, S. Y., & Lee, J. S. (2002). Characterization of physiological functionalities in Korean traditional liquors. *Korean Journal of Food Science and Technology, 34*(1), 118–122.

Kim, N. Y., Song, E. J., Kwon, D. Y., Kim, H. P., & Heo, M. Y. (2008). Antioxidant and antigenotoxic activities of Korean fermented soybean. *Food and Chemical Toxicology, 46*(3), 1184–1189.

Korea Agro-Fisheries & Food Trade Corporation (2017). *Newsletter of food market – Fermented milks.* aT Food Information Statistics System.

Lee, H. J., Baek, J. H., Yang, M., Han, H. U., Ko, Y. D., & Kim, H. J. (1993). Characterizations of lactic acid bacterial community during kimchi fermentation by temperature downshift. *Korean Journal of Microbiology, 31*(4), 346–353.

Lee, M. E., Jang, J. Y., Lee, J. H., Park, H. W., Choi, H. J., & Kim, T. W. (2015). Starter cultures for kimchi fermentation. *Journal of Microbiology and Biotechnology, 25*(5), 559–568.

Lee, S. H., Jung, B. H., Kim, S. Y., Lee, E. H., & Chung, B. C. (2006). The anti-stress effect of ginseng total saponin and ginsenoside Rg3 and Rb1 evaluated by brain polyamine level under immobilization stress. *Pharmacological Research, 54*(1), 46–49.

Lee, D. K., Kim, S. J., Cho, J. H., & Kim, J. H. (2008). Microbial population dynamics and temperature changes during fermentation of kimjang kimchi. *The Journal of Microbiology, 46* (5), 590–593.

Lee, Y. S., Seol, J. N., Jeong, D. Y., & Kim, S. Y. (2016). Application of functional microbial strains isolated from traditional rice wine in Korea. *Microbiology and Biotechnology Letters, 44*(3), 229–235.

Lee, C. H., Yang, E. I., Song, G. S., Chai, O. H., & Kim, Y. S. (2006). Effects of Cheonhhukjang on immune responses and gastrointestinal functions in rats. *Food Science and Biotechnology, 15*(1), 19–23.

Lim, C. T., Park, H. K., & Han, H. U. (1989). Reevaluation of isolation and identification of gram positive bacteria in kimchi. *Korean Journal of Microbiology, 27*(4), 404–414.

Markets and Markets Research (2019). *Probiotic market by application (functional food & beverages [dairy products, non-dairy beverages, infant formula, cereals], dietary supplements, feed), ingredient (bacteria, yeast), form (dry, liquid), end user, and region-global forecast to 2023.* Markets and Markets Research Private Ltd..(2019). *https://www.marketsandmarkets.com/Market-Reports/probiotic-market-advanced-technologies-and-global-market-69.html.*

Ministry of Food and Drug Safety (2018). *Standards for probiotic food. In Code of Health Functional Food.* Korea Ministry of Food and Drug Safety(2018). *https://www.mfds.go.kr/eng/index.do.*

Ministry of Food and Drug Safety (2019a). *Report for annual production of health functional foods.* Ministry of Food and Drug Safety.(2019a). *https://www.mfds.go.kr/eng/index.do.*

Ministry of Food and Drug Safety (2019b). *Standards for fermented milks. In Food code.* Korea Ministry of Food and Drug Safety(2019b). *https://www.mfds.go.kr/eng/index.do.*

Nam, Y. R., Won, S. B., Chung, Y. S., Kwak, C. S., & Kwon, Y. H. (2015). Inhibitory effects of doenjang, Korean traditional fermented soybean paste, on oxidative stress and inflammation in adipose tissue of mice fed a high-fat diet. *Nutrition Research and Practice, 9*(3), 235–241.

National Food Safety Information Service (2020). *Ministry of Food and Drug Safety. (2020). https://www.mfds.go.kr/eng/index.do.*

Nile, S. H. (2015). The nutritional, biochemical and health effects of makgeolli - a traditional Korean fermented cereal beverage. *Journal of the Institute of Brewing, 121*(4), 457–463.

Park, K. Y., Jeong, J. k., Lee, Y. E., & Daily, J. W. (2014). Health benefits of kimchi (Korean fermented vegetables) as a probiotic food. *Journal of Medicinal Food, 17*(1), 6–20.

Park, J. H., Moon, H. J., Oh, J. H., Lee, J. H., Jung, H. K., Choi, K. M. , et al. (2014). Changes in the functional components of *Lactobacillus acidophilus*-fermented red ginseng extract and its application to fresh cheese production. *Korean Journal of Dairy Science and Technology, 32*(1), 47–53.

Park, E. K., Shin, Y. W., Lee, H. U., Kim, S. S., Lee, Y. C., Lee, B. Y. , et al. (2005). Inhibitory effect of ginsenoside Rb1 and compound K on NO and prostaglandin E2 biosyntheses of RAW264.7 cells induced by lipopolysaccharide. *Biological & Pharmaceutical Bulletin, 28*(4), 652–656.

Park, J. S., Song, S. H., Choi, J. B., Kim, Y. S., Kwon, S. H., & Park, Y. S. (2014). Physicochemical properties of Korean rice wine (Makgeolli) fermented using yeasts isolated from Korean traditional nuruk, a starter culture. *Food Science and Biotechnology, 23*(5), 1577–1585.

Patra, J. K., Das, G., Paramithiotis, S., & Shin, H. S. (2016). Kimchi and other widely consumed traditional fermented foods of Korea: A review. *Frontiers in Microbiology, 7*, 1493. https://doi.org/10.3389/fmicb.2016.01493.

Quan, L. H., Liang, Z., Kim, H. B., Kim, S. H., Kim, S. Y., Noh, Y. D. , et al. (2008). Conversion of ginsenoside Rd to compound K by crude enzyme extracted from *Lactobacillus brevis* LH8. *Journal of Ginseng Research, 32*(3), 226–231.

Ryu, H. Y., Kum, E. J., Bae, K. H., Kim, Y. K., Kwun, I. S., & Sohn, H. Y. (2007). Evaluation for the antimicrobial, antioxidant and antithrombosis activity of Korean traditional liquors. *Korean Journal of Microbiology and Biotechnology, 35*(3), 238–244.

Ryu, M. S., Yang, H. J., Kim, J. W., Jeong, S. J., Jeong, S. Y., Eom, J. S. , et al. (2017). Potential probiotics activity of *Bacillus* spp. from traditional soybean pastes and fermentation characteristics of Cheonggukjang. *Korean Journal of Food Preservation, 24*(8), 1168–1179.

Shin, Y. S. (2010). Fermentation of red ginseng using CKDHC 0801 and CKDHC 0802. *Korean Journal of Food and Cookery Science, 26*(4), 469–474.

Shin, D. W., & Jeong, D. Y. (2015). Korean traditional fermented soybean products: Jang. *Journal of Ethnic Foods, 2*(1), 2–7.

Shin, D. H., Kim, M. S., Han, J. S., Lim, D. K., & Bak, W. S. (1996). Changes of chemical composition and microflora in commercial kimchi. *Korean Journal of Food Science and Technology, 28*(1), 37–145.

Song, S. H., Lee, C., Lee, S., Park, J. M., Lee, H. J., Bai, D. H. , et al. (2013). Analysis of microflora profile in Korean traditional nuruk. *Journal of Microbiology and Biotechnology, 23*(1), 40–46.

Surh, J., Kim, Y. H., & Kwon, H. (2008). Korean fermented foods, Kimchi and Doenjang. In E. R. Farnworth (Ed.), *Handbook of fermented functional foods* (pp. 333–351). Boca Raton, FL: CRC Press.

CHAPTER

6

Probiotic beverages in Thailand: Health attributes and future trends

Sudsai Trevanich

Department of Food Science and Technology, Faculty of Agro-Industry, Kasetsart University, Bangkok, Thailand

6.1 Introduction

Currently, probiotics are one of the most important and frequently used functional food compounds. Probiotic beverages have become popular as functional drinks for consumers in many countries including Thailand. Probiotic beverages may contain either a single strain or a mixture of two or more strains. Some studies have shown that such probiotic beverages provide some health benefits for humans, such as cholesterol reduction, gastrointestinal system improvement, immune system enhancement, allergy reduction, antagonistic activity toward intestinal pathogens, and lower risk of colon cancer development (Manas, Marimuthu, Ramesh, & Rizwana, 2014). Probiotic beverages in Thailand can be simply classified into two main categories based on the type of raw materials and the process used (Fig. 6.1) (Kumar, Vijayendra, and Reddy (2015); Kwanmuang, 2018). There are dairy-based probiotic beverage and non-dairy-based probiotic beverages (with or without fermentation).

In Thailand, dairy probiotic beverages are still the main products that serve as carriers of probiotics in the diet of the consumer. However, lactose intolerance, cholesterol content, milk protein allergy, and vegetarianism trend have increased research and development in the scope of non-dairy probiotic beverage products. Therefore, non-dairy-based probiotic beverages such as plant probiotic beverages have become attractive to Thai consumers. Most probiotic vegetable and fruit juices developed in Thailand

Probiotic Beverages
https://doi.org/10.1016/B978-0-12-818588-9.00007-3

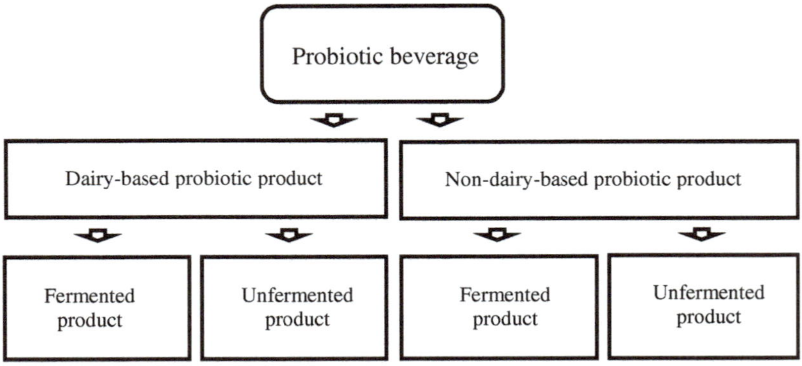

FIG. 6.1 Classification and category of probiotic beverages in Thailand. *Modified from Kumar, B.V., Vijayendra, S.V.N., & Reddy, O.V.S. (2015). Trends in dairy and non-dairy probiotic products-review.* Journal of Food Science and Technology, *52(10), 6112–6124; Kwanmuang, P. (2018). Plant probiotic beverages: Alternative for functional beverages.* Journal of Industrial Education, *17(1), 212–221.*

use lactic acid bacteria as the probiotic. Generally, there are three main types of processing of probiotic beverages in Thailand: processing by direct addition of probiotic microorganisms into vegetable and fruit juices, fermentation by probiotic microorganisms as starter cultures that are inoculated into the starting raw materials, and fermentation of heat-treated raw materials along with inoculation of probiotics as starter cultures.

6.2 Current and future trends in research development of probiotic beverages in Thailand

Interest in developing probiotic beverage products by Thai researchers is rising, driven by various reasons including consumers' needs, government support, collaboration with entrepreneurs, and the market potential for these beverages to improve consumer health. Beverages based on fruits, vegetables, and cereals using as major raw materials have been proposed as new potential probiotic products; in particular, fruit juices have been known as a novel, promising, and appropriate vehicle for probiotic agents, especially probiotic bacteria, as fruits contain most of the essential nutrients. However, several major limits including the survivability of the probiotics in fruit juice products throughout storage and the deterioration, and the effect of the probiotic on overall quality acceptance could preclude their production at the industrial scale. This communication addresses the inoculation of probiotics in juices, with a special focus on the following traits: the kinds of probiotics and their stability and health benefits;

fortification with prebiotics, sensory challenges, and shelf life. There has been research on the development of probiotic beverages in Thailand with most being carried out by academic researchers from different universities or research institutes in collaboration with the research and development departments in food companies. Some publications of this research on probiotic beverages over the past 10 years are provided below. They consider the human health benefit impacts of using probiotics in beverage products and how to increase their survivability, as well as their sensory stability, and evaluation of the product during storage.

6.2.1 Dairy-based probiotic beverages of Thailand

Saengthong and Sirimunee (2011) used *Lactobacillus casei* BGP93 as a probiotic starter culture for the production of a fermented drinking yoghurt. They reported that the finished drinking yoghurt consisted of a final population of *L. casei* BG93 of 1.8×10^7 CFU/mL, which met the Thai Industrial Standard for drinking yoghurt (TISI 2146–2546). The product had a pH of approximately 3.76 ± 0.02 and a lactic acid content of $1.07 \pm 0.01\%$. The shelf life of the product stored at 4–8°C was 7 days and the product was in precipitated form with a sour taste after storage for 7 days.

6.2.2 Fruit- and vegetable-based probiotic beverages of Thailand

Waiwong (2007) isolated probiotic bacteria from three commercial fermented milk products marketed in Thailand. Each probiotic bacterium was used as a single starter culture or mixture for the fermentation of probiotic drink using different raw materials from herbs, green apples, and soymilk. Many herbs were used including safflower, ye ju hua, celery, and lemongrass. Liquid prepared from different ratios of herbs, green apple, and soymilk was inoculated with a starter culture, at the appropriate concentration, for *in vitro* fermentation at 37°C up to 72 h. Samples were taken at different time intervals for chemical and microbiological analyses. From the results obtained, the probiotic bacteria in *Lactobacillus* genus they tested grew well in the four formulas (herbs, green apple, and soymilk) especially when supplemented with soymilk (10% *v*/*v*) and brown sugar (5% *w*/*v*). *Lactobacillus casei* strain YK 5001 had the highest viable cell count (about 8.62×10^7 CFU/mL) after 48 h when incubated at 37°C. Based on sensory evaluation, the probiotic drinks from the herbs, green apple, and soymilk supplemented with honey, were considered satisfactory by most consumers. Storage stability of probiotic drinks after 4 weeks at 5–7°C was also tested and the viable cell counts of YK 5001 and a mixed culture of YK 5001, BG 5001, and FM 5001 were 1.62×10^8

and 1.86×10^8 CFU/mL, respectively, which had decreased less than 1 log cycle. Waiwong concluded that herbs, green apple, and soymilk could all be used as a starting raw material for the fermentation of probiotic drink products.

Lertcanawanichakul, Thaiauer, Chaopongpan, and Petchnajak (2010) studied the survival of a specific type of probiotic bacterium isolated from various natural sources including vegetables, fruits, pasteurized milk, Nham, and fruit juices. Using an API 50 CHL Test Kit, one isolate obtained from tomato was identified as *Lactobacillus plantarum* 1, using colonization as the selection criteria. This bacterium showed appropriate properties for a probiotic bacterium, namely that it inhibited the growth of other types of bacteria including *Micrococcus luteus* TISTR 884, *Bacillus subtilis* ATCC 6633, *Salmonella* Typhimurium TISTR 292, *Staphylococcus aureus* TISTR 517, *Escherichia coli* TISTR 887, and *Pseudomonas aeruginosa* TISTR 1467. It could survive and grow at pH 2–10 and was resistant to some antibiotics such as Oxacillin and Nitrofurantoin. The results of the survival study indicated that an initial amount of 8 log CFU/mL of this bacterium decreased to 5.0–5.4 log CFU/mL at the end of the 21st day after storage at 4°C. However, its survival was very poor in coconut juice and there was no survival on day 9 of storage at 4°C. Interestingly, fruit juices with or without a prebiotic showed no significant ($p \leq 0.05$) difference on the survivability of this bacterium.

Chaiyasut (2010) and Chaiyasut, Sirilun, Pheerachan, and Kumar (2011) reported that fermented plant juice or bioextract juice could be obtained from fermentation parts of a single plant or from mixed plants (*Great morinda, Chebulic myrobalans,* Black galingale rhizome, or Indian gooseberry) or extract juice from plants with lactic acid-producing cultures including *Lactobacillus delbrueckii* subsp. *bulgaricus, L. casei, L. acidophilus* as well as *Bifidobacterium.* Bioextract juice can be divided into two groups, namely fermented plant juice without water dilution and flavoring addition and fermented plant juice with water dilution and flavoring fortification. The nature of the fermented plant juice is a liquid with a final pH of 4.3 or less, which may still have turbidity and sediment caused by the ingredients coming from a piece of plant tissue and the microbial cells in the fermentation process. In addition, the product had good natural color, aroma, and flavor originating from the components in the plant used and it's processing. If a preservative is used in the product, then it must be used according to the type and quantity prescribed by food additive legislation. Bioextract juice obtained after 30 or more days of fermentation exhibited effective antimicrobial activity against standard microorganisms tested including *Bacillus cereus, Candida albicans* ATCC 90028, *Escherichia coli* ATCC 25922, *Pseudomonas aeruginosa* ATCC 27853, and *Staphylococcus aureus* ATCC 25923. A possible explanation was that this was due to the lactic acid, ethanol, and bacteriocin produced during the fermentation process.

Kwanmuang (2013, 2014) studied the fermentation of different plants using lactic acid bacteria isolated from fermented food products. Fermented carrot juice is a liquid beverage, with a sour taste, an orange color, and a little alcohol and carbon dioxide gas. The product is produced using a mixture of carrot juice and pineapple juice and then the total solid solubility is adjusted to 10–15 °Brix using sucrose. After pasteurization, the product is left to cool at room temperature and *Lactobacillus pentosus* and *Saccharomyces cerevisiae* are inoculated for a 24–48 h fermentation. The fermented carrot juice contains beta-carotene, which has antioxidant properties and gives a natural color to the product.

Kwanmuang (2014) developed a fermented Jerusalem artichoke (*Helianthus tuberosus* known in Thai as Kaentawan) juice. This plant is in the sunflower family and contains high amounts of prebiotics, including inulin that has benefits as dietary fiber. The fermented Kaentawan juice was prepared using a mixture of Kaentawan juice, carrot juice, beetroot juice, pineapple juice, and distilled water in the ratio of 40:10:20:20:10 (by volume), respectively, and then the total amount of total dissolved solids was adjusted to 15°Brix using sucrose. The mixture was pasteurized and left to cool. *L. pentosus* was used as the starter culture for the fermentation. The resulting product was sour and sweet with a purple color, turbidity, and sediment. The finished product had a unique odor resulting from a combination of the Kaentawan, the beetroot, and the fermentation.

Kaeitsast and Kwanmuang (2016) developed a probiotic beverage from Gac fruit (*Momordica cochinchinensis*), a type of perennial melon. The beverage was prepared from the pulp and seed membrane, using *L. pentosus* for fermentation. The fermented juice produced a high final population level of lactic acid bacteria (about $1.5–2.0 \times 10^{12}$ CFU/mL).

Gae-in, Deetae, Kingkaew, and Sawhasan (2014) developed a fermented probiotic beverage from sweet potato (*Ipomoea batatas*) as a new alternative drink for consumers. Ten potential probiotic lactic acid bacteria strains were isolated from yoghurt, sour milk, and homemade Kimchi. Their probiotic potentials were preliminarily evaluated by testing for resistance to a low pH (pH 2.5) in a stimulant gastric model at 37°C for 3 h, by an antimicrobial activity test against three major foodborne bacterial pathogens (*Escherichia coli*, *Salmonella* Enteritidis, and *Listeria monocytogenes*) using a well diffusion assay, and by an antibiotic resistance test against five representative antibiotics (Ampicillin, Penicillin G, Kanamycin, Streptomycin, and Tetracycline) using a disc diffusion assay. They found that among the 10 lactic acid bacteria isolates, the KN2 strain isolated from homemade Kimchi had the highest probiotic performance, as this bacterial strain was more resistant to the low pH and had a strong inhibitory effect against all three bacterial pathogens tested. Therefore, KN2 was used as the probiotic starter culture for the fermentation process of yellow and purple sweet potatoes. The sweet potatoes were cut into small pieces and steamed at 100°C for 20 min. Drinking water was added into the steamed sweet potatoes at a ratio of 1:3 (*v*/*w*) and mixed well. The resulting suspension was filtered, and the obtained filtrate was heated at 121°C for 15 min. Amylase enzyme was added into the filtrate and the filtrate was inoculated with KN2 for fermentation at 37°C for 48 h. After the fermentation process, the viable counts of KN2 from fermented filtrates of yellow and purple sweet potatoes were 2.80×10^9 and 7.10×10^8 CFU/mL, respectively. Gae-in et al. also determined the total phenolic content and free radical scavenging of ABTS from fermented yellow sweet potatoes, resulting in 30.14 mg of gallic acid equivalents (GAEs)/100 mL and 16.79 mg of vitamin C equivalent antioxidant capacity (VCEAC)/100 mL, respectively. The total phenolic content and free radical scavenging of ABTS from fermented purple sweet potatoes were 41.25 mg of GAE/100 mL and 16.83 mg of VCEAC/100 mL, respectively. They also performed a sensory evaluation with 60 panelists using a paired preference test to compare the probiotic drinks obtained from yellow or purple sweet potatoes and found that the panelists preferred the beverages made from the fermented purple sweet potato.

Chaikham and Apichartsrangkoon (2012) used the dynamic Simulator of the Human Intestinal Microbial Ecosystem (SHIME) in a controlled *in vitro* condition setting for their research on simulation of oral administration of the encapsulated *Lactobacillus acidophilus* LA5 or *Lactobacillus casei* 01 mixed with pressurized longan juice. While testing in the SHIME reactors, they observed that both encapsulated probiotics led to increase in the viable colon *Lactobacillus* spp. Both encapsulated probiotics combined with pressurized longan juice significantly increased the production of lactic acid and some short chain fatty acids (SCFA: propionate, butyrate, and acetate), whereas toxic ammonia decreased. The results also showed that encapsulated probiotic *Lactobacillus,* combined with pressurized longan juice, produced a significant increase in *Bifidobacterium* spp. and a decrease in fecal coliforms and *Clostridium* spp. Chaikham (2015) also investigated the impact of alginate encapsulation with some Thai herbal extracts from the cashew flower (*Anacardium occidentale* L.), pennywort (*Centella asiatica* (Linn.) Urban), and yanang (*Tiliacora triandra*) on the stability and survivability of three probiotic bacteria strains (*L. casei* 01, *L. acidophilus* LA5, and *Bifidobacterium lactis* BB-12) in various fruit juices (mulberry, maoberry, longan, and melon juices) and stirred yoghurt, during refrigerated storage at 4 °C for 30 days. After this storage period, there was a noticeable surviving number of *L. casei* 01 cells entrapped with the 0.05% (*w*/*v*) cashew flower extract, which was stored under normal atmosphere and vacuum environments. Levels of surviving *L. casei* 01 were significantly higher than those encapsulated with pennywort and yanang extracts, after refrigerated storage for 30 days. Cashew flower extract at 0.05% was chosen to be used for immobilization of the probiotic cells before adding into fruit juices and stirred yoghurt, for comparison with green tea extract as a standard plant extract. Following storage at 4°C, the cashew flower and green tea extracts noticeably increased the stability of the probiotic beads in the fruit juices and stirred yoghurt, compared to the controls. Encapsulated *L. casei* 01 and *B. lactis* BB-12 had better survival in the products during the refrigerated storage compared to encapsulated *L. acidophilus* LA5. Recently, Chaikham, Kemsawasd, and Seesuriyachan (2017) applied two potential probiotic bacteria, *L. casei* 01 and *L. acidophilus* LA5, in dehydrated fruit juices, as this product could be an alternative for consumers interested in functional beverages. Chaikham investigated the impact of yanang gum on the survivability of both probiotic cultures combined with maoluang juice after spray drying and their activities in a simulated gastrointestinal (SGI) model, compared to the supplement of inulin. The obtained results exhibited that probiotic-maoluang juice powders, as immobilized by yanang gum and inulin, gave similar protection levels for probiotic bacteria against the adverse conditions in the SGI model. After 6h incubation in the SGI model, the spray-dried *L. casei* 01 and *L. acidophilus* LA5, with maoluang juice and yanang gum or inulin, showed higher the survival rates than that for the free cells, with increases of about 15%–20% and 20%–21%, respectively. According to the *in vitro* colon experiments, yanang gum and inulin significantly increased the accumulation of lactic acid, SCFA, and groups of useful colon bacteria (*Lactobacillus* spp. and *Bifidobacterium* spp.), whereas the amount of toxic ammonium compounds and the number of harmful bacteria (*Clostridium* spp. and fecal coliforms) were noticeably reduced. In addition, they examined the stability of the probiotic *Lactobacillus* encapsulated with maltodextrin plus yanang gum and maltodextrin plus inulin in maoluang juice powder. A similar ability of protection on probiotic *Lactobacillus* tested against adverse conditions of simulated stomach and small intestinal fluids was found. Spray-dried probiotic combined with maoluang juice containing yanang gum also increased the concentrations of lactic acid, SCFA, *Lactobacillus* spp., and *Bifidobacterium* spp. while decreasing toxic ammonia, *Clostridium* spp., fecal coliforms, and total anaerobes. Their research indicated that yanang gum showed prebiotic effects on microorganisms in the human colon and therefore yanang gum could be used as effective and promising co-encapsulating material for spray drying probiotics.

Researchers working on an innovative development prototype for a value-added sugar cane beverage project (Innovative development prototype for value added sugar cane beverage project, 2015) developed fermented sugar cane juice (fermented sugar cane punch with probiotics), which was made from sugar cane juice fermented using a probiotic lactic acid bacterium (*Lactobacillus johnsonii*). The fermented sugar cane juice had the natural color of sugar cane juice, or the colors of the raw materials added to the mixture, such as orange from carrot juice, purple from mulberry or beet juice, or green from green vegetables and fruit juices. There was an aroma caused by the microbial fermentation or obtained from the addition of herbal juices such as ginger and lemon grass. The product had a sour taste due to the lactic acid from the fermentation. The final product produced met the Thai Community Products Standard for Fermented Plant Juice (TCPS 481/2547). Various plant species were used as a mix with the sugar cane juice and the nutrients and bioactive compounds found in such plants (phenolic compounds, flavonoids, and prebiotics) are beneficial for consumer health. The product's claims of health benefits include the improvement of immune system, and amelioration in constipation, allergies, and reducing diarrhea.

Saengdee, Vangpikul, and Itsaranuwat (2016) developed a fermented corn milk synbiotic product (i.e., combining probiotics and prebiotics in a form of synergism) supplemented with the probiotic bacteria, *Lactobacillus acidophilus* LA-5 (2% starter) and tuber plant powder (3% and 5%) and with the inclusion of Jerusalem artichoke (also called Kaentawan) and Gobo (Burdock root). After incubation at 37°C for 24h, the pH and total acidity generally decreased during the period of fermentation, whereas the amount of the probiotic *L. acidophilus* LA-5 generally increased following incubation. After 9h of incubation, the total acidity ranged between 0.7% and 0.9% and the pH was approximately 4. Fermented corn milk supplemented with 3% Kaentawan and Gobo powder produced the highest probiotic levels (9.18 log CFU/mL). The shelf life of the synbiotic product after storage at 4°C with *L. acidophilus* LA-5 tended to increase at the beginning of refrigerated storage. After 15days of storage, the amount of probiotic ranged between 8.78 and 9.20 log CFU/mL. Fermented corn milk supplemented with 5% Gobo powder had the highest amount of probiotic growth (9.38 log CFU/mL). The pH was observed to decrease until 6days of storage and then remained stable to day 15. The pH of the control sample of fermented corn milk, without addition of Kaentawan or Gobo, was the lowest (pH3.56) after 15days of storage. They found that the total acidity level of fermented corn milk supplemented with 3% Kaentawan and 3% Gobo powder was the highest at 1.46% after 15days of refrigerated storage. The survival of total viable bacteria increased at the initial time of storage, tended to decrease slightly, and then was constant after longer storage. The total bacteria present in the synbiotic products ranged between 8.70 and 9.38 log CFU/mL at the initial time of storage. The fermented corn milk supplemented with 3% Kaentawan and 3% Gobo powder had the highest total bacteria (9.23 log CFU/mL) after storage at 4°C for 15days. No pathogenic bacteria (*E. coli*) were found in any of the synbiotic products. The results of the sensory examination showed that most consumers accepted the taste of the fermented corn milk (control) and the product with supplementation of 3% Kaentawan powder produced the highest sensory scores (5.93 and 5.80); however, there was no significant ($P > 0.05$) difference in the overall acceptance. Fermented corn milk supplemented with 3% Gobo powder produced the highest amount of γ-aminobutyric acid (GABA) at 166.10 μg/mL.

Kantachote, Ratanaburee, Hayisama-ae, Sukhoom, and Nunkaew (2017) studied a fermented functional beverage made from mature coconut water (MCW), a by-product from a coconut milk factory, using the potential probiotic *Lactobacillus plantarum* DW12 as the starter culture to contribute health benefits, as this potential probiotic is known for producing GABA, vitamin B12, antioxidants, and antibacterial substances. After fermentation with *L. plantarum* DW12 for 48 h, MCW mixed with 0.5% monosodium glutamate (MSG) showed a probiotic growth of 8.4 log CFU/mL, and contained 128 μg/mL of GABA, 14 μg/mL of vitamin B12 and several essential minerals (3312 μg/mL of potassium, 235 μg/mL of calcium, and 2,214 μg/mL of sodium). In addition, the fermented MCW with added 0.5% MSG, had antioxidant activity for scavenging of 75% of 2,2′-azino-bis (3-ethylbenzothiazoline-6-sulfonic acid), 55% of 2,2-diphenyl-1-picrylhydrazyl. This fermented MCW supplemented with 0.5% MSG gave a total phenolic content of 134 μg/mL GAE. Furthermore, this fermented MCW showed antimicrobial activity against all six tested food pathogenic bacteria (*Bacillus cereus* TISTR 2687, *Escherichia coli* PSSCMI 0001, *Listeria monocytogenes* PSSCMI 0001, *Salmonella* Typhi ATCC 19430, *Staphylococcus aureus* PSSCMI 0004, and *Vibrio parahaemolyticus* PSSCMI 0064). The fermented MCW combined with 0.5% MSG and 1% sugarcane by *L. plantarum* DW12 gave similar properties to the fermented MCW combined with 0.5% MSG only. The researchers found that the fermented MCW with an addition of 20% honey had a better taste than without honey addition. The fermented MCW with *L. plantarum* DW12 has high potential as novel functional beverage by having not only probiotic cells but also other useful compounds (i.e., minerals from the MCW, GABA, vitamin B12, antioxidants, and antimicrobial compounds) for promoting good health for consumers. To date, it is believed that this is the first published research for using MCW as an inexpensive raw material to produce value-added functional beverage containing GABA produced from *L. plantarum* DW12.

6.2.3 Cereal-based probiotic beverages of Thailand

Nakkarach and Withayagiat (2018) developed a non-dairy synbiotic drink product for lactose-intolerant consumers and vegetarians using riceberry malt extract (RME) as the starting raw material. Five potential probiotic lactic acid bacteria (*Enterococcus faecalis* N1–33, *Lactobacillus acidophilus* TISTR450, *Lactobacillus johnsonii* KUN119–2, *Lactobacillus plantarum* TC24, and *Lactobacillus reuteri* KUB-AC5) were used and investigated as starter cultures in the form of free probiotic cells and encapsulated probiotic cells for production of the RME-based synbiotic beverage. The researchers found that *L. plantarum* TC24 showed the greatest probiotic potential among the five tested lactic acid bacteria under SGI tract conditions. Their viability was about 9 log CFU/mL. The obtained results showed that the five selected lactic acid bacteria strains could tolerate the acidic condition in the stimulated gastrointestinal tract. All of the lactic acid bacteria tested exhibited antimicrobial activity against all four bacteria strains (*Bacillus subtilis* TISTR025, *Escherichia coli* 010, *Salmonella* Enteritidis DMST17368, and *Staphylococcus aureus* TISTR118), whereas *L. plantarum* TC24 had the strongest antibacterial effect. The researchers found that encapsulation of calcium alginate significantly enhanced the survival of *L. plantarum* TC24 under the stimulated gastrointestinal tract conditions. Therefore, *L. plantarum* TC24 encapsulated with calcium alginate could be used to improve human gastrointestinal tract health. However, such an encapsulated form of *L. plantarum* TC24 may not be stable for long periods of refrigerated storage. The researchers recommended that appropriate conditions for the developed synbiotic beverage products, containing high populations of *L. plantarum* TC24, should include less than 2 weeks of storage at refrigeration temperature. From the results, RME showed high potential to be used as a nutritious raw material for making a novel non-dairy synbiotic drink that enhances health benefits in balancing the human gastrointestinal system.

Kemsawasd and Chaikham (2018) examined the impact of mulberry leaf extract (MLE) on the survivability of *Lactobacillus casei* 01 and *Lactobacillus acidophilus* LA5 in soyoghurt (a yoghurt made from protein-rich soybean as the main ingredient) during refrigerated storage at 4°C for 30 days. The physiochemical characteristics and sensory attributes of probiotic soyoghurts with added MLE were investigated. The researchers found that probiotic soyoghurts combined with MLE increased the antioxidative effects and reduced viable probiotic cell loss during extended refrigerated storage. Studies on sensory attributes indicated that all probiotic-soyoghurt samples had similar scores for all sensory attributes, regardless of the probiotic strain or MLE. Interestingly, overall likeability was slightly less in the probiotic-soyoghurt products after refrigerated storage for 30 days. They found that both *L. casei* 01 and *L. acidophilus* LA5 in soyoghurt products, with and without addition of MLE, exhibited no significant differences in their survival and tolerance to gastric and bile fluids under *in vitro* gastrointestinal conditions. Soyoghurt, using *L. casei* 01 and MLE, had the greatest antioxidative effects and the highest survival of the probiotic cells throughout storage under refrigeration temperatures. MLE appears to have potential to be used as a healthy ingredient in novel probiotic-based products with improvement of health benefits for consumers.

6.3 Commercial probiotic beverage market in Thailand and health benefits of these beverages

Like many countries around the world, Thailand has a wide variety of probiotic beverages, which are either produced originally by local Thai manufacturers or by foreign companies. In this section, some examples of commercial probiotic beverages that have been recently available nationwide through major retail chains or online stores are described.

6.3.1 Probiotic-based milk beverage products

The development of probiotic beverages in Thailand is increasing, as the market expands. There are now many probiotic-based milk beverage products available on the Thai market and this section provides a few examples of these probiotic-based milk beverages.

6.3.1.1 Dutch Mill Delight

Dutch Mill Co., Ltd. was founded by a group of Thai food scientists from Kasetsart University, Bangkok, who wished to maintain the good health of Thai people by providing them with the best quality dairy products. The company was formerly known under the name "Pro Food Co., Ltd." on 27 January 1984. The company has been managed by Thais and is best known for a yoghurt drink made from high-quality fresh cow's milk, real fruit juice, and cultured probiotics, under an aseptic fermentation process. The Thai brand product "Dutch Mill Delight Imulus" is one of a variety of milk-based products produced by this company. "Imulus" was derived from the two words "immunity" and "stimulus," to reflect the probiotic microbes stimulating the immune system in the body of the consumer. The product is described as helping to decrease diarrhea, constipation, and lactose intolerance.

The company is well known for their yoghurt drink, which contains high-quality fresh cow's milk, less sugar, vitamin B, 0% fat and cholesterol, real fruit juice, and cultured probiotics. This product is fermented by two well-known probiotics, *Lactobacillus bulgaricus* and *Streptococcus thermophilus*. The Dutch Mill product is not only nutritious but is also considered to be delicious. Currently, the company is introducing new Dutch

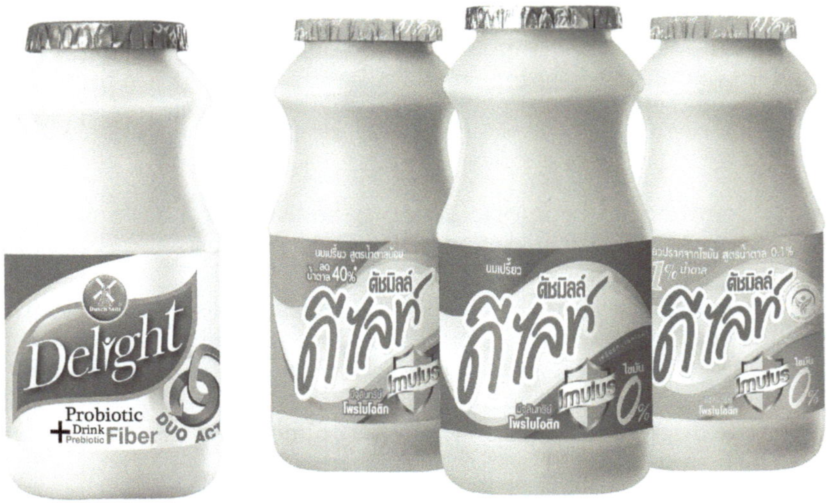

FIG. 6.2 Some examples of Dutch Milk probiotic beverages. *With permission courtesy of Dutch Mill Co., Ltd., Thailand.*

Mill product lines, including pasteurized and ultra-high temperature drinking yoghurts. Following the company success in Bangkok, Dutch Mill Co., Ltd. expanded to provincial markets via direct sales using the "Dutch Mill ladies" who worked and introduced Dutch Mill products to local customers. Presently, various Dutch Mill products are routinely exported to other ASEAN countries (Brunei, Burma, Cambodia, China, Indonesia, Laos, Malaysia, Philippines, Singapore, and Vietnam). In addition, the company plans to expand to other regions of the world. Fig. 6.2 shows one of Dutch Mill's beverages.

6.3.1.2 Dairy Home Synbiotic Drinking Yoghurt

Dairy Home was established as Thailand's first organic dairy family business in order to produce excellent dairy products in a sustainable way and to help in the improvement of consumer health in the community. Dairy Home Synbiotic Drinking Yoghurt is one of company's milk-based products, which is judged to be delicious and also healthy. The product contains prebiotics (Oligomate: a commercial prebiotic galacto-oligosaccharide) and four different types of beneficial probiotic bacteria (*Bifidobacterium* spp., *Lactobacillus acidophilus*, *Lactobacillus delbrueckii* subsp. *bulgaricus*, and *Streptococcus thermophilus*). The probiotics in the product keep consumers healthy by inhibiting the harmful bacteria, improving their gastrointestinal system, reducing inflammation,

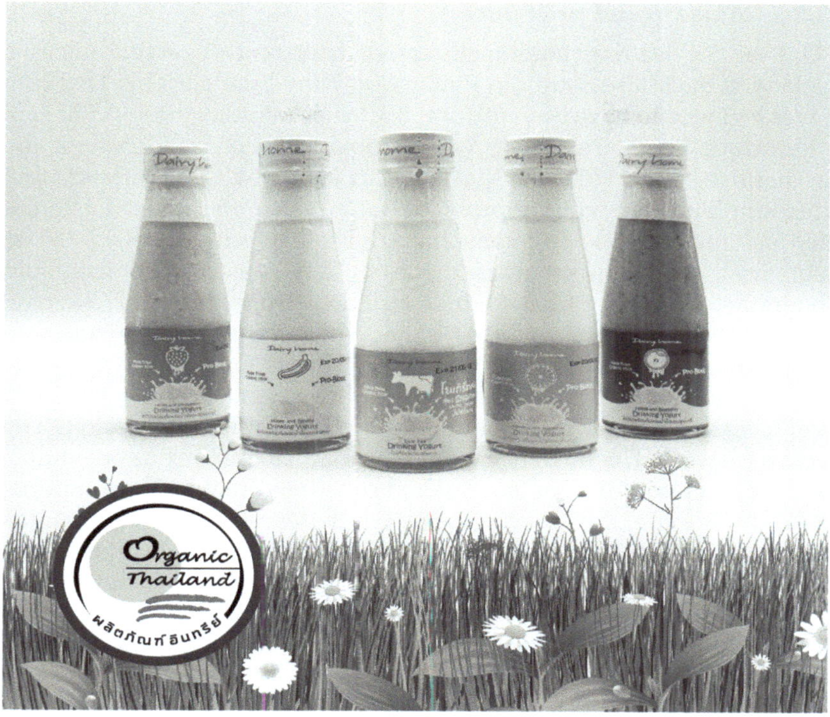

FIG. 6.3 Some examples of Dairy Home Synbiotic Drinking Yoghurts. *With permission courtesy of Dairy Home Co., Ltd., Thailand.*

and preventing digestion-related diseases. Specific prebiotics supplemented in the product support the growth and activity of those beneficial probiotics and also improve bowel function. Such prebiotics used may also have beneficial effects on appetite and weight control. The Dairy Home Synbiotic Drinking Yoghurt contains up to 2 billion CFU of beneficial probiotics per bottle and six flavors are available in the market (plain without added sugar, honey lemon, strawberry, blueberry, banana, and wheatgrass). Fig. 6.3 shows some examples of their products.

6.3.2 Probiotic based-plant beverage products

There are a small number of probiotic-based plant beverage products on the Thai market. This section discusses a few of these examples of probiotic-based fruit beverages in Thailand.

6.3.2.1 Malee brand fruit juice

One of the leading manufacturers of fruit and vegetable juices in Thailand is the Malee Sampran Public Company Limited. This Thai company is believed to have been the first fruit juice manufacturer in Thailand to introduce 100% fruit juice with probiotic lactic acid bacteria into the Thai market. In 2015, the Malee brand launched three different fruit juices supplemented with the probiotic bacteria *Lactobacillus paracasei* marketed as "for health-loving consumers." These products, called "Malee Probiotics," were marketed as the first 100% pasteurized fruit juice containing probiotics, to help in consumers' digestive and excretory systems. All three products (100% mandarin orange juice mixed with orange pulp and orange sacs, 100% white grape juice mixed with *Aloe vera* pulp, and 100% prune juice mixed with apple juice and white grape juice) were alternatives for consumers allergic to milk protein and to vegetarians (Fig. 6.4) The three new recipes contained as many as one million live probiotics per 1 mL of juice. When consumed regularly for a period of 14 days or more, this lactic acid bacterium is reputed to help maintain a balance between good bacteria and bad bacteria in the gastrointestinal tract, with a consequent improvement of the digestive, excretory, and immune system. Malee Probiotics also contain a variety of beneficial ingredients from the fruit juices, such as vitamins and fiber, which contribute to a healthy body.

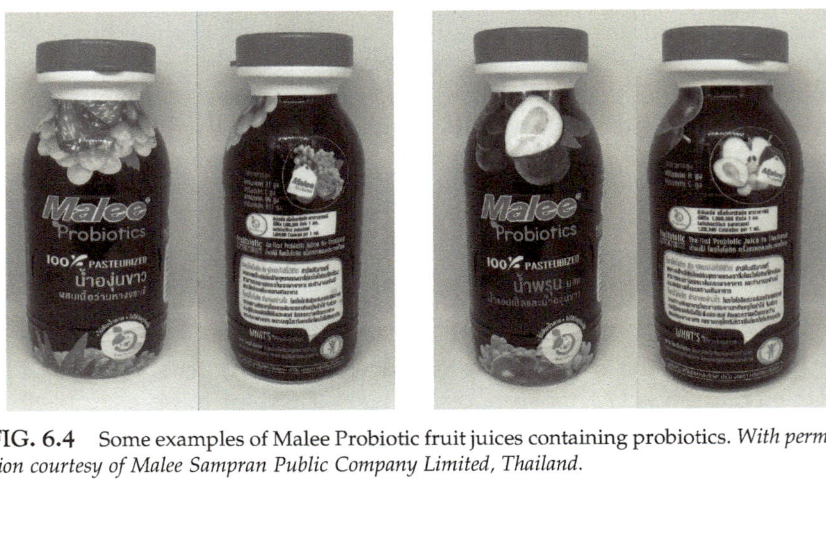

FIG. 6.4 Some examples of Malee Probiotic fruit juices containing probiotics. *With permission courtesy of Malee Sampran Public Company Limited, Thailand.*

6.4 Future considerations

Currently, probiotic beverage products are a multi-million-dollar food industry product in Thailand. Their development, popularity, and acceptance in Thailand are expanding as a result of the rising awareness of the probiotic health benefits combined with the high spending power of Thai consumers on new natural products. However, these newer ingredients (i.e., probiotics) are not familiar to the consumer; therefore, probiotic beverage manufacturers still have to educate consumers more in order to increase their knowledge with respect to these products. Moreover, there are not enough scientific and justifiable studies validating many of the health benefits claimed by some probiotic beverage manufacturers, where claims are only based on consumer feedback and focus groups. Currently, many reputable academic universities and institutions, as well as manufacturers, are undertaking detailed scientific research in order to validate the health benefits of probiotics.

Currently, only general health claims are allowed on food and beverage products containing probiotics in Thailand. Because of the growing probiotic product market and discrepancies in probiotic product marketing, the Thai Food and Drug Administration should urgently take a closer look at probiotic product labeling. Recently, guidelines have been established to evaluate and regulate claims by probiotic and prebiotic manufacturers. It is recommended that specific health claims on food and beverage products should be allowed relating to the use of probiotics providing that sufficient and strong scientific evidence is made available. Such specific health claims of probiotics should be permitted on the product label and in promotional material. Furthermore, the future success of functional probiotic beverages in the Thai marketplace depends on consumer acceptance and awareness of such products. Thai consumers must be convinced of the associated health benefit claims through simple, clear, honest, and definitive messages and be willing to pay the higher costs associated with probiotic beverage production. The development of probiotic beverage products with addition of prebiotics (namely synbiotic beverages, which are mainly based on fruits and vegetables as well as milk) is a key research priority for beverage design and has been a recent challenge for both industry scientists and academics in Thailand. A challenge for Thai researchers in the future will be the use of newer and more effective probiotic strains and natural prebiotics in Thailand's beverage industry.

References

Chaikham, P. (2015). Stability of probiotics encapsulated with Thai herbal extracts in fruit juices and yoghurt during refrigerated storage. *Food Bioscience*, *12*, 61–66.

Chaikham, P., & Apichartsrangkoon, A. (2012). Comparison of bioactive components in pressurized and pasteurized longan juices fortified with encapsulated *Lactobacillus casei* 01. *High Pressure Research: An International Journal, 32*(2), 316–322.

Chaikham, P., Kemsawasd, V., & Seesuriyachan, P. (2017). Spray drying probiotics along with maoluang juice plus *Tiliacora triandra* gum for exposure to the in vitro gastrointestinal environments. *LWT-Food Science and Technology, 78*, 31–40.

Chaiyasut, C. (2010). *Bioextracts: Book series health and beauty begin from internal*: (p. 88). Book Center NSTDA. National Science and Technology.

Chaiyasut, C., Sirilun, S., Pheerachan, S., & Kumar, N. (2011). *Handbook of bioextract for consume*: (p. 56). National Science and Technology Capability.

Gae-in, S., Deetae, P., Kingkaew, J., & Sawhasan, P. (2014). Production of potentially probiotic beverages using sweet potatoes fermented by lactic acid bacteria. *Agricultural Science Journal, 45*(2, Suppl), 237–240.

Innovative development prototype for value added sugar cane beverage project (2015). *Handbook of fermented sugar cane punch probiotic*: (p. 18). King Mongkut's Institute of Technology Ladkrabang Corporate with Office of the Cane and Sugar Board.

Kaeitsast, S., & Kwanmuang, P. (2016). Fermentation of probiotic beverage Gac fruit prepared from pulp and seed membrane with *Lactobacillus pentosus*. In: *Education national conference 6th "Development experiences on learning STEM and lifelong learning skills in the 21st century"*, pp. 812–821.

Kantachote, D., Ratanaburee, A., Hayisama-ae, W., Sukhoom, A., & Nunkaew, T. (2017). The use of potential probiotic *Lactobacillus plantarum* DW12 for producing a novel functional beverage from mature coconut water. *Journal of Functional Foods, 32*, 401–408.

Kemsawasd, V., & Chaikham, P. (2018). Survival of probiotics in soyoghurt plus mulberry (cv Chiang Mai 60) leaf extract during refrigerated storage and their ability to tolerate gastrointestinal transit. *LWT-Food Science and Technology, 93*, 94–101.

Kumar, B. V., Vijayendra, S. V. N., & Reddy, O. V. S. (2015). Trends in dairy and non-dairy probiotic products-review. *Journal of Food Science and Technology, 52*(10), 6112–6124.

Kwanmuang, P. (2013). Carrot juice fermentation with mixed cultures of *Lactobacillus pentosus* and *Saccharomyces cerevisiae*. In: *The 2nd agro-industry conference, 30 August 2013, Windsor Suites Hotel, Sukhumvit Road, Bangkok, Thailand*, pp. 9–15.

Kwanmuang, P. (2014). *Processing of Jerusalem artichoke juice with alcoholic and lactic fermentation. Research report, 2014.* Thailand: Faculty of Industrial Education, King Mongkut's Institute of Technology Ladkrabang.

Kwanmuang, P. (2018). Plant probiotic beverages: Alternative for functional beverages. *Journal of Industrial Education, 17*(1), 212–221.

Lertcanawanichakul, M., Thaiauer, K., Chaopongpan, P., & Petchnajak, W. (2010). Survival of probiotic bacteria in different kinds of fruit juices. *Thailand Journal of Health Promotion and Environmental Health*, 97–109.

Manas, R. S., Marimuthu, A., Ramesh, C. R., & Rizwana, P. R. (2014). Fermented fruits and vegetables of Asia: A potential source of probiotics. *Biotechnology Research International, 2014*, 1–19.

Nakkarach, A., & Withayagiat, U. (2018). Comparison of symbiotic beverages produced from riceberry malt extract using selected free and encapsulated probiotic lactic acid bacteria. *Agriculture and Natural Resources, 52*, 467–476.

Saengdee, W., Vangpikul, S., & Itsaranuwat, P. (2016). *Development of synbiotic fermented corn milk product. Research report from the faculty of science and technology*: (p. 83). Rajamangala University of Technology Suvarnabhumi, Thailand.

Saengthong, S., & Sirimunee, M. (2011). *The use of* Lactobacillus casei *for probiotic drinking yoghurt production. Research report from the faculty of home economics technology*: (p. 75). Rajamangala University of Technology Phra Nakhon, Thailand.

Waiwong, T. (2007). *Production of probiotic drink from herbs, green apple and soymilk. Report from the faculty of liberal arts and science*: (p. 111). Bangkok, Thailand: Kasetsart University.

Further reading

Kwanmuang, P. (2016). Fermentation of mixed beetroot juice with lactic acid bacteria and recycling starter. *Journal of Industrial Education*, *15*(1), 143–149.

Thai Community Products Standard. TCPS 481/2547. Fermented Plant Juice. Thai Industrial Standard Institute (cited 15 September 2019). Available from http://app.tisi.go.th/otop/pdf_file_47.pdf.

CHAPTER

7

Probiotic beverages: Health benefits and current trends in the Middle East

Neda Mollakhalili Meybodi[a,b], *Sarah Sanaei Nasab*[a], *Nasim Khorshidian*[c], *and Amir M. Mortazavian*[d]

[a]Department of Food Sciences and Technology, School of Public Health, Shahid Sadoughi University of Medical Sciences, Yazd, Iran, [b]Research Centre for Food Hygiene and Safety, Shahid Sadoughi University of Medical Sciences, Yazd, Iran, [c]Food Safety Research Center (Salt), Semnan University of Medical Sciences, Semnan, Iran, [d]Department of Food Science and Technology, National Nutrition and Food Technology Research Institute, Faculty of Nutrition Sciences, Food Science and Technology, Shahid Beheshti University of Medical Sciences, Tehran, Iran

7.1 Introduction

The Middle East region extends from Morocco to Iran horizontally (west to east) as depicted in Fig. 7.1. It consists of Africa and Bahrain, Iran, Iraq, Israel, Jordan, Kuwait, Lebanon, Oman, Palestine, Qatar, Saudi Arabia, Syria, the United Arab Emirates, and Yemen. The population has been estimated to be around 300 million. Urbanization development, modern lifestyle adaption, and affluence provided in oil-producing countries have changed eating habits in the Middle East. This nutrition transition has resulted in a prevalence of obesity, cardiovascular disease, and strokes, with a high proportion of mortality and it has been estimated this will have tripled during 1990–2020 (Aljefree & Ahmed, 2015; Farrag, Cheskin, & Farag, 2017). Consequently, concerns exist about health and well-being, leading to an increased desire for health promoting foods called "functional foods."

Probiotic Beverages
https://doi.org/10.1016/B978-0-12-818588-9.00011-5

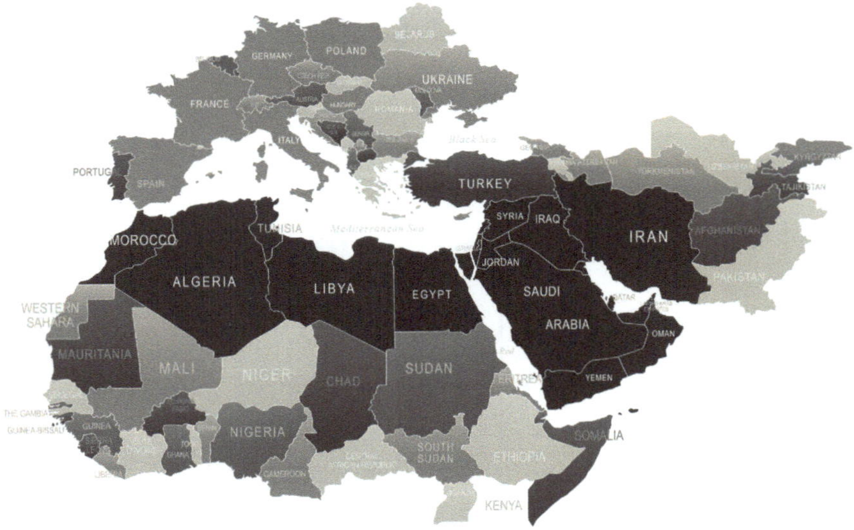

FIG. 7.1 The Middle East region (Hotez, Savioli, & Fenwick, 2012).

Functional foods are defined as foodstuffs providing beneficial bioactive ingredients (such as dietary fiber, antioxidant agents, and active microorganisms) either naturally or in a supplemented manner (Altay, Karbancıoglu-Güler, Daskaya-Dikmen, & Heperkan, 2013). Active microorganisms, which adjust the balance of the intestinal bacteria, are known as "probiotic." Probiotic functionality is attributed to their beneficial effects in improving gut immunity, preserving gut functionality and digestion, and preventing bacterial and yeast infections (Shori, 2016). The main probiotic species existing in the food market are *Lactobacillus* and *Bifidobacterium*. From the *Lactobacillus* species, the more commonly used strains are *L. crispatus, L. acidophilus, L. gallinarum, L. amylovarus, L.gasseri, L. helveticus, L. johnsonii, L. delbrueckii* subsp. *bulgaricus, L. salivarius* subsp. *salivarius, L. paracasei* subsp. *paracasei, L. casei, L. paracasei* subsp. *tolerans, L. rhamnosus, L. plantarum, L. fermentum, L. reuteri and from the Bifidobacterium spp., B. bifidum, B. infanti, B. longum, B. breve, B. animalis, and B. adolescentis* (Kandylis, Pissaridi, Bekatorou, Kanellaki, & Koutinas, 2016). The fastest growth in demand is reported for functional drink/beverages using probiotics (Corbo, Bevilacqua, Petruzzi, Casanova, & Sinigaglia, 2014).

The probiotic beverage market is a growing sector of the food industry, since modern health-conscious consumers have an increased desire fora beneficial foods that reduce the risk of disease. However, although some fermented beverages may have enough probiotic species to be categorized as probiotic; it is also possible to have supplemented beverages.

Considering the importance of the probiotic nature and the inoculated matrix in a consumer's acceptance of a product, this chapter aims to introduce probiotic beverages available in the Middle East and North Africa while considering their potential health benefits.

7.2 Health benefits of probiotic beverages

Good nutrition is considered as the most effective way to develop human health and comfort. Different types of beverages are consumed in large amounts including water, coffee, tea, fruit juice, milk, or any combination of ingredients found on the basis of water. Humans started to drink water even before birth. The consumption of beverages continues after birth, frequently with breast milk, and continues until death. However, the mechanisms by which the ingredients mixed with the water affect our nutritional health is poorly understood (Wilson & Temple, 2016). It is clear that beverages, whether from animal, plant, or natural sources, have assisted humans well through the years. The health-promoting effects of beverages are related to their nutraceutical content, which is dependent on their origin (Nickolas & Stewart, n.d.).

Throughout the world, fermentation is considered to be an economical way to protect and improve the nutritional quality and sensory properties of the raw ingredients. Fermentation is used to convert milk, cereals, and other substrates to health-promoting beverages in many regions of Asia, Africa, Europe, the Middle East, and South America (Marsh, Hill, Ross, & Cotter, 2014). Fermented food products are greatly consumed since they accomplish functional food requirements (German et al., 2009). Using fermentation, products can be made ready to consume, dense in nutritional components, and with lower unacceptable factors. Fermented products can also have a lower fat content with different flavor and aroma compounds and improved texture characteristics and volume (Behera, Bal, Das, Panda, & Mohanty, 2018; Praagman et al., 2015; Swain, Anandharaj, Ray, & Parveen Rani, 2014). Therefore, fermented beverages are potentially a good vehicle to deliver probiotics to humans (Kandylis et al., 2016).

A wide and day-by-day increasing number of health benefits have been acclaimed for probiotic-containing foods, such as antimicrobial activity, prevention of gastrointestinal infection, anti-mutagenic/anti-carcinogenic activity, anti-diarrheal activity, serum cholesterol reduction and prevention of cardiovascular disease, nutritional enhancement, intestinal microflora modulation, anti-IBS effect, anti-osteoporosis impact, prevention of non-alcoholic fatty liver disease, glycemic control of type 2 diabetes and immune response enhancement (Meybodi, Mortazavian, da Cruz, & Mohammadi, 2017; Shah, 2007). In this regard, probiotic beverages could

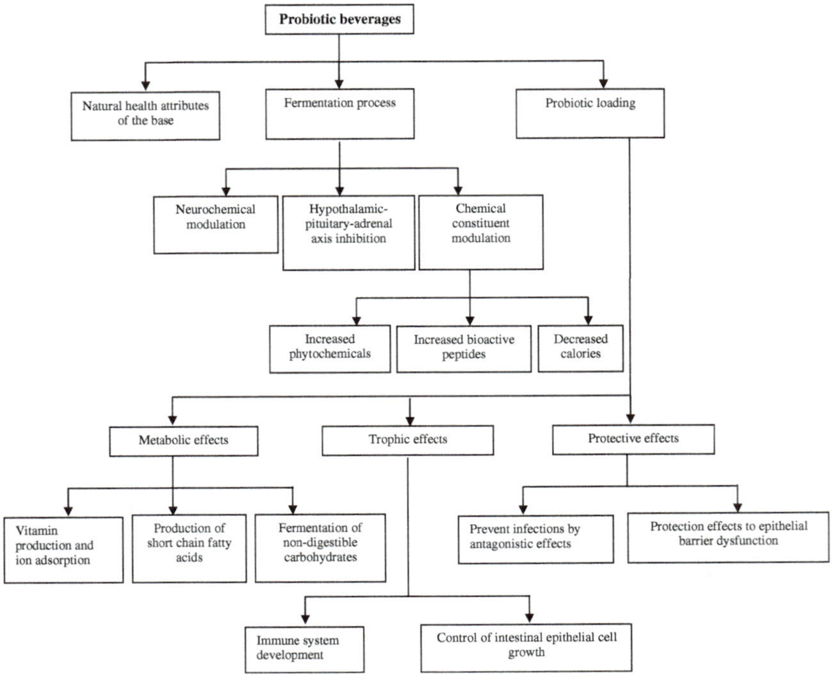

FIG. 7.2 Potential health benefits of probiotic beverages. *Adapted from Kim, B., Hong, V.M., Yang, J., Hyun, H., Im, J.J., Hwang, J., et al. (2016). A review of fermented foods with beneficial effects on brain and cognitive function.* Preventive Nutrition and Food Science, 21*(4), 297–309; Niba, A., Beal, J., Kudi, A., & Brooks, P. (2009). Bacterial fermentation in the gastrointestinal tract of non-ruminants: influence of fermented feeds and fermentable carbohydrates.* Tropical Animal Health and Production, 41*(7), 1393. http://doi.org/10.1007/s11250-009-9327-6.*

render multi-factorial beneficial effects for three reasons as previously mentioned: (1) The nutritional and nutraceutical nature in their bases, (2) favorable added effects to the bases by the fermentation process, and (3) the considerable health impacts of probiotic loading. The potential health effects of probiotic beverages are depicted in Fig. 7.2.

7.3 Types of probiotic beverage

Probiotic-containing beverages can be categorized based on different points of view (i.e., the involved probiotic species, the commodities or supposed health effects, the originating countries, and the food matrix). Three prerequisites that should be considered in probiotic-containing food products include viability, dose, and induced health effects. Providing beneficial health effects will be influenced by the number of probiotic microorganisms passed through the gastrointestinal tract intact and viable

(Meybodi et al., 2017). In this regard, the beverage-incorporated probiotic microorganisms need to be able to tolerate the harsh conditions of processing, such as mechanical conditions, thermal processing, and acidity. Beverage conditions, such as nutrient/anti-nutrient existence, titratable acidity, fermentations involving bacteria, as well as available oxygen and titratable acidity and the bile of the gastrointestinal tract play a part. The nature of the beverage plays an important role in the maintenance of the probiotic microorganisms, either during the processing or storage stage (i.e., chemical composition of beverage, presence of organic acid and pH, accompanying microbes in fermented beverages, etc). The basis of probiotic beverage categorization is illustrated in Fig. 7.3. The main publications in the realm of probiotic beverages of the Middle East are summarized in Table 7.1. Different types of probiotic beverages are discussed in two main categories, namely, dairy-based and non-dairy-based probiotic beverages.

7.3.1 Dairy-based probiotic beverages

Dairy-based probiotic beverages can be categorized into two main groups; fermented and non-fermented beverages. The fermentation process is an old treatment used in food processing and is induced either by naturally occurring native microorganisms and/or inoculated starter cultures (selected microorganisms such as bacteria and yeast). Fermentation is used as a preservation approach, mainly due to organic acid production. It also provides pleasing sensory characteristics and additional nutritional values. The fermentation process is not compulsory in probiotic beverage development. Despite the prevalence of probiotic fermented dairy products in the market, their physicochemical properties differ according to the type of probiotic microorganism incorporated, the milk type, and the use of other starter cultures in the product. Microorganisms incorporated as starter cultures are very important in the flavor and textural improvement of the final fermented product. In probiotic fermented beverages, different probiotic microorganisms can be added in addition to the starter culture microorganisms, which may afford benefits as well as some drawbacks. For example, yogurt starter culture bacteria are generally recognized as oxygen scavengers, which may be valuable in improving the growth and viability of anaerobic probiotics. However probiotic dairy beverages are mainly in the category of fermented products, non-dairy probiotic products, such as fruit/vegetable-based beverages, are often produced without a fermentation process due to adverse sensory characteristics (Umer, 2014).

Three main strategies can be used for probiotic additions to fermented dairy beverages; first, added together with a starter culture (most typical method); second, parallel incorporation into two different batches; third,

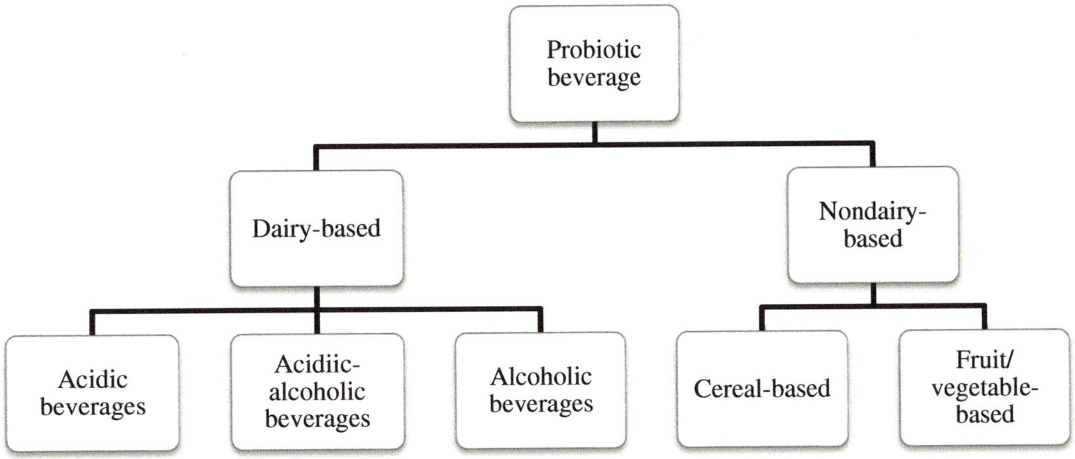

FIG. 7.3 Classification of probiotic beverages in the Middle East.

TABLE 7.1 Selected publications on probiotic beverages.

Beverage	Base	Probiotic strains	Conclusion	Reference
Doogh	Dairy-based	*Lactobacillus acidophilus* LA-5, *Bifidobacterium lactis* BB-12	Viability of both probiotic microorganisms increased by using standardization after fermentation	Mortazavian, Khosrokhavar, Rastegar, and Mortazaei (2010)
Ayran	Dairy-based	*Lactobacillus acidophilus*	Probiotic culture addition improved the functional characteristics of Ayran	Ayar and Burucu (2013)
Kefir	Dairy-based	*Lactococcus lactis* spp. *lactis*, *Lactococcus lactis* spp. *cremoris*, *Lactococcus lactis* spp. *diacetylactis*, *Leuconostoc mesenteroides* spp. *cremoris*, *Lactobacillus kefir*, *Kluyveromyces marxianus, and Saccharomyces unisporus*	The consumption of kefir even at short-term decreased high levels of salivary mutans streptococci and lactobacilli	Cogulu et al. (2010)
Probiotic flavored fermented milk	Dairy-based	*L. acidophilus* LA-5, *L. casei* L01, L. casei LAFTI L26, *L. paracasei* Lcp37, and *L. rhamnosus* HN001	*L. casei* LAFTI L26 and L. *acidophilus* LA-5 showed the highest viability retention and viability loss during refrigerated storage	Sadaghdar, Mortazavian, & Ehsani (2012)
Koumiss	Dairy-based	*Lactobacillus acidophilus* RRAM-01and *Lactococcus lactis* RRAM-01	Inoculation of goat milk with probiotic bacteria restrains coliform growth and has strong inhibition activity against *Escherichia coli* ATCC 25922	Nuraeni, Arief, and Soenarno (2014)

Continued

TABLE 7.1 Selected publications on probiotic beverages—cont'd

Beverage	Base	Probiotic strains	Conclusion	Reference
Boza	Cereal-based	*Weisella paramesenteroides*, *L. casei* Shirota and *Lactobacillus acidophilus*	Total counts of *boza* lactic acid bacteria ranged from 9.09 to 10.48 log cfu/ml with the lowest pH (4.08 ± 0.02) in samples produced with *L. acidophilus* and *L. casei* Shirota. *Boza* samples showed non-Newtonian pseudo plastic behaviors	Tornuk, Ozturk, Karaman, Sagdic, and Yetim (2014)
Beer	Cereal-based	*S. cerevisiae var. boulardii*	The predominant yeast was *S. cerevisiae* strain (with a range of 8 × 106 to 7.0 × 107/mL) in almost all samples. Probiotic inclusion did not negatively affect beer aroma but did increase the antioxidant activity and polyphenol content	Capece et al. (2018)
Beer	Cereal-based	*Lactobacillus acidophilus* LA-5 and *Bifidobacterium lactis* BB-12	The viability of the probiotic bacteria was not retained in beer during the cold storage period	Sohrabvandi, Razavi, Mousavi, and Mortazavian (2010)
Grape drink	Fruit-based	*L. delbrueckii*, *L. plantarum* and *L. rhamnosus*	Probiotic grape juice production using *L. rhamnosus* was suggested due to its higher viability and desirable organoleptic properties	Malganji, Sohrabvandi, Jahadi, Nematollahi, and Sarmadi (2016)

TABLE 7.1 Selected publications on probiotic beverages—cont'd

Beverage	Base	Probiotic strains	Conclusion	Reference
Carrot juice	Fruit-based	*Lactobacillus acidophilus* NRRL-B-4495, *Lactobacillus plantarum-C3, Lactobacillus casei B-442* and *Bifidobacterium longum 35,624*	Fermented carrot juice was considered to be a suitable media for delivering probiotics	Rafiq, Sharma, Nazir, Rashid, and Sofi (2016)
Apple juice	Fruit-based	*Lactobacillus paracasei* ssp. *paracasei*	The turbidity of apple juice increased by probiotic inoculation, but total acceptance did not change significantly	Pimentel, Madrona, and Prudencio (2015)
Apple/blueberry yogurt mixes	Fruit-based	*L. acidophilus and L. rhamnosus*	The fruit type and probiotic bacteria used were effective on the microbiological and sensory properties of the fermented beverage	Ozcan, Yilmaz-Ersan, Akpinar-Bayizit, Delikanli, and Barat (2015)

using the probiotic microorganisms as the starter culture (Paquin, 2009). The probiotic dairy drinks available in the market are generally in the category of fermented products, with three main subgroups (acidic, acidic-alcoholic, and alcoholic) based on the type of microorganisms involved in the fermentation and the desired final product. Lactic acid fermentation and alcoholic fermentation are considered to be two main respiration methods that occur in an anaerobic environment. Lactic acid is produced from pyruvate in an acidic fermentation process; ethyl alcohol and carbon dioxide are produced in an alcoholic fermentation as illustrated in Fig. 7.4. Dairy-based beverages are considered to be an excellent medium to carry or generate live and active cultures. *L. acidophilus* and *Bifidobacterium lactis* are the main probiotic species incorporated in dairy products. *Streptococcus thermophilus* is also important, as the aforementioned species are unable to show appropriate proteolysis activity (Fijan, 2014). The main probiotic dairy beverages consumed in the Middle East region are summarized in the next sections.

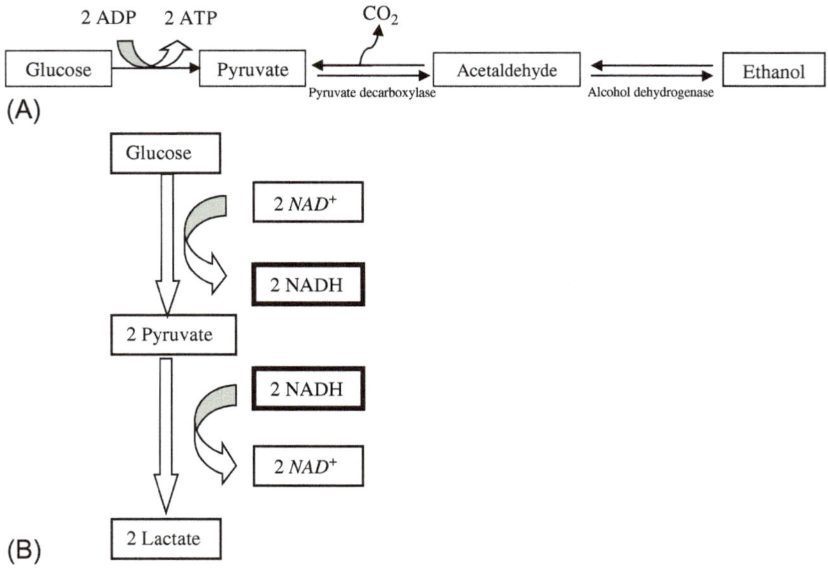

FIG. 7.4 Schematic pathway of (A) an alcoholic fermentation and (B) a lactic acid fermentation (Doyle, Steenson, & Meng, 2013).

7.3.1.1 Doogh

According to Codex Alimentarius (CXS 332R-2018), *doogh* is a "drink based on fermented milk" provided either by mixing yogurt with drinking water and sodium chloride (not compulsory) or by direct addition of drinking water and salt to the milk before heating and the fermentation process (Codex alimentarius (FAO), 2018). *Doogh* has been produced and consumed in Iran and the surrounding countries for thousands of years. The word *doogh* is derived from Doo (a very ancient Iranian world, meaning milk) and the term Dootar (used as daughter in present times), means a person who milks the cow (normally, females at that time) (ISIRI, 2008a).

Doogh is a fermented beverage and it is typically classified as plain (without flavoring agent addition)/flavored, carbonated/un-carbonated, and heat-treated/un-heated (Codex alimentarius (FAO), 2018). Carbonated *doogh* is produced by either injection or fermentation, on the basis of the carbon dioxide addition state (i.e., either directly added or by the use of gas producing harmless microorganisms) (ISIRI, 2008b). Permitted ingredients for use in *doogh* production are sodium chloride, natural flavoring agents, dietary fiber, and dairy derived ingredients (milk powder, milk fat, or milk protein) (Codex alimentarius (FAO), 2018). *Doogh* is generally categorized by the content of the milk fat (max 25% w/v of total dry non-fat in final product), milk solid non-fat (min 3% *w*/w), pH (max 4.5), titratable acidity (min 0.3% w/w lactic acid), milk protein (min 1.8% w/w), salt (0.2%–1.0% w/w), carbon dioxide (min 0.4% w/w), and optional thickening agents (Codex alimentarius (FAO), 2018; Mortazavian et al., 2008). The main starter culture of both traditionally and/or commercially produced *doogh* includes *Streptococcus thermophilus* and *L. delbrueckii subsp. bulgaricus* (Bagheri poor Fallah, SAM, Hosseini, Shahraz, & Bahadori Monfared, 2016). Alongside other harmless microorganisms, probiotic inclusion may also be added for acidification, aroma/gas production, texture improvement, as well as other functional product characteristics. The inoculated probiotic microorganisms should also be present minimally at 10^7 cfu/g in the final product. Ieachstrain.n traditionally produced types of beverages, further microorganism loading can come from the applied water, from Mashk (a traditional container made of goat skin), or from the equipment used, which may result in a final microbial composition that is complex and varies locally (Sayevand et al., 2018).

The possibility of *doogh* to deliver active and live probiotic bacteria has been considered in different studies. Since the beneficial health effects of probiotic products are determined by the number of viable cells at the time of consumption (minimum 10^7 cfu/mL or g) (Ahmadi et al., 2019), the survival of probiotic bacteria should be investigated. It has been reported that the ability of probiotic bacteria to endure severe conditions in food products, such as pH, titratable acidity, and oxygen toxicity, is species- and strain-specific (Mortazavian, Mohammadi, & Sohrabvandi, 2012). In his regard, *Lactobacillus* strains, especially *L. acidophilus,* have been found to be more resistant when compared to *Bifidobacteria* at low pH, considering their high cytoplasmic buffering capacity (pH 3.72–7.74) (Tamime, Saarela, Sondergaard, Mistry, & Shah, 2005). For industrial production of probiotic *doogh* (available on the market), acid stable probiotic strains have been used. Furthermore, since the sensory properties of functional food products are of high importance, for preference by the consumer, the characteristics of conventional *doogh* should not be adversely affected by probiotic inclusions (Rahmdar, Rahmati Roudsari, Javanmard, Mortazavian, & Sohrabvandi, 2013).

7.3.1.2 *Ayran*

Ayran is a non-alcoholic, yogurt-based beverage consumed in Turkey and is produced either traditionally or industrially. Traditionally, yogurt is diluted by salt containing water (at a level of 1% in final product) to decrease the dry matter content to 50% (the microbiota is similar to its originating yogurt). *Ayran* constituents include protein, dry matter, salt, and fat, their content varying in different studies depending on the type of milk, dilution ratio, and fat removal efficiency. Industrially, milk with attuned solid content is fermented by *Streptococcus thermophilus* and

L. delbrueckii subsp. bulgaricus (Ivanovska, Zhivikj, Bogdanovska, Mladenovska, & Petrushevska-Tozi, 2018). In the Turkish Food Codex (Turkish Food Codex, 2009), *Ayran* is defined as a fresh product with a shelf-life of 10–15 days, which has protein (min 2.8 g), non-fat solids (6 g/100 mL), and fat (min 1.8, 0.8 and 0.15 g for full fat, semi-fat, and non-fat product, respectively). *Ayran* differs from other beverages based on fermented milk, as it has salt added (up to 1% *w*/w) and is without any fruit flavoring agents.

Two different methods can be used for the industrial production of *Ayran*, in which the dilution (at a level of 30%–50%) can be accomplished either with the milk or with the final fermented product. Similar to other acidic milk beverages (e.g., *doogh*), textural instability is present in *Ayran* during storage, owing to its low pH. The main textural problems in *Ayran* are low viscosity and phase separation during storage, which negatively affect consumer acceptability (Koksoy & Kilic, 2004). *Ayran* is an easily digestible and highly nutritious beverage, whose functional properties can be improved by prebiotic or probiotic inclusions. Since lactic acid bacteria are inherently connected to dairy products, probiotic *Ayran* is easily accepted by consumers (Altay et al., 2013; Ayar & Burucu, 2013). The potential application of *Ayran* to deliver probiotics has been investigated in a number of studies (Ayar & Burucu, 2013; Ivanovska et al., 2018; Kuş, 2010; Taş & Güzel-Seydim, 2010).

7.3.1.3 Leben

Leben is a traditional fermented dairy product, widely consumed in the Middle East region, and prepared from buffalo, cow, or goat milk. However, in the Levant region, *Leben* is a type of yogurt. This beverage in Arabia and North Africa is also known as Laban, Lben, Maghre, Labankhad, and Laban Kherbah. Leben beverages were traditionally produced by deliberately souring milk for around 24 h using Mashk (a sack made of goat's skin). The butter is removed after churning and the remaining buttermilk is termed *Leben*, after storage at room temperature for several days (Samet-Bali, Felfoul, Lajnaf, Attia, & Ayadi, 2017). The physico-chemical characteristics of *Leben* are as follows: protein 2.5% (*w*/w), lactic acid 0.81% (w/w), total solids 6.5% (w/w), fat 0.9% (w/w), lactose 2.7% (w/w), and pH 4.25. Microbiological characteristics reveal that lactic acid bacteria are the main microflora in different traditionally fermented milk-based beverages with Lactic streptococci as the predominant organism in *Leben* (National Research Council, 1992). *Leben* has been used therapeutically long before the existence of microorganisms was discovered (Makinen, Berger, Bel-Rhlid, & Ananta, 2012). To normalize *Leben* characteristics, low- or non-fat milk is now fermented industrially by selected bacterial species and probiotic cultures, similar to bio-stirred yogurt, and in developed countries is commercially available (e.g., Activia Laban).

The resulting beverage is usually tarter in flavor and thicker compared to the traditional ones (Anon, n.d.).

7.3.1.4 *Qatiq*

Qatiq is a yogurt-based beverage, thicker than *Ayran,* which is consumed by Turkic peoples (Perry, 1997). Locally, it is also known as Katik, атыҮ, Айран, Gatyk, Къатыкъ and Қатик. It is produced by fermenting pasteurized milk for 6–10 h and red beets or cherries are used as a coloring agent. No published information was found on the microbiological and physicochemical characteristics of *Qatiq*. However, a probiotic *Qatiq* is produced by some companies (Marsh et al., 2014).

7.3.1.5 *Koumiss*

Koumiss, which is also known as *kumiss, kumis, kymis, kymmyz, coomys,* and *airag,* is an acidic-alcoholic beverage heavily consumed in the Middle East. This product is unique compared to other dairy foods, due to its mare's milk origin. The starter cultures used in a *koumiss* fermentation include different lactic acid bacteria and yeasts. Both lactic acid and alcoholic fermentations occur in *koumiss* similar to *kefir*. *Koumiss* is categorized into three main groups according to its lactic acid content: strong (pH 3.3–3.6), moderate (pH 3.9–4.5), and light (pH 4.5–5). Studies have investigated the participation of different microorganisms in *koumiss* fermentation and despite the diversity of the microbial composition in the original *koumiss,* three main groups have been reported to be involved. The main microflora is L. *delbrueckii subsp. bulgaricus, L. acidophilus,* and lactose-fermenting yeasts (*Torula koumiss* and *Saccharomyces lactis*). However, *Streptococcus lactis* is also a species used to produce good-quality *koumiss*. Physicochemical and organoleptic characteristics of finished *koumiss* include milk fat less than 10% (w/w), ash 0.4%–0.5% (w/w), carbon dioxide 0.5%–0.9% (w/w), ethanol 0.6%–2.5% (w/w), lactic acid 0.7%–1.8% (w/w), lactose 3.5%–4.3% (w/w), lipid 0.6%–1.3% (w/w), protein 1.7%–1.9% (w/w), specific gravity 1.03, pH 3.8–4.0, a milky-gray color, natural carbonation, and a sharp acidic-alcoholic taste (Dhewa, Mishra, Kumar, & Sangu, 2015). It is worthy to mention that mare's milk does not coagulate at its isoelectric point and therefore a curdle is not formed in the final product (Centeno & Carballo, 2014). Due to the higher sugar content of mare's milk, *koumiss* is higher in lactic acid and alcohol content compared to other fermented dairy products (made from sheep, goat, cow, buffalo, and other animal milks) (Uniacke-Lowe, Huppertz, & Fox, 2010). However, with increasing demand for *koumis,* other animal milks may be used in *koumiss* production, due to the limited supply of mare's milk.

7.3.1.6 *Kefir*

Kefir is a white/yellowish, acidic-alcoholic fermented beverage with a balanced and yeasty aroma with high consumption in the Middle East. It is one of the oldest fermented milk beverages and originated from the Caucasus region and was first manufactured in bags made of animal hides (Mashk). With the repeated use of Mashk, a thin layer and cluster are formed on the surface of the containers (called "kefir grain") (Tamime, 2008). Kefir is prepared by kefir grains or is derived from a mother culture inoculation into any type of milk (cow, goat, sheep, coconut, or soy) for 18–24h at 20–25°C.

The main ingredients affecting the organoleptic characteristics of kefir include volatile acids, carbon dioxide, and ethanol. Physicochemical characteristics of kefir are as follows: protein min 2.7% (*w*/w), milk fat less than 10% (w/w), titratable acidity min 0.6% (w/w), pH 4.27–4.42, viscosity 543.83–651.00cp, ethyl alcohol variable, but normally 0.05%–0.22% (w/w), acetic acid 0.22–0.25mg/mL, and lactic acid 1.73–1.82mg/mL (Behera, Panda, Kayitesi, & Mulaba-Bafubiandi, 2017; Temiz & Kezer, 2014).

Kefir has recently attracted much research interest due to its probiotic properties (Tamime, 2008). Natural different probiotic species, especially *L. acidophilus* and *Bifidobacterium bifidum*, are provided by *kefir* in enough quantity to be beneficial (Guzel-Seydim, Kok-Tas, Ertekin-Filiz, & Seydim, 2011). See Chapter 16 for detailed information on the history of Kefir and production details.

7.3.1.7 *Shubat*

Shubat, also known as *chaal*, is a camel milk probiotic beverage with high consumption and is considered a "healing food" in Africa, Asia, and the Middle East (Rahman, Xiaohong, Meiqin, & Mingsheng, 2009). It is produced by a semi-continuous or fed-batch fermentation process. Traditionally, the camel milk (diluted with warm water at a ratio of 1:1), and with added previously soured milk, is left at 25–30°C to produce coagulates with a typical taste. The main lactic acid bacteria isolated and identified in *shubat* are as follows: *L. sakei, L. helveticus, Enterococcus feacium, E. feacalis, L. brevis, Leuconstoc lactis, and Weissella hellenica* (Rahman, Dirar, & Osman, 2009). *Shubat* can be improved by adding starter cultures, such as *L. casei, S. thermophilus,* and lactose-fermenting yeasts, inoculated into the milk and incubated for 8h at 25°C, and then for 16h at 20°C (Kuliev, 1959). The physicochemical characteristics of *shubat* are as follows: fat 4.3% (*w*/w), protein (not specified in references), ash 0.75% w/w, titratable acidity 0.17–0.24, lactose 1.32% (w/w), ethyl alcohol 1.1% (w/w), ascorbic acid 4.8mg/mL, carbohydrate 2.5%–5% (w/w), and CO_2 0.05%–1.2% (w/w) (Shori, 2012).

7.3.1.8 Sameel milk

Sameel milk is a traditional Saudi Arabian fermented milk, generally consumed by nomadic herders. It is a type of sour buttermilk, which is produced by the removal of butter from the fermented milk. Different types of milk (cow, goat, sheep, or camel) are used in its production. The microorganism species of *sameel milk* have been isolated and identified recently as *L. plantarum, L. paracasei* subsp. *paracasei, Candida lusitania, L. pentosus, Cryptococcus laurentii,* and *Saccharomyces cerevisiae (S. cerevisiae* subsp. *cerevisiae)* (Al-Otaibi, 2012). Although some of the mentioned microorganisms have probiotic potential, this is necessary to be verified by further research into their use in *sameel milk,* as currently no scientific research has been published about the physicochemical and industrial production of *sameel milk.*

7.3.1.9 Matzun

Matzun, also known as *Matsoun, Madzoon, Madzoun, Mancun, Matson, Matsoni, Matsoon, Matsun,* and *Matxoun,* is a fermented dairy beverage prepared from buffalo, goat, or cow milk, or their combinations. It has high consumption in West Asia, especially Armenia. Traditionally, *Matzun* is prepared using a back-slopping fermentation, with known commercial starter cultures commonly used for industrial production. *L. delbrueckii* subsp. *Bulgaricus,* and *S. thermophilus* are the main production species used. Traditionally produced *Matzun* differs greatly on the basis of its microbiota, which is determined by its biogeographic conditions. The physico-chemical characteristics of *Matzun* are as follow: pH 3.6–4.2, volatile acids 0.11%–16% (*w*/w), ethyl alcohol 0.16–0.4% (w/w), and titratable acidity 150–200°D. Matzun can also be used in *Tan* beverage production (by its dilution and salt addition) (Keryan, Bazukyan, & Trchounian, 2017).

7.3.2 Non-dairy-based probiotic beverages

The prevalence of consumer vegetarianism throughout the developed countries and the inability of consumers to tolerate lactose have resulted in an increased demand for non-dairy-based beverages (Soccol et al., 2012). Tradition and economic reasons, especially in developing countries, has challenged the food industry to select less expensive vehicles for probiotics. However, traditional non-dairy-based beverages are already found around the world and their probiotic origin and ability to deliver probiotic microorganisms needs further investigation for implementation in the Middle East. Non-dairy beverages are generally produced in the absence of a fermentation process, due to the creation of undesirable sensory characteristics that can develop, such as acidity enhancement and detrimental effects in terms of texture, color, and viscosity. Non-dairy-based probiotic beverages of the Middle East and North Africa will be discussed in two main categories—cereal-based and fruit/vegetable-based beverages.

7.3.2.1 Cereal-based probiotic beverages

Cereals have recently gained popularity in food product development due to their high essential vitamins, dietary fiber, and mineral content (Charalampopoulos, Wang, Pandiella, & Webb, 2002). However, their low protein and essential amino acid (lysine) content, low starch availability, and the presence of anti-nutrients decrease their suitability compared to milk and its derived products (Blandino, Al-Aseeri, Pandiella, Cantero, & Webb, 2003). Fermentation is considered a strategy to overcome these problems. The use of oat, wheat, sorghum, barley, and malt have been investigated to produce non-alcoholic and functional drinks, preferred in the Middle East due to religious beliefs about alcohol consumption. Cereal-based fermented beverages, which are generally produced as depicted in Fig. 7.5, are commonly homogeneous suspensions, with a light to dark beige color, and a slightly sweet-sour taste and with distinct enhanced sensory characteristics due to probiotic incorporation. Furthermore, these cereal-based fermented functional beverages can be effectively and safely consumed as a meal alternative for weight conscious consumers, as the fiber and protein result in decreased digestion and extended satiety (Vander Wal, McBurney, Cho, & Dhurandhar, 2007). Lactic acid bacteria have been broadly investigated for the production of non-alcoholic fermented functional cereal-based beverages. Though these products can be denoted as a new generation of cereal-based beverages, traditional cereal-based fermented beverages also fall into this category due to their inherent probiotic nature (Roberfroid, 2002). The main traditional fermented functional cereal-based beverages consumed in the Middle East are discussed below.

Beer (low alcohol and no alcohol)

Beer is consumed globally and is a very popular beverage made using malt (germinated barley), water, and yeast. The popularity of beer is generally induced by its pleasant sensory characteristics, constructive nutritional and medicinal properties, and its low cost (Ahvenainen & Kuhanen, 1993).

The main beneficial health effects that have been reported for beer consumption include anti-carcinogenic/antimutagenic, anti-microbial/anti-viral, anti-osteoporosis, prevention of cardiovascular disease, anti-diabetes, immunomodulation, aging retardation, tension reduction, and relieving abdominal constipation symptoms (Sohrabvandi, Mortazavian, & Rezaei, 2011). However, while the consumption of beer at light to moderate contents results in both nutritional and medicinal health benefits, excessive

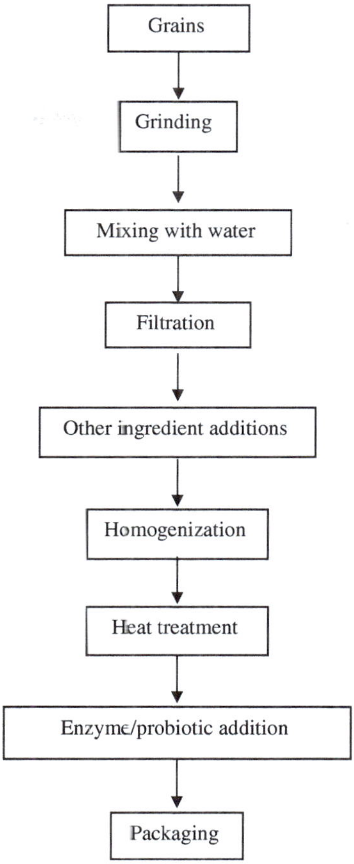

FIG. 7.5 General process flow diagram of probiotic cereal-based beverages. *Adapted from Gadaga, T., Mutukumira, A., Narvhus, J., & Feresu, S. (1999). A review of traditional fermented foods and beverages of Zimbabwe.* International Journal of Food Microbiology, 53*(1), 1–11.*

consumption (especially of those products with a high alcohol amount) results in adverse health impacts. Most of the popular beers produced worldwide have an alcohol content of 2.5%–13%. However, recently there is an increased demand for non-alcoholic or alcohol-free beers, with the definition varying from country to country, but usually less than 1% alcohol (Sohrabvandi, Mousavi, Razavi, Mortazavian, & Rezaei, 2010).

Today, "specialty beers" are considered as new beer products derived from regular ones. The differences may be induced by new flavor additions, changing the fermentation process or using alternative fermentable substrates (Bellut & Arendt, 2019).

In this regard, specialty beers can be categorized to five main groups: low-calorie beer, low- or non-alcohol, newly flavored beer, gluten free beer, and functional beer (Nachel & Ettlinger, 2012). Probiotic microorganism addition can be considered as a strategy to warrant the properties of functional beer in the final product. Considering the importance of probiotic viability to deliver beneficial effects, "craft beer" (i.e., un-pasteurized and unfiltered beer) may be more suitable compared to other beers, since probiotics may be killed by heat treatments and/or removed by filtration. The production of lactic acid by probiotic microorganisms may improve their stability in the final beer. The β-glucan content of beer has been reported to convalesce the stress (pH, ethanol, and hop acids inhibitory effects) tolerance of probiotic species (Stack, Kearney, Stanton, Fitzgerald, & Ross, 2010; Suharja, Henriksson, & Liu, 2014). It has been also reported that the presence of yeast in beer enhances the survival of probiotic bacteria (Liu & Tsao, 2010). A well-known probiotic yeast strain, *S. cerevisiae* var. *boulardii*, may also have possible use (Capece et al., 2018).

Boza

Boza is an acidic-alcoholic beverage, rich in probiotic lactic acid bacteria and is widely consumed in Bulgaria, Albania, Turkey, and Romania (Todorov et al., 2008). It is often consumed daily due to its pleasant taste and high nutritional content. This yellow, thick, and sour beverage is consumed principally in Egypt, Turkey, and in some Eastern European countries. It is also known as *braga, brascha, busa, buha, merissa*, and *bouza* (Arici & Daglioglu, 2002). Microorganisms isolated and identified in *boza* include L. *plantarum, L. acidophilus, L. fermentum, L. coprophilus, Leu. reffinolactis, Leu. Mesenteroides, and* L. *brevis.* The yeasts isolated were *S. cerevisiae, Candida tropicalis, C. glabrata, Geotrichum penicillatum*, and *G. candidum* (Blandino et al., 2003; Gotcheva, Pandiella, Angelov, Roshkova, & Webb, 2000). *Boza* is produced from rye, wheat, millet, maize, and other cereals mixed with sugar or saccharine. Traditionally, the milled grains are cooked with water in an open or steam-jacketed vessel. After cooking, *boza* is cooled in a way to prevent cream accumulation on its surface and then it is percolated. The fermentation occurs at 30°C for 24 h using a back-slopping process. The physicochemical characteristics of *boza* are as follows: protein 0.50%–1.61% (*w*/w), carbohydrate 12.3% (w/w), moisture 75–85% (w/w), pH 3.16–4.02, and ethyl alcohol less than 0.5% w/w. Despite the presence of lactic acid bacteria, there is some alcohol produced by yeast activity in *boza* production (Blandino et al., 2003).

Sobia

Sobia is a fermented beverage based on cereal, with high consumption in the western region of Saudi Arabia. This sweet-sour beverage, which is consumed cold, has a 24 h fermentation process and is traditionally produced by suspending malt and wheat flour in an equal ratio in water (2–2.5 L/100 g whole wheat flour). Then, sugar at 7%–10% (w/w) and spices (cinnamon and cardamom) are added to the mixture and it is left for 24 h at 30–40°C to be inoculated by chance from the environment. Differences exist in type of flour used and the soaking process. *Sobia* consumption is especially popular during the month of Ramadan. Its microbial composition is composed of lactic acid bacteria and yeast as the main species (Gassem, 2003). The lactic acid bacteria consist of *L. cellobiosus, L. buchneri, L. plantarum, L. brevis, L. delbrueckii* subsp. *delbrueckii, Leu. Lactis,* and *Pediococcus pentosaceus.* The yeasts encompass *S. cerevisiae, Candida tropicalis, C. ciferrii, C. guilliermondii, C. lipolytica, Kloeckera japonica,* and *Rhodotorula rubra* (Gassem, 2002).

7.3.2.2 *Fruit/vegetable-based beverages*

Today, there is growing product research devoted to the development of functional fruit/vegetable-based beverages, due to their high content of beneficial nutrients (minerals, vitamins, dietary fibers, and antioxidants), a pleasing taste profile for all age groups, as well as healthy and refreshing characteristics (Pereira, Maciel, & Rodrigues, 2011). In this regard, the fortification of fruit/vegetable-based beverages with probiotic and prebiotic ingredients has been investigated in different studies despite potential sensory challenges, especially the potential use of beverages, such as apple, orange, pomegranate, grape, tomato, berries, and mixed fruits to deliver probiotics. Despite the suitability of the aforementioned media, a limited number of probiotic fruit/vegetable juices are commercially available. Probiotic addition to the vegetable/fruit juices is more complicated compared to the production of probiotic dairy products, which is attributed to the necessity of bacteria requiring more protection against the acidic conditions. Microencapsulation technologies have been used to deliver probiotics successfully into functional foods and there is now increasing use of this technology outside of the pharmaceutical and supplement industries (Del Piano et al., 2006). Probiotic fruit/vegetable beverages available in the marketplace can be categorized into fermented and non-fermented products. Their production is similar except for the one additional step in fermented beverage production as represented in Fig. 7.6. The main probiotic fermented fruit/vegetable juices are described below.

Hardaliye

Hardaliye is a non-alcoholic probiotic beverage produced from a grape (*Vitis vinifera*) juice fermentation (Dlusskaya, Jänsch, Schwab, & Gänzle, 2008). It has been widely consumed in Turkey since ancient times. Traditionally, it is produced in wooden (or now plastic) containers as follows: washing and pressing of the grape seeds, addition of crushed raw mustard seeds, 0.2% (*w*/w) for flavor improvement, 0.1% (w/w) benzoic acid addition to prevent alcohol formation, and fermentation for 5–10 days at room temperature. Once fermented, it is kept at 4 °C to be consumed either fresh or after aging. The physicochemical characteristics of *hardaliye* are as

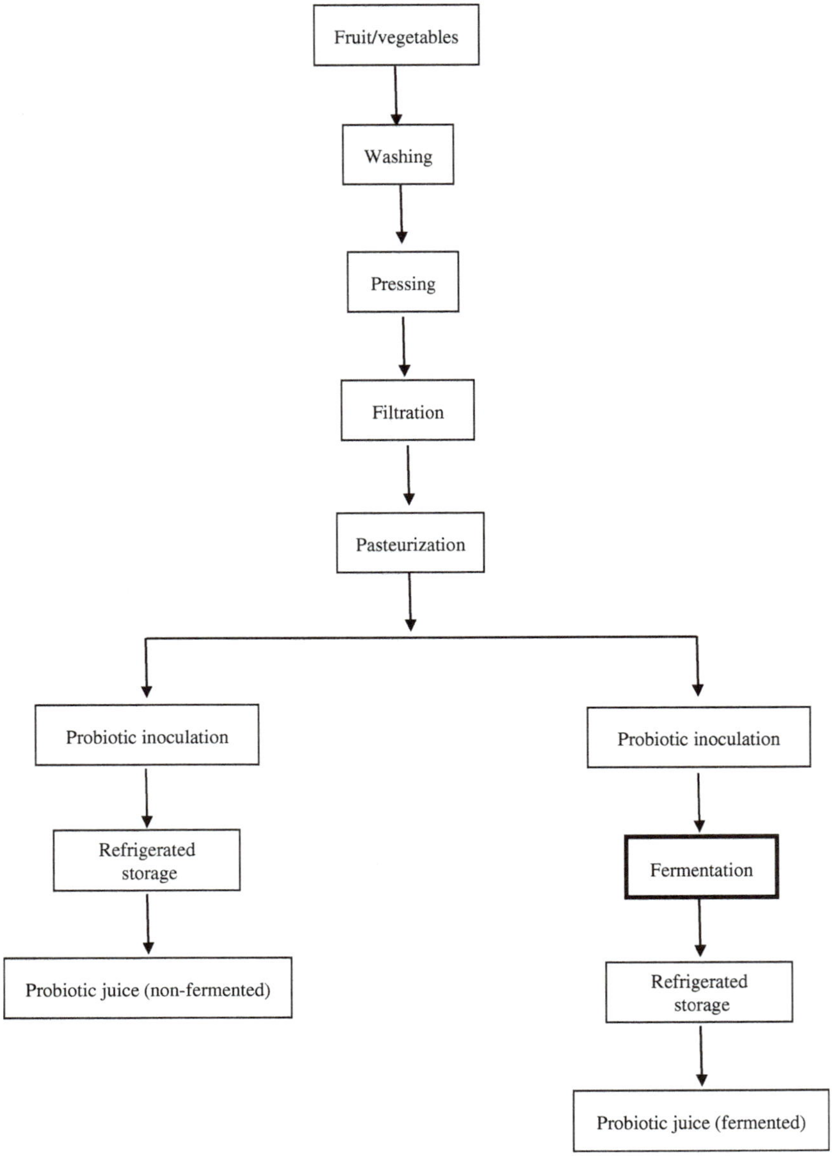

FIG. 7.6 Process flow diagram of the production of probiotic fermented and non-fermented fruit/vegetable juices. *Adapted from Grassin, C., & Coutel, Y. (2010). Enzymes in fruit and vegetable processing and juice extraction.* Enzymes in Food Technology, *236–263.*

follows: pH3.21–3.97, titratable acidity 0.38%–0.91% (w/w), total phenolics 368.8–2647.5 mg/L, and ethanol 0.4–6.0% (w/w). The lactic acid bacteria in the beverage are *L. paracasei subsp. paracasei, L. casei* subsp. *pseudoplantarum, L. brevis, L. pontis, L. acetotolerans, L. sanfransisco,* and L. *vaccinostercus* (Arici & Coskun, 2001).

Wine and malolactic fermentation

Wine as an alcoholic beverage is generally produced from a fermentation of grapes (*Vitis vinifera*). Non-grape based wines, such as rice and fruit wines (plum, cherry, pomegranate, currant, and elderberry), are also available. Traditionally, the substrate has been fermented by a yeast and lactic acid bacteria fermentation, with organisms originating from the grapes and/or winery apparatus. Yeasts of the genera *Kloeckera, Hansensiaspora, Candida, Pichia,* and *Hansenula* have been reported to be present in the early stages of fermentation with *S. cerevisiae* as the dominant species to complete the fermentation process (Fleet, Lafon-Lafourcade, & Ribéreau-Gayon, 1984). Alcohol is produced by the ability of the yeast to convert sugars to ethanol, carbon dioxide, and heat. The lactic acid bacteria involved in the wine-making process generally belong to the genera *Oenococcus, Pediococcus,* and *Lactobacillus. Oenococcus oeni* is the main species capable of malolactic fermentation (MLF) (García-Ruiz et al., 2014; Muller & Fugelsang, 1997). These bacteria are able to maintain growth during harsh conditions provided during the wine elaboration (high acid and ethanol content, poor nutrient availability, etc.) (Neeley, Phister, & Mills, 2005; Spano & Massa, 2006). High resistance, and their resemblance in both structural and functional properties with other conventional probiotic species, introduces them as potential probiotic candidates that are beneficial to human health. The probiotic characteristics of wine-derived lactic acid bacteria have been investigated for in-vitro immuno-modulatory activities (Foligné et al., 2010) and a measurable immuno-modulatory potential reported for *O. oeni.* The in-vivo consideration confirmed the lysozyme resistance of *Lactobacillus* and *Pediococcus* strains and their ability to survive at low pH values (pH1.8) and in the presence of bile salts (García-Ruiz et al., 2014).

Salgam

Salgam (*shalgam*) is a non-alcoholic fermented beverage, widely consumed with food, in Turkey and especially in the cities of Istanbul, Ankara, and Izmir. The main raw ingredients used in *salgam* production are black carrot (*Daucus carota* subsp. *sativus var. atrorubens* Alef), turnip (*Brassica rapa* L.), salt, sourdough, bulgur flour, and water (Erten, Tanguler, & Canbaş, 2008). Considering the presence of flour as the main raw ingredient, this product can also be categorized in the cereal-based beverage group. However, no standard methods exist for *salgam* production. It is traditionally produced in separate fermentation stages. The first fermentation stage is carried out with the aim of lactic acid bacteria and yeast enrichment. The mixture of bulgur flour 3% (*w*/w), salt 1%–2% (w/w), sourdough 0.2% (w/w), and water is fermented for 3–5 days at 25 °C. The extracted mixture obtained from the first fermentation is then mixed with chopped black carrot at 10%–20% (w/w), and turnip 1%–2% (w/w), and water. This mixture is left in a tank for a second fermentation of 3–10 days storage at 25 °C. This fermented juice is then removed from the vessel and marketed. The physicochemical characteristics of *salgam* are as follows: total solids 2.3–2.9% (w/w), protein 0.09–0.18% (w/w), ash 1.46–2.06% (w/w), salt 1.4–2.0% (w/w), titratable acidity 0.6–0.9% (w/w), lactic acid 0.5–0.8% (w/w), alcohol 0.1–0.6% (*v*/v), and total phenolic content 0.49–0.53% (w/w) (Canbas & Deryaoglu, 1993). Lactic acid bacteria are speculated to be one of the main microorganisms in *salgam* production with L. *plantarum, L. paracasei* subsp. *Paracasei,* and L. *brevis* as the predominant species. Despite the obvious impact of lactic acid bacteria in *salgam* preparation, there is currently no published information about their probiotic impact.

Kombucha

Kombucha, also known as *tea mushroom, tea fungus, tea kwaas,* or *Manchurian mushroom* (botanical name *Medusomyces gisevii*), is an alcoholic beverage originating from China and now widely consumed in Russia and Eastern Europe as an alternative beverage. It is produced by a tea fungus inoculation of black tea, sweetened with sucrose (Lončar, Djurić, Malbaša, Kolarov, & Klašnja, 2006). The amounts of raw ingredients used in kombucha preparation differ according to where it is produced. Please see Chapter 16 for additional details of *kombucha* production.

7.3.3 Regulatory and application of probiotic microorganisms in the Middle East

The regulatory prerequisite of probiotic microorganisms differs greatly according to their proposed use either as a drug or as a dietary supplement. Food products are preferred considering its effect to satisfy hunger or for hedonistic reasons (Meybodi et al., 2017). However, the viability of probiotic microorganisms in the product until the consumption date and via delivery through the gastrointestinal tract (efficiency), sensory properties of final product, and the cost-benefit outlook of the final products are all important parameters and should be considered in determining the customer's consumption patterns. The effectiveness of probiotic incorporation into food products is determined by their safety, the compatibility of the products ingredients and incorporated microorganisms with probiotics, and the viability of probiotics during food processing, packaging, and storage conditions. Despite difficulties in the formulation of probiotic incorporated beverages to maintain stability and viability, contemporary technological improvements will provide ways to offer new media and address growing consumer demand. In the selection of potential new probiotic strains to develop probiotic beverages, their safety and their potential effect on final products' sensory characteristics are of critical importance.

7.4 Conclusions

The Middle East is a region with wide food diversity, its market recently moving toward the increased production of functional beverages, especially probiotic types. Probiotic beverages in the market can be categorized based on the microorganisms involved, beneficial health effects, and the matrix. Considering the matrices of these beverages, there are two major groups: dairy- and non-dairy-based beverages. The beneficial health effects of probiotic beverages can be attributed to the nutraceutical content of their substrates, the potential health effects of the fermentation process, as well as the beneficial effects of probiotic loading. Probiotic participation can be obtained either directly (belonging to the natural flora) or indirectly (added furthermore with the aim of increasing nutrient content and beneficial health effects). Despite the commercial production of different probiotic beverages, traditional fermented types with their probiotic origins are also present. Future work should focus on the industrialization of native (ethnic) probiotic beverages and on the setting of regulations and standards, as well as producing defined probiotic beverages with specific health claims.

References

Ahmadi, E., Mohammadi, R., Hasanvand, S., Rouhi, M., Mortazavian, A. M., & Sarlak, Z. (2019). Effects of fermentative factors on biochemical, microbiological and sensory characteristics of probiotic Iranian fermented milk (Doogh). *Current Nutrition & Food Science, 15*(1), 40–47.

Ahvenainen, J., & Kuhanen, J. (1993). *Method for the fermentation of beer.* US Patent 5,273,762.

Aljefree, N., & Ahmed, F. (2015). Association between dietary pattern and risk of cardiovascular disease among adults in the Middle East and North Africa region: A systematic review. *Food & Nutrition Research, 59*(1), 27486. https://doi.org/10.3402/fnr.v59.27486.

Al-Otaibi, M. (2012). Isolation and identification of lactic acid bacteria and yeasts from Sameel milk: A Saudi traditional fermented milk. *International Journal of Dairy Science, 7*, 73–83.

Altay, F., Karbancıoglu-Güler, F., Daskaya-Dikmen, C., & Heperkan, D. (2013). A review on traditional Turkish fermented non-alcoholic beverages: Microbiota, fermentation process and quality characteristics. *International Journal of Food Microbiology, 167*(1), 44–56.

Anon. n.d. Available from https://www.alsafidanone.com/activia-laban.

Arici, M., & Coskun, F. (2001). Hardaliye: Fermented grape juice as a traditional Turkish beverage. *Food Microbiology, 18*(4), 417–421.

Arici, M., & Daglioglu, O. (2002). Boza: A lactic acid fermented cereal beverage as a traditional Turkish food. *Food Reviews International*, *18*(1), 39–48.

Ayar, A., & Burucu, H. (2013). Effect of whey fractions on microbial and physicochemical properties of probiotic ayran (drinkable yogurt). *International Food Research Journal*, *20*(3), 1409–1415.

Bagheri poor Fallah, N., SAM, M. F., Hosseini, H., Shahraz, F., & Bahadori Monfared, A. (2016). Identification of microorganisms in industrial Iranian Doogh. *Food Science and Technology*, *13*(57), 185–202.

Behera, S. S., Bal, P., Das, S., Panda, S. H., & Mohanty, N. (2018). Advances in microbial fermentation and fermented food for health. In S. K. Panda, & P. H. Shetty (Eds.), *Innovations in technologies for fermented food and beverage industries* (pp. 53–69). Cham: Springer International Publishing.

Behera, S. K., Panda, S. K., Kayitesi, E., & Mulaba-Bafubiandi, A. F. (2017). Kefir and Koumiss origin. In R. C. Ramesh, & D. Montet (Eds.), *Health benefits and current status of knowledge. Fermented foods—Part II: Technological interventions* (pp. 400–417). Baco Raton, FL: CRC Press. (Chapter 18).

Bellut, K., & Arendt, E. K. (2019). Chance and challenge: Non-Saccharomyces yeasts in nonalcoholic and low alcohol beer brewing—A review. *Journal of the American Society of Brewing Chemists*, *77*(2), 77–91.

Blandino, A., Al-Aseeri, M., Pandiella, S., Cantero, D., & Webb, C. (2003). Cereal-based fermented foods and beverages. *Food Research International*, *36*(6), 527–543.

Canbas, A., & Deryaoglu, A. (1993). A research on the processing techniques and characteristics of shalgam beverage. *Doga*, *17*, 119–129.

Capece, A., Romaniello, R., Pietrafesa, A., Siesto, G., Pietrafesa, R., Zambuto, M. , et al. (2018). Use of *Saccharomyces cerevisiae* var. boulardii in co-fermentations with S. cerevisiae for the production of craft beers with potential healthy value-added. *International Journal of Food Microbiology*, *284*, 22–30.

Centeno, J. A., & Carballo, J. (2014). *Starter and adjunct microbial cultures used in the manufacture of fermented and/or cured or ripened meat and dairy products. Beneficial microbes in fermented and functional foods*: (pp. 35–54). New York: CRC Press.

Charalampopoulos, D., Wang, R., Pandiella, S., & Webb, C. (2002). Application of cereals and cereal components in functional foods: A review. *International Journal of Food Microbiology*, *79*(1–2), 131–141.

Codex alimentarius (FAO) (2018). *Regional standard for doogh. CXS 332R-2018. (2018).* http://www.fao.org/fao-who-codexalimentarius/committees/codex-regions/ccne/regional-standards/en/.

Cogulu, D., Topaloglu-Ak, A., Caglar, E., Sandalli, N., Karagozlu, C., Ersin, N. , et al. (2010). Potential effects of a multistrain probiotic-kefir on salivary Streptococcus mutans and Lactobacillus spp. *Journal of Dental Sciences*, *5*(3), 144–149.

Corbo, M. R., Bevilacqua, A., Petruzzi, L., Casanova, F. P., & Sinigaglia, M. (2014). Functional beverages: The emerging side of functional foods: Commercial trends, research, and health implications. *Comprehensive Reviews in Food Science and Food Safety*, *13*(6), 1192–1206.

Del Piano, M., Morelli, L., Strozzi, G., Allesina, S., Barba, M., Deidda, F. , et al. (2006). Probiotics: From research to consumer. *Digestive and Liver Disease*, *38*, 248–255.

Dhewa, T., Mishra, V., Kumar, N., & Sangu, K. (2015). *Koumiss: The nutritional and therapeutic values. Fermented foods and beverages series. Fermented milk and dairy products*: (pp. 483–494). *2015*. CRC Press.

Dlusskaya, E., Jänsch, A., Schwab, C., & Gänzle, M. G. (2008). Microbial and chemical analysis of a kvass fermentation. *European Food Research and Technology*, *227*(1), 261–266.

Doyle, M. P., Steenson, L. R., & Meng, J. (2013). Bacteria in food and beverage production. In E. Rosenberg, D. L. EF, S. Lory, E. Stackebrandt, & F. Thompson (Eds.), *The prokaryotes:*

Applied bacteriology and biotechnology (pp. 241–256). Berlin, Heidelberg: Springer Berlin Heidelberg.

Erten, H., Tanguler, H., & Canbaş, A. (2008). A traditional Turkish lactic acid fermented beverage: Shalgam (Salgam). *Food Reviews International*, *24*(3), 352–359.

Farrag, N. S., Cheskin, L. J., & Farag, M. K. (2017). A systematic review of childhood obesity in the Middle East and North Africa (MENA) region: prevalence and risk factors meta-analysis. *Advances in Pediatric Research. 4*, https://doi.org/10.12715/apr.2017.4.8.

Fijan, S. (2014). Microorganisms with claimed probiotic properties: An overview of recent literature. *International Journal of Environmental Research and Public Health*, *11*(5), 4745–4767.

Fleet, G., Lafon-Lafourcade, S., & Ribéreau-Gayon, P. (1984). Evolution of yeasts and lactic acid bacteria during fermentation and storage of Bordeaux wines. *Applied and Environmental Microbiology*, *48*(5), 1034–1038.

Foligné, B., Dewulf, J., Breton, J., Claisse, O., Lonvaud-Funel, A., & Pot, B. (2010). Probiotic properties of non-conventional lactic acid bacteria: Immunomodulation by Oenococcus oeni. *International Journal of Food Microbiology*, *140*(2–3), 136–145.

García-Ruiz, A., de Llano, D. G., Esteban-Fernández, A., Requena, T., Bartolomé, B., & Moreno-Arribas, M. V. (2014). Assessment of probiotic properties in lactic acid bacteria isolated from wine. *Food Microbiology*, *44*, 220–225.

Gassem, M. (2002). A microbiological study of Sobia: A fermented beverage in the Western province of Saudi Arabia. *World Journal of Microbiology and Biotechnology*, *18*(3), 173–177.

Gassem, M. A. A. (2003). Physico-chemical properties of sobia: A traditional fermented beverage in western province of Saudi Arabia. *Ecology of Food and Nutrition*, *42*(1), 25–35.

German, J. B., Gibson, R. A., Krauss, R. M., Nestel, P., Lamarche, B., Van Staveren, W. A. , et al. (2009). A reappraisal of the impact of dairy foods and milk fat on cardiovascular disease risk. *European Journal of Nutrition*, *48*(4), 191–203.

Gotcheva, V., Pandiella, S. S., Angelov, A., Roshkova, Z. G., & Webb, C. (2000). Microflora identification of the Bulgarian cereal-based fermented beverage boza. *Process Biochemistry*, *36*(1–2), 127–130.

Guzel-Seydim, Z., Kok-Tas, T., Ertekin-Filiz, B., & Seydim, A. (2011). Effect of different growth conditions on biomass increase in kefir grains. *Journal of Dairy Science*, *94*(3), 1239–1242.

Hotez, P. J., Savioli, L., & Fenwick, A. (2012). Neglected tropical diseases of the Middle East and North Africa: Review of their prevalence, distribution, and opportunities for control. *PLoS Neglected Tropical Diseases. 6*(2) e1475 https://doi.org/10.1371/journal.pntd.0001475.

ISIRI (2008a). *Doogh–Specifications ans test method. 2453. (2008a).* http://ssu.ac.ir/cms/fileadmin/user_upload/Mtahghighat/tfood/file/aeen_nameh_meli/dough.pdf.

ISIRI (2008b). *Doogh-code of practice and production. 10528. (2008b).* http://www.isiri.gov.ir/portal/files/std/10528.PDF.

Ivanovska, T. P., Zhivikj, Z., Bogdanovska, L., Mladenovska, K., & Petrushevska-Tozi, L. (2018). Application of Lactobacillus casei 01 and oligofructose-enriched inulin in ayran. *Macedonian Journal of Chemistry and Chemical Engineering*, *37*(1), 43–52.

Kandylis, P., Pissaridi, K., Bekatorou, A., Kanellaki, M., & Koutinas, A. A. (2016). Dairy and non-dairy probiotic beverages. *Current Opinion in Food Science*, *7*, 58–63.

Keryan, A., Bazukyan, I., & Trchounian, A. (2017). Lactobacilli isolated from the Armenian fermented milk product matsoun: Growth properties, antibacterial and proteolytic activity and their dependence on pH. *International Journal of Dairy Technology*, *70*(3), 389–398.

Koksoy, A., & Kilic, M. (2004). Use of hydrocolloids in textural stabilization of a yoghurt drink, ayran. *Food Hydrocolloids*, *18*(4), 593–600.

Kuliev, K. (1959). Utilisation of camel's milk. *Molochnaya Promyshlennost*, *2*, .

Kuş, H. (2010). *Production of probiotic buttermilk using probiotic bacteria of human origin.* Namık Kemal University.

Liu, S.-Q., & Tsao, M. (2010). Enhancing stability of lactic acid bacteria and probiotics by Williopsis saturnus var. saturnus in fermented milks. *Nutrition & Food Science, 40*(3), 314–322.

Lončar, E., Djurić, M., Malbaša, R., Kolarov, L., & Klašnja, M. (2006). Influence of working conditions upon kombucha conducted fermentation of black tea. *Food and Bioproducts Processing, 84*(3), 186–192.

Makinen, K., Berger, B., Bel-Rhlid, R., & Ananta, E. (2012). Science and technology for the mastership of probiotic applications in food products. *Journal of Biotechnology, 162*(4), 356–365.

Malganji, S., Sohrabvandi, S., Jahadi, M., Nematollahi, A., & Sarmadi, B. (2016). Effect of refrigerated storage on sensory properties and viability of probiotic in grape drink. *Applied Food Biotechnology, 3*(1), 59–62.

Marsh, A. J., Hill, C., Ross, R. P., & Cotter, P. D. (2014). Fermented beverages with health-promoting potential: Past and future perspectives. *Trends in Food Science & Technology, 38*(2), 113–124.

Meybodi, N. M., Mortazavian, A. M., da Cruz, A. G., & Mohammadi, R. (2017). Probiotic supplements and food products: Comparison for different targets. *Applied Food Biotechnology, 4*(3), 123–132.

Mortazavian, A., Ehsani, M., Azizi, A., Razavi, S., Mousavi, S., Sohrabvandi, S. , et al. (2008). Viability of calcium-alginate-microencapsulated probiotic bacteria in Iranian yogurt drink (Doogh) during refrigerated storage and under simulated gastrointestinal conditions. *Australian Journal of Dairy Technology, 63*(1), 25–30.

Mortazavian, A., Khosrokhavar, R., Rastegar, H., & Mortazaei, G. (2010). Effects of dry matter standardization order on biochemical and microbiological characteristics of freshly made probiotic Doogh (Iranian fermented milk drink). *Italian Journal of Food Science, 22*(1), 98–104.

Mortazavian, A. M., Mohammadi, R., & Sohrabvandi, S. (2012). *Delivery of probiotic microorganisms into gastrointestinal tract by food products. New advances in the basic and clinical gastroenterology*: (pp. 121–146). InTech.

Muller, C., & Fugelsang, K. (1997). Red wine but not white: The importance of fully characterizing wines used in health studies. *The American Journal of Clinical Nutrition, 66*(2), 447. https://doi.org/10.1093/ajcn/66.2.447.

Nachel, M., & Ettlinger, S. (2012). *Beer for dummies: Wiley brand-making everything easier.*

National Research Council (1992). *Moroccan traditional fermented dairy products*: (pp. 75–80). By Panel on the Applications of Biotechnology to Traditional Fermented Foods, Office of International Affairs, Policy and Global Affairs, National Research Council.. (1992). *https://books.google.com/books?hl=en&lr=&id=x3khQLIr8IwC&oi=fnd&pg=PA75&dq=Moroccan+Traditional+Fermented+Dairy+Products&ots=KRgMqe7uhR&sig=VX3cShbkHUfbUl1iiIhy67K7U#v=onepage&q=Moroccan%20Traditional%20Fermented%20Dairy%20Products&f=false.*

Neeley, E. T., Phister, T. G., & Mills, D. A. (2005). Differential real-time PCR assay for enumeration of lactic acid bacteria in wine. *Applied and Environmental Microbiology, 71*(12), 8954–8957.

Nickolas S, Stewart A. Process for addition of a nutraceutical to a beverage. U.S. Patent No. 6,855,358. Washington, DC: U.S. Patent and Trademark Office.

Nuraeni, E., Arief, I., & Soenarno, M. (2014). Characteristics of probiotic koumiss from goat milk with addition of Roselle extract (Hibiscus sabdariffa Linn). *Journal of the Indonesian Tropical Animal Agriculture, 39*(2), 117–125.

Ozcan, T., Yilmaz-Ersan, L., Akpinar-Bayizit, A., Delikanli, B., & Barat, A. (2015). Survival of Lactobacillus spp. in fruit based fermented dairy beverages. *International Journal of Food Engineering, 1*(1), 44–49.

Paquin, P. (2009). *Functional and speciality beverage technology.* Elsevier.

Pereira, A. L. F., Maciel, T. C., & Rodrigues, S. (2011). Probiotic beverage from cashew apple juice fermented with *Lactobacillus casei*. *Food Research International*, *44*(5), 1276–1283.

Perry, C. (1997). *The horseback kitchen of Central Asia. Food on the move. In: Proceedings of the Oxford symposium on food and cookery, 1996*, Editor Harlan Walker(1997). *https://archive.org/stream/bub_gb_uYqTiD7SbcQC/bub_gb_uYqTiD7SbcQC_djvu.txt*.

Pimentel, T. C., Madrona, G. S., & Prudencio, S. H. (2015). Probiotic clarified apple juice with oligofructose or sucralose as sugar substitutes: Sensory profile and acceptability. *LWT - Food Science and Technology*, *62*(1, Part 2), 838–846.

Praagman, J., Dalmeijer, G. W., van der Schouw, Y. T., Soedamah-Muthu, S. S., Verschuren, W. M., Bueno-de-Mesquita, H. B. , et al. (2015). The relationship between fermented food intake and mortality risk in the European prospective investigation into cancer and nutrition-Netherlands cohort. *British Journal of Nutrition*, *113*(3), 498–506.

Rafiq, S., Sharma, V., Nazir, A., Rashid, R., & Sofi, S. (2016). Development of probiotic carrot juice. *Journal of Nutrition & Food Sciences*, *6*(534), 2.

Rahman, I. E. A., Dirar, H. A., & Osman, M. A. (2009). Microbiological and biochemical changes and sensory evaluation of camel milk fermented by selected bacterial starter cultures. *African Journal of Food Science*, *3*(12), 398–405.

Rahman, N., Xiaohong, C., Meiqin, F., & Mingsheng, D. (2009). Characterization of the dominant microflora in naturally fermented camel milk shubat. *World Journal of Microbiology and Biotechnology*, *25*(11), 1941–1946.

Rahmdar, S. R., Rahmati Roudsari, M., Javanmard, A., Mortazavian, A. M., & Sohrabvandi, S. (2013). The impact of inoculation rate and order on physicochemical, microstructural and sensory attributes of probiotic doogh. *Iranian Journal of Pharmaceutical Research*, *12*(4), 917–924.

Roberfroid, M. B. (2002). Functional foods: Concepts and application to inulin and oligofructose. *British Journal of Nutrition*, *87*(S2), S139–S143.

Sadaghdar, Y., Mortazavian, A. M., & Ehsani, M. R. (2012). Survival and activity of 5 probiotic lactobacilli strains in 2 types of flavored fermented milk. *Food Science and Biotechnology*, *21*(1), 151–157.

Samet-Bali, O., Felfoul, I., Lajnaf, R., Attia, H., & Ayadi, M. (2017). Enumeration and identification of microflora in" Leben ', a traditional Tunisian dairy beverage. *International Food Research Journal*, *24*(3), 927–932.

Sayevand, H. R., Bakhtiary, F., Pointner, A., Remely, M., Hippe, B., Hosseini, H. , et al. (2018). Bacterial diversity in traditional Doogh in comparison to industrial Doogh. *Current Microbiology*, *75*(4), 386–393.

Shah, N. P. (2007). Functional cultures and health benefits. *International Dairy Journal*, *17*(11), 1262–1277.

Shori, A. B. (2012). Comparative study of chemical composition, isolation and identification of micro-flora in traditional fermented camel milk products: Gariss, Suusac, and Shubat. *Journal of the Saudi Society of Agricultural Sciences*, *11*(2), 79–88.

Shori, A. B. (2016). Influence of food matrix on the viability of probiotic bacteria: A review based on dairy and non-dairy beverages. *Food Bioscience*, *13*, 1–8.

Soccol, C., De Dea, J., Yamaguishi, C., Spier, M., de Souza, L., & Soccol, V. (2012). Probiotic nondairy beverages. In *Handbook of plant-based fermented food and beverage technology* (pp. 707–728). (second ed.). CRC Press.

Sohrabvandi, S., Mortazavian, A., & Rezaei, K. (2011). Advanced analytical methods for the analysis of chemical and microbiological properties of beer. *Journal of Food and Drug Analysis*, *19*(2), 202–222.

Sohrabvandi, S., Mousavi, S. M., Razavi, S. H., Mortazavian, A. M., & Rezaei, K. (2010). Alcohol-free beer: Methods of production, sensorial defects, and healthful effects. *Food Reviews International*, *26*(4), 335–352.

Sohrabvandi, S., Razavi, S. H., Mousavi, S. M., & Mortazavian, A. M. (2010). Viability of probiotic bacteria in low alcohol-and non-alcoholic beer during refrigerated storage. *Philippine Agricultural Scientist*, *93*(1), 24–28.

Spano, G., & Massa, S. (2006). Environmental stress response in wine lactic acid bacteria: Beyond Bacillus subtilis. *Critical Reviews in Microbiology*, *32*(2), 77–86.

Stack, H. M., Kearney, N., Stanton, C., Fitzgerald, G. F., & Ross, R. P. (2010). Association of beta-glucan endogenous production with increased stress tolerance of intestinal lactobacilli. *Applied and Environmental Microbiology*, *76*(2), 500–507.

Suharja, A. A., Henriksson, A., & Liu, S. Q. (2014). Impact of Saccharomyces cerevisiae on viability of probiotic Lactobacillus rhamnosus in fermented milk under ambient conditions. *Journal of Food Processing and Preservation*, *38*(1), 326–337.

Swain, M. R., Anandharaj, M., Ray, R. C., & Parveen Rani, R. (2014). Fermented fruits and vegetables of Asia: A potential source of probiotics. *Biotechnology Research International*,250424 19 pages(2014). https://doi.org/10.1155/2014/250424.

Tamime, A. Y. (2008). *Fermented milks*. John Wiley & Sons.

Tamime, A., Saarela, M., Sondergaard, A. K., Mistry, V., & Shah, N. (2005). Production and maintenance of viability of probiotic microorganisms in dairy products. *Probiotic Dairy Products*, 39–72.

Taş, T., & Güzel-Seydim, Z. (2010). Determination of effects of using fat replacers and probiotic on ayran quality. *GIDA-Journal of Food*, *35*(2), 105–111.

Temiz, H., & Kezer, G. (2014). Effects of fat replacers on physicochemical, microbial and sensorial properties of kefir made using mixture of cow and goat's milk. *Journal of Food Processing and Preservation*, *39*(6), 1421–1430.

Todorov, S., Botes, M., Guigas, C., Schillinger, U., Wiid, I., Wachsman, M. , et al. (2008). Boza, a natural source of probiotic lactic acid bacteria. *Journal of Applied Microbiology*, *104*(2), 465–477.

Tornuk, F., Ozturk, I., Karaman, S., Sagdic, O., & Yetim, H. (2014). Rheological and some physicochemical properties of probiotic boza beverage fermented with Lactobacillus casei Shirota: Application of principal component analysis for the characterisation. *Quality Assurance & Safety of Crops and Food*, *6*(2), 237–247.

Turkish Food Codex (2009). *Fermented milk products*. Turkey: Ministry of Food, Agriculture and Livestock.(2009). https://members.wto.org/crnattachments/2016/SPS/TUR/16_4756_00_e.pdf.

Umer, K. S. (2014). Probiotics in dairy foods: A review. *Nutrition & Food Science*, *44*(1), 71–88.

Uniacke-Lowe, T., Huppertz, T., & Fox, P. F. (2010). Equine milk proteins: Chemistry, structure and nutritional significance. *International Dairy Journal*, *20*(9), 609–629.

Vander Wal, J., McBurney, M. I., Cho, S., & Dhurandhar, N. V. (2007). Ready-to-eat cereal products as meal replacements for weight loss. *International Journal of Food Sciences and Nutrition*, *58*(5), 331–340.

Wilson, T., & Temple, N. J. (2016). *Beverage impacts on health and nutrition*. New York, NY: Human Press.

CHAPTER

8

Current trends and opportunities of plant-based non-alcoholic probiotic beverages: A European and African perspective

Juliana Mandha[a,b], Habtu Shumoy[a], Athanasia O. Matemu[b], and Katleen Raes[a]

[a]Ghent University Campus Kortrijk, Kortrijk, West Flanders, Belgium, [b]Nelson Mandela African Institution of Science and Technology, Arusha, Tanzania

8.1 Introduction

Probiotics are defined as "live microorganisms which, when administered in adequate amounts, confer a health benefit on the host" (FAO/WHO, 2002). Probiotic beverages exert beneficial effects and/or improve body functions beyond the traditional nutritional effects (Perricone, Bevilacqua, Altieri, Sinigaglia, & Corbo, 2015). Probiotics are well known to improve human gut health by resisting the colonization of pathogenic microorganisms and synthesizing nutrients such as B vitamins (Lee, Song, Do Nam, & Lee, 2018). Moreover, they are also known to prevent and/or treat allergies, possess anti-mutagenic effects, lower serum cholesterol, strengthen the immunity, control inflammatory bowel diseases, control irritable bowel syndrome, reduce risk of colon cancer, and suppress endogenous or exogenous pathogens that cause diarrhea (Bajaj, Claes, & Lebeer, 2015; Parvez, Malik, Ah Kang, & Kim, 2006).

Dairy products, such as yoghurt and cheese, have been the conventional vehicles of probiotics (Marsh, Hill, Ross, & Cotter, 2014; Shori, 2016). However, animal products are associated with various health-related problems

Probiotic Beverages
https://doi.org/10.1016/B978-0-12-818588-9.00013-9

such as high cholesterol levels that increase risk of cardiovascular diseases, milk proteins that cause allergic reactions, and about 75% of the world population are lactose intolerant, manifesting symptoms, such as gas/flatulence, bloating, abdominal pain, or diarrhea on dairy consumption (De Vrese, Stegelmann, Richter, Fenselau, & Laue, 2001; Granato, Branco, Nazzaro, Faria, & Cruz, 2010; Perricone et al., 2015). Hence, the number of vegetarians/veganists is growing. Windows of opportunities have been opened for plant-based foods as ideal choices for delivering probiotics and the consumer demand for new inspired product innovations has increased. A recent Lancet report calls upon a global shift toward a planetary health diet that largely consists of vegetables, fruits, whole grains, legumes, nuts, and unsaturated oil, in order to meet the United Nations Sustainable Development Goals (SDGs) (Willett et al., 2019).

Fruits, vegetables, and cereals are rich sources of carbohydrates, fibers, proteins, essential minerals and vitamins (Bhat, Gupta, Andrabi, & Bajaj, 2017). Recent studies have demonstrated their suitability as probiotic substrates (Fayemi, Taylor, & Buys, 2017; Jaiswal & Abu-Ghannam, 2013; Kort et al., 2015; Lorusso, Coda, Montemurro, & Rizzello, 2018; Perricone, Corbo, Sinigaglia, Speranza, & Bevilacqua, 2014) and various probiotic beverages are currently on the market. However, different dynamics in Europe and Africa affect their production, regulation, and marketing. Africa has a long history of using traditionally fermented foods, but the use of beneficial microorganisms has received little attention, whereas in Europe, extensive research and development have been performed but the strict regulations hinder marketing of plant-based probiotic beverages. This chapter aims to highlight the current trends of plant-based probiotic beverages. Specifically, this article will highlight the recently developed and commercialized non-alcoholic plant-based probiotic beverages in Europe and Africa from 2010 to 2019.

8.2 Plant-based non-alcoholic beverages in Europe

Although probiotics have appeared as part of the human diet as starter cultures in fermented foods, the term functional food was first introduced in the 21st century (1980) in Japan under the regulatory approval of Foods for Specified Health Use (FOSHU) (Sanders, 1998). In the European region, the concept of functional foods as a whole was first explored in the 1990s. The European Commission formed a project called the "Functional Food Science in Europe (FuFoSE)" to use an evidence-based approach to explore the concept (Corbo, Bevilacqua, Petruzzi, Casanova, & Sinigaglia, 2014). The outcome of this project was that foods can be regarded as functional if they can be satisfactorily demonstrated to affect beneficially one or more target functions in the body, beyond adequate nutritional effects, in a way relevant to an improved state of health and well-being and/or reduction of risk of disease"(Contor, 2001).

European Food Safety Authority (EFSA) (2005) scientific committee created a system known as Qualified Presumption of Safety (QPS), which provides prior knowledge and ensures adequate safety assessment of microorganisms used in food (EFSA, 2005). The QPS is similar to the concept of Generally Recognized As Safe (GRAS) used by the Food and Drug Authority (FDA) in the United States of America (USA) (U.S. Food & Drug Administration FDA, 2019), whereby microorganisms that are assigned the QPS status are safe and can be used in food (Salvetti & Toole, 2017). Probiotic strains may be assigned QPS status after review. Since 2007, the number of scientific research articles and innovations on probiotic beverages has increased reflecting the growing attention to this area. Currently, the European Union (EU) has neither EU-wide legal framework defining probiotics nor is there a harmonized EU legal framework with guidelines to consider a strain as probiotic (International Probiotics Association (IPA) Europe, 2016).

Health and nutritional claims enable the transfer of significant and relevant information from producers to consumers facilitating marketing in the long run. A nutrition claim implies or suggests that a food has beneficial properties, whereas a health claim implies or suggests that there is a relationship between a food or its components and health (Verhagen, Vos, Francl, Heinonen, & Van Loveren, 2012). The EU established the Nutrition and Health Claims Regulation (The European Parliament and Council of the European Union (EU), 2006) to ensure allegations made are precise, clear, and rooted in scientific evidence. Currently, to the best of our knowledge, there are no health claims approved in the EU, as the EFSA has not yet permitted the use of the term "probiotics" on any of the products available on the EU market (Reid, 2016). But different member states in the EU have different policies for the regulation of nutritional health claims (Van & Brouns, 2015). This variance has slowed down the rate of development of probiotic beverages in the region.

Nevertheless, the probiotics market was valued at 35.95 billion USD worldwide in 2015 and is projected to increase to 65.87 billion USD by the end of 2024 and probiotic foods and beverages are the main significant segment in the overall probiotics market (Grand View Research, 2019). The growth rate of probiotic beverages in Europe is around 20% per year (Zielinska & Kolozyn-Krajewska, 2018) and the market is driven by consumer awareness of linkages between probiotics and health, changing lifestyles and need for convenience foods and the rising costs of health care (Grand View Research, 2019). Continuous growth is expected in this area as new innovations are being developed to meet consumer demands.

The European industry landscape has several companies, such as Chr. Hansen, Danisco A/S, Nestle, Lesaffre Human Care, Biosearch Life,

Bifodan Inc., and Probi AB that commercially provide probiotic strains (Table 8.1), thereby enabling research and development. The majority of probiotics commercially used in foods belong to the genera of *Lactobacillus* and *Bifidobacterium* (Prasad, Gill, Smart, & Gopal, 1999), which are safe and able to dominate the human intestine. Other species, such as *Streptococcus thermophilus, Saccharomyces cerevisiae var. boulardii, Pediococcus pentosaceus* and *Leuconostoc mesenteroides* have also been used as probiotic microorganisms. These strains are obtained from natural niches ranging from fermented foods, human milk, and human gastrointestinal tracts, to vegetable and fruit by-products. Probiotics used in food must demonstrate the ability to survive in the human gastrointestinal tract

TABLE 8.1 Commercial probiotic strains produced in Europe

Company	Strains
Chr. Hansen	*L. acidophilus* LA-5, *L. reuteri* RC-14 *L. rhamnosus* GR-1, *B. animalis subsp. lactis* Bb12 *L. rhamnosus* LGG, *L. casei* 431 *L.* F-19, *L. fermentum* PCC *Streptococcus thermophilus* TH-4
Danisco A/S	*B. bifidum* Bb-06, Bb-02, *B. breve* Bb-03 *B. lactis* Bi-07, Bl-04, Bb-02, *B. longum* Bl-05 *B. longum* subsp. infantis Bi-2 6, *B. lactis* HN019 *L. acidophilus* L a-14, *L. brevis* Lbr-35 *L. bulgaricus* Lb-87, *L. casei* L c-11 *L. fermentum* S B S -1, *L. gasseri* Lg-36 *L. paracasei* Lpc-37, *L. plantarum* L p -115 *L. reuteri* 1E1, *L. rhamnosus* (ATCC 53103) GG, Lr-32 *L. salivarius* Ls-33, *Lactococcus lactis* L l-23 *S. thermophilus* St-21, *L. rhamnosus* HN001 *L. acidophilus* NCFM
Nestle	*L. reuteri* SD2112
Probi AB	*L. plantarum* 299v, *L. plantarum* HEAL9, HEAL19 *L. paracasei* 8700:2
Lesaffre Human Care	*S. cerevisiae* CNCM I-3856, *S. cerevisiae var. boulardii* CNCM I-3799 *B. subtilis* CNCM I-2745 *L. rhamnosus* GG
Biosearch Life	*L. fermentum* CECT5716, *L. salivarius* CECT5713 HM6 *L. coryniformis* CECT5711 K8
Bifodan Inc	*B. animalis, subsp. lactis* BIFOLAC 12, *B. longum* BIFOLAC 536 *L. acidophilus* BIFOLAC 5, *L. rhamnosus* BIFOLAC GG *L. rhamnosus* BIFOLAC PB01, *L. gasseri* BIFOLAC EB01 *L. curvatus* BIFOLAC EB10

Adapted from Tripathi, M. K., & Giri, S. K. (2014). Probiotic functional foods: Survival of probiotics during processing and storage. Journal of Functional Foods, *9(1), 225–241. https://doi.org/10.1016/j.jff.2014.04.030.*

by being tolerant to harsh acidic environments, bile, digestive enzymes, adhere to mucosal lining, and inhibit pathogenic bacteria (FAO/WHO, 2002). Recent studies have demonstrated the suitability of cereals, vegetables, and fruits as substrates for probiotics (Perricone et al., 2014; Salmerón, Thomas, & Pandiella, 2015). Plant-based probiotic beverages currently commercialized in the EU market include: Yosa, Proviva, Gelifus, Biola, Fiscus, Jovita Probiotisch, Velle, Biola, and Rela.

8.2.1 Cereal-based beverages

Wheat and rye are the most common cereals consumed in Europe, mainly as sourdough-based food products. Cereals have been traditionally fermented (spontaneously) to produce beverages, such as *boza* and *kvass,* which have probiotic properties (Blandino, Al-Aseeri, Pandiella, Cantero, & Webb, 2003). *Boza* is a sour tasting beverage common in the Balkan Peninsula, Turkey, and Caucasus. It is produced by fermentation of a slurry mixture of pulses and maize, oats, wheat, bulgur, millet, chickpea, or rice and uses a combination of yeast (*S. cerevisiae*) and lactic acid bacteria (*Leu. mesenteroides* and *Lactobacillus spp.*) (Gotcheva, Pandiella, Angelov, Roshkova, & Webb, 2001; Todorov et al., 2008). *Kvass* is another fermented non-alcoholic beverage consumed in Eastern Europe (Dlusskaya, Jänsch, Schwab, & Gänzle, 2008). *Leuconostoc mesenteroides, Lactobacillus casei,* and *S. cerevisiae* are the most dominant probiotics in the fermentation of *Kvass,* which contains rye and barley as raw materials (Dlusskaya et al., 2008). Although, use of specific starter cultures that impart sustainable nutritional and sensory quality is a preferred alternative, the prevailing fermentation of traditionally fermented beverages is initiated by either back slopping or occurs spontaneously.

Several studies have investigated the potential of cereals as substrates for probiotics (Table 8.2). Gelatinized emmer flour (30% (wt/wt)), an ancient wheat cereal harbored autochthonous *Lactobacillus rhamnosus* at a cell density > 8 log CFU/mL during cold storage (4°C) for 30 days (Coda et al., 2011). Charalampopoulos and Pandiella (2010) demonstrated growth of human-derived *Lactobacillus plantarum* (initial concentration 7 log CFU/mL) in sterile wheat, barley, and malt slurry extracts and the germinated cereals (malt) reported higher cell counts (9.5–10.3 log CFU/mL) than their non-germinated counterparts (8.2–9.6 log CFU/mL) upon incubation at 37°C for 24 h. Similarly, single cultures of *Lactobacillus acidophilus, L. plantarum,* and *Lactobacillus reuteri* increased from 7 to 7.73–8.20 log CFU/mL in starch free oat, barley and malt water suspensions (5% w/w), and the highest probiotic (*L. reuteri*) growth (8.20 log CFU/mL) was registered in a malt beverage after fermentation at 37°C for 10 h (Salmerón et al., 2015). During germination, hormones are produced that stimulate

TABLE 8.2 Overview of plant-based probiotic beverages studied in Europe

Beverage	Probiotic strain	Reference
Cereal-based beverages		
Malt, wheat, and barley extracts	*L. plantarum* NCIMB 8826	Charalampopoulos and Pandiella (2010)
Emmer beverages	*L. rhamnosus* SP1	Coda, Rizzello, Trani, and Gobbetti (2011)
Oat flakes beverage	*L. plantarum* LP09	Luana et al. (2014)
Oats, barley, and malt beverages	*L. plantarum* NCIMB 8826, *L. acidophilus* NCIMB 8821, *L. reuteri* NCIMB 11951	Salmerón, Thomas, and Pandiella (2014) and Salmerón et al. (2015)
Oats and fruit beverage	*S. thermophiles* TKM3 KKP 2030p	Goncerzewicz, Misiewicz, Owczarek, Jasińska, and Skąpska (2016)
Quinoa based beverage	*L. plantarum* Q823	Vera-Pingitore et al. (2016)
Oat based beverage	*L. plantarum* UFG 121	Russo et al. (2017)
Quinoa beverages	*L. rhamnosus* SP1, *W. confusa* DSM 20194 *L. plantarum* T6B10	Lorusso et al. (2018)
Vegetable- and legume-based beverages		
Cabbage juice	*L. plantarum* ATCC 8014, *L. rhamnosus* ATCC 9595, *L. brevis* ATCC 8287	Jaiswal and Abu-Ghannam (2013)
Carrot juice, tomato juice,	*L. plantarum*	Filannino et al. (2014)
Carrot juice	*L. casei* 01	Petreska-Ivanovska et al. (2014)
Blend of beetroot, carrot and celery, mixed with honey	*L. acidophilus* LA-5, *L. casei* 431 *S. boulardii*	Profir, Neagu, and Camelia (2015)
Blend of carrot juice and orange juice	*L. plantarum* CECT 220 (LP)	Valero-Cases and Frutos (2017)
Tomato juice	*L. plantarum* DSM20205 (ATCC 8014)	Valero-Cases et al. (2017)
Fruit-based beverages		
Orange, grapefruit, blackcurrant, pineapple, pomegranate and strawberry juices	*B. longum* NCIMB 8809	Nualkaekul, Salmeron, and Charalampopoulos (2011)

TABLE 8.2 Overview of plant-based probiotic beverages studied in Europe—cont'd

Beverage	Probiotic strain	Reference
Peach and orange juices	*L. paracasei* L26	Rodrigues et al. (2012)
Pomegranate fruit juice	*L. plantarum* C2, POM1 or LP09	Filannino et al. (2013)
Green apple, pineapple, orange juices, and red fruit juice	*L. reuteri DSM* 20016	Perricone et al. (2014)
Apple juice	*L. plantarum* PCS 26	Dimitrovski, Velickova, Langerholc, and Winkelhausen (2015)
Apricot fruit juice	*B. lactis* Bb-12, *B. longum* Bb-46 *L. casei* 01, *L. acidophilus* La-5	Mai, Dam, Bujna, and Annama (2018)
Cornelian cherry	*L. plantarum ATCC 14917*	Mantzourani et al. (2018)

the release of enzymes, such as β-amylases, α-amylases, dextrinases, proteases, and peptidases, which break down starch and proteins increasing the concentration of fermentable sugars and nitrogenous compounds (Salmerón et al., 2014).

However, about 1% of the European population have restricted their diets to gluten-free foods due to celiac disease and/or an allergy (White, Bannerman, & Gillett, 2016). There is a niche market for gluten-free probiotic beverages from oats, corn, sorghum, teff, millet, and pseudo-cereals; amaranth, buckwheat, and quinoa. A quinoa-based beverage favored the growth of *L. plantarum* to 10.4 log CFU/mL after fermentation at 30°C for 8h and this cell concentration remained constant during storage (4°C) for 7 days (Vera-Pingitore et al., 2016). In another study, a quinoa suspension (20-30% (w/w)) increased strains of *L. plantarum, L. rhamnosus*, and *Weissella confusa* from 6.9 to 9.2 CFU/mL when fermented at 30°C for 20h (Lorusso et al., 2018).

Oats have also been reported as good substrates for probiotics and are known for their soluble fibers. A *L. plantarum* strain, with anti-fungal properties, grew in a whole grain oat slurry increasing from 8 to 9 log CFU/mL after incubation at 30 °C for 16h and remained viable (~8 log CFU/mL) for 21 days during cold storage (4°C), with no off flavors/odors (Russo et al., 2017) reflecting the preservation capacity of probiotics. Beverages from oat flakes (25% wt/wt) were a suitable media for the growth of *L. plantarum* (from 7 to 8 log CFU/mL) after 12h of fermentation at 30°C (Luana et al., 2014). Probiotic microorganisms especially *Lactobacilli* exhibit good adaption to cereal substrates and the cell populations in the cereal beverages reach satisfactory probiotic values.

The use of probiotics in cereal beverages improves their product sensory quality, as the strains produce high amounts of volatile compounds, especially acetaldehyde, which optimize the beverage's flavor making it more desired by consumers (Salmerón et al., 2015). However, over-fermentation may lead to undesirable taste characteristics that can be limited by using natural preservatives such as nisin (NIS) alone or combination with lysozyme (LYS), to decrease lactic acid bacteria activity (Sozbilen, Korel, & Yemenicioğlu, 2018). Probiotics also have antagonistic activity and inhibitory substances, especially organic acids, that increase the shelf life of beverages (Russo et al., 2017).

Some of the current commercialized cereal-based probiotic beverages in Europe are summarized in Table 8.3. Proviva (5% oatmeal and fruit juices; strawberry, black currant, rosehip, banana, grape, lime, and lemon) is an oat-based beverage produced by Skane in Sweden with *L. plantarum 299* (~10 log CFU/L) as the probiotic component (Nyanzi & Jooste, 2012). Yosa is also an oat-based probiotic beverage produced by Frazerin Finland, with active components of *L. acidophilus* LA5 and *Bifidobacterium lactis* Bb12 (Nyanzi & Jooste, 2012). It is marketed as an "organic oat-based, with probiotic bacteria, 100% vegetarian beverage." Velle probiotic beverage is produced from a fermentation of oats and fruits with probiotic strains, such as *Bifidobacterium bifidum,* and *L. acidophilus*. Jovita Probiotish is a blend of cereals, fruit, and probiotic yoghurt. The average shelf life of these commercial probiotic beverages is 30 days during storage at refrigeration conditions (4°C) Fig. 8.1 (Panghal et al., 2018; Vasudha & Mishra, 2013).

TABLE 8.3 Examples of commercially available plant-based probiotic beverages in Europe

Product brand	Composition	Company, country	Probiotic strain
Cereal-based beverages			
Proviva	Oatmeal 5%, strawberry, black current, rosehip, tropical fruits (banana, grape, lime and lemon)	Skane, Sweden	*L. plantarum* 299
Yosa	Oat, fruit and berries	Fazer, Finland	*L acidophilus* LA5, *B. lactis* Bb12
Jovita Probiotisch	Blend of cereals and fruit	H&J Bruggen, Germany	Probiotic yoghurt
Velle	Oat base and fruit	VelleOats, St. Petersburg, Russia	*B. bifidum*, *L. acidophilus*

TABLE 8.3 Examples of commercially available plant-based probiotic beverages in Europe—cont'd

Product brand	Composition	Company, country	Probiotic strain
Vegetable-based beverages			
Sauerkraut juice	100% Organic sauerkraut juice, sea salt	Biotta, Switzerland	Lacto-fermented
Fruit-based beverages			
Biola	Apples, grapes and passion fruit Orange and tangerine	Tine SA, Norway	*L. rhamnosus* GG
Probi Bravo Friscus	Orange juice 100% Apple juice 100%	Skanemejerier, Sweden	*L. plantarum* HEAL9, *L. paracasei* 8700:2
Gefilus	Apple juice 80%, grape juice 20% Orange, grape, mango, peach, passion fruit juice concentrates Cranberry juice 20%, grape and pineapple juice Mango puree 39%, orange juice 27.5%, apple juice 21.5% banana puree 10%, passion fruit juice 2% Bilberry 10%, raspberry 6% Pineapple juice 50%, carrot juice 10% Orange juice 53%, peach juice 7%	Valio Ltd., Finland	*L. rhamnosus* GG
Proviva Lemonade	Lemon	Skane, Sweden	*L. plantarum* 299
Proviva Mango	Mango		
Rela	Multi fruit	Arla Ingman Ou Ab, Finland	*L. reuteri* MM53
SHOT	Raspberry, black current and grape	Skanemejerier, Sweden	*L. plantarum* 299

Modified from Hardy, N. (2010). Future innovations in food and drinks to 2015, Report No. BI00014-024. *London: Business Insights; Patel, A. R. (2017). Probiotic fruit and vegetable juices- recent advances and future perspective.* International Food Research Journal, *24(5), 1850–1857.*

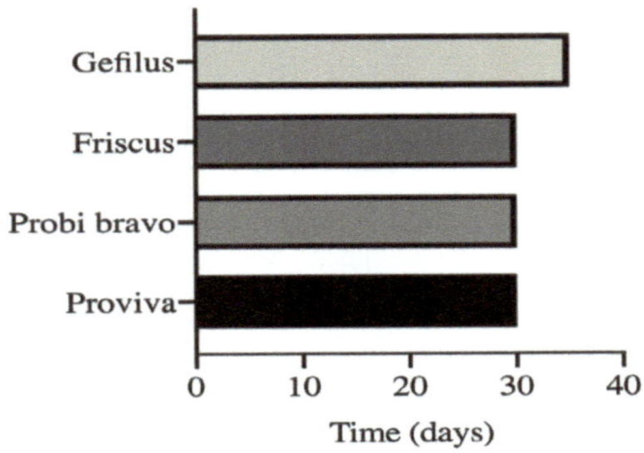

FIG. 8.1 Shelf life of commercial plant-based probiotic beverages in Europe (Panghal et al., 2018; Vasudha & Mishra, 2013).

8.2.2 Vegetable based beverages

Vegetable based beverages in Europe are mainly from asparagus, broccoli, carrot, cucumber, kale, onion, lettuce, parsley, pumpkin, tomato, and beetroot (CBI Ministry of Foreign Affairs, 2018). These juices have unique health benefits as they are rich sources of bioactive compounds, such as lycopene, β-carotene, dietary fiber, and polyphenols (Koh, Kim, Hwang, & Lim, 2013). The EU supports the World Health Organization recommendation of consumption of 400 g/day of vegetables and fruits for a healthier life (Tennant et al., 2014).

Olive, cucumber, tea, and shredded white cabbage are the most popular fermented vegetables consumed in Europe, some as pickles and sauerkraut. Traditional vegetable beverages include kombucha and shalgam. Kombucha is produced from fermented black tea and sugar using a symbiotic association of yeast and bacteria (Dufresne & Farnworth, 2000). It has a pleasant fruity sour-like sparkling flavor that changes to a vinegar-like taste with an increment of fermentation time and the most dominant microorganisms are acetic acid bacteria and yeasts, such as *S. cerevisiae* (Jayabalan, Malbaˇ, Lonˇ, Vitas, & Sathishkumar, 2014).(Note - Further details on kombucha fermentations can be found in Chapter 16).

Shalgam, a Turkish fermented beverage common in the European market, is produced from a natural fermentation of black carrot, turnip root, and bulgur flour at 10–35°C for 3–10 days, with *L. plantarum* spp. *arabinosus*, *L. fermentum*, *L. brevis*, and *S. cerevisiae* as the probiotic strains (Coskun, 2017a). Probiotics in naturally traditional fermented beverages occur in competition with other microorganisms for nutrients. Therefore, surviving probiotic organisms may not be present in sufficient amounts at the time of consumption.

Use of probiotics as starter cultures gives an assurance to cell viability in adequate amounts (> 6 log CFU/mL) in beverages. In a previous study, it was found that *L. brevis*, *L. plantarum*, and *L. rhamnosus* grew rapidly in sterilized cabbage juice without additional supplementation, reaching nearly 10.6 log CFU/mL after 24h of fermentation at 37°C (Jaiswal & Abu-Ghannam, 2013). Similarly, tomato juice as a media increased the concentration of *L. plantarum* inoculum from 6 log CFU/mL to 8.73 log CFU/mL after incubation at 37°C for 24h (Valero-Cases et al., 2017). Other authors have also found tomato and carrot juices to be favorable substrates for growth and survival of *L. plantarum* strains (Filannino et al., 2014) and *L. casei* (Petreska-Ivanovska et al., 2014).

Vegetable beverages may be blended with fruits to improve color, taste, and odor. Carrot juice (67% (v/v)) mixed with orange juice (33% (v/v)) at a pH of 4.9 enabled the growth of *L. plantarum* to 9.13 log CFU/mL after fermentation at 37°C for 24h (Valero-Cases & Frutos, 2017). Honey has also been blended with vegetable juices to increase sugar levels for probiotic growth. A vegetable pulp mixture (beetroot, carrot, and celery (2.16–3 g/100 mL)) and honey (7.5 g/100 mL) increased the growth of a mixed culture of *L. acidophilus*, *L. casei*, and *Saccharomyces boulardii* to 7–8 log CFU/mL after incubation at 37°C for 8–9h (Profir et al., 2015).

Commercially, sauerkraut juice, ideal for digestion, is produced in Switzerland by Biotta, as a main fermented beverage with probiotics from the natural fermentation of white cabbage. However, commercial vegetable-based probiotic beverages in Europe are still limited.

8.2.3 Fruit-based beverages

Fruits have been reported as good sources of bioactive components, such as phenolic compounds, anthocyanins, organic acids, and ascorbic acid, which give them antibacterial, antioxidant, anti-inflammatory, and radioprotective properties that prevent fatal chronic diseases such as cardiovascular diseases and cancer. Fruits are also high in water soluble vitamins (B and C), essential minerals, and sugars (glucose, fructose and sucrose) needed for probiotics' growth (Guergoletto, Saori, Mauro, & Garcia, 2017).

Given their health value, fruits are proposed delivery vehicles for probiotics. A few fruits are naturally fermented in Europe to produce fermented fruit-based beverages. For example, *gilaburu* is a traditionally fermented beverage from cranberry-bush fruit with the predominant probiotic strains *L. plantarum* (52.1%), *L. casei* (15.7%), *L. brevis* (7.2%), and *Leu. mesenteroides* (6.0%) (Sagdic, Ozturk, Yapar, & Yetim, 2014). *Hardaliye* is another a lactic acid fermented beverage consumed in the European part of Turkey, produced from grapes (juice and crushed) and blended with different concentrations of whole/ground or heat-treated mustard seeds and sour cherry leaves (Coskun, 2017b).

Recently, various experimental studies have shown varying results on the growth and/or survival of probiotic starter cultures in different fruit-based substrates. The survival of *L. reuteri,* at an initial cell density of 8.15–8.60 log CFU/mL, was higher in green apple, pineapple, orange fruit beverages (36.30–52.52 days reduction time to decrease 1 log CFU/mL) than in red fruit beverages (0.47 days) during storage (4°C) and the authors attributed the hindrance in red fruit beverages to high phenolic content (Perricone et al., 2014). Likewise, *B. longum* extremely decreased (~ 8 logs) from an initial inoculum of 8 log CFU/mL in pomegranate and strawberry juices after only 1 and 4 weeks of cold storage (4°C), respectively, contrary to orange, grapefruit, blackcurrant and pineapple juices (Nualkaekul et al., 2011). Fruits such as pomegranate have polyphenols, especially tannins, which affect probiotics but these effects are species and strain-specific (Bialonska, Kasimsetty, Schrader, & Ferreira, 2009). For example, growth of *Bifidobacterium brevis* and *Bifidobacterium infantis* was enhanced to 275% and 241%, respectively, whereas growth of *B. bifidum* and *Lactobacilli* was inhibited to 83% and by ~10–20% respectively, in pomegranate juice (Bialonska et al., 2009).

Fermentation favors growth of probiotics in fruit beverages. *L. plantarum* strains isolated from fruits and vegetables showed an increasing trend in pomegranate beverages from 7 to 9 log CFU/mL as fermentation time increased reaching the climax after 120h at 30°C (Filannino et al., 2013). The use of mixed cultures, rather than monocultures for fermentation, may increase probiotic growth as favorable symbiotic effects are developed between two or more types of bacteria. Mai et al. reported higher cell counts (9–10 log CFU/mL) of mixed cultures composed of *Bifidobacteria* (*B. lactis, B. longum*) and *Lactobacilli (L. casei, L. acidophilus*) in pH adjusted (6.5) apricot beverages than their respective monocultures (8 log CFU/mL), after 24h of fermentation at 37°C, from an initial inoculum of 6 log CFU/mL without any nutrient supplementation (Mai et al., 2018).

The acidity of fruit juices is one of the main challenges in the development of probiotic fruit beverages. Apple juice supported the growth of *L. plantarum* cells (from 7 to 10 log CFU/mL, incubation 37°C for 48h) only after the pH was adjusted from 3.5 to 5.1 (Dimitrovski et al., 2015). However, Rodrigues et al. demonstrated the survival of *L. paracasei* cells of counts up to 7 log CFU/mL in peach and orange fruit drinks, with low pH ranging from 3.7 to 2.9, during cold storage for 30 days (Rodrigues et al., 2012). During storage, a gradual declining trend of *L. plantarum* from an initial 11.15 to 10.28 log CFU/mL and finally to 7.36 log CFU/mL after 4 weeks of cold storage (4°C) was reported in cornelian cherry juice (Mantzourani et al., 2018). Cell counts in probiotics beverages after storage are recommended to be at a minimum count of 6–7 log CFU/mL at the time of consumption (FAO/WHO, 2001).

Today, a variety of fruit-based probiotic beverages are available on the European market (Table 8.3). Valio Ltd. produces a wide range of Gelifus fruit-based beverages from apple, grape, orange, mango, peach, passion fruit juice, cranberry juice, pineapple, banana puree, passion fruit, bilberry, and raspberry. Gefilus fruit beverages contain *L. rhamnosus* GG along with calcium and vitamin D that helps to strengthen natural immunity. Skane in Sweden also produces a range of probiotic fruit drinks, with the brand name Proviva, made from orange, mango, blueberry, red currant, and raspberry fruit juices and inoculated with *L. plantarum* 299. Biola is a brand from Tine SA, Norway made from apples, grapes, and passion fruit and the active component is *L. rhamnosus* GG. Mixed cultures of *L. plantarum* and *L. paracasei* are used to produce Probi Bravo Friscus from orange and apple juices.

8.3 Plant-based non-alcoholic beverages in Africa

Probiotic application in Africa is an evolving area that has not yet been fully exploited. Probiotics generated 11.47 billion USD in 2018 and are projected to increase to 14.77 billion USD by 2023 in Africa and the Middle East, with a compound annual growth rate of 5.5% (Market Data Forecast, 2018). This exceptional growth is driven by an ageing population and awareness of the potency and efficacy of probiotics, self-care, and online purchasing (Market Data Forecast, 2018). The market success of probiotic foods in the African marketplace will depend on mass-market positioning, sensory appeal, effective communication of health benefits to potential consumers, price and convenience, industrial management and quality control, brand loyalty and legislation (Granato et al., 2010).

The development, use, and regulation of probiotic legislation and health claims are still limited in developing countries. A majority of African countries use the United States Food and Drug Administration (FDA) guidelines to ensure food safety and quality control. Therefore, as per the FDA, probiotics are Generally Recognized As Safe (GRAS) (U.S. Food & Drug Administration FDA, 2019). At different national levels, some countries have set up commissions or laws to regulate the use and marketing of probiotics, such as the South African regulations in the Foodstuffs, Cosmetics, and Disinfectants Act (Act No. 54 of 1972) (Government Gazette, 2014). However, manpower, structures, and systems for surveillance and marketing of probiotic products are still inadequate. A study conducted in South Africa showed that the information of probiotic strains on the product labels did not correspond to recovered strains in terms of cell viability and type of strains in the probiotic products (Elliott & Teversham, 2004). Effective regulations of probiotic foods are needed.

In Africa, probiotics are mainly consumed as food supplements in the form of capsules and tablets (Table 8.4) to boost immunity and gut health.

TABLE 8.4 Examples of probiotic sources available in Africa

Brand	Strain	Country of distribution	Company, country of manufacture	References
Probiotic liquid concentrates				
Probyo Digestive	*Lactobacillus spp. Bifidobacterium spp.*	South Africa	Probyo and The Noakes Foundation, South Africa	Spence and Spence (2016)
Probyo Sports	*Lactobacillus, Bifidobacterium,*			
Probyo Immune	*Lactobacillus, Bifidobacterium,*			
Probiotic 15 Liquid	*B. lactis, B. longum, B. bifidum, L. bulgaricus, L. casei, L. delbrueckii, L. fermentum, L. lactis, L. plantarum*	South Africa	Naturefresh, South Africa	NatureFresh Health Products (2019)
Internal Microbial Stabilizer Pre & Probiotic Liquid	*Lactobacillus, Bifidobacterium,*	South Africa	Imsyser Health products, South Africa	Imsyser Healthy Products, 2019
12 Strain Liquid Probiotic	*L. rhamnosus, L. acidophilus, B. lactis, B. longum*			
Probiotic capsules and tablets				
Entiro	*L. plantarum, Enterococcus mundtii*	South Africa	Cipla Pharmaceutical company, South Africa	Cipla (2019)
Nativa Digestive	*L. acidophilus, B. longum, B. bifidum, B. infantis*	South Africa	Nativa, South Africa	Nativa (2016)

TABLE 8.4 Examples of probiotic sources available in Africa—cont'd

Brand	Strain	Country of distribution	Company, country of manufacture	References
Trilac	*L. acidophilus, L. bulgaricus, B. animalis*	Kenya	Allergon AB, Sweden	
Kalsis	*Lactobacillus acidophilus*	Kenya	Catalysis Lab, Spain	Catalysis (2019)
Lacteol Fort	*L. fermentum, L. delbrueckii*	South Africa	Rameda, Egypt	Rameda Pharmaceutical (2015)
Combiforte, Comb 15	*L. acidophilus, B. longum, B. bifidum*	South Africa	Bioflora CC, South Africa	Bioflora (2017)
BioproMulti	*L. acidophilus*	South Africa	Akacia HealthCare (Pty) Ltd, South Africa	Akacia HealthCare (Pty) (2019)
Culturelle	*B. longum, L. acidophilus, L. rhamnosus* GG, *S. thermophilus*	South Africa	Culturelle, UK	Culturelle (2018)
Probiotic 10	*L. acidophilus*	Egypt	Puritan, Egypt	Puritan Healthy (2016)
Forever Active Probiotic	*B. lactis, B. longum, L. rhamnosus, L. acidophilus, L. bulgaricus, L. plantarum*	Kenya	Forever Living Products, USA	Forever Living (2017)
Reuterina	*L. reuteri (*DSM 17938*)*	South Africa	Ascendis Health, South Africa	Ascendis Pharma (2017)
UltraFlora	*B. lactis B-420*	South Africa	Amipro, South Africa	Amipro (2016)
Daily Flora, Metakids Probiotic	*L. acidophilus NCFM, B. lactis Bi-07*			
Lp299	*L. plantarum 299v*	South Africa	Adcock Ingram, South Africa	Adcock Ingram (2015)
Probio Flora	*Lactobacillus, Bifidobacterium*			
Bestum	*B. longum, L. rhamnosus*			

Probiotic liquid concentrates, such as Probyo Digestive, Probyo Sports, Probyo Immune, Probiotic 15 Liquid, Internal Microbial Stabilizer, Pre & Probiotic Liquid and 12 Strain Liquid, are consumed at a recommended dosage per day. These products are mainly imported from overseas companies with multinational sales reach, such as Cipla, Allergon AB, Seeking Health, Wellington Pharmaceuticals, Bioflora, Danisco, or obtained from national companies, such as Adcock Ingram, Amipro, Ascendis Health, and Nativa. Consequently, the high costs for importation and storage incurred make the probiotic products expensive and unaffordable to the majority of the African population (Westerik, Kort, Sybesma, & Reid, 2018). The use of locally available foods would be a less expensive alternative of providing probiotics.

Probiotic microorganisms, such as *L. fermentum, W. confuse, P. pentosaceus,* and *L. plantarum* have been identified in fermented foods (Lei & Jakobsen, 2004; Turpin, 2011). Fermented foods from cereals, starchy foods,and vegetables have been part of the African diet for a very long time (Franz et al., 2014). Fermentation is carried out spontaneously or by back slopping to improve flavor, preserve the food, improve its digestibility, and increase the nutritional value. However, probiotic strains in traditionally fermented foods occur in competition with other microorganisms such as yeasts and other bacteria (Madoroba et al., 2011; Okeke et al., 2015). Therefore, they may not occur in sufficient amounts to provide health benefits to the host as per the FAO/WHO consultation guidelines (FAO/WHO, 2001).

In 2005, the Western Heads East program for people living with HIV in Mwanza, Tanzania spearheaded the use and distribution of probiotic foods in Africa by producing yoghurt from milk using *Lactobacillus rhamnosus* (Reid, 2010) as a small social enterprise. In 2011, the Yoba for Life Foundation developed sachets containing *L. rhamnosus* GG and *S. thermophilus* C106 where 1 g of sachet was used to make 100 L of probiotic yoghurt from milk (Kort et al., 2015). The East African Yoba production operation units consist of local dairy farmers who include the Yoba logo on their brand packaging. At the moment, over 20,000 L of probiotic yoghurt are produced per week in Uganda (Reid et al., 2018). However, animal products are associated with dietary diseases, such as cardiovascular diseases and diabetes, which are responsible for 80% of all deaths in developing countries (World Health Organization (WHO), 2013). In addition, high medical costs are incurred in the treatment of these chronic diseases. Plant-based functional foods, such as probiotic beverages, could be a preventive strategy to protect public health. Some studies have been carried out to demonstrate the potential of cereals, fruits, and vegetables as probiotic carriers (Kassim, Baijnath, & Odhav, 2014; Kort et al., 2015; Niyibituronsa et al., 2019).

8.3.1 Cereal-based beverages

Cereals, such as maize, teff, millet, and sorghum are of economic importance as they are staple foods in most African communities. These cereals are traditionally fermented to produce beverages, gruels, and porridges, such as *bogobe, ben saalga, degue, hussuwa, koko, kenkey, kunu-zaki, kisra, injera, mahewu, mawe, ogi, obusera, potopoto,* and *uji* (Franz et al., 2014). Traditional fermentation involves different steps and often a combination of soaking, washing, milling, water addition, sieving, fermentation, and cooking (Achi & Ukwuru, 2015). Fermented cereal-based beverages are consumed as weaning/complementary foods to improve digestion or are preferred for their taste and flavor (Mouquet-Rivier, Guyot, Tou, & Tre, 2008).

Various strains of lactic acid bacteria with probiotic properties have been identified in traditional cereal-based fermented beverages. Probiotics, such as *Lactobacillus fermentum* and *Lactobacillus plantarum*, with resistance to low pH (2.5), bile salts (0.3% w/v), antibiotics, and adhesion capacity to the HT29 cell line have been isolated from traditionally fermented cereal beverages (Oguntoyinbo & Narbad, 2015; Owusu-Kwarteng, Tano-Debrah, Akabanda, & Jespersen, 2015). *Ben-saalga*, a fermented millet gruel in Ghana and Burkina Faso, normally consumed as a complementary food had the most dominant strains as *L. fermentum, P. pentosaceus,* and *L. plantarum* (Turpin, 2011). Similarly, *L. fermentum* and *L. plantarum* were the predominant *Lactobacilli* in *mkarango*, a roasted fermented maize flour in western Kenya (Mwizerwa et al., 2018). Other probiotic species such as *S. cerevisiae* were identified in *togwa*, a sorghum, or millet or sorghum/millet mix beverage consumed in Tanzania (Hellström, Vázques-Juárez, Svanberg, & Andlid, 2010; Mugula, Nnko, Narvhus, & Sørhaug, 2003). Traditional cereal-based fermented beverages have been the main food source of probiotics in Africa.

However, traditional cereal-based fermented beverages usually have array of mixed microbial populations including yeasts (*S. cerevisiae, Saccharomyces chevalieri, Candida spp., Pichia anomala*), molds (*Fusarium, Aspergillus, Cladosporium* and *Penicillium*), and bacteria (*Leuconostoc, Lactobacillus, Lactococcus, Pediococcus, Corynebacterium, Enterococcus, Escherichia coli, Acetobacter,* and *Streptococcus)* (Achi & Ukwuru, 2015), which vary product quality and stability. The use of beneficial probiotic strains as starter cultures in African cereal beverages, as shown in Table 8.5, could produce improved products. Kort et al. demonstrated the growth of *L. rhamnosus* from an initial inoculum of 6–9 log CFU/mL in *obusera* (sorghum) and *uji* (maize or sorghum or a blended mixture) beverages after incubation at 25°C and 45°C respectively for 16–24h (Kort et al., 2015). Similarly, the number of *L. rhamnosus* cells increased to 9 log CFU/mL in *kwete*, a maize slurry (2% v/v) after 24h of fermentation at 30°C and remained viable ($\geq$ 8 log CFU/mL) during 4 weeks of cold

TABLE 8.5 Overview of recent studies on plant-based probiotic beverages in Africa

Beverage	Composition	Probiotic strain	Reference
Cereal-based beverages			
Mageu	Maize	*L. delbrueckii* subsp *lactis, L. acidophilus, L. casei, L. rhamnosus*	Nyanzi et al. (2010)
Probiotic beverage	Rice or millet blended with pumpkin seed 10% v/v and sesame seed 10% v/v	*S. thermophilus ST-20Y L. acidophilus LA-5, Bifidobacterium BB-12*	Hassan, Aly, and El-Hadidie (2012)
Obushera	Sorghum	*L. rhamnosus yoba* 2012, *S. thermophilus* C106	Kort et al. (2015)
Uji	Maize, sorghum or a blend mixture	*L .rhamnosus yoba* 2012, *S. thermophilus* C106	Kort et al. (2015)
Maize gruel	Maize	*L. plantarum* B411	Fayemi et al. (2017)
Kunun-aya	Maize	*L. plantarum*	Olaoye, Ndife, and Raymond (2017)
Kwete	Maize	*L. rhamnosus yoba* 2012, *S. thermophilus* C106	Wacoo et al. (2019)
Vegetable- and legume-based beverages			
Ginger, garlic, and honey	Rhizomes	*L. plantarum, L. bulgaricus*	Adeniran, Abiose, and Ukeyima (2010)
Soymilk	Soybean	*Bifidobacterium longum, Bifidobacterium adolescentis*	Ebhodaghe, Abiose, and Adeniran (2012)
Solanum nigrum, Amaranthus spinosus, Amaranthus hybridus, Ceratotheca triloba, Asparagus sprengeri, Tulbaghia violacea, Cleome monophylla, Asystasia gangetica, Senna occidentalis	Leaf	*L. lactis, L. bulgaricus,*	Kassim et al. (2014)

TABLE 8.5 Overview of recent studies on plant-based probiotic beverages in Africa—cont'd

Beverage	Composition	Probiotic strain	Reference
Momordica balsamina, Amarantus dubius, Justucia flava, Galinsoga parviflora, Oxyginum sinuatum, Centella asiatica	Leaf	*L. bulgaricus*	Kassim et al. (2014)
Sonchu soleraceus	Leaf, root	*L. lactis, L. bulgaricus, L. reuteri*(ATCC 55730), *B. longum* (Rosell-175 ME)	Kassim et al. (2014)
Tarraxacum officinale	Leaf, root	*L. lactis, L. bulgaricus, B. longum* (Rosell-175 ME)	Kassim et al. (2014)
Chenopodium album		*B. longum*(Rosell-175 ME)	Kassim et al. (2014)
Bambara milk and soymilk	Bambara groundnuts, soybean	*L. delbrueckii* subsp. *bulgaricus, S. salivarus* subsp. *thermophilus*	Falade, Ogundele, Ogunshe, Fayemi, and Ocloo (2015)
Soymilk	Soybean	*L. plantarum, L. brevis, L. reuteri*	Niyibituronsa et al. (2019)
Fruit-based beverages			
Mutandabota	Baobab fruit juice (4%wt/wt) and milk	*L. rhamnosus yoba*	Mpofu et al. (2016, 2014)
Pineapple beverage	Natural pineapple fruit juice	*P. pentosaceus* LaG1, *P. pentosaceus* LBF2, *L. rhamnosus* GG	AdebayoTayo and Akpeji (2016)

storage (Wacoo et al., 2019). In another study, autochthonous *L. plantarum* grew from 6 log CFU/mL in steeped maize gruel to a cell concentration of 8 log CFU/mL after fermentation at 37°C for 24h (Fayemi et al., 2017). However, some strains such as *S. thermophilus* did not multiply in cereal matrices (Kort et al., 2015).

Blending of cereals with other foods may increase the probiotic cell viability. Sorghum blended with tiger-nut milk to improve protein, mineral, and dietary fiber content had higher *L. plantarum* growth (8.5 log CFU/

mL) than the non-blended sorghum beverage (6.5 log CFU/mL) (Olaoye et al., 2017). Addition of pumpkin and sesame seed milk (10%) to a fermented rice beverage increased *L. acidophilus* cell counts (from 9.66 to 9.73–9.80 log CFU/mL) and decreased *Bifidobacterium BB* (from 9.87 to 9.66–9.74 log CFU/mL) but had no effect on *S. thermophilus* (9.78 log CFU/mL) during cold storage (4°C) (Hassan et al., 2012).

Probiotics are mainly delivered into cereal beverages through fermentation and this process is associated with numerous benefits. For instance, previous studies have shown the ability of *L. rhamnosus* to bind with aflatoxins, commonly found in cereals, to non-detectable limits (Ahlberg, Joutsjoki, & Korhonen, 2015; Wacoo et al., 2019; Westerik, Wacoo, Sybesma, & Kort, 2016). Long fermentation time increases the bioavailability of minerals (iron and zinc) in cereals given it favors the degradation of phytic acid, a mineral binder (Gabaza, Muchuweti, Vandamme, & Raes, 2017), and cereal protein concentration and bioavailability of essential amino acids are increased by the activity of microbial enzymes during fermentation (Chelule, Mbongwa, Carries, & Gqaleni, 2010).

8.3.2 Vegetable and legume-based beverages

The presence of diverse wild and/or cultivated edible plants (Van Wyk, 2011) in Africa creates a huge potential for developing new products. A wide range of vegetables (dark green, red, orange, and starchy) and legumes (beans and peas) are regularly consumed as they are inexpensive and readily available (Mensah, Okoli, & Eifediyi, 2008). Leafy vegetables are usually eaten fresh, cooked, sun-dried, or fermented (Ayua & Omware, 2013; Oguntoyinbo et al., 2016). A combination of sun-drying and fermentation reduces the level of anti-nutrients (nitrates, oxalates, and phenols) in vegetables such as cowpea leaves (Muchoki, Imungi, & Lamuka, 2010) thus increasing the bioavailability of micronutrients. Micronutrients (essential vitamins and minerals), non-digestible carbohydrates and phytochemicals in vegetables are responsible for their antioxidant, antibacterial, and anti-inflammatory properties (Septembre-Malaterre, Remize, & Poucheret, 2018).

In Africa, fermented vegetables are mainly consumed as condiments, sauces, and soups (Ayua & Omware, 2013; Oguntoyinbo et al., 2016) but rarely as beverages. Common traditionally fermented vegetable foods produced by mainly cleaning, mixing with water, boiling (varies), dehulling (for seeds), fermentation, steaming and drying include; *ntobambodi* (Congo), *bikalga* (Burkina Faso), *soumbala* (Burkina Faso), or*iru* (Nigeria), *ugba* (Nigeria), *okpehe* (Nigeria), and *kawal* (Sudan) from cassava leaves, roselle seeds, African locust bean seeds, Africa oil bean cotyledon, *Prosopis Africana* seeds, and sicklepod leaves, respectively (Ballogun & Oyeyiola, 2011; Lawane, Aly, François, Flibert, & Yves, 2016; Olasupo, Okorie, &

Oguntoyinbo, 2016; Ouoba, Parkouda, Sawadogo, Kobawila, & Keleke, 2010; Town, State, & State, 2018). *Bacillus* species (*Bacillus subtilis, Bacillus pumilus, Bacillus licheniformis*, and *Bacillus megaterium*) have high protease activity and have been found to be the most dominant strains in the majority of spontaneously fermented vegetable foods (Lawane et al., 2016; Tamang, Watanabe, & Holzapfel, 2016; Town et al., 2018). Among the lactic acid bacteria, *W. confuse* was reported to be the most dominant and other strains include the following: *L. plantarum, P. pentosaceus, W. confuse, L. brevis, L. fermentum*, and *L. casei* (Lawane et al., 2016; Ouoba et al., 2010; Town et al., 2018). Unfavorable conditions during vegetable fermentations such as increment of pH (from 5 to 8.3) and reduction of fermentable sugars inhibit (Oguntoyinbo, Cho, et al., 2016; Ouoba et al., 2010; Town et al., 2018) growth of probiotics in vegetable media. However, a study in Kenya reported rapid growth of *L. plantarum* and *L. fermentum* (from an initial concentration of 7 log CFU/mL to >8 log CFU/mL) when used as single starter cultures on kale leaves with 24 h of fermentation at 25°C (Oguntoyinbo, Fusco, et al., 2016).

Some experiments have been carried out to investigate probiotic growth or survival in vegetable beverages (Table 8.5). Vegetables are high in inulin, which is known to stimulate the growth of *Lactobacilli* and *Bifidobacteria* (Roberfroid, 2007). A study in South Africa showed that vegetable infusions from dried vegetable leaves and roots enabled the growth of pure cultures of *L. lactis, L. bulgaricus*, and *L. reuteri* from an initial cell concentration of 5 log CFU/mL (Kassim et al., 2014). Ginger and garlic are valued for their medicinal abilities (Baliga, Arora, & Baliga, 2013) and addition of probiotics would increase their health promoting characteristics. *L. plantarum* (initial cell concentration 8–9 log CFU/mL) remained viable at 7–8 log CFU/mL in sterile ginger and ginger with garlic beverages sweetened with honey, at ambient and refrigeration temperatures, after 4 weeks but *L. bulgaricus* decreased to <5 log CFU/mL from an initial inoculum of 6–7 log CFU/mL after only 3 weeks of storage under similar conditions (Adeniran et al., 2010). Although survival of probiotic strains in the beverages varied within the probiotic species, the use of honey increased the amount of fermentable sugars for probiotic survival.

Legumes are well known to improve nutritional value and the majority of African communities consume more legumes than meat for their protein. Legumes are rich sources of protein, oil, fiber, vitamins, and minerals, in fact, 40% of soybean is high-quality protein (Gandhi, 2009; Sanchez-Zapata, Fernandez-Lopez, & Perez-Alvarez, 2012). Soybean also contains bioactive compounds, such as isoflavones (0.1–5 mg/g), which reduce the incidence of fatal diseases (cancer, heart disease, and osteoporosis) (Vij, Hati, & Yadav, 2011). Soybean, tiger nut, and bambara groundnuts can be processed to soymilk, tiger-milk, and bambara milk, respectively, by cleaning, mixing with water, milling, filtration, and then fermented to produce plant-based yoghurts (Amponsah, Golly, Endeme, Derigubah, &

Sarpong, 2017; Falade et al., 2015; Niyibituronsa et al., 2019). Different probiotic strains, such as *L. plantarum, L. acidophilus, L. brevis, L. reuteri, L. rhamnosus, Lactococcus cremoris*, and *L. casei* strains, have been tested for their ability to ferment soymilk and the ones with the best capacity were *L. plantarum, L. reuteri*, and *L. brevis* at 9.02, 8.92, and 8.88 log CFU/mL, respectively, after incubation at 30°C for 24h (initial 6 log CFU/mL) (Niyibituronsa et al., 2019). Fermentation (42°C, 6h) of soymilk and bambara milk beverages with mixed culture (*L. delbrueckii* subsp. *bulgaricus* and *Streptococcus salivarus* subsp. *thermophilus)* increased the initial inoculum from 6–7 log CFU/mL and strains further grew to 8.7 log CFU/mL during storage at ambient temperature (Falade et al., 2015). No significant differences were observed between probiotic soymilk, tiger-nut milk beverages, and non-fermented milk beverages in terms of their sensory characteristics (Amponsah et al., 2017). Plant-based yoghurts are low cost favorable substitutes to dairy yoghurts and are suitable for vegetarians and persons with allergies or cholesterol restricted diets as a source of probiotics.

Probyo immune is a commercial liquid concentrate produced from the fermentation of a combination of herb extracts (chamomile flowers, rose hips, olive leaf, elderberry, ginseng, and astragalus) and marketed as an "immune-boosting punch."

8.3.3 Fruit-based beverages

Africa has conducive environmental conditions of temperature and rainfall that encourage the growth of over 1200 fruit tree species (Sthapit, Rao, & Sthapit, 2012). Cultivated fruits include mango, pineapple, papaya, banana, melons, guava, lemon, orange, passion fruit, and avocado among others (Awodoyin et al., 2015; Crane, 2009). Fruits contain considerable amounts of sugars, fibers, essential vitamins, and minerals (Islam, Afrin, Khan, & Howlader, 2015) that may boost the growth of probiotics. However, fruits also possess organic acids, low pH, and phenolic compounds (Mustafa, Chua, El-Enshasy, Majid, & Malek, 2016) that may hinder cell viability.

Traditionally, fruits in Africa have been fermented to produce alcoholic beverages, such as *mudetemwa* (sand apple), *marula* (marula fruits), *masau* (buffalo thorn fruits), and *mutandavira* (*Uapacakirkiana* fruits) (Gadaga, Mutukumira, Narvhus, & Feresu, 1999). Non-alcoholic probiotic fruit beverages have not been a part of the African diet and are unavailable on the African market to the best of our knowledge. However, the use of only fruit as a medium for probiotic cell growth is an emerging area in Africa. Single and mixed cultures of *P. pentosaceus and L. rhamnosus* increased to 9 from 7 log CFU/mL after incubation for 72h at 37°C in pineapple fruit juice and survived (7 log CFU/mL) for 4 weeks in cold storage (AdebayoTayo & Akpeji, 2016).

Fruits are nowadays usually mixed with other foods, especially milk, to develop probiotic beverages. Locally available baobab fruit pulp (4% wt/vol), mixed with heat treated full-fat cow milk promoted the increase of *L. rhamnosus yoba* from 5.8 to 8.8 log CFU/mL after 24h of fermentation at 23–37°C (Augustine et al., 2016; Mpofu et al., 2014). The probiotic strain inhibited the growth of the bacterial pathogens *B. cereus* and *Campylobacter jejuni* (Augustine et al., 2016). Furthermore, probiotics produce different metabolites, such as vitamins, bacteriocin, hydrogen peroxide, diacetyl, glutathione, butyrate, folate, acetaldehyde, lactic acid, and other bioactive compounds (Rezac, Kok, Heermann, & Hutkins, 2018) during fermentation that have antioxidant characteristics signifying the health value of these probiotic beverages (Mai et al., 2018).

Commercially produced by the Probyo Company and the Noakes foundation, Probyo is a liquid concentrate rich in live lactic acid bacteria. Probyo Sports is produced from a lacto-fermentation of honey-bush, aronia berries, blackcurrant, cranberries, goji berries, beetroot, sour cherry, turmeric, cocoa, Siberian ginseng, guarana, and spirulina and marketed as "an ideal product for an active lifestyle, enhancing the body's natural energy supply." A daily dose of 15 ml of Probyo added into water or fruit juice is recommended (Spence & Spence, 2016).

8.4 Conclusions

The main strains used in plant-based beverages are *Lactobacillus* and *Bifidobacteria* strains and fermentation enables the increment of cell populations to satisfactory probiotic values (> 6–7 log CFU/mL). Today, cereals are the main plant beverages used as substrates for probiotics and the use of fruits and vegetables for probiotic beverages is yet to be fully exploited, especially in Africa.

Acknowledgments

This work, within the PhD of J. Mandha, has been financed by the BOF Special Research Fund of Ghent University, Centre for Research, Agricultural Advancement, Teaching Excellence and Sustainability (CREATES) Fellowship at the Nelson Mandela African Institution of Science and Technology and L'OREAL–UNESCO for Women in Science Sub-Saharan regional fellowship.

References

Achi, O. K., & Ukwuru, M. (2015). Cereal-based fermented foods of Africa as functional foods. *International Journal of Microbiology and Application*, *2*(4), 71–83.

Adcock Ingram (2015). *Products*. http://www.adcock.co.za/. Accessed 4/04/2019.

AdebayoTayo, B., & Akpeji, S. (2016). Probiotic viability, physicochemical and sensory properties of probiotic pineapple juice. *Fermentation*, *2*(4), 20–31. https://doi.org/10.3390/fermentation2040020.

Adeniran, A. H., Abiose, S. H., & Ukeyima, M. T. (2010). Microbiological assessment of probioticated ginger-based beverages. *Nutrition and Food Science*, *40*(2), 209–220. https://doi.org/10.1108/00346651011029246.

Ahlberg, S. H., Joutsjoki, V., & Korhonen, H. J. (2015). Potential of lactic acid bacteria in aflatoxin risk mitigation. *International Journal of Food Microbiology*, *207*, 87–102. https://doi.org/10.1016/j.ijfoodmicro.2015.04.042.

Akacia HealthCare (Pty) (2019). *L. Biopro Multi.* http://www.biopromulti.com/about.htm. Accessed on 14/04/2019.

Amipro. Probiotics (2016). https://www.amipro.co.za/store/c17/Probiotics. Accessed 4/04/2019

Amponsah, A. S., Golly, M. K., Endeme, M., Derigubah, B., & Sarpong, F. (2017). Proximate and sensory evaluation of non-diary probiotic beverages made from tiger - nuts (*Cyperus esculentus* L.) and soy bean (*Glycine max*). *International Journal of Innovative. Food Science and Technology*, *1*(1), 9–17. http://doi.org/10.25218/ijifst.2017.01.001.02.

Ascendis Pharma (2017). *Reuterina.* http://www.reuterina.co.za/. Accessed on 03/04/2019.

Augustine, M., Anita, R., Martinus, J. R., Marcel, H., Eddy, J. S., & den Besten, H. M. W. (2016). Inactivation of bacterial pathogens in yoba mutandabota, a dairy product fermented with the probiotic *Lactobacillus rhamnosus yoba*. *International Journal of Food Microbiology*, *217*, 42–48. https://doi.org/10.1016/j.ijfoodmicro.2015.09.016.

Awodoyin, R. O., Olubode, O. S., Ogbu, J. U., Balogun, R. B., Nwawuisi, J. U., & Orji, K. O. (2015). Indigenous fruit trees of tropical Africa: Status, opportunity for development and biodiversity management. *Agricultural Sciences*, *6*(1), 31–41. https://doi.org/10.4236/as.2015.61004.

Ayua, E., & Omware, J. (2013). Assessment of processing methods and preservation of African Leafy Vegetables in Siaya County, Kenya. *Global Journal of Biology, Agriculture & Health Sciences*, *2*(2), 46–48.

Bajaj, B. K., Claes, I. J. J., & Lebeer, S. (2015). Functional mechanisms of probiotics. *Journal of Microbiology, Biotechnology and Food Sciences*, *04*(04), 321–327. http://doi.org/10.15414/jmbfs.2015.4.4.321-327.

Baliga, M. S., Arora, R., & Baliga, M. S. (2013). A review ginger in the prevention of nausea and vomiting : A review. *Critical Reviews in Food Science and Nutrition*, *53*(7), 669–689. https://doi.org/10.1080/10408398.2011.553751.

Ballogun, M., & Oyeyiola, G. (2011). Microbiological and chemical changes during the production of okpehe from *Prosopis africana* seeds. *Journal of Asian Scientific Research*, *1*(8), 390–398.

Bhat, B., Gupta, M., Andrabi, S. T., & Bajaj, B. K. (2017). Growth and viability of probiotic *Weissella kimchi* R-3 in fruit and vegetable beverages. *Indian Journal of Biochemistry & Biophysics*, *54*, 191–199.

Bialonska, D., Kasimsetty, S. G., Schrader, K. K., & Ferreira, D. (2009). The effect of pomegranate (*Punica granatum* l.) byproducts and ellagitannins on the growth of human gut bacteria. *Journal of Agricultural and Food Chemistry*, *57*(18), 8344–8349. https://doi.org/10.1021/jf901931b.

Bioflora, C. C. (2017). *Forte range.* https://www.bioflora.co.za/category/forterange/>. Accessed 06/04/2019.

Blandino, A., Al-Aseeri, M. E., Pandiella, S. S., Cantero, D., & Webb, C. (2003). Cereal-based fermented foods and beverages. *Food Research International*, *36*(6), 527–543. https://doi.org/10.1016/S0963-9969(03)00009-7.

Catalysis (2019). *Food supplements.* https://www.catalysis.es/en/products>. Accessed 06/04/2019.

CBI Ministry of Foreign Affairs (2018). *Exporting vegetable juices to Europe.* https://www.cbi.eu/node/2161/pdf/.

Charalampopoulos, D., & Pandiella, S. S. (2010). Survival of human derived *Lactobacillus plantarum* in fermented cereal extracts during refrigerated storage. *LWT - Food Science and Technology*, *43*(3), 431–435. https://doi.org/10.1016/j.lwt.2009.09.006.

Chelule, P. K., Mbongwa, H. P., Carries, S., & Gqaleni, N. (2010). Lactic acid fermentation improves the quality of amahewu, a traditional South African maize-based porridge. *Food Chemistry*, *122*(3), 656–661. https://doi.org/10.1016/j.foodchem.2010.03.026.

Cipla (2019). *Entiro.* http://entiro.co.za/. Accessed on 06/04/2019.

Coda, R., Rizzello, C. G., Trani, A., & Gobbetti, M. (2011). Manufacture and characterization of functional emmer beverages fermented by selected lactic acid bacteria. *Food Microbiology*, *28*(3), 526–536. https://doi.org/10.1016/j.fm.2010.11.001.

Contor, L. (2001). Functional Food Science in Europe. *Nutrition, Metabolism, and Cardiovascular Diseases: NMCD*, *11*(4 Suppl), 20–23.

Corbo, M. R., Bevilacqua, A., Petruzzi, L., Casanova, F. P., & Sinigaglia, M. (2014). Functional beverages: The emerging side of functional foods: Commercial trends, research, and health implications. *Comprehensive Reviews in Food Science and Food Safety*, *13*(6), 1192–1206. https://doi.org/10.1111/1541-4337.12109.

Coskun, F. (2017a). A traditional Turkish fermented non-alcoholic beverage, "Shalgam" *Beverages*, *3*(49), 1–13. https://doi.org/10.3390/beverages3040049.

Coskun, F. (2017b). A traditional Turkish fermented non-alcoholic grape-based beverage. "Hardaliye" *Beverages*, *3*(1), 1–11. https://doi.org/10.3390/beverages3010002.

Crane, J. H. (2009). In J. Janick, & R. E. Paull (Eds.), *The Encyclopedia of fruit and nuts.* Vol. 46. Oxfordshire, UK: Cambridge University Press. https://doi.org/10.5860/CHOICE.46-5375.

Culturelle (2018). *Culturelle products.* https://www.culturelle.com/. Accessed 09/04/2019.

De Vrese, M., Stegelmann, A., Richter, B., Fenselau, S., & Laue, C. (2001). Probiotics—compensation for lactase insufficiency. *American Journal of Clinical Nutrition*, *73*(2 suppl), 421S–429S. https://doi.org/10.1093/ajcn/73.2.421s.

Dimitrovski, D., Velickova, E., Langerholc, T., & Winkelhausen, E. (2015). Apple juice as a medium for fermentation by the probiotic *Lactobacillus plantarum* PCS 26 strain. *Annals of Microbiology*, *65*(4), 2161–2170. https://doi.org/10.1007/s13213-015-1056-7.

Dlusskaya, E., Jänsch, A., Schwab, C., & Gänzle, M. G. (2008). Microbial and chemical analysis of a kvass fermentation. *European Food Research and Technology*, *227*(1), 261–266. https://doi.org/10.1007/s00217-007-0719-4.

Dufresne, C., & Farnworth, E. (2000). Tea, kombucha, and health : A review. *Food Research International*, *33*(6), 409–421. https://doi.org/10.1016/S0963-9969(00)00067-3.

Ebhodaghe, S. O., Abiose, S. H., & Adeniran, H. A. (2012). Assessment of physico-chemical characteristics, viability and inhibitory effect of bifidobacteria in soymilk. *Journal of Food Research*, *1*(2), 159–170. https://doi.org/10.5539/jfr.v1n2p159.

Elliott, E., & Teversham, K. (2004). An evaluation of nine probiotics available in South Africa. *South African Medical Journal*, *94*(2), 121–124.

European Food Safety Authority (EFSA) (2005). *EFSA scientific colloquium summary report. OPS qualified presumption of safety of micro-organisms in food and feed, 13–14 December 2004, Brussels, Belgium.* http://www.efsa.eu.int/science/colloquium_series/no2_qps/948_en.html/. Accessed 03/04/2019.

Falade, K. O., Ogundele, O. M., Ogunshe, A. O., Fayemi, O. E., & Ocloo, F. C. K. (2015). Physico-chemical, sensory and microbiological characteristics of plain yoghurt from bambara groundnut (*Vigna subterranea*) and soybeans (*Glycine max*). *Journal of Food Science and Technology*, *52*(9), 5858–5865. https://doi.org/10.1007/s13197-014-1657-3.

FAO/WHO (2001). *Evaluation of health and nutritional properties of probiotics in food including powder milk with live lactic acid bacteria.* http://www.fao.org/3/a-a0512e.pdf. Accessed 03/03/2019.

FAO/WHO (2002). *"Guidelines for the evaluation of probiotics in foods", report of a joint FAO/ WHO working group on drafting guidelines for the evaluation of pro- biotics in food, Geneva, Switzerland.* .

Fayemi, O. E., Taylor, J. R. N., & Buys, E. M. (2017). Potential for prevention of non-O157 Shiga toxin-producing *Escherichia coli* contamination in traditionally fermented African maize gruel by fermentative probiotic *Lactobacillus plantarum*. *International Journal of Food Science and Technology, 52*(4), 1064–1071. https://doi.org/10.1111/ijfs.13373.

Filannino, P., Azzi, L., Cavoski, I., Vincentini, O., Rizzello, C. G., Gobbetti, M. , et al. (2013). Exploitation of the health-promoting and sensory properties of organic pomegranate (*Punica granatum* L) juice through lactic acid fermentation. *International Journal of Food Microbiology, 163*(2–3), 184–192. https://doi.org/10.1016/j.ijfoodmicro.2013.03.002.

Filannino, P., Cardinali, G., Rizzello, C. G., Buchin, S., De Angelis, M., Gobbetti, M. , et al. (2014). Metabolic responses of *Lactobacillus plantarum* strains during fermentation and storage of vegetable and fruit juices. *Applied and Environmental Microbiology, 80*(7), 2206–2215. https://doi.org/10.1128/AEM.03885-13.

Forever Living (2017). *Products.* https://foreverliving.com/page/products/all-products/2-nutrition/610/usa/en. Accessed 04/04/2019.

Franz, C. M. A. P., Huch, M., Maina, J., Abriouel, H., Benomar, N., Reid, G. , et al. (2014). African fermented foods and probiotics. *International Journal of Food Microbiology, 190*, 84–96. https://doi.org/10.1016/j.ijfoodmicro.2014.08.033.

Gabaza, M., Muchuweti, M., Vandamme, P., & Raes, K. (2017). Can fermentation be used as a sustainable strategy to reduce iron and zinc binders in traditional African fermented cereal porridges or gruels? *Food Reviews International, 33*(6), 561–586. https://doi.org/10.1080/87559129.2016.1196491.

Gadaga, T. H., Mutukumira, A. N., Narvhus, J. A., & Feresu, S. B. (1999). A review of traditional fermented foods and beverages of Zimbabwe. *International Journal of Food Microbiology, 53*(1), 1–11. https://doi.org/10.1016/S0168-1605(99)00154-3.

Gandhi, A. P. (2009). Review paper quality of soybean and its food products. *International Food Research Journal, 16*(1), 11–19.

Goncerzewicz, A., Misiewicz, A., Owczarek, L., Jasińska, U., & Skąpska, S. (2016). The effect of a newly developed oat-banana fermented beverage with a beta-glucan additive on ldhL gene expression in Streptococcus thermophilus TKM3 KKP 2030p. *Current Microbiology, 73*(6), 773–780. https://doi.org/10.1007/s00284-016-1126-5.

Gotcheva, V., Pandiella, S. S., Angelov, A., Roshkova, Z., & Webb, C. (2001). Monitoring the fermentation of the traditional Bulgarian beverage boza. *International Journal of Food Science and Technology, 36*(2), 129–134. https://doi.org/10.1046/j.1365-2621.2001.00429.x.

Government Gazette (2014). *Foodstuffs, cosmetics and disinfectants act, 1972 (Act No. 54 of 1972) Regulations relating to the labelling and advertising of foods amendment. South Africa. Retrieved from*www.gpwonline.co.za.

Granato, D., Branco, G. F., Nazzaro, F., Faria, A. F., & Cruz, A. G. (2010). Functional foods and nondairy probiotic food development: trends, concepts, and products. *Comprehensive Reviews in Food Science and Food Safety, 9*(3), 292–302. https://doi.org/10.1111/j.1541-4337.2010.00110.x.

Grand View Research (2019). *Probiotics market size, share & trends analysis report by application (food & beverages, dietary supplements, animal feed), by end-use, by region, and segment forecast, 2018–2024.* Retrieved February 19, 2019, from https://www.zionmarketresearch.com/report/probiotics-market.

Guergoletto, K. B., Saori, C., Mauro, I., & Garcia, S. (2017). Juçara (*Euterpe edulis*) pulp as a substrate for probiotic bacteria fermentation : Optimisation process and antioxidant activity. *Emirates Journal of Food and Agriculture, 29*(12), 949–959. https://doi.org/10.9755/ejfa.2017.v29.i12.1565.

Hassan, A. A., Aly, M. M. A., & El-Hadidie, S. T. (2012). Production of cereal-based probiotic beverages. *World Applied Sciences Journal, 19*(10), 1367–1380. https://doi.org/10.5829/idosi.wasj.2012.19.10.2797.

Hellström, A. M., Vázques-Juárez, R., Svanberg, U., & Andlid, T. A. (2010). Biodiversity and phytase capacity of yeasts isolated from Tanzanian togwa. *International Journal of Food Microbiology, 136*(3), 352–358. https://doi.org/10.1016/j.ijfoodmicro.2009.10.011.

Imsyser Healthy Products (2019). *Probiotics.* https://imsyser.co.za/. Accessed April 6, 2019.

International Probiotics Association (IPA) Europe (2016). *Probiotics in the EU.* http://www.ipaeurope.org/probiotics.php?ID=4. Accessed April 11, 2019.

Islam, M. R., Afrin, S., Khan, T. A., & Howlader, Z. H. (2015). Nutrient content and antioxidant properties of some popular fruits in Bangladesh. *International Journal of Pharmaceutical Sciences and Research, 6*(4), 1407–1414. https://doi.org/10.13040/IJPSR.0975-8232.6(4).1407-14.

Jaiswal, A. K., & Abu-Ghannam, N. (2013). Kinetic studies for the preparation of probiotic cabbage juice: Impact on phytochemicals and bioactivity. *Industrial Crops and Products, 50,* 212–218. https://doi.org/10.1016/j.indcrop.2013.07.028.

Jayabalan, R., Malbaˇ, R. V., Lonˇ, E. S., Vitas, J. S., & Sathishkumar, M. (2014). A review on kombucha tea—Microbiology, composition , fermentation, beneficial effects, toxicity, and tea fungus. *Comprehensive Reviews in Food Science and Food Safety, 13*(4), 538–550. https://doi.org/10.1111/1541-4337.12073.

Kassim, M. A., Baijnath, H., & Odhav, B. (2014). Effect of traditional leafy vegetables on the growth of lactobacilli and bifidobacteria. *International Journal of Food Sciences and Nutrition, 65*(8), 977–980. https://doi.org/10.3109/09637486.2014.945155.

Koh, J. H., Kim, N., Hwang, D., & Lim, Y. H. (2013). Effect of water-soluble fraction of cherry tomatoes on the adhesion of probiotics and Salmonella to intestinal epithelial cells. *Journal of the Science of Food and Agriculture, 93*(15), 3897–3900. https://doi.org/10.1002/jsfa.6255.

Kort, R., Westerik, N., Mariela Serrano, L., Douillard, F. P., Gottstein, W., Mukisa, I. M. , et al. (2015). A novel consortium of *Lactobacillus rhamnosus* and *Streptococcus thermophilus* for increased access to functional fermented foods. *Microbial Cell Factories, 14*(195), 1–14. https://doi.org/10.1186/s12934-015-0370-x.

Lawane, A. I., Aly, S., François, T., Flibert, G., & Yves, T. (2016). Identification and biochemical analysis of microorganisms involved in the fermentation of kawal-A traditional fermented sicklepod leaves (*Senna obtusifolia*). *International Journal of Current Microbiology and Applied Sciences, 5*(9), 261–270. http://doi.org/10.20546/ijcmas.2016.509.029.

Lee, E. S., Song, E. J., Do Nam, Y., & Lee, S. Y. (2018). Probiotics in human health and disease: From nutribiotics to pharmabiotics. *Journal of Microbiology, 56*(11), 773–782. https://doi.org/10.1007/s12275-018-8293-y.

Lei, V., & Jakobsen, M. (2004). Microbiological characterization and probiotic potential of koko and koko sour water, African spontaneously fermented millet porridge and drink. *Journal of Applied Microbiology, 96*(2), 384–397. https://doi.org/10.1046/j.1365-2672.2004.02162.x.

Lorusso, A., Coda, R., Montemurro, M., & Rizzello, G. C. (2018). Use of selected lactic acid bacteria and quinoa flour for manufacturing novel yogurt-like beverages. *Foods, 7*(4), 51–71. https://doi.org/10.3390/foods7040051.

Luana, N., Rossana, C., Curiel, J. A., Kaisa, P., Marco, G., & Rizzello, C. G. (2014). Manufacture and characterization of a yogurt-like beverage made with oat flakes fermented by selected lactic acid bacteria. *International Journal of Food Microbiology, 185,* 17–26. https://doi.org/10.1080/01418639408240221.

Madoroba, E., Steenkamp, E. T., Theron, J., Scheirlinck, I., Cloete, T. E., & Huys, G. (2011). Diversity and dynamics of bacterial populations during spontaneous sorghum fermentations used to produce ting, a South African food. *Systematic and Applied Microbiology, 34*(3), 227–234. https://doi.org/10.1016/j.syapm.2010.11.016.

Mai, A., Dam, M. S., Bujna, E., & Annama, N. (2018). Lactic acid fermentation of apricot juice by mono- and mixed cultures of probiotic *Lactobacillus* and *Bifidobacterium strains. Food Science and Biotechnology, 27*(12), 547–554. https://doi.org/10.1007/s10068-017-0269-x.

Mantzourani, I., Nouska, C., Terpou, A., Alexopoulos, A., Bezirtzoglou, E., Panayiotidis, M. , et al. (2018). Production of a novel functional fruit beverage consisting of cornelian cherry juice and probiotic bacteria. *Antioxidants, 7*(11), 163–173. https://doi.org/10.3390/antiox7110163.

Market Data Forecast, I. (2018). *Middle-East and Africa probiotics market (2018-2023).* https://www.marketdataforecast.com/market-reports/middle-east-and-africa-probiotics-market.

Marsh, A. J., Hill, C., Ross, R. P., & Cotter, P. D. (2014). Fermented beverages with potential : Past and future perspectives. *Trends in Food Science & Technology, 38*(2), 113–124. https://doi.org/10.1016/j.tifs.2014.05.002.

Mensah, J. K., Okoli, R. I., & Eifediyi, K. (2008). Phytochemical, nutritional and medical properties of some leafy vegetables consumed by Edo people of Nigeria. *African Journal of Biotechnology, 7*(14), 2304–2309. https://doi.org/10.5897/AJB08.062.

Mouquet-Rivier, C., Guyot, J., Tou, E. L. H., & Tre, S. (2008). Consumption pattern, biochemical composition and nutritional value of fermented pearl millet gruels in Burkina Faso. *International Journal of Food Sciences and Nutrition, 59*(7–8), 716–729. https://doi.org/10.1080/09637480802206389.

Mpofu, A., Linnemann, A. R., Nout, M. J. R., Zwietering, M. H., Smid, E. J., & den Besten, H. M. W. (2016). Inactivation of bacterial pathogens in yoba mutandabota, a dairy product fermented with the probiotic *Lactobacillus rhamnosus yoba. International Journal of Food Microbiology, 217*, 42–48. https://doi.org/10.1016/j.ijfoodmicro.2015.09.016.

Mpofu, A., Linnemann, A. R., Sybesma, W., Kort, R., Nout, M. J., & Smid, E. J. (2014). Development of a locally sustainable functional food based on mutandabota, a traditional food in southern Africa. *Journal of Dairy Science, 97*(5), 2591–2599. https://doi.org/10.3168/jds.2013-7593.

Muchoki, C. N., Imungi, J. K., & Lamuka, P. O. (2010). Reduction of nitrates, oxalates and phenols in fermented solar-dried stored cowpea (*Vigna unguiculata* L.) leaf vegetables. *Scientific Research, 10*(11), 4398–4412. https://doi.org/10.4236/fns.2012.33054.

Mugula, J. K., Nnko, S. A. M., Narvhus, J. A., & Sørhaug, T. (2003). Microbiological and fermentation characteristics of togwa, a Tanzanian fermented food. *International Journal of Food Microbiology, 80*(3), 187–199. https://doi.org/10.1016/S0168-1605(02)00141-1.

Mustafa, S. M., Chua, L. S., El-Enshasy, H. A., Majid, F. A. A., & Malek, R. A. (2016). A review on fruit juice probiotication : Pomegranate. *Current Nutrition & Food Science, 12*(1), 4–11. https://doi.org/10.2174/1573401311666151015213508.

Mwizerwa, H., Abong, G. O., Mbugua, S. K., Okoth, M. W., Gacheru, P., Muiru, M. , et al. (2018). Profiling of microbial content and growth in fermented maize based products from western Kenya. *Current Research in Nutrition and Food Science, 06*(2), 509–519. https://doi.org/10.12944/CRNFSJ.6.2.25.

Nativa (2016). *Nutritional supplements.* http://www.nativa.co.za/.Accessed April 4, 2019.

NatureFresh Health Products (2019). *NF 047 probiotic-15 liquid: 200ml amber bottle.* http://naturefresh.co.za/products/nf-047-probiotic-15-liquid-200ml-amber-bottle/. Accessed April 14, 2019.

Niyibituronsa, M., Onyango, A. N., Gaidashova, S., Imathiu, S., De Saeger, S., Neirnck, E. , et al. (2019). The growth of different probiotic microorganisms in soymilk from different soybean varieties and their effects on anti-oxidant activity and oligosaccharide content. *Journal of Food Research, 8*(1), 41–51. https://doi.org/10.5539/jfr.v8n1p41.

Nualkaekul, S., Salmeron, I., & Charalampopoulos, D. (2011). Investigation of the factors influencing the survival of *Bifidobacterium longum* in model acidic solutions and fruit juices. *Food Chemistry, 129*(3), 1037–1044. https://doi.org/10.1016/j.foodchem.2011.05.071.

Nyanzi, R., & Jooste, P. J. (2012). Cereal-based functional foods. In E. C. Rigobelo (Ed.), *Probiotics* (pp. 162–188). (3rd ed.). Rijeka, Croatia: IntechOpens.

Nyanzi, R., Jooste, P. J., Abu, J. O., Beukes, E. M., Nyanzi, R., Jooste, P. J. , et al. (2010). Consumer acceptability of a synbiotic version of the maize beverage mageu consumer acceptability of a synbiotic version of the maize beverage mageu. *Development Southern Africa, 27* (3), 447–463. https://doi.org/10.1080/0376835X.2010.498955.

Oguntoyinbo, F. A., Cho, G. S., Trierweiler, B., Kabisch, J., Rösch, N., Neve, H. , et al. (2016). Fermentation of African kale (*Brassica carinata*) using *L. plantarum* BFE 5092 and L. fermentum BFE 6620 starter strains. *International Journal of Food Microbiology, 238*, 103–112. https://doi.org/10.1016/j.ijfoodmicro.2016.08.030.

Oguntoyinbo, F. A., Fusco, V., Cho, G. S., Kabisch, J., Neve, H., Bockelmann, W. , et al. (2016). Produce from Africa's gardens: Potential for leafy vegetable and fruit fermentations. *Frontiers in Microbiology*, *7*(981), 1–14. https://doi.org/10.3389/fmicb.2016.00981.

Oguntoyinbo, F. A., & Narbad, A. (2015). Multifunctional properties of *Lactobacillus plantarum* strains isolated from fermented cereal foods. *Journal of Functional Foods, 17*, 621–631. https://doi.org/10.1016/j.jff.2015.06.022.

Okeke, C. A., Ezekiel, C. N., Nwangburuka, C. C., Sulyok, M., Ezeamagu, C. O., Adeleke, R. A. , et al. (2015). Bacterial diversity and mycotoxin reduction during maize fermentation (steeping) for Ogi production. *Frontiers in Microbiology*, *6*(1402), 1–12. https://doi.org/10.3389/fmicb.2015.01402.

Olaoye, O. A., Ndife, J., & Raymond, V. I. (2017). Use of *Lactobacillus plantarum* as Starter Culture and Its Influence on Physicochemical , Microbiological, and Sensory Characteristics of Kunnu-Aya Produced from Sorghum and Tigernut. *Journal of Food Quality*, *2017*(Article ID 6738137), 1–8. https://doi.org/10.1155/2017/6738137.

Olasupo, N. A., Okorie, C. P., & Oguntoyinbo, F. A. (2016). The biotechnology of Ugba, a Nigerian traditional fermented food condiment. *Frontiers in Microbiology*, *7*(1153), 1–10. https://doi.org/10.3389/fmicb.2016.01153.

Ouoba, L. I. I., Parkouda, C., Sawadogo, H., Kobawila, S. C., & Keleke, S. (2010). Genotypic diversity of lactic acid bacteria isolated from African traditional alkaline-fermented foods. *Journal of Applied Microbiology*, *108*(6), 2019–2029. https://doi.org/10.1111/j.1365-2672.2009.04603.x.

Owusu-Kwarteng, J., Tano-Debrah, K., Akabanda, F., & Jespersen, L. (2015). Technological properties and probiotic potential of *Lactobacillus fermentum* strains isolated from West African fermented millet dough. *BMC Microbiology*, *15*(1), 261–271. https://doi.org/10.1186/s12866-015-0602-6.

Panghal, A., Janghu, S., Virkar, K., Gat, Y., Kumar, V., & Chhikara, N. (2018). Potential non-dairy probiotic products – A healthy approach. *Food Bioscience*, *21*(December 2017), 80–89. https://doi.org/10.1016/j.fbio.2017.12.003.

Parvez, S., Malik, K. A., Ah Kang, S., & Kim, H. Y. (2006). Probiotics and their fermented food products are beneficial for health. *Journal of Applied Microbiology*, *100*(6), 1171–1185. https://doi.org/10.1111/j.1365-2672.2006.02963.x.

Perricone, M., Bevilacqua, A., Altieri, C., Sinigaglia, M., & Corbo, M. R. (2015). Challenges for the production of probiotic fruit juices. *Beverages*, *1*(2), 95–103. https://doi.org/10.3390/beverages1020095.

Perricone, M., Corbo, M. R., Sinigaglia, M., Speranza, B., & Bevilacqua, A. (2014). Viability of *Lactobacillus reuteri* in fruit juices. *Journal of Functional Foods*, *10*, 421–426. https://doi.org/10.1016/j.jff.2014.07.020.

Petreska-Ivanovska, T., Petrushevska-Tozi, L., Grozdanov, A., Petkovska, R., Hadjieva, J., Popovski, E. , et al. (2014). From optimization of synbiotic microparticles prepared by spray-drying to development of new functional carrot juice. *Chemical Industry and Chemical Engineering Quarterly*, *20*(4), 549–564. https://doi.org/10.2298/CICEQ130218036P.

Prasad, J., Gill, H., Smart, J., & Gopal, P. K. (1999). Selection and characterisation of *Lactobacillus* and *Bifidobacterium* strains for use as probiotics. *International Dairy Journal*, *8*(12), 993–1002. https://doi.org/10.1016/S0958-6946(99)00024-2.

Profir, G. A., Neagu, V. C., & Camelia, V. (2015). Impact of Nutrients on the Probiotic Survival and Sensory Properties of Vegetables Juice. *Romanian Biotechnological Letters*, *20*(6), 11041–11048.

Puritan Healthy (2016). *Products*. http://puritan-egypt.com/Product.aspx?ID=53. Accessed April 6, 2019.

Rameda Pharmaceutical (2015). https://www.ramedapharma.com/gastro-intestinal-tract/15-products/gastro-intestinal-tract/64-lacteol-fort. Accessed April 11, 2019.

Reid, G. (2010). The potential role for probiotic yogurt for people living with HIV/AIDS. *Gut Microbes*, *1*(6), 411–414. https://doi.org/10.4161/gmic.1.6.14079.

Reid, G. (2016). Probiotics : Definition, scope and mechanisms of action. *Best Practice & Research Clinical Gastroenterology*, *30*(1), 17–25. https://doi.org/10.1016/j.bpg.2015.12.001.

Reid, G., Kort, R., Alvarez, S., Bourdet-Sicard, R., Cunningham, M., Saulnier, D. , et al. (2018). Expanding the reach of probiotics through social enterprises. *Beneficial Microbes*, *9*(5), 707–715. https://doi.org/10.3920/BM2018.0015.

Rezac, S., Kok, C. R., Heermann, M., & Hutkins, R. (2018). Fermented foods as a dietary source of live organisms. *Frontiers in Microbiology*, *9*(1785), 1–29. https://doi.org/10.3389/fmicb.2018.01785.

Roberfroid, M. (2007). Prebiotics : The concept revisited. *The Journal of Nutrition*, *137*(3), 830S–837S. https://doi.org/10.1093/jn/137.3.830S.

Rodrigues, D., Sousa, S., Gomes, A. M., Pintado, M. M., Silva, J. P., Costa, P. , et al. (2012). Storage stability of *Lactobacillus paracasei* as free cells or encapsulated in alginate-based microcapsules in low pH fruit juices. *Food and Bioprocess Technology*, *5*(7), 2748–2757. https://doi.org/10.1007/s11947-011-0581-z.

Russo, P., Pia, M., Fiocco, D., Capozzi, V., Drider, D., & Spano, G. (2017). *Lactobacillus plantarum* with broad antifungal activity : A promising approach to increase safety and shelf-life of cereal-based products. *International Journal of Food Microbiology*, *247*, 48–54. https://doi.org/10.1016/j.ijfoodmicro.2016.04.027.

Sagdic, O., Ozturk, I., Yapar, N., & Yetim, H. (2014). Diversity and probiotic potentials of lactic acid bacteria isolated from gilaburu, a traditional Turkish fermented European cranberry bush (*Viburnum opulus* L.) fruit drink. *Food Research International*, *64*, 537–545. https://doi.org/10.1016/j.foodres.2014.07.045.

Salmerón, I., Thomas, K., & Pandiella, S. S. (2014). Effect of substrate composition and inoculum on the fermentation kinetics and flavour compound profiles of potentially non-dairy probiotic formulations. *LWT - Food Science and Technology*, *55*(1), 240–247. https://doi.org/10.1016/j.lwt.2013.07.008.

Salmerón, I., Thomas, K., & Pandiella, S. S. (2015). Effect of potentially probiotic lactic acid bacteria on the physicochemical composition and acceptance of fermented cereal beverages. *Journal of Functional Foods*, *15*, 106–115. https://doi.org/10.1016/j.jff.2015.03.012.

Salvetti, E., & Toole, P. W. O. (2017). When regulation challenges innovation : The case of the genus *Lactobacillus*. *Trends in Food Science & Technology*, *66*, 187–194. https://doi.org/10.1016/j.tifs.2017.05.009.

Sanchez-Zapata, E., Fernandez-Lopez, J., & Perez-Alvarez, J. A. (2012). Tiger Nut (*Cyperus esculentus*) commercialization : Health aspects , composition, properties, and food applications. *Comprehensive Reviews in Food Science and Food Safety*, *11*(4), 366–377. https://doi.org/10.1111/j.1541-4337.2012.00190.x.

Sanders, M. E. (1998). Overview of functional foods : Emphasis on probiotic bacteria. *International Dairy Journal*, *8*(5–6), 341–347. https://doi.org/10.1016/S0958-6946(98)00056-9.

Septembre-Malaterre, A., Remize, F., & Poucheret, P. (2018). Fruits and vegetables, as a source of nutritional compounds and phytochemicals: Changes in bioactive compounds during lactic fermentation. *Food Research International, 104*(September 2017), 86–99. https://doi.org/10.1016/j.foodres.2017.09.031.

Shori, A. B. (2016). Influence of food matrix on the viability of probiotic bacteria : A review based on dairy and non-dairy beverages. *Food Bioscience, 13,* 1–8. https://doi.org/10.1016/j.fbio.2015.11.001.

Sozbilen, G. S., Korel, F., & Yemenicioğlu, A. (2018). Control of lactic acid bacteria in fermented beverages using lysozyme and nisin: test of traditional beverage boza as a model food system. *International Journal of Food Science and Technology, 53*(10), 2357–2368. https://doi.org/10.1111/ijfs.13828.

Spence, C., & Spence, C. (2016). *The Noakes Foundation's Newest Affiliate : Probyo.* Retrieved March 21, 2019, from https://thenoakesfoundation.org/news/media/the-noakes-foundations-newest-affiliate-probyo.

Sthapit, B., Rao, V., & Sthapit, S. (2012). *Tropical fruit tree species and climate change. Bioversity international.* New Delhi, India: Bioversity International. Retrieved from http://www.ecoagriculture.org/documents/files/doc_420.pdf.

Tamang, J. P., Watanabe, K., & Holzapfel, W. H. (2016). Review: Diversity of microorganisms in global fermented foods and beverages. *Frontiers in Microbiology, 7*(377), 1–28. https://doi.org/10.3389/fmicb.2016.00377.

Tennant, D. R., Davidson, J., Day, A. J., Limited, A. U. K., Anne, S., Drive, C. L. , et al. (2014). Phytonutrient intakes in relation to European fruit and vegetable consumption patterns observed in different food surveys. *British Journal of Nutrition, 112*(7), 1214–1225. https://doi.org/10.1017/S0007114514001950.

The European Parliament and Council of the European Union (EU) (2006). Regulation (EC) No 1924/2006 of the European parliament and of the council on nutrition and health claims made on foods. *Official Journal of the European Union, L*(404), 9–25. Retrieved from http://eur-lex.europa.eu/legal-content/EN/TXT/PDF/?uri=CELEX:32006R1924&from=en.

Todorov, S. D., Botes, M., Guigas, C., Schillinger, U., Wiid, I., Wachsman, M. B. , et al. (2008). Boza, a natural source of probiotic lactic acid bacteria. *Journal of Applied Microbiology, 104*(2), 465–477. https://doi.org/10.1111/j.1365-2672.2007.03558.x.

Town, O., State, O., & State, O. (2018). Microbial interaction in selected fermented vegetable condiments in Nigeria. *International Food Research Journal, 25*(1), 439–446.

Turpin, W. (2011). Genetic screening of functional properties of lactic acid bacteria in a fermented pearl millet slurry and in the metagenome of fermented starchy foods. *Applied and Environmental Microbiology, 77*(24), 8722–8734. https://doi.org/10.1128/AEM.05988-11.

U.S. Food & Drug Administration (FDA) (2019). *GRAS notice inventory. U.S. Food & Drug Administration.* Silver Spring, MD: U.S. Food & Drug Administration. Retrieved from https://www.fda.gov/Food/IngredientsPackagingLabeling/GRAS/NoticeInventory/default.htm.

Valero-Cases, E., & Frutos, M. J. (2017). Effect of inulin on the viability of *L. plantarum* during storage and in vitro digestion and on composition parameters of vegetable fermented juices. *Plant Foods for Human Nutrition, 72*(2), 161–167. https://doi.org/10.1007/s11130-017-0601-x.

Valero-Cases, E., Roy, N. C., Frutos, M. J., Anderson, R. C., Frutos, M. J., & Anderson, R. C. (2017). Influence of the fruit juice carriers on the ability of *Lactobacillus plantarum* DSM20205 to improve in vitro intestinal barrier integrity and its probiotic properties. *Journal of Agricultural and Food Chemistry, 65*(28), 5632–5638. https://doi.org/10.1021/acs.jafc.7b01551.

Van, V. J., & Brouns, F. J. P. H. (2015). Nutrition and health claims as marketing tools nutrition and health claims as marketing tools. *Critical Reviews in Food Science and Nutrition, 55*(11), 1552–1560. https://doi.org/10.1080/10408398.2012.754738.

Van Wyk, B. E. (2011). The potential of South African plants in the development of new food and beverage products. *South African Journal of Botany, 77*(4), 857–868. https://doi.org/10.1016/j.sajb.2011.08.003.

Vasudha, S., & Mishra, H. N. N. (2013). Non dairy probiotic beverages. *International Food Research Journal, 20*(1), 7–15. https://doi.org/10.1109/MWSCAS.2007.4488836.

Vera-Pingitore, E., Jimenez, M. E., Dallagnol, A., Belfiore, C., Fontana, C., Fontana, P. , et al. (2016). Screening and characterization of potential probiotic and starter bacteria for plant fermentations. *LWT - Food Science and Technology, 71*, 288–294. https://doi.org/10.1016/j.lwt.2016.03.046.

Verhagen, H., Vos, E., Francl, S., Heinonen, M., & Van Loveren, H. (2012). Status of nutrition and health claims in Europe. *Archives of Biochemistry and Biophysics, 501*(1), 6–15. https://doi.org/10.1016/j.abb.2010.04.012.

Vij, S., Hati, S., & Yadav, D. (2011). Biofunctionality of probiotic soy yoghurt. *Food and Nutrition Sciences, 2*(5), 502–509. https://doi.org/10.4236/fns.2011.25073.

Wacoo, A. P., Mukisa, I. M., Meeme, R., Byakika, S., Wendiro, D., Sybesma, W. , et al. (2019). Probiotic enrichment and reduction of aflatoxins in a traditional African maize-based fermented food. *Nutrients, 11*(2), 265–280. https://doi.org/10.3390/nu11020265.

Westerik, N., Kort, R., Sybesma, W., & Reid, G. (2018). *Lactobacillus rhamnosus* probiotic food as a tool for empowerment across the value chain in Africa. *Frontiers in Microbiology, 9* (1501), 1–6. https://doi.org/10.3389/fmicb.2018.01501.

Westerik, N., Wacoo, A. P., Sybesma, W., & Kort, R. (2016). Novel production protocol for small-scale manufacture of probiotic fermented foods. *Journal of Visualized Experiments, 115*(e54365), 1–8. https://doi.org/10.3791/54365.

White, L. E., Bannerman, E., & Gillett, P. M. (2016). Coeliac disease and the gluten-free diet : A review of the burdens ; factors associated with adherence and impact on health-related quality of life, with specific focus on adolescence. *Journal of Human Nutrition and Dietetics, 29*(3), 593–606. https://doi.org/10.1111/jhn.12375.

Willett, W., Rockström, J., Loken, B., Springmann, M., Lang, T., Vermeulen, S. , et al. (2019). Food in the anthropocene: the EAT-Lancet Commission on healthy diets from sustainable food systems. *The Lancet, 393*(10170), 447–492. https://doi.org/10.1016/S0140-6736(18)31788-4.

World Health Organization (WHO) (2013). *A global brief on hypertension.* https://apps.who.int/iris/bitstream/handle/10665/79059/WHO_DCO_WHD_2013.2_eng.pdf;jsessionid=2BAAA779A2BA6155E42DEB413E68FA98?sequence=1.

Zielinska, D., & Kolozyn-Krajewska, D. (2018). Food-origin lactic acid bacteria may exhibit probiotic properties: Review. *BioMed Research International, 2018*(5063185), 1–15. https://doi.org/10.1155/2018/5063185.

CHAPTER

9

The Americas

Inge Russell

ICBD, Heriot Watt University, Edinburgh, United Kingdom

9.1 Introduction

The Americas, encompassing both North and South America, produce a large number of probiotic beverages. Some of these beverages are produced by large global manufacturers and others by smaller local companies or even produced in the home. Local regulations on what is a probiotic beverage and how is its production and safety monitored vary greatly. This chapter explores probiotic beverage production, regulation, and some historical indigenous beverages, with a primary focus on the USA, Canada, Mexico, Brazil, and Argentina. According to the World Health Organization (WHO) and the Food and Agriculture Organization (FAO), for microorganisms to be considered probiotic, they must be "live microorganisms that, when administered in adequate amounts, confer a health benefit on the host." Although not all countries have detailed rules and regulations around probiotics, this definition is widely accepted. Regulations around the advertised health benefits of probiotic beverages is where countries diverge in their different approaches to what claims are allowed and how they are communicated.

In both North America and Latin America, cardiovascular health, digestive health, and weight management are high on the list of consumer concerns (Euromonitor, 2018).

Mintel (2018) reports that from 2013 to 2017, there were 4378 products launched globally (this includes new products, line extensions, new packaging, relaunches, and new formulations) on which packaging included claims for "functional-digestive properties." The highest number of these launches was in the USA (51% in 2017), followed by China, Russia, Canada, and Brazil. Packaging claims specifically related to dairy products with a label declaring a "functional digestive property," came most often from the countries of Japan, China, Canada, and the USA, in that order.

Probiotic Beverages
https://doi.org/10.1016/B978-0-12-818588-9.00021-8

9.2 The USA and probiotic beverages

Increasing demand for probiotic fortified foods to replace pharmaceutical products is an emerging trend in the global marketplace. In North America, there has been a rise in lifestyle-related diseases, such as diabetes and obesity, which is generating growing interest in disease prevention through healthy eating, and with the COVID-19 global pandemic in 2020, the desire to boost one's immune status through a range of approaches, including healthy eating, has been heightened as a priority for consumers.

In 2019, the overall global probiotics market was valued at USD 48.9 billion (Fortune Business Insights, 2020). The US probiotic food and beverage market was valued at about USD 2.8 billion in 2017 (Grandview Research, 2018). Beverages represent a growing share of the probiotic market. The rise in the sale of digestive health beverages has been significant, with retail sales rising from USD 17 million in 2013 to USD 37 million in 2017 to a projected USD 65 million in 2022. A 2012 National Health Interview Survey reported that 4 million US adults had used probiotics or prebiotics, in various forms, in the past month (NCCIH, 2020). Probiotics in a drink form have a unique appeal to time-pressed consumers who are looking for convenience and Millennials who are looking for innovative new drinks that offer a variety of taste and flavor options. Middle-aged adults interested in maintaining their digestive health are an increasing market segment, as probiotic drink marketing materials emphasize both the drink's health benefits and its convenience. The probiotic drink market is dominated by a few major companies (e.g., Amul, Yakult, PepsiCo-Kevita Inc., Lifeway, and Goodbelly), with small and regional players maintaining local popularity through innovative drink introductions.

9.3 Regulation of use in the USA

The US government's regulation of probiotics is complex and is focused on the probiotic's intended use.

If sold as a dietary supplement, then it does not require FDA approval before being marketed. Claims about how the product affects the structure or function of the body are allowed, but health claims such as "the supplement will lower your risk of a specific disease" are not allowed without FDA approval.

If sold as a drug for treating a disease or disorder, then there are stricter requirements that must be met. It must be proven to be safe and effective for the intended use through clinical trials and the FDA must approve the product before it can be sold.

If a probiotic is an ingredient in a food product, then the probiotic must either be approved by the FDA as a "food additive" or be a "GRAS" (generally recognized as safe) organism.

Probiotics currently on the US market are foods or dietary supplements. To date, no probiotic products have been approved by the FDA to treat, lessen, cure, or prevent specific diseases.

All probiotic strains are not created equal. Even within the same species, there will be variations. The particular strains used in probiotic drinks should be easily discernable by the consumer, especially when consumers today are demanding more transparency regarding product ingredients (e.g., non-GMO), and they also want to know about a manufacturing company's adherence to sustainability and the company's social conscience.

A recent publication by Binda et al. (2020) recommends four simple criteria that could be used to conclude whether a specific strain of microorganism qualifies as a probiotic for use in foods and dietary supplements, as the term probiotic is too often misused. They recommend the following:

> 1. *Sufficiently characterized*
> 2. *Safe for the intended use*
> 3. *Supported by at least one positive human clinical trial conducted according to generally accepted scientific standards*
> 4. *Alive in the product at an efficacious dose throughout the product's shelf life.*
>
> **Binda et al. (2020)**

There are many probiotic drinks on the market ranging from Kombuchas, to sparkling waters, to sodas, to drinkable yogurts, to shots. A new beverage was launched in the summer of 2020 by Chobani. It is a plant-based line of probiotic drinks called Chobani probiotic, which caters to the rise in health-consciousness and the emerging veganism trend. This new line is marketed as a fermented, plant-based drink made with organic fruit juice, botanicals, and immunity-supporting probiotics. The product line includes variations, such as their "Pineapple Turmeric," with ingredients such as oats, various juices, apple cider vinegar, turmeric, and probiotic bacteria (Chobani, 2020). In this example, one can see that health claims on the product are limited to the wording "Probiotics for Immunity" and the statement that the cultures "stay live" in the product. The probiotics in this probiotic drink product would fall under the classification of "ingredient in a food product," and the health benefit on the packaging is limited to "for immunity."

9.4 Canada

The Canadian probiotic market was USD 660 million in 2019 and is forecast to reach USD 1027 million by 2025 (Researchandmarkets, 2020b). Canada has a population of almost 38 million people, with 90% of Canadians living within 160 km of the US border, and food products that flow easily in both directions across the Canada/US border.

During a recent survey by Health and Wellness Canada (AAFC, 2018), when asked which food product features were important for their health, 40% of Canadian respondents identified "contains probiotics," and 29% identified "contains prebiotics." The top product feature identified most frequently in the survey as important to the respondents was fiber (66%).

In 2019, the most popular probiotic drink products in Canada were yogurt and sour milk drinks, with three major players accounting for 75% of retail value sales (Groupe Danone, General Mills, and Agropur Co-operative Agro-Alimentaire). Newer probiotic drink entrants into the Canadian market include probiotic sparkling waters, iced teas, plant-based drinks, and various kefir drinks, such as Ryazhenka, an unsweetened Russian style kefir with a creamy caramel taste, made with baked whole milk (Euromonitor, 2019).

With a plethora of probiotic drinks on the market, selecting one for a consumer's specific needs can be difficult. In Canada, a useful example of how to make an informed purchase choice on a probiotic beverage can be found in a report called the "2020 Clinical Guide to Probiotic Products Available in Canada, Indications, Dosage Formats, and Clinical Evidence to Date, 12th edition." Products are included on the list only if four strict criteria are met:

> 1. *The product must be commercially available in Canada (supplement or probiotic-containing food).*
> 2. *Have FDA GRAS status (FDA) or a Health Canada Natural Product Number for the probiotic strains used.*
> 3. *There is favorable published clinical evidence for the strains used in the product.*
> 4. *Results must be for the specified combination (not an extrapolation from evidence for separate probiotic strains).*
>
> ***AEProbio (2020)***

With these strict criteria, the list of functional foods with probiotics that meet all four criteria is currently relatively short, with the largest number focused on products for babies and toddlers, where more extensive research is historically available. For adults, one can find probiotic beverages on the list. For example, Goodbellys' Probiotic Juice Drinks is a listed product with the following relevant information: *L. plantarum229v*, 20 billion CFU/8 oz. serving, one serving/day recommended, and with the specific areas targeted as the prevention of antibiotic-associated diarrhea

(AAD—evidence level 3) and irritable bowel syndrome (IBS—evidence level 1). The paper describes what the level of evidence means (1 is highest level) and gives the reader references to the relevant publications/studies. In a similar manner, a Yakult bottled product is described as: *L. casei* Shirota, 88 billion CFU/80 mL bottle, 1–2 servings/day, recommended for constipation (evidence level 1), common infectious disease—community acquired (CID—evidence level 1), mood and affect (symptoms related to stress/anxiety)—(M/A-evidence level 2). For fermented milk liquids, products from Activia and DanActive are listed with species *B. (animalis) lactis* CNCM I-2494 and *L. casei* sp. Paracasei CNCM I-1518, respectively, and similar to the two previous examples, additional specific information is provided as well.

The value of this particular report is the fact-based guidance on Canadian probiotic products that it provides. There is transparency in terms of information on what the product contains, the dose, and the effectiveness claims are backed up with scientific studies in a manner that is accessible to the reader and generally understandable. Hopefully, this type of listing will become more common and continue in the future to guide both prescribers and consumers through the often-bewildering claims on probiotic drink products, helping to match a drink's benefit with the particular health issue the consumer is seeking to address.

9.5 Canadian regulations governing claims on probiotics

In 2009, the Canadian Government Food Directorate, Health Products and Food Branch issued a guidance document on the use of probiotic microorganisms in food (probiotic beverages being included in this group), which defines health claims, function claims, and therapeutic claims. (Canadian Food Directorate, Health Products and Food Branch (Government of Canada), 2009).

Currently, there are clear guidelines from the Canadian Food Inspection Agency (CFIA, 2019) on definitions, strain-specific and nonstrain-specific claims, including a table of acceptable nonstrain specific claims for probiotics. This table lists eligible species and minimum levels in the product. One serving of a stated size of a product should contain a minimum level of 1.0×10^9 CFUs of one or more of the eligible microorganism(s) that is (are) the subject of the claim.

In Canada, the use of the term prebiotic is well defined in how and when it can be used. The CCFIA is responsible for compliance and enforcement of labeling requirements related to food. However, it is Health Canada that carries out this role for Natural Health Products, and it is Health Canada that determines a product's classification as a food or a Natural Health Product.

The following is an excerpt from the Health Canada website to clarify the status of a probiotic: "Food products containing probiotic microorganisms are generally classified as food. Where a food product is represented as having a therapeutic use or purpose (e.g., carrying claims about disease risk reduction or treatment), the product is generally classified as a natural health product, depending on the nature of and risks associated with the microorganism and taking into consideration the product's represented therapeutic use, as well as the history of use and public perception of the product's intended use" (Health Canada, 2009).

An example of a recent approval for a natural health product with a therapeutic use claim is Kaneka's Floradapt Cardio, a patented probiotic solution of *L. plantarum* strains, which is aimed at reducing cardiovascular health hazards. They received a Health Canada Class III approval under the Natural Health Products Directorate and can identify using the Natural Product Number (NPN) 80096187. They are allowed to advertise in Canada with the claim that Floradapt is a "source of probiotics that can promote favorable gut flora and support cardiovascular health" (Floradapt Press Release, 2020).

Although this product is not sold as a probiotic beverage, but rather as a once a day capsule, one can envisage beverage product applications in the future applying for similar government approval for therapeutic claims with well-studied strains, especially knowing that the trend is for consumers to move from probiotics in capsules to probiotics in beverages. More and more consumers are moving away from high-sugar sodas and looking for nutrient-filled drinks that are convenient, that can act as a health-promoting snack or meal, and that are made with all-natural ingredients that are ethically sourced or locally produced.

In Canada, there has been a rise in the sales of beverages tied to cardiovascular health in terms of retail sales, from USD 32 million in 2013 to USD 38 million in 2017, to a projected USD 46 million in 2022. These sales have been in the area of heart-healthy ingredients, such as omegas, plant sterols, and complex carbohydrates, as well as in the area of digestive health, with a focus on maintaining a healthy gut flora (AAFC, 2018).

9.6 Mexico

With its population of 129 million, Mexico shares a border of over 3000 km with the USA. Despite the influences of multinationals distributing similar probiotic beverages in North America, there are significant differences in awareness of probiotics and in government regulations between Mexico, the USA, and Canada. Currently, Mexico does not have an approved health claim regulation associated with probiotics, but a proposal named Draft NOM-086 (2015) was published in 2015 to allow health claims related to probiotics to be used on food and supplements.

A 2017 survey looked at factors influencing eating and drinking decisions in Mexico. It identified the top three factors that influence consumer purchase decisions as low in sugar (52%), GMO-free (49%), and low in fat (49%), with contains prebiotics or probiotics (33%) in eighth place in terms of influence (GFK Insights, 2017). Mexico has a lower awareness of the benefits of probiotics than the USA (Mintel, 2018). A survey by Valdovinos-García, Abreu, and Valdovinos-Díaz (2019) examined the use of probiotics in Mexico and assessed knowledge by gastroenterologists and nutritionists. The survey indicated that overall, the concept of probiotics was well understood by health professionals, that they frequently recommended probiotics, and that they considered them to be safe.

Mexico also has an abundance of locally produced traditional probiotic beverages. Many of these beverages were traditionally used for nutritional, medicinal, and ceremonial purposes. These include Atole agrio, Pozol, Tejuino, Tepache, and Pulque (Pérez-Armendáriz & Cadoso-Ugarte, 2020; Romero-Luna, Hernández-Sánchez, & Dávila-Ortiz, 2017). A long shelf life, consistency, and quality are not easy to achieve when products are produced on a very small scale, however microbial (probiotic) viability is probably still high because the beverage is consumed shortly after the fermentation is complete. Although refrigeration can extend the shelf life somewhat, refrigeration is not sufficient to identify the product as a shelf-stable drink. The lessons that commercial producers of traditional products, such as Kombucha, have learned about maintaining shelf life as production moved from a craft product to a mainstream probiotic beverage in North American grocery stores, will prove useful for other locally produced drinks (Behera & Panda, 2020).

Atole agrio is a typical Mexican fermented maize porridge/thin gruel beverage connected to the Mazateche indigenous community in the north of Sierra Madre de Oazaca. Sour atole is a drink consumed during festive occasions as a refreshing, nonalcoholic sour drink (Väkeväinen et al., 2018). Usually consumed from May to September, tender maize is used to prepare it. Tender maize (called maize de dobla) is used as the raw material in a simple process. The maize is not soaked or boiled prior to a very short spontaneous fermentation (mainly lactic acid bacteria, LAB), with the end product boiled before consumption. The final product can be consumed unflavored or flavored (cinnamon, cocoa, and sugar).

Pozol is a whitish porridge drink prepared by fermenting a corn dough. It is consumed in Southeastern Mexico with origins in Pre-Columbian Mexico. The drink has a slightly acidic taste and is nonalcoholic. Variations of pozol include added sugar, honey, cocoa, chili, salt, or lemon. Historically, the fermented corn doughs (corn balls) were used as a provision for long journeys through the jungle as they are rich in nutrients, amino acids, vitamins, and fiber. The drink is made by soaking the dough ball in water (Fig. 9.1). In addition to its use as a refreshing drink, it

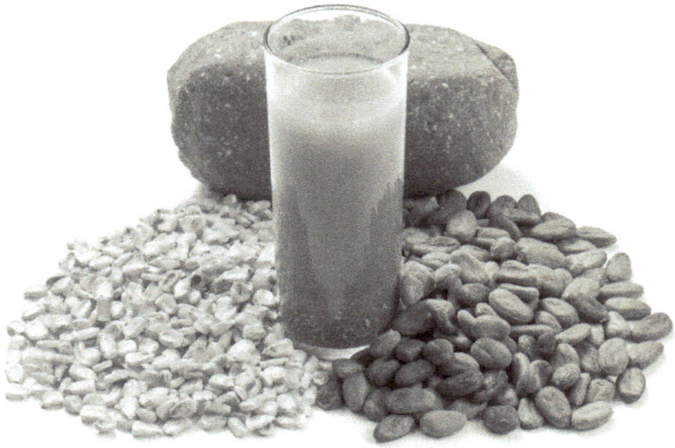

FIG. 9.1 Pozol beverage showing dough ball, corn kernels, and raw cacao beans (Shutterstock).

is also used for religious ceremonies and as a medicine. It is primarily a LAB natural fermentation (up to 4 days), and it is speculated that pozol's medicinal properties to control diarrhea and reduce fever are due to the mix of microflora present in the fermentation (Väkeväinen et al., 2018).

Tejuino is a drink that dates back to pre-Columbian times. It is very popular in the Mexican state of Jalisco. It is traditionally made from corn dough (masa used for tortillas) mixed with water and unrefined cane sugar (piloncillo), boiled, and this is followed by a short (3 day) spontaneous fermentation in a clay pot, which results in a very low alcohol content drink. The beverage is served cold, often with lime juice, a pinch of salt, and shaved ice. *Weissella cibaria* and *Leuconostoc citreum* have been isolated from Tejuino fermentations and provide some of the probiotic properties of the drink (Silva et al., 2017).

Tepache uses the peel and rind of pineapples as the raw material, with cane sugar (piloncillo) or brown sugar as a sweetener and powdered cinnamon as the seasoning. The fermentation is short (up to 3 days), so the drink is very low in alcohol and is sold cold, mainly by street vendors. It is a drink easily produced at home. Fermented fruit beverages in Mexico are often fermented with starters called tibicos, and these are similar in function to kefir grains.

Pulque is a nondistilled alcoholic beverage produced by fermenting the sap of the agave plant. The drink has a sour yeast-like/buttermilk-like taste. It is a traditional beverage of central Mexico (Fig. 9.2), and it is a rapid fermentation (3–6 h) that produces 2%–6% alcohol. The product has a very short shelf life and spoils within a few days. A diverse number

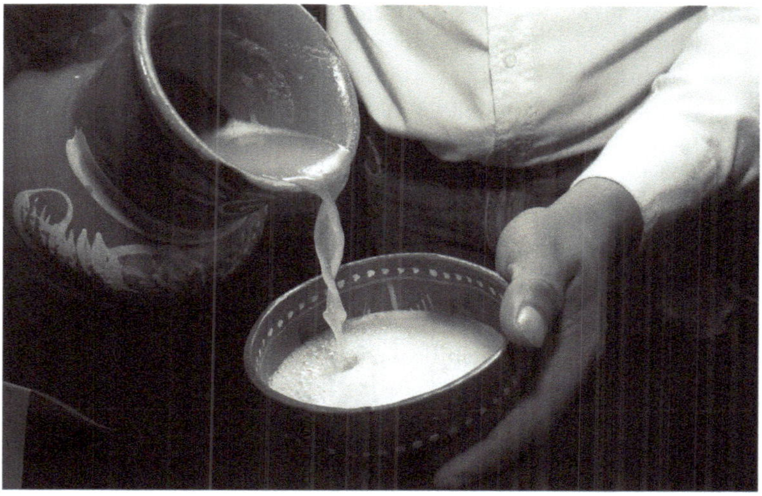

FIG. 9.2 Pulque being poured into drinking cup from the fermentation vessel (Shutterstock).

of probiotic/LAB have been identified in samples examined (Giles-Gómez et al., 2016). The drink is reputed to have various health benefits due to the presence of different probiotic bacteria. It is rich in nutrients, containing minerals, and amino acids, as well as vitamins B and C. It is also said to reduce cholesterol since it contains the enzyme, bile salt hydrolase.

9.7 Latin America

With almost 600 million inhabitants, Latin America is one of the most dynamic and diverse regional markets in the world, with large economic, political, cultural, and social differences. Regulatory statuses vary widely as regulations for probiotics are usually determined at national levels, but there is increased global and regional harmonization occurring in Latin America. The regulatory status and generic claims in 2018, for a number of Latin American countries, are well summarized by Morán (2018).

Comparing per capita consumption of probiotics, Latin America places fourth (USD 1.98/year) after Europe (USD 12.87/year) and the USA (USD 6.34/year), with Asia (USD 2.16/year) and Africa (USD 0.45/year) in third and fifth place. The highest probiotic retail value sales per year are in Brazil (USD 3034), Mexico (USD 680), and Argentina (USD 207) (Euromonitor, 2018).

A Mintel survey of Latin American consumer health concerns lists aging, eye health, and intestinal regularity as the top concerns. Growth drivers are health and wellness trends, recommendations from doctors, friends, and family, and consumer education on probiotics. The COVID-19 pandemic is adding a new level of attention to health with consumers searching for products that promote a healthy body, boost immunity, contribute to digestive health, and are part of a sustainable lifestyle, sometimes described as "clean and green."

The number of plant-based beverage launches has doubled over the past 3 years (Innova Database, September 2019). The value of the probiotic market in Latin America (encompassing Central and South America and Mexico) in 2018 was USD 5.58 billion, and in 2023, it is expected to be USD 7.73 billion (Marketdataforecast, 2020). However, retail sales of probiotic milk formula products decreased in sales value from USD 1037 million in 2013 to USD 763 million in 2017 (AAFC, 2018).

Brazil. In the Latin American probiotic product market, Brazil is the fastest growing market and represents 52% of the market (followed by Mexico at 28%). Brazil's probiotic market is still developing and claims benefiting digestion are the main benefit sought by consumers (Mordor Intelligence, 2019). The overall Brazilian probiotic market has an estimated value of USD 1495 million and is expected to reach a market size of USD 2245 million by 2025, at a CAGR of 7% (Researchandmarkets, 2020a).

In order to claim that a dietary supplement is good for the digestive system on a product's packaging, the Brazilian health regulatory agency Agência Nacional de Vigilância Sanitária (ANVISA), regulates that the claim must be scientifically proven (Resolution RDC No. 241/2018). ANVISA evaluates applications based on unequivocal proof of the identity of the probiotic microorganism's lineage, safety, and beneficial effect. An example of such an approval by ANVISA was for the 2018 *Bifidobacterium lactis* HN019 probiotic strain from the company DuPont Nutrition & Health, where it was ruled that the scientific data supported this probiotic strain's gastrointestinal health and immune function benefits. This meant that the company could then include the claim "Bifidobacterium lactis HN019™ may contribute to gastrointestinal health" on their product packaging. In 2019, ANVISA approved claims for a psychobiotic (a term used to refer to live bacteria that, when ingested, may confer a mental health benefit by affecting the microbiota of the host organism). The approved psychobiotic is a combination of Lallemand's *Lactobacillus helveticus* Rosell®-52 and *Bifidobacterium longum* Rosell®-175 with the following approved wording "May contribute to a reduction of feelings of anxiety in healthy individuals and the reduction of gastrointestinal complications such as abdominal pain and nausea/vomit brought on by light to moderate stress in healthy individuals." This product statement had also, with similar claims, been approved earlier for use by Health Canada's NNHPD.

Argentina. Attempts at harmonized probiotic guidelines for products in Latin America have been a work in progress (Binda et al., 2020; FAO/WHO, 2002). FAO/WHO guidelines have not been widely implemented and only a few countries have regulations on probiotics. Argentina incorporated into its food regulatory framework a definition of probiotics, a guide for evaluating a probiotic as a food ingredient, and a definition of food with probiotics.

Argentina offers an interesting example of a government program to improve children's health with a focus on a probiotic food/drink. Government actions by the Social Development Ministry in Argentina implemented a social program to improve the health and nutrition of children using a probiotic fermented milk in the form of a yogurt called "Yogurito," which contains the probiotic bacteria *L. rhamnosus* CRL1505. This probiotic bacteria had been found to have a positive influence on children's health in trials conducted in Argentina (Villena et al., 2012). Since 2008, the "Yogurito Social Program" has been providing a daily probiotic product to more than 300,000 school children in Tucumán and some 50,000 in other provinces and municipalities of Argentina. The product moved from just a yogurt (Yogurito) to "Chocolet," a chocolate-flavored probiotic drink, whose distribution was alternated with the yogurt, and finally with the addition of "Biosec," a dehydrated probiotic that could be reconstituted in milk or juice, thus avoiding the issue of having to provide the product in a refrigerated form (Bortz, Becerra, & Thomas, 2018).

9.8 Concluding thoughts

With such complex diversity in regulations, it is difficult to ensure that national regulations are being adhered to when launching new probiotic beverages across a number of countries in the Americas. Local producers will have an advantage in terms of the "buy local movement" and their closeness to their country market and regional products should continue to thrive despite the ongoing internationalization of probiotic drinks marketed and distributed by large global companies.

Local producers can also form cooperations for improved market linkage and raw material sourcing. National food laboratories in the Americas could facilitate more research on indigenous American probiotic beverages, which could be useful to establish health claims and validations, as well as increase the shelf-life period. Universities and research centers could align with the indigenous producers of probiotic beverages to impart knowledge and skills on the application of defined starters for the internationalization of these probiotic products. Apart from the traditional dairy and nondairy beverage products, novel food products such as probiotic ice cream and chocolates have gained the attention of young consumers. Product development will continue to be very important to ensure that there are always new probiotic products available to the consumer with proven health and safety benefits as well as innovative, flavorful, and exciting options.

References

AAFC (Agriculture and Agri-Food Canada). (2018). *Health and wellness series—Metabolic health products and trends—December 2018.* https://www.agr.gc.ca/eng/international-trade/market-intelligence/reports/health-and-wellness-series-metabolic-health-products-and-trends/?id=1543607941377.

AEProbio. (2020). *The 2020 clinical guide to probiotic products available in Canada, indications, dosage formats, and clinical evidence to date* (12th ed.). www.probioticchart.ca.

Behera, S. S., & Panda, S. K. (2020). Ethnic and industrial probiotic foods and beverages: Efficacy and acceptance. *Current Opinion in Food Science, 32*, 29–36.

Binda, S., Hill, C., Johansen, E., Obis, D., Pot, B., Sanders, M. E., et al. (2020). Criteria to qualify microorganisms as "probiotic" in foods and dietary supplements. *Frontiers in Microbiology, 11*. https://doi.org/10.3389/fmicb.2020.01662.

Bortz, G., Becerra, L., & Thomas, H. (2018). From technology transfer to local development strategies. Sociotechno-cognitive dynamics in the case of the Yogurito Escolar (Argentina, 1984-2015). *Apuntes. Revista de Ciencias Sociales, 45*(82), 33–69.

Canadian Food Directorate, Health Products and Food Branch (Government of Canada). (April 2009). *Guidance document—The use of probiotic microorganisms in food.* https://www.canada.ca/en/health-canada/services/food-nutrition/legislation-guidelines/guidance-documents/guidance-document-use-probiotic-microorganisms-food-2009.html.

CFIA (Canadian Food Inspection Agency). (2019). *Health claims on food labels.* https://www.inspection.gc.ca/food-label-requirements/labelling/industry/health-claims-on-food-labels/eng/1392834838383/1392834887794.

Chobani. (2020). https://www.chobani.com/probiotic/.

DRAFT. (2015). *NOM-08.* https://www.lumina-intelligence.com/blog/probiotics/report-preview-overview-of-regulation-for-the-use-of-the-term-probiotics/.

Euromonitor. (2018). *The world market for health and wellness packaged food.* https://www.euromonitor.com/world-market-for-health-and-wellness-packaged-food/report.

Euromonitor. (September 2019). *Yoghurt and sour milk products in Canada.* https://www.euromonitor.com/yoghurt-and-sour-milk-products-in-canada/report.

FAO/WHO. (2002). *Guidelines for the evaluation of probiotics in food.* https://www.who.int/foodsafety/fs_management/en/probiotic_guidelines.pdf.

Floradapt Press Release. (January 28, 2020). *Kaneka receives NPN license approval for Floradapt™ cardio.* https://www.newswire.ca/news-releases/kaneka-receives-npn-license-approval-for-floradapt-tm-cardio-808782535.html.

Fortune Business Insights. (2020). https://www.fortunebusinessinsights.com/industry-reports/probiotics-market-100083.

GFK Insights. (2017). *Factores de Decisión Sobre qué Comer o Beber, Octubre 2017* (p. 103).

Giles-Gómez, M., García, J. G. S., Matus, V., Quintana, I. C., Bolívar, F., & Escalante, A. (2016). In vitro and in vivo probiotic assessment of *Leuconostoc mesenteroides* P45 isolated from pulque, a Mexican traditional alcoholic beverage. *Springerplus, 5*(1), 708. https://doi.org/10.1186/s40064-016-2370-7.

Grandview Research. (2018). *Probiotics market size...2019–2025.* https://www.grandviewresearch.com/industry-analysis/probiotics-market.

Health Canada. (2009). *Food labelling health claims.* https://www.canada.ca/en/health-canada/services/food-nutrition/food-labelling/health-claims/questions-answers-probiotics.html.

Innova Database. (September 2019). https://www.innovamarketinsights.com/all-press-releases/.

Marketdataforecast. (2020). *Latin America probiotics market... (2020-2025).* https://www.marketdataforecast.com/market-reports/latin-america-probiotics-market.

Mintel. (July 2018). *Tap into the self-care market with food and drink.* www.mintel.com.

Morán, J. (2018). Probiotics in Latin America—Regulation, market and trends. In *PROBIOTA 2018. PANEL DEBATE, Barcelona, February 8th, 2018.* http://www.foodconsulting.es/wp-content/uploads/probiota18.pdf.

Mordor Intelligence. (2019). *Brazil probiotics market—Growth, trends, and forecast (2020–2025).* https://www.mordorintelligence.com/industry-reports/brazil-probiotics-market-industry.

NCCIH. (2020). *National center for complementary and integrative health. Probiotics what you need to know.* https://www.nccih.nih.gov/health/probiotics-what-you-need-to-know.

Pérez-Armendáriz, B., & Cadoso-Ugarte, G. A. (2020). Traditional fermented beverages in Mexico: Biotechnological, nutritional, and functional approaches. *Food Research International, 136,* 109307.

Researchandmarkets. (2020a). *Brazil probiotics market—Forecasts from 2020 to 2025.* https://www.researchandmarkets.com/. Report ID: 4858193. (June 2020 Brazil Probiotics Market—Forecasts from 2020 to 2025).

Researchandmarkets. (2020b). *Canada probiotics market—Forecasts from 2020 to 2025.* June 2020. https://www.researchandmarkets.com/reports/4858271.

Resolution RDC No. 241/2018. (2018). https://www.gov.br/anvisa/pt-br. https://www.nutraingredients-latam.com/Article/2019/04/04/ANVISA-probiotics-in-food-application-RDC-241-2018-guidance.

Romero-Luna, H. E., Hernández-Sánchez, H., & Dávila-Ortiz, G. (2017). Traditional fermented beverages from Mexico as a potential probiotic source. *Annals of Microbiology, 67*(9), 577–586.

Silva, M. S., Ramos, C. L., González-Avila, M., Gschaedler, A., Arrizon, J., Schwan, R. F., et al. (2017). Probiotic properties of *Weissella cibaria* and *Leuconostoc citreum* isolated from tejuino—A typical Mexican beverage. *LWT, 86,* 227–232.

Väkeväinen, K., Valderrama, A., Espinosa, J., Centurión, D., Rizo, J., Reyes-Duarte, D., et al. (2018). Characterization of lactic acid bacteria recovered from Atole agrio, a traditional Mexican fermented beverage. *LWT, 88,* 109–118.

Valdovinos-García, L. R., Abreu, A. T., & Valdovinos-Díaz, M. A. (2019). Probiotic use in clinical practice: Results of a national survey of gastroenterologists and nutritionists. *Revista de Gastroenterología de México (English Edition), 84*(3), 303–309.

Villena, J. C., Salva, M. S., Nuñez, M. S., Corzo, J., Tolaba, R., Faedda, J., et al. (2012). Probiotics for everyone! The novel immunobiotic *Lactobacillus rhamnosus* CRL1505 and the beginning of Social Probiotic Programs in Argentina. *International Journal of Biotechnology for Wellness Industries.* https://ri.conicet.gov.ar/handle/11336/77651.

PART III

Health and genomics

CHAPTER

10

Probiotics: Emerging functional ingredients for healthy aging and age-related diseases

Pei Lei Tan and Sae Hun Kim

College of Life Science and Biotechnology, Korea University, Seoul, South Korea

10.1 Introduction

People are expected to live longer in the future. According to the World Health Organization (WHO), the older population is increasing dramatically on a global scale. The number of people aged 60 years or older is expected to rise to over double, from 900 million in 2015 to 2 billion by 2050, representing 22.5% of the world's overall population (WHO, 2018). Despite the lifespan being convolved with healthspan, an increase in life expectancy does not always coincide with an increase in healthspan. With time, aging leads to a rise in the deleteriome that is adjusted by genetic, stochastic, and environmental processes; resulting in progressively increased frailty and susceptibility to age-related diseases (Gladyshey, 2016). It has thus become imperative to promote healthful aging and to dampen the potentially unsustainable rise in health care costs.

With the advance in translational geroscience, it has become possible to better disentangle the intricacies of biological phenomena underlying healthy aging and age-related diseases in humans (Sierra, 2016). Accumulated evidence has proposed that the decline of fitness in mammals results from the functional interconnections between the nine hallmarks of aging, which can be further subdivided into three categories, namely, primary hallmarks (genomic instability, telomere attrition, epigenetic alterations, and loss of proteostasis); antagonistic hallmarks (deregulated nutrient

https://doi.org/10.1016/B978-0-12-818588-9.00002-4

sensing, mitochondrial dysfunction, and cellular senescence); and integrative hallmarks (stem cell exhaustion and altered intercellular communication) (López-Otín, Blasco, Patridge, Serrano, & Kroemer, 2013). Although the current mechanistic findings in these categories may not thoroughly define aging, ameliorating any of these hallmarks could potentially impact healthspan.

Aging is a malleable process. In contrast to disease-specific approaches, geroscience-oriented approaches have the capacity to prevent multiple age-related diseases simultaneously, thereby promoting healthy aging, and delaying the onset of dependency and disability (Kaeberlein, 2017). Several geroprotective interventional studies that target the hallmarks of aging have been demonstrated to have high translational potential. Generally, mTOR inhibits autophagy and promotes protein synthesis, which may lead to mitochondrial dysfunction and stem cell exhaustion (Stallone, Infante, Prisciandaro, & Grandaliano, 2019). These mTOR activation events ultimately promote tissue dysfunction and accelerate the pathogenesis of various aging diseases. Meanwhile, rapamycin, an FDA-approved mTOR inhibitor, is not only capable of extending health span but also mitigates any undesirable immune functions relevant to aging and inflammation (Hurez et al., 2015; Johnson, Rabinovitch, & Kaeberlein, 2013). Metformin, a first-line applied for the treatment of type 2 diabetes (T2D), has also been shown to prolong lifespan and slow down the onset of age-related diseases. *Caenorhabditis elegans* is a powerful model system in behavioral and molecular aging research, primarily due to the presence of lifespan-regulating genes associated with metabolic pathways, short lifespan, and clear physiological changes (Gao, Bos et al., 2018; Son, Altintas, Kim, Kwon, & Lee, 2019). Molecular mechanistic studies have shown that metformin inhibits TORC1 and activates AMPK through the v-ATPase-regulator lysosomal pathway, leading to the extension of lifespan in *C. elegans* (Chen, Ou, Hu, Shao, & Liu, 2017). Thirty-week metformin-supplemented dietary treatment also improved physical performance, insulin sensitivity and lipid profile, and reduced oxidative stress- and chronic-inflammatory markers that promote healthy aging in middle-aged C57BL/6 mice (Martin-Montalvo et al., 2013). Despite these drugs being associated with promising geroprotective properties, the chronic use of rapamycin and metformin has the potential to cause metabolic impairment and gastrointestinal complications, respectively; which may further preclude their deployment as anti-aging alternatives in older adults (Salmon, 2015; Schlender et al., 2017).

Dietary pattern is an important modifiable risk factor for disease prevention, and it is inextricably linked to healthspan in older adults (Govindaraju, Sahle, McCaffrey, McNeil, & Owen, 2018). Some nutrient ingredients have been identified to consistently target biomarkers of healthy aging and aging-related pathologies in humans (Kiefte-de Jong,

Mathers, & Franco, 2014). Moreover, non-nutrient ingredients such as probiotics, in particular, have received increasing attention and are thus becoming a promising tool for ongoing antiaging research. Although the antiaging potential of probiotics remains understudied, compelling evidence has demonstrated that live probiotics and/or probiotic-derived components augment a healthy lifestyle by modulating the gut microbiota, which play a pivotal role in orchestrating integrative physiology (Eloe-Fadrosh et al., 2015; Han et al., 2017; Leulier et al., 2017). This chapter documents up-to-date preclinical and clinical evidence of proposed beneficial roles of probiotics in promoting healthy aging and delaying age-related disease and discusses their possible molecular and cellular mechanisms of action.

10.2 Hallmarks of aging as a potential target for probiotics intervention

Recent advances in next-generation sequencing (NGS) technologies have paved the way for greater investigatory capabilities to read the complex human microbiome. This rapid advancement has led to an explosion of microbiome research over the past few years, to the extent that the gut microbiota has been proposed to be a key determinant of human health, including healthy aging (Ding et al., 2019). The gut harbors diverse microorganisms, including fungi, viruses, archaea and, predominantly, bacteria that live symbiotically within the host. Studies using gnotobiotic models have demonstrated that the microbiota influences host immune development and homeostasis (El Aidy et al., 2012), metabolism and adiposity (Cox et al., 2014), intestinal morphology and functions (Hayes et al., 2018), as well as behavior, brain function, and development (Sampson & Mazmanian, 2016).

The characterization of the microbiome features in healthy populations is notably an essential step prior to any preclinical and clinical studies that attempt to modulate dysbiotic microbial communities or promote health. King et al. (2019) have recently generated a healthy human reference microbiome list (GutFeelingKB) that involves 157 organisms, and they successfully identified a total of eight phyla, 18 families, 23 classes, 38 orders, 59 genera, and 109 species. The authors also highlight that the gut microbiome in these healthy individuals represents higher taxonomic levels, and is predominantly composed of 63 (40%), 32 (20%), and 31 (19.7%) bacterial members belonging to Firmicutes, Actinobacteria, and Bacteroidetes, respectively. In contrast, lower microbial diversity and species have been reproducibly observed in several age-related pathological conditions, including type 2 diabetes, obesity, as well as neurodegenerative diseases (Lambeth et al., 2015; Turnbaugh et al., 2009; Vogt et al.,

2017), suggesting that the reduction in gut microbial diversity could possibly be a novel hallmark of aging. Therefore, the gut microbiota is not only viewed as a key component for revolutionizing age-related disease etiology but can even be a potential therapeutic target.

The composition of the gut microbiota changes with age and the core microbiota associated with health in elderly individuals is distinct from that of younger adults. Current clinical evidence suggests that elderly individuals (~ 65 y and above) have a reduced level of microbiota diversity that is accompanied by a lower abundance level of Firmicutes (*Clostridium* cluster XIVa, *Faecalibacterium prausnitzii*), Actinobacteria (Bifidobacteria), a higher abundance level phylum Bacteroidetes (genera *Bacteroides, Alistipes, Parabacteroides*), *Clostridium* cluster IV, and Proteobacteria (Enterobacteriaceae), compared to that of younger adults (Claesson et al., 2011; O'Toole & Claesson, 2010; Odamaki et al., 2016; Woodmansey, 2007).

Furthermore, changes in the core microbiota of aging hosts, as described above, undoubtedly leads to the modification of metabolism and physiology. Metagenomic analysis revealed that the gut microbiota in elderly subjects may enrich them with genes linked to pathobionts (e.g., *Escherichia*), resulting in the loss of abundant genes responsible for short-chain fatty acid (SCFA) production, and shifting from saccharolytic fermentation to putrefactive metabolism that eventually causes physiological inflammation (Rampelli et al., 2013). The aging population is also associated with an increased abundance of gut microbial genes involved in tryptophan metabolic pathways and proteolytic functions, potentially leading to an increased risk of age-related complications, including dementia and sarcopenia (Collino et al., 2013; Rampelli et al., 2013). Correcting nutritional status and metabolic activities through the restoration of microbial balance in the elderly may thus reduce the pace of aging and age-associated diseases.

Interestingly, dietary adjustment by incorporating probiotic beverages into our daily life could be a feasible way to promote a healthier aging process. Probiotic bacteria are most often used as dietary adjuncts in the pediatric and adult population, owing to their immunomodulatory properties that promote healthy digestive functions (Tan, Eor, Chun, & Kim, 2015). In recent years, many research findings have also proposed that the beneficial impact of probiotics is not only limited to gastrointestinal disease but is also linked to extraintestinal disease by shaping the highly dynamic and functional microbiome (Kiousi et al., 2019; Sanders, Merenstein, Reid, Gibson, & Rastall, 2019). Furthermore, given that a growing body of evidence corroborated the critical impact of the microbiome during aging and later life, extensive probiotic intervention research is ongoing, with the aim of discovering the gut microbiota-modulating potential for health promotion and disease prevention in older adults.

10.3 Probiotics for healthy aging

As life span increases, the immune system undergoes a dynamic process termed "immunosenescence," which continuously increases the susceptibility of the elderly to diseases. It has been suggested that impaired immune surveillance accelerates the accumulation of senescent cells and increases tissue fibrosis, eventually compromising the functionality of human organs (Ovadya et al., 2018). Nonetheless, probiotics and its components can exert beneficial effects on the rejuvenation of organ functions, and thereby, promoting longevity and healthy aging. Despite in vitro and animal trials suggesting various promising antiaging mechanisms of probiotics, currently available clinical evidence highlights that the principal claimed benefits of probiotics in healthy elderly people are merely attributed to immunomodulatory functions (Table 10.1). A most recent systemic review and meta-analysis of controlled studies further conclude that short-term (3 to 12 weeks) probiotic supplementation effectively enhances cellular immune function in healthy elderly adults (Miller, Lehtoranta, & Lehtinen, 2019). Taken together, further clinical studies are crucial to justify the other putative mechanisms of probiotics in promoting overall healthy aging and longevity.

10.3.1 Longevity extension

Regarding lifespan extension, one in vitro study proposed that a cell-free supernatant (CFS) of *Lactobacillus* strains, including *L. fermentum* DR9, *L. paracasei* OFS 0291, and *L. helveticus* OFS 1515, exhibited antisenescence potential by activating a highly conserved intracellular energy sensor and prolongevity target, namely, adenosine monophosphate–activated protein kinase (AMPK) (Hor et al., 2019). Another study demonstrated that the cell wall component of *B. longum* BB68, instead of its cell wall–free extract, extended longevity in *C. elegans* via activation of TIR-1-JNK-DAF16 stress-response pathways (Zhao et al., 2017). The feeding of live *L. rhamnosus* CNCM I-3690, associated with anti-inflammatory properties, is also capable of modulating DAF-16/insulin-like signaling pathways, thereby extending the lifespan of *C. elegans* by 20% (Grompone et al., 2012). In addition to the highly conserved DAF-16-dependent lifespan regulator, probiotics may also stimulate longevity via the nuclear hormone receptor (NHR) superfamily, a class of ligand-activated and small lipophilic hormone-regulated transcription factors that govern diverse biological activities such as metabolism, development, and aging (Mangelsdorf et al., 1995; Park et al., 2018). Whole transcriptional analysis revealed that *C. elegans* fed with *L. fermentum* JDFM216 up-regulated C-type lectin-, F-box protein-, and NHR-family-related genes (*nhr*-172, *nhr*-127, *nhr*-221,

TABLE 10.1 Clinical trials involving probiotic strains that demonstrate the promotion of healthy aging in middle-aged and elderly populations.

Treatment (country)	Probiotic strain	Subject	Dose and duration (intervention)	Result	Reference
Enhancement of the T-cell-mediated immune defense in healthy elderly (China)	*L. paracasei* N1115	103 healthy Chinese volunteers (aged ≥ 45 y)	300 mL of yogurt supplemented with *L. paracasei* N1115, 2.3 × 10^7 CFU/mL; daily for 12 weeks (Randomized, controlled, open-label trial)	- $CD3^+$ cells ↑ - risk and frequency of URTI ↓ - no significant change in the total protein, albumin, globulin, and prealbumin levels	Pu et al. (2017)
Reduction of the duration of CID (France)	*L. casei* DN-114001	537 free-living health elderly (aged ≥ 70 y)	100 g of fermented dairy drink (Actimel®) containing *L. casei* DN-114001 (~10^{10} CFU/100g), *S. thermophilus* and *L. delbrueckii* subsp. *bulgaricus* (~10^9 CFU/100g yogurt) (Multicenter, randomized, double-blind, and controlled trial)	- Number of *L. casei* species in stool ↑ - average duration per episode for CID↓ - episode and cumulative duration for URTI and rhinopharyngitis ↓	Guillemard, Tondu, Lacoin, and Schrezenmeir (2010)
Enhancement of systemic immunity in the elderly (Spain)	*L. delbrueckii* subsp. *bulgaricus* 8481	26 elderly, 23 females and 3 males, (aged ≥ 65 y)	Capsule containing 3 × 10^7 CFU *L. delbrueckii* subsp. *bulgaricus*; trice/day for 6 months (Multicenter, double-blind, placebo-controlled trial)	- NK cells ↑ - improved immune risk profile ($CD8^+$ T cells, CD^+CD28^{null} T cells ↓) - naïve $CD4^+$ T cells) ↑ - IL-8 ↓ - antimicrobial peptide hBD2 ↑	Moro-Garcia et al. (2013)

Restoration of bifidobacterial and protection against inflammaging in elderly (Italy, Germany, France)	VSL#3	31 healthy elderly, (aged 65–85 y)	Optimized diet supplemented with capsule containing 1.12×10^{11} CFU of VSL#3; twice capsules/daily for 8 weeks (Open-label, randomized, multicenter trial)	- Fecal bifidobacterial ↑ - Folate and vitamin B12 - level s ↑ - Homocysteine level ↓	Valentini et al. (2015)
Restoration of bifidobacterial and lactobacilli populations in elderly (United Kingdom)	*B. bifidum* BB-02 *and B. lactis* BL-01	9 healthy elderly (aged 68–90 y)	Synbiotic supplement containing $\sim 3.5 \times 10^{10}$ CFU of *B. bifidum* BB-02 and *B. lactis* BL-01, with 6 g of Raftilose synergy I (inulin-based prebiotic); twice daily for 3 weeks (Randomized, double-blind, controlled feeding trial)	- total number of fecal bifidobacteria ↑ - total number of fecal lactobacilli ↑ - total number of *B. bifidum* (during feeding) ↑	Bartosch, Woodmansey, Paterson, McMurdo, and Macfarlane (2005)
Stimulation of immune responses during the winter period (France)	*Bacillus subtilis* CU1	50 healthy free-living elderly (aged of 60–74 y)	Probiotic capsule containing 2.10^9 spores of *B. subtilis* CU1/daily; 10 days intermittently, 18 days course of a break (4 cycles) (Randomized double-blind placebo-controlled clinical trial)	- No improvement in the duration of CID symptoms - Stool and salivary IgA ↑ - Frequency of respiratory infections ↓	Lefevre et al. (2015)
Reduction of URTI risk in healthy middle-aged office workers (Japan)	*L. casei* Shirota	49 healthy office workers (aged 30–49 y)	One bottle of fermented milk containing 1.0×10^{11} CFU *L. casei* Shirota; daily for 12 weeks (randomized, controlled trial)	- URTI-free rate ↑ - Incidence of URTI ↓ - NK cell activity ↑ - Salivary cortisol level ↑	Shida et al. (2017)

Continued

TABLE 10.1 Clinical trials involving probiotic strains that demonstrate the promotion of healthy aging in middle-aged and elderly populations—cont'd

Treatment (country)	Probiotic strain	Subject	Dose and duration (intervention)	Result	Reference
Modulation of anti-inflammatory cytokine profile in elderly (United Kingdom)	*L. casei* Shirota	16 healthy volunteers (aged of 55–74 y)	Probiotic drink containing 1.3×10^{10} CFU *L. casei* Shirota; daily for 4 weeks (Randomized placebo-controlled, single-blind crossover trial)	- NK cell activity ↑ - $CD25^-$ T cells ↓ - IL-10/IL-12 ↑	Dong, Rowland, Thomas, and Yaqoob (2013)
Modulation of bone metabolism and gut microbiota in healthy postmenopausal women (Japan)	*B. subtilis* C-3102	38 healthy postmenopausal women (aged 50–69 y)	Three tablets containing 3.4×10^9 CFU *B. subtilis* C-3102 spore; daily for 12 weeks (Randomized placebo-controlled, double-blind clinical trial)	- urinary type I collagen cross-linked N-telopeptide ↓ - tartrate-resistant acid phosphatase isoform 5b ↓ - relative abundance of genus Bifidobacterium ↑ - relative abundance of genus Fusobacterium ↓	Takimoto et al. (2018)
Modulation of pro- and anti-inflammatory cytokine profile in elderly (USA)	*L. rhamnosus* GG ATCC 53103	15 healthy volunteers, (aged of 66–80 y)	Capsule containing 1×10^{10} CFU *L. rhamnosus* GG ATCC 53103; twice daily for 28 days and were followed through day 56 (Phase 1 open label clinical trial)	- IL-8 ↓, and returning to baseline 1 month after discontinuation - No significant effects on IFN-γ, IL-1β, IL-2, IL-4, IL-5, IL-10, IL-12p70, - IL-13, and TNF-α, IL-6)	Hibberd et al. (2014)

URTI = upper respiratory tract infection; CID = common infectious disease; VSL#3 = Probiotic mixture of *L. plantarum* DSM 24730, *L. delbrueckii* subsp. *bulgaricus* DSM 24734, *L. paracasei* DSM 24733, *L. acidophilus* DSM 24735, *B. breve* DSM 24732, *B. longum* DSM24736, *B. infantis* DSM 24737, *S. salivarius* subsp. *thermophilus* DSM 24731.

nhr-25, *nhr*-150, *nhr*-165, *nhr*-209), while *L. fermentum* JDFM216 had no life-prolonging effect on worms with deleted *nhr*-25, *nhr*-127, or *nhr*-209. These in vivo studies thus far indicate that probiotics and their components hold great potential to stimulate host longevity and immune response, but in a specific pathway-dependent manner.

10.3.2 Aging muscle

Mitochondria are the energy-producing organelles responsible for maintaining the homeostasis and plasticity of skeletal muscle. However, the mitochondrial function of skeletal muscle declines with advancing age. It has been demonstrated that aging results in an enhanced detection level of biomarkers of DNA oxidative damage (8-oxo-deoxy-guanosine), as well as a reduction in the content of nine mitochondrial proteins in older human muscle (Short et al., 2005). These phenomena can ultimately lead to skeletal muscle dysfunction, which is common in the elderly.

Chen et al. (2019) examined the potential of *L. paracasei* PS23 in preventing muscle loss in 28-week-old senescence-accelerated prone-8 (SAMP8) mice. They found that administration of 1×10^9 CFU/day for 12 weeks significantly up-regulated genes related to mitochondrial biogenesis (*PGC1α, NRF1, TFAM*), anti-inflammatory cytokine IL-10, enzymatic antioxidant activities *(SOD, GPx)*, and attenuated age-related decrease in muscle mass and strength, thereby preserving mitochondrial function and decelerating age-related muscle loss in SAMP8 mice.

Furthermore, despite no research ever reporting that probiotics may preserve musculoskeletal functionality in the elderly via modulation of the gut microbiota-muscle axis, several findings have underlined such potential. Siddharth et al. (2017) initially demonstrated that age-related change in the *Sutterella* to *Barnesiella* ratio was associated with a physiological decline in the musculoskeletal functionality of aged rats. The authors also proposed that *Sutterella* is correlated with the loss of gastrocnemius muscle and contributed to the sarcopenic phenotype in aged rats by counteracting the favorable response of *Barnesiella* against skeletal muscle damage. Similarly, Fielding et al. (2019) found that abundant levels of bacterial genus-level *Barnesiella* and *Prevotella*, and *Barnesiella intestinihominis* were significantly higher in high-functioning older adults, while the grip strength of mice colonized with microbiota from high-functioning older adults significantly increased by 6.4%, compared to mice colonized with microbiota from low-functioning older adults. Therefore, these findings propose that probiotics may preserve muscle function in the elderly by increasing the abundance levels of *Barnesiella* and/or reducing abundance levels of *Sutterella*. It is worthy to note that the gut microbiota–modulating potential of probiotics in the prevention of muscle loss warrants further in-depth investigation, prior to clinical trials.

10.3.3 Aging brain

With advancing age, the human brain undergoes a series of neuroanatomical and neurophysiological changes that disrupt cognitive function. Cognitive decline is an inevitable hurdle to healthy aging. Both dopamine and serotonin neurotransmitter activities modulate synaptic transmission that influences on cerebral functions, including learning and episodic memory persistence in old age (Chowdhury, Guitant-Masip, Bunzeck, Dolan, & Düzel, 2012; González-Burgos & Feria-Velasco, 2008). By using a pharmacological fMRI approach, Abdulrahman, Fletcher, Bullmore, and Morcom (2017) found that memory specificity in the hippocampus and prefrontal cortex was significantly reduced in older adults compared to younger adults, while memory specificity in the hippocampus was modulated by dopamine signaling in an age-dependent manner.

Furthermore, human studies have continuously emphasized the influence of the gut microbiota on cognitive function. Activation of microglia, brain-resident macrophages in cortical white matter, can elevate neuroinflammatory responses leading to cognitive decline during aging (Gefen et al., 2019). Whereas, the microbiota-derived short chain fatty acids, such as butyrate, can cross the blood-brain barrier and are able to attenuate microglial inflammatory responses, as well as promote serotonin production in the gut (Logsdon, Erickson, Rhea, Salameh, & Banks, 2018; Huuskonen, Suuronen, Nuutinen, Kyrylenko, & Salminen, 2004; Reigstad et al., 2015). However, gut microbiota analysis across the elderly population is associated with a reduced relative abundance of butyrate-producing communities, family Lachnospiraceae, Ruminococcaceae, genera *Roseburia* and *Faecalibacterium* (Biagi et al., 2010; Wang et al., 2015). These findings collectively suggest that decreased level of butyrate may limit the production of colonic serotonin and induce microglial activation, thereby promoting the cognitive decline in the elderly. Furthermore, elderly subjects with cognitive impairment were also found to have an elevated level of peripheral inflammation that could possibly be attributed to the increased relative abundance of the proinflammatory genera *Escherichia/Shigella* and the decreased relative abundance level of the anti-inflammatory species *Eubacterium rectale* (Cattaneo et al., 2017). This finding implies that altered gut microbiota can influence the state of peripheral inflammation and exacerbate the process of neuroinflammation, ultimately leading to neurodegeneration. Moreover, Bajaj et al. (2016) investigated the gut microbiota composition and their correlation with cognitive performance in an elderly population with cirrhosis. Interestingly, cognitively unimpaired elderly subjects had a higher abundance level of *Faecalibacterium* and butyrate-producing genus *Butyricicoccus*, and a relative abundance of the order Lactobacillales, including family

Streptococceae, Lactobacillaceae, and Carnobacteriaceae, which were positively correlated with good cognition in elderly cirrhotic patients. Considering that most of the probiotic strains belong to Lactobacillales and are capable of producing butyrate and modulating immune responses, probiotics may well maintain cognitive functioning in healthy elderly.

Indeed, several studies have suggested the potential use of probiotic strains in preventing cognitive decline in both aged mice and rats. Corpuz et al. (2018) evaluated the potential of long-term diets supplemented with *L. paracasei* K7 to prevent age-related cognitive decline in SAMP8 mice. The authors found that 14-week-old female SAMP8 mice, fed with a standard diet containing 0.05 % (w/w) *L. paracasei* K7 for 43 weeks, had significantly improved cognitive performance in passive avoidance and Barnes maze tests. The hippocampus, prefrontal cortex, and striatum are the brain regions densely innervated by dopaminegeric and serotonergic neurons, which can influence both behavioral and cognitive functions including episodic and procedural memory (González-Burgos & Feria-Velasco, 2008; Sasaki-Adams & Kelley, 2001). Long-term administration of *L. paracasei* K7 was found to activate a cyclic AMP response element–binding protein (CREB) and subsequently upregulate the expression of brain-derived neurotropic factors (BDNF) that modulate memory formation in the hippocampus, but not in the cortex. Hence, prolonged administration of a diet supplemented with *L. paracasei* K7 may rejuvenate aged-dependent cognitive decline by activating the CREB-BDNF pathway in the hippocampus. Similarly, Huang et al. (2018) also found that male and female SAMP8 mice, orally administered with *L. paracasei* PS23 for 12 weeks, improved memory and anxiety-like behaviors. Specifically, *L. paracasei* PS23 was capable of increasing levels of BDNF, neurotransmitter serotonin and dopamine in the striatum and hippocampus, as well as enhancing the antioxidant activities of superoxide dismutase (SOD) and glutathione peroxidase (GPx) in the serum and hippocampus. In addition, decreased levels of proinflammatory tumor necrosis factor-alpha (TNF-α) and monocyte chemoattractant protein-1 (MCP-1), and an increased level of anti-inflammatory IL-10 was also found in the serum, suggesting that *L. paracasei* PS23 may delay age-related cognitive decline via the gut–brain axis. In addition to *L. paracasei* strains, a 12-week administration of 1×10^{10} CFU *L. casei* LC122 or *B. longum* BL896 also improved learning and memory ability in aged mice by upregulating expression levels of neurodegenerative and neurotrophic factors in the hippocampus (Ni et al., 2019).

Several studies have also evaluated the effect of multistrain probiotics on cognitive function. Distrutti et al. (2014) evaluated the effect of probiotic VSL#3, a mixture of eight probiotic strains (*Streptococcus thermophilus* DSM24731, *B. breve* DSM24732, *B. longum* DSM24736, *B. infantis* DSM24737,

L. acidophilus DSM24735, *L. plantarum* DSM24730, *L. paracasei* DSM24733, and *L. delbrueckii* subspecies *bulgaricus* DSM24734) on long-term potentiation (LTP) deficits in both middle-aged and aged rats. Daily oral administration of 1.286×10^{10} CFU/kg VSL#3 for 6 weeks modulated the expression of genes related to neuronal and inflammatory processes, suppressed microglial activation, and enhanced synapsin and BDNF, thereby reverting LTP deficits and synaptic loss in aged rats. Recently, Yang, Yu, Xue, Li, and Du (2020) suggested that administration of a ProBiotic-4 cocktail containing 50 % *B. lactis*, 25 % *L. casei*, 12.5 % *B. bifidum*, and 12.5 % *L. acidophilus*, at a dose of 2 $\times 10^9$ CFU/day for 12 weeks, may synergistically improve memory deficit and counteract a series of age-associated pathologies, including altered microbiota composition, cerebral synaptic and neuronal injuries, glial activation, and disrupted blood–brain barrier and intestinal barrier in 9-month-old SAMP8 mice. The authors also highlighted that ProBiotic-4 may exert these beneficial effects via the inhibition of the activated toll-like receptor 4/NF-κB and the retinoic acid–inducible gene-I/NF-κB signaling pathways, that are attributed to changes in gut microbiota composition associated with cognitive impairment and inflammation.

On the other hand, Romo-Araiza et al. (2018) attempted to investigate the cognitive improving effect of a synbiotic supplementation in a model of the middle-aged rat. Daily oral administration of a synbiotic formulation, containing 4×10^8 CFU *E. faecium* and 860 mg/kg inulin for 5 weeks, significantly attenuated proinflammatory responses and increased the fecal butyrate level and the hippocampal BDNF content. A reduced level of proinflammatory IL-1β was also correlated with improved spatial learning performance in the Morris water maze test. The electrophysiological analysis further suggested that the synbiotic formulation containing *E. faecium* and inulin could favorably influence the glutamatergic components of the excitatory transmission, namely the N-methyl-D-aspartate receptor (NMDA) and α-amino-3-hydroxy-5-methyl-4-isoxazolepropionic acid (AMPA). Enhanced synaptic transmission subsequently facilitates the induction of LTP in the pyramidal cells of hippocampal CA, which could ultimately enhance memory function.

To our knowledge, only a very limited number of clinical trials have been conducted to evaluate the effect of probiotic supplements in promoting cognitive functioning in healthy elderly subjects. Inoue et al. (2018) conducted a randomized, double-blind, placebo-controlled trial involving 38 healthy Japanese elderly participants to examine whether a combination of moderate resistance training and bifidobacteria supplementation (*B. longum* BB536, *B. infantis* M-63, *B. breve* M-16V, and *B. breve* B-3; approximately 1.25×10^{10} CFU/strain) for 12 weeks improved age-related cognitive decline. The authors found significantly decreased depression–anxiety scores and increased flanker task scores, suggesting that moderate resistance training and a probiotic bifidobacterial supplementation cocktail promoted cognitive function in these healthy Japanese elderlies. In addition, it is also worth noting that Sanborn, Azcarate-Peril, Updegraff, Manderino, and Gunstad (2018) are conducting a double-blinded and randomized study to determine the influence of 3-month *L. rhamnosus* GG (LGG) probiotic supplementation (1×10^{10} CFU/capsule/day) on cognitive function and mood in healthy middle-aged and older American adults (aged 55–75, $n = 200$). Owing to the well-documented health beneficial effects of probiotic LGG, the authors are expecting that the LGG group will demonstrate greater improvements in processing speed and executive functioning during neuropsychological tests, compared to the placebo group. Despite preclinical animal studies showing promising results, more global large scale clinical trials are needed to further evaluate the effectiveness of probiotics in improving cognitive functioning in healthy elderly subjects.

10.4 Probiotics for age-related diseases

10.4.1 Macular degeneration

Age-related macular degeneration (AMD) is a late onset problem and is among the leading causes of vision impairment and irreversible blindness in the elderly. The global population affected by AMD is anticipated to rise from 8.4 million in 2015, to 8.9 million by 2020 (Flaxman et al., 2017). AMD is characterized by photoreceptor cell death and retinal pigment epithelium (RPE) cell degeneration in the central retina, with the accumulation of lipofuscin (Inana et al., 2018). Owing to the significant link between unhealthy dietary patterns and poor vision health, increasing evidence suggests that altered gut microbiota could interact with the retina via the "gut–retina axis," to drive the development and progression of AMD (Rinninella et al., 2018). It has been suggested that altered gut microbiota may trigger autoimmunity in the eyes via the activation of autoreactive T-cell receptor–dependent retina-specific T-cells and induce chronic low-grade inflammation, which in turn accelerates AMD progression in the elderly (Horai et al., 2015; Rinninella et al., 2018). Indeed, the gut microbiota profile of patients with AMD has been found to be enriched with genera that are associated with proinflammatory events, including *Anaerotruncus*, *Oscillibacter*, *Ruminococcus torques*, and *Eubacterium ventriosum* (Zinkernagel et al., 2017). Furthermore, the gut microbiome of these patients is also enriched with genes associated with glutamate degradation and arginine biosynthesis pathways, which may result in the exacerbation of excitatory neurotransmitter deficiency in the retina and chorioretinal atrophy. Probiotic intervention may thus be a promising strategy to prevent the progression of AMD by reducing the abundance level of these detrimental bacteria.

To our knowledge, despite no prior studies describing that probiotics can modulate the gut microbiota in patients with AMD, Morita et al. (2018) attempted to investigate the potential of probiotics that activated the retinal M2 macrophage anti-inflammatory response in attenuating pathophysiological events of AMD. They reported that 5-week-old male BALB/c mice fed with a diet containing approximately 1 mg/day heat-killed *L. paracasei* KW3110 for 2 weeks, could attenuate blue light–induced retinal inflammation and degeneration by retaining the thickness of the retinal outer nuclear layer containing photoreceptor cells, and the amplitude of a- and b-wave in the photopic electroretinography that represents the cone and rod photoreceptor functions. Furthermore, Morita et al. (2018) evaluated the effect of a 6-month administration of this heat-killed probiotic diet in physiological-aged mice. The results demonstrated that the long-term intake of heat-killed *L. paracasei* KW3110 attenuated small intestinal and retinal immunosenescence by decreasing interferon-gamma (IFN- γ)-producing inflammatory $CD4^+$ cells in the lamina propia and expression of IFN- γ, IL-6, as well as TNF-α in $CD11b^+$ $F4/80^+$ retinal macrophages, respectively, in 11-month old C57BL/6N female mice. Moreover, the intake of a heat-killed *L. paracasei* KW3110 diet also modulated the gut microbiota composition that orchestrated a Th1/Th2 cell cytokine response by reducing the relative abundance level of Streptococcaceae and increasing the relative abundance level of Peptostreptococcaceae and Bifidobacteriaceae. These results imply that components of probiotic bacteria may mitigate retinal chronic inflammation and retinal cell death in AMD via the gut–retina axis. However, more clinical trials are required to further justify such potentials.

10.4.2 Osteoporosis

With aging, the bone deteriorates in microarchitecture, mass, and function that together predisposes one to osteoporotic fractures. Despite a higher prevalence of osteoporosis in postmenopausal women than in men, the mortality rate after an osteoporotic hip fracture in institutionalized men is higher than in women in the last 17 years (Guzon-Illescas et al., 2019). Estrogen deficiency plays a prominent role in contributing to the pathogenesis of primary osteoporosis in both sexes. Age-associated estrogen deficiency increases the production of proinflammatory TNF-α by bone marrow T-cells, which increase both the macrophage colony-stimulating factor (M-CSF)-induced osteoclastic bone resorption, and the receptor activator of nuclear factor kappa-B ligand (RANKL)–induced osteoclastic bone resorption, and bone loss in postmenopausal women and elderly men (Cenci et al., 2000). Furthermore, estrogen deficiency has altered intricate stromal T-lymphocytes crosstalk that stimulates stromal cells to further produce pro-osteoclastogenic cytokines, and also indirectly reduced vitamin D–mediated intestinal calcium absorption associated with bone metabolism (Khosla & Pacifici, 2013).

Interestingly, the correlation analysis between fecal microbiome and urinary estrogen metabolites suggests that fecal microbiota composition may influence estrogen metabolism, where the relative abundance of the class *Clostridia* was positively correlated with systemic estrogen metabolites in both postmenopausal women and men, whereas the relative abundance of the genus *Bacteroides* was negatively correlated with estrogen metabolites in postmenopausal women (Flores et al., 2012; Fuhrman et al., 2014). In addition to estrogen metabolism, altered gut microbiota composition has been associated with reduced bone mineral density, bone strength, and tissue material properties (Guss et al., 2017). The genera *Roseburia*, *Lactobacillus*, and *Bifidobacterium* have also recently been shown to be positively correlated with bone mineral density in the elderly Chinese population with low mineral density (Li et al., 2019), suggesting that supplementation of probiotic bacteria, including *Lactobacillus* and *Bifidobacterium*, may positively impact bone mineral density and prevent age-related bone loss.

An increasing number of animal studies have investigated the potential use of probiotics for age-related osteoporosis (Table 10.2). In general, the current data suggests that probiotics and/or their fermented products may increase bone mineral density and bone mineral content at osteoporotic fracture sites (distal femur, tibia, spine) and bone strength, primarily by suppressing osteoclastogenesis in animal models of osteoporosis including spontaneously hypertensive male rats, ovariectomized mice, and ovariectomized rats. There is still no strong evidence that probiotics may interfere with gut-bone signaling, a promising new therapeutic target, for effective treatment of osteoporosis. It is also worth highlighting that many aspects of their mechanism of action remain poorly answered and may vary depending on sex and female hormonal status. *Lactobacillus reuteri* 6475 is a promising osteoprotective strain that has been shown to attenuate bone loss in multiple osteoporosis models via different mechanisms of action (Britton et al., 2014; Collins et al., 2016; McCabe, Irwin, Scharfer, & Britton, 2013; Nilsson, Sundh, Bäckhed, & Lorentzon, 2018; Schepper et al., 2019; Zhang et al., 2015). By using healthy male and female mice, McCabe et al. (2013) emphasized that 4-week administration of *L. reuteri* 6475 significantly increased the trabecular bone volume in male, but not in female mice, whereas Collins et al. (2016) demonstrated that 8-week administration of *L. reuteri* 6475 is only capable of increasing bone density under the elevated inflammatory status in estrogen-sufficient healthy female mice. With regard to the mechanism of action, *L. reuteri*

TABLE 10.2 Overview of animal studies investigating the effect of probiotic administration on age-associated osteoporosis.

Model	Probiotic strain	Sex	Dose and duration	Result	Reference
Ovariectomized mice	*L. reuteri* 6475	Female	13-week old ovariectomized Balb/c mice were administered gavagely with 1×10^9 CFU *L. reuteri* 6475, three times per week for 4 weeks; and fed *ad libitum* volume of drinking water containing 1.5×10^8 CFU of *L. reuteri* 6475	- Bone marrow CD4+ T-lymphocytes ↓ - Osteoclast bone resorption markers and activators (Trap5 and RANKL) in tibia ↓ - BMD and BMC in the femur distal trabecular bone ↑ - No significant effects on osteoblast and osteoclast markers - Gut bacterial richness ↑ - Jejunal Clostridiales ↑ - Jejunal Bacteriodales ↓	Britton et al. (2014)
Ovariectomized mice	*L. plantarum* NTU 101	Female	18-week old ovariectomized C57BL/6J mice were administered gavagely with 0.1 g of freeze-dried powder of soy skim milk fermented by *L. plantarum* NTU 101, once daily for 8 weeks	- Trabecular bone volume of the distal femur ↑ - Trabecular number of the distal femur ↑ - Bone network density and thickness of the distal metaphyseal trabecular ↑	Chiang and Pan (2011)
Ovariectomized rat	*L. casei* 393	Female	11-week old Sprague-Dawley ovariectomized rats were fed *ad libitum* with diet containing 1 % (w/w) *L. casei 393* fermented milk product for 6 weeks	- Body weight ↑ - BMD ↑ - Bone breaking force ↑ - tartrate resistant acid phosphatase activity ↓	Kim et al. (2009)

Ovariectomized rat	*L. helveticus* ATCC 27558	Female	14-week old ovariectomized Sprague-Dawley rats were administered gavagely with 1×10^8-10^9 CFU/day of *L. helveticus* ATCC 27558 once daily for 16 weeks	- Serum osteocalcin ↓ - Bone volume and trabecular thickness ↑ - Total porosity percentage in the femur ↓ - Serum C-terminal telopeptide ↓ - BMD, bone strength ↑ - mRNA expression level of *Runx2* and *Bmp2* in the femur ↑	Parvaneh et al. (2018)
Ovariectomized rat	*B. longum* ATCC 15707	Female	14-week old ovariectomized Sprague-Dawley rats were administered gavagely with 1×10^8-10^9 CFU/day of *B. longum* ATCC 15707 once daily for 16 weeks	- Serum osteoblasts ↑ - Serum osteocalcin ↓ - Serum C-terminal telopeptide ↓ - BMD ↑ - mRNA expression level of *Sparc* and *Bmp-2* in the femur ↑	Parvaneh et al. (2015)
Ovariectomized rat	*L. paracasei* DSM 13434 *L. plantarum* DSM 15312 *L. plantarum* DSM 15313	Female	Eight-week old C57BL/6N mice were fed *ad libitum* volume of drinking water containing 10^9 CFU of single *L. paracasei* DSM 134134 or L. mix for 6 weeks, starting 2 weeks before ovariectomy surgery	- Cortical BMC ↑ - Serum C-terminal telopeptides ↓ - Urinary calcium ↓ - Pro-inflammatory TNF-α and IL-1β↓ - OPG ↑ - Treg cells in bone marrow ↑	Ohlsson et al. (2014)

Continued

TABLE 10.2 Overview of animal studies investigating the effect of probiotic administration on age-associated osteoporosis.—cont'd

Model	Probiotic strain	Sex	Dose and duration	Result	Reference
Spontaneously hypertensive rat	*L. helveticus* LBK-16H	Male	Six-week old spontaneously hypertensive rat were fed *ad libitum* with *L. helveticus* LBK-16 H fermented milk 14 weeks	- BMC ↑ - BMD ↑	Narva, Collin, et al., 2004
Ovariectomized rat	*L. acidophilus* *L. casei* *L. reuteri*	Female	13-15-week old Sprague-Dawley rats were administered gavagely with 1×10^9 CFU/day of monospecies for 4 weeks	- Serum Ca and ALP ↑ (LA, LC) - Serum phosphorus ↓ (LA, LC) - BMD ↑ (LA, LC) - BMC (LA, LR, LC)	Montazeri-Najafabady et al. (2019)
Ovariectomized rat	*L. rhamnosus* HN001	Female	5.5-month old Sprague-Dawley rats were fed *ad libitum* with diet containing 1×10^9 CFU/day *L. rhamnosus* HN001 for 12 weeks	- rate of bone loss ↓ - lumbar spine BMD and BMC ↑ - femur BMD and BMC ↑	Kruger, Fear, Chua, Plimmer, and Schollum (2009)

BMD = bone mineral density; BMC = bone mineral content; LA = *L. acidophilus*; LC = *L. casei*; LR = *L. reuteri* ; L. mix = *L. paracasei* DSM 13434 + *L. plantarum* DSM 15312 + *L. plantarum* DSM 15313 ; OPG = osteoprotegerin.

6475 may increase bone mineral density in healthy male mice by secreting T-lymphocyte regulated factors that enhanced osterix, a transcription factor involved in osteoblast differentiation (Collins et al., 2019). Whereas, Quach, Parameswaran, McCabe, and Britton (2019) suggested that *L. reuteri* 6475 produced lactobacillic acid that potentially has activated long-chain fatty acid receptors, GPR120-mediated signaling pathways, thereby inhibiting osteoclastogenesis and preventing ovariectomized-induced bone loss in mice. *L. reuteri* 6475 may also prevent postantibiotic femoral and vertebral trabecular bone loss by decreasing Firmicutes: Bacteroidetes ratio and intestinal permeability (Schepper et al., 2019). These findings suggest that a single probiotic strain may employ different mechanisms of osteoprotective action in different models of osteoporosis. The efficiency of osteoprotective strain should be evaluated in age- and sex-specific groups and clinical trial participants should be representative of the patient population.

Several clinical trials have suggested that probiotics may favorably interfere with bone metabolism in both osteopenic postmenopausal women and older women with low bone mineral density. Nilsson et al. (2018) conducted a double-blind, randomized, placebo-controlled, single-center trial study to examine the effect of *L. reuteri* 6475 on bone loss in older Swedish women (age, 75–80 years; $n = 70$) with low bone mineral density. The authors have found that women ($n = 34$) who received 5×10^9 CFU of *L. reuteri* 6475 twice daily for 12 months had significantly reduced loss of total volumetric bone mineral density in the tibia, compared to the placebo group ($n = 36$). Angiotensin-converting enzyme (ACE) inhibitors are one class of antihypertensive drugs that may have a positive impact on bone mineral density in elderly men and women (Lynn, Kwok, Wong, Woo, & Leung, 2006). In a small randomized double-blind crossover study involving 20 postmenopausal Finnish women (aged of 50–78 years), Narva, Nevala, Poussa, and Korpela (2004) evaluated the effects of both *L. helveticus* LBK-16H fermented milk and juice containing *L. helveticus* LBK-16H-derived ACE inhibitory peptides (isoleucyl-prolyl-proline [IPP] and valyl-propyl-proline [VPP]) for acute changes in bone resorption and calcium metabolism. The results have demonstrated that *L. helveticus* LBK-16H fermented milk significantly increased serum calcium levels and reduced parathyroid hormone (PTH) that could attenuate bone resorption and calcium release from the bone. Whereas higher levels of PTH and lower levels of ionized calcium have been observed in postmenopausal women consuming juice containing *L. helveticus* LBK-16H-derived ACE inhibitory peptides, indicating that the osteoprotective effect was not attributed to the *L. helveticus* LBK-16H-derived IPP and VPP, but other unidentified osteoprotective bioactive substances released in milk fermented by *L. helveticus* LBK-16H. Furthermore, Jafarnejad et al. (2017) evaluated the effects of multispecies probiotic supplementation on bone metabolism in a 6-month randomized, double-blind, controlled trial involving 50 postmenopausal women (aged 50–72 years) with osteopenia in Iran. The postmenopausal women ($n = 25$) who received probiotic capsule, GeriLact containing 7 bacterial species (5×10^{10} CFU *B. longum*, 1×10^{10} CFU *B. breve*, 1.5×10^{8} CFU *S. thermophilus*, 2.5×10^{8} CFU *L. bulgaricus*, 3.5×10^{9} CFU *L. rhamnosus*, 1.5×10^{10} CFU *L. acidophilus*, and 1.3×10^{10} CFU *L. casei* per 500 mg) once daily before any meal for 6 months had significantly reduced levels of bone-specific alkaline phosphatase, collagen type 1 cross-linked C-telopeptide (CTX), PTH, and TNF-α in the serum, compared to the placebo group. However, no significant differences have been observed in the bone mineral density of the spine and have exerted favorable effects in osteopenic postmenopausal women by slowing down bone turnover rate. On the other hand, bioavailable isoflavones with selective estrogen receptor affinity have been shown to dampen estrogen-deficient bone resorption in postmenopausal women (Yamori et al., 2002). Interestingly, Lambert, Thorup, Hansen, and Jeppesen (2017) examined the effect of a novel red clover extract (RCE)–rich bioavailable isoflavone aglycones and a probiotic strain capable of promoting isoflavone uptake and enhancing isoflavone bioavailability, on bone and estrogen metabolism in a 12-month, double-blind, parallel design, placebo-controlled, randomized controlled trial involving 78 osteopenic postmenopausal women in Denmark. Compared to RCE supplementation alone, administration of RCE (60 mg isoflavone aglycones/day) and probiotic-supplemented with calcium (1200 mg/day), magnesium (550 mg/day), and calcitriol (25 mg/day) for 12 months effectively reduced bone resorption marker (collage type 1 cross-linked-C-telopeptide), improved the estrogen metabolite profile (2-OH: 16α-OH), promoted equal production, and mitigated bone mineral density decline at the L2–L4 lumbar spine vertebra, trochanter, and femoral neck, in osteopenic postmenopausal women. It should be noted that despite preclinical and clinical studies have shown the potential of probiotic bacteria to protect against age-related bone loss, further in-depth clinical investigations are needed to understand their mechanism of action.

10.4.3 Cardiovascular disease

The prevalence of cardiovascular disease (CVD) increases dramatically with age in both men and women. The most recent update from the American Heart Association reported that the incidence rates of CVD in older adults, aged 60–79 years, were 78.2% and 77.2% in females and males, respectively (Benjamin et al., 2019). Atherosclerosis is the dominant cause of CVD, in which the lipid and fibrous elements deposit in the inner arterial wall (atheromatous plaques) promoting cardiac remodeling that impairs cardiac function. It is also commonly involved in the development of several major age-related cardiac pathologies, including heart failure, coronary artery disease, atrial fibrillation, and myocardial infarction (Frostegård, 2013). Animal studies have shown that probiotics may attenuate atherosclerosis and provide protection against CVD (Table 10.3). Overall, apolipoprotein-E knockout (ApoE(-/-)) mice administered with probiotic strains for 4–16 weeks have reduced atherosclerotic lesion, vascular and systemic inflammation, improved antioxidant capacity and cholesterol metabolism, and altered the microbial profile. However, there have been some conflicting results on the antiatherosclerotic effect of probiotics (Fåk & Bäckhed, 2012).

Interestingly, probiotics may counteract myocardial infarction that greatly contributes to the development of cardiac hypertrophy and heart failure, which are highly prevalent in elderly populations. Male Sprague-Dawley rats with left main coronary artery ligated heart and fed *ad libitum* with drinking water containing 1×10^9 CFU *L. rhamnosus* GR-1 for 6 weeks exhibited significant attenuation of left ventricular hypertrophy, reduced plasma concentrations of the leptin:adiponectin ratio, as well as improved systolic and diastolic left ventricular function (Gan et al., 2014). Furthermore, an in vitro study using neonatal rat ventricular cardiomyocytes revealed that the cardioprotective effect of *L. rhamnosus* GR-1 was not attributed to its major secreted protein 1 (MSP-1), but to the other unknown factors (Ettinger, Burton, Gloor, & Reid, 2017). In addition to *Lactobacillus* sp., Danilo et al. (2017) have demonstrated that the administration of *B. animalis* subsp. *lactis* 420, at 10^9 CFU/day for 10 or 28 days, mediated the activation of T regulatory cells, thereby attenuating cardiac injury and proinflammatory cytokines in mice following ischemia/reperfusion. Moreover, the daily administration of a viable probiotic cocktail containing *B. breve, L. casei, L. bulgaricus,* and *L. acidophilus,* at a dose of 2×10^6 CFU/mL for 14 days, has also been shown to protect rats against myocardial injury via suppression of the proinflammatory TNF-α level and lipid peroxidation (Sadeghzadeh et al., 2017). Myocardial infarction may also trigger intestinal barrier defects, stimulate the translocation of intestinal microbiota products, such as lipopolysaccharide and D-lactate, into the systemic circulation and induce inflammation that may induce postmyocardial infarction depression and apoptosis in the limbic system (Girard et al., 2009; Zhou et al., 2018). In particular, the administration of *L. helveticus* RR052 and *B. longum* R0175 has been found to reduce proapoptotic (caspase-3 and Bax), increase antiapoptotic (Akt) activities in the lateral and medial amygdala and dentate gyrus, attenuate depressive symptoms, as well as restore intestinal barrier integrity in the rat after myocardial infarction (Arseneault-Bréard et al., 2012; Girard et al., 2009). Recently, Tang et al. (2019) also highlighted that myocardial infarction is associated with reduced abundance level of *Lactobacillus*, while supplementation with *Lactobacillus* shifted the balance of short-chain fatty acids toward propionate and promoted postinfarction cardiac repair

TABLE 10.3 Overview of animal studies investigating the effect of probiotic administration on atherosclerosis.

Model	Probiotic strain	Sex	Dose and duration	Result	Reference
ApoE (-/-) mice	*L. acidophilus* ATCC 4356	Male	8-week old $ApoE^{-/-}$ mice were administered gavagely with 1×10^9 CFU *L. acidophilus* ATCC 4356 per day for 16 weeks	- Plasma cholesterol level ↓ - Cholesterol absorption (NPC1L1↓ - PPAR/LXR pathway ↑ - Fecal *Lactobacillus* and - *Bifidobacterium* count ↑	Huang et al. (2014)
ApoE (-/-) mice	*L. rhamnosus GG*	Female	7-week old $ApoE^{-/-}$ mice were administered gavagely with 1×10^8 CFU *L. rhamnosus GG* per day for 12 weeks	- Atherosclerotic plaque size at aortic sinus and aortic tree ↓ - Serum endotoxin ↓ (A-FABP, cholesterol, sE-selectin, sICAM-1, sVCAM-1 ↓) - No significant effect on microbial diversity	Chan et al. (2016)
ApoE (-/-) mice	VSL#3	Female	6-week old $ApoE^{-/-}$ mice were administered gavagely with 2.78×10^{11} CFU VSL#3 per day for 12 weeks	- Atherosclerotic plaques ↓ - Polypeptide YY hormone ↑ - Vascular inflammation ↓ (sICAM-1, sVCAM-1, sE-selectin ↓, - TNF-α: MCP-1, fibrinogen, MMP-9↓) - Intestinal microbial diversity ↑	Chan, El-Nezami, Chen, Kinnunen, and Kirjavainen (2016)
Cholesterol-fed New Zealand white rabbit	*E. faecium* CRL183	Male	9 to 10-week old rabbit were administered gavagely with 1×10^8 CFU *E.faecium* CRL183 per day for 60 days	- HDL-cholesterol level ↑ - No effect on atherosclerotic lesion	Cavallini, Bedani, Bomdespacho, Vendramini, and Rossi (2009)

ApoE (-/-) mice	*L. acidophilus* ATCC 4356	Male	9-week old ApoE$^{-/-}$ mice were administered gavagely with 5 × 10^7 /10^8 CFU *L. acidophilus* ATCC 4356 per day for 12 weeks	- No effect on serum lipid profile - atherosclerotic lesion size ↓ - Serum MDA, oxLDL, TNF-α ↓ - Serum IL-10 and SOD activities ↑ - Inhibited translocation of NF-κB p65 from cytoplasm to nucleus - Degradation of aortic IκB-α ↓ - Colonic *E. coli* ↓ - Colonic *Enterococcus*, *Lactobacillus*, and *Bifidobacterium* count ↑	Chen et al. (2013)
ApoE (-/-) mice	*L. reuteri* ATCC PTA 4659	-	8-week old ApoE$^{-/-}$ mice were administered gavagely with 1 × 10^9 CFU *L. reuteri* ATCC PTA 4659 per day for 12 weeks	- Serum insulin ↓ - No effect on atherosclerotic biomarkers	Fåk and Bäckhed (2012)
ApoE (-/-) mice	*L. paracasei* *NFBC338 +* *Gtf* *L. mucosae* DPC6426	Male	12 to 14-week old ApoE$^{-/-}$ mice fed *ad libitum* with drinking water containing ~10^9 CFU of each strain per day for 12 weeks	- Serum cholesterol and triglycerides ↓ - GTF: Fecal cholesterol excretion ↑ - DPC6426: Relative abundance of Porphyromonadaceae, Prevotellaceae ↑ - DPC6426: Relative abundance of Clostridiaceae, Peptococcaceae, and Staphylococcaceae ↓	London et al. (2014)

Continued

TABLE 10.3 Overview of animal studies investigating the effect of probiotic administration on atherosclerosis—cont'd

Model	Probiotic strain	Sex	Dose and duration	Result	Reference
ApoE (-/-) mice	*L. acidophilus* K301	-	8-week old ApoE$^{-/-}$ mice were administered gavagely with 1 × 10^{8} CFU *L. acidophilus* K301 twice a week for 8 weeks	- Accumulation of lipoprotein in the arterial lumen ↓ - Induce squalene reductase and oxidosqualene cyclase - Cholesterol efflux ↑	Hong et al. (2016)
ApoE (-/-) mice	*Pediococcus acidilactici* R037	Female	6-week old ApoE$^{-/-}$ mice were fed ad libitum with diet containing 1.8 × 10^{11} CFU (viable) and 0.4 × 10^{11} CFU (heat-killed) *P. acidilactici* R037 six times a week for 12 weeks	- Atherosclerotic lesions in the aortic root ↓ - Expression of Ki-67 in CD4^{+} T cells ↓ - Population of IFN-γ-producing CD4+ T cells ↓ - Pro-inflammatory cytokines ↓	Mizoguchi et al. (2017)
ApoE (-/-) mice	*L. plantarum* ZDY04	Male	7 to 9-week old ApoE$^{-/-}$ mice were administered gavagely with 1 × 10^{9} CFU *L. plantarum* ZDY04 for 4 weeks	- serum TMAO ↓ - cecal TMA ↓ - relative abundance of families - Lachonospiraceae, - Erysipelotrichaceae, Bacteroidaceae↓ - relative abundance of genus *Mucispirillum* ↑	Qiu, Tao, Xiong, Yu, and Wei (2018)

VSL#3= Probiotic mixture of *L. plantarum* DSM 24730, *L. delbrueckii* subsp. *bulgaricus* DSM 24734, *L. paracasei* DSM 24733, *L. acidophilus* DSM 24735, *B. breve* DSM 24732, *B. longum* DSM24736, *B. infantis* DSM 24737, *S. salivarius* subsp. *thermophilus* DSM 24731.

Overall, current evidence has shown that probiotic bacteria not only protect against myocardial infarction but also protect against inflammation-mediated events following myocardial infarction.

To date, there is limited evidence for the efficacy of probiotics in older adults with CVD. In a small randomized controlled trial, Karlsson et al. (2010) found that Swedish men ($n = 9$; aged 60–75 years) with an atherosclerotic plaque on the carotid artery wall, who consumed 100 mL of fermented oat drink containing 10^{11} CFU of *L. plantarum* DSM 9843 per day for 4 weeks, had significantly increased gut microbial diversity and viable counts of lactobacilli in the fecal matter, while a reduced concentration of cytotoxic carboxylic acids, including isovaleric acid and valeric acid, was observed in the fecal matter. Meanwhile, Malik et al. (2018) evaluated the effect of *L. plantarum* 299v supplementation for vascular endothelial function and systemic inflammation in a nonrandomized study involving 20 men (aged of 40–75 years) with stable coronary artery disease. Patients who consumed a drink containing 2×10^{10} CFU once daily for 6 weeks had significantly improved brachial flow-mediated dilation, reduced levels of circulating proinflammatory markers (IL-8, IL-12), leptin, and plasma acetate, while there was increased plasma propionate without significant changes in trimethylamine oxide (TMAO) accelerated development of atherosclerosis. Recently, Farrokhian et al. (2019) also conducted a randomized, double-blind, placebo-controlled trial to evaluate the effects of synbiotic supplementation in 60 Iranian adults (aged 50–85 years) with coronary heart disease, who were also overweight and diabetic. However, patients ($n = 30$) who received synbiotic capsules containing *L. acidophilus* strain T16 (IBRC-M10785), *L. casei* strain T2 (IBRC-M10783), and *B. bifidum* strain T1 (IBRC-M10771) (2×10^9 CFU/g each) and 800 mg inulin for 12 weeks had reduced serum high-sensitivity C-reactive protein, plasma nitric oxide, and malondialdehyde, but no effect was observed on both carotid intima-media thickness and oxidative stress. These contradictory results warrant further major international cohort studies. On the other hand, Moludi, Alizadeh, Davari, Golmohammadi, and Maleki (2019) conducting a randomized, double-blinded, placebo-controlled trial ($n = 46$) to evaluate the safety and efficacy of 3-months of *L. rhamnosus* (1.6×10^9 CFU/day) intervention on cardiac remodeling in Iranian patients with myocardial infarction. The results of this study will provide preliminary clinical evidence about the potential use of probiotics in attenuating cardiac remodeling after myocardial infarction.

10.4.4 Diabetes mellitus

Diabetes mellitus is a global health problem that not only undermines the quality of life and family relationships but also imposes a substantial financial burden on patients. International Diabetes Federation (IDF) Diabetes Atlas has estimated that the prevalence of diabetes among subjects aged 65 years or older will increase to 195.2 million by 2030 and 276.2 million by 2045 from 135.6 million in 2019 (IDF, 2019). Type 2 diabetes (T2D), characterized by hyperglycemia, insulin resistance with relative insulin deficiency, is the most common type of diabetes in older adults (Beaudry & Devries, 2019). Interestingly, mounting evidence proposes that probiotic supplementation could treat T2D and its complications, such as diabetic foot ulcers and nephropathy in aging adults (Miraghajani, Zaghian, Dehkohneh, Mirlohi, & Ghiasvand, 2019; Mohseni et al., 2018; Tao, Gu, Mao, Zhang, & Pei, 2020).

The results of many studies using T2D animal models have suggested that treatment with live probiotics can modulate antioxidant capacity, insulin sensitivity, beta cell function, lipid and glucose metabolisms, as well as attenuating systemic inflammation, resulting in an alleviation of symptoms of T2D (Dang et al., 2018; Everard, Matamoros, Geurts, Delzenne, & Cani, 2014; Li et al., 2016; Zeng et al., 2019). Even though the exact mechanism of antidiabetic action of probiotics is still not entirely clear, accumulating evidence suggests that these bacteria may modulate gut microbiota that plays a key role in orchestrating pathological events that contribute to the onset and progression of T2D. By using high fat and streptozotocin-induced C57BL/6J mice, Wang Li, Zhao, Zhang, and Chen (2017) investigated whether a 12-week daily administration of 10^8–10^{10} CFU of *L. casei* CCFM419 could attenuate diabetes symptoms and modulate altered gut microbiota. 12-week administration of *L. casei* CCFM419 at a daily dose of 10^9 CFU significantly attenuated inflammatory markers (TNF-α, IL-6), enhanced intestinal glucagon-like peptide-1 (GLP-1), and increased the abundance levels of SCFA-producing bacteria (*Allobaculum, Bacteroides*), *Lactobacillus* and *Bifidobacterium*, suggesting that *L. casei* CCFM419 could ameliorate T2D via a gut microbiota-SCFA-inflammation/GLP-1 dependent mechanism. Furthermore, Wang et al. (2020) have also reported that a 6-week administration of a probiotic cocktail (10 *Lactobacillus* strains (1×10^{10} CFU/mL) and four yeast strains ($1 \text{x} 10^8$ CFU/mL) augmented SCFA-producing bacteria (*Bifidobacterium, Clostridium leptum*, and Roseburia) and decreased the abundance level of *E. coli*, and thereby enhancing insulin secretion, preventing pancreatic apoptosis. and improving blood glucose level in db/db mice, a mouse model of T2D. Despite the antidiabetic effect of probiotics being potentially mediated by SCFA-producing bacteria, more mechanistic studies are needed to examine the interaction between probiotics and these bacteria in improving glycemic control and insulin sensitivity.

Several studies have also evaluated the antidiabetic effects of probiotic fermented beverages in type 2 diabetic rats. Li et al. (2014) found that 5-week administration of carrot juice fermented with *L. plantarum* NCU116 (10^9 CFU/mL, 10 mL/kg/day) not only significantly decreased blood glucose levels and favorably modulated mRNA expression levels of glucose and lipid metabolism–associated genes (low-density lipoprotein (LDL) receptors, glucose transporter-4 (GLUT-4), peroxisome proliferator-activated receptor-γ (PPAR- γ), cholesterol 7α-hydroxylase (CYP7A1) and peroxisome proliferator–activated receptor-α (PPAR-α), but also increased antioxidant capacity and the concentration of SCFAs in the colon, thereby ameliorating low dose streptozotocin- and high-fat–induced type 2 diabetes in rats. Microbiota-derived SCFAs, including butyrate and propionate, have been shown to stimulate GLP-1 and gut hormone peptide YY (PYY) that play an important role in regulating insulin secretion and appetite and are of promising therapeutic targets for T2D (Psichas et al., 2015). Six-week administration of fermented yogurt containing 2.3×10^9 CFU/mL *L. casei* Q14 significantly increased the relative abundance of SCFA-producing bacteria, along with an elevated concentration of SCFAs (acetate and butyrate) that subsequently stimulated GLP-1 and PYY secretion, resulting in an improvement of the lipid profile, insulin and glucose levels in the blood of T2D rats (Qu et al., 2018).

Noteworthy, in addition to live probiotics, probiotic bacteria-derived components and bioactive have also been associated with antidiabetic properties. Plovier et al. (2017) discovered that a purified outer member protein (Amuc_1100) from *Akkermansia muciniphila* is capable of improving insulin resistance, lipid metabolism, and gut barrier function in diabetic mice. On the other hand, it has been reported that high fat- and streptozotocin-induced type 2 diabetic rats administered with polysaccharides extracted from *Momordica charantia* L., fermented with *L. plantarum* NCU116 for 4 weeks, significantly enhanced antidiabetes effects (hyperlipidemia, hyperglycemia, hyperinsulinemia), enhanced colonic SCFAs production, increased microbial diversity and abundance levels of *Lactococcus laudensis* and *Prevotella loescheii,* as compared with nonfermented *M. charantia* L. -fed rats (Gao, Wen, et al., 2018). Hence, *L. plantarum* NCU116 may metabolize *Momordica charantia* polysaccharides during fermentation, and subsequently mediates antidiabetic activities either directly through the production of bioactive polysaccharides or indirectly via the generation of a structure of polysaccharides that favors gut microbial balance and SCFAs production.

Regarding human studies, several systematic reviews and meta-analyses of randomized controlled trials in adults with T2D suggested that the potential of probiotic supplementation in improving glycemic control is promising, but controversial (Hendijani & Akbari, 2018; Barengolts, Smith, Reutrakul, Tonucci, & Anothaisintawee, 2019; Tiderencel, Hutcheon, & Ziegler, 2020; Sum et al., 2020). Although the antidiabetic potential of probiotics has been demonstrated primarily in the animal models and middle-aged adults (36–55 years) of T2D, the role of gut microbiota and probiotic in elderly patients with T2D, is currently lacking. Interestingly, Gunung et al. (2020) recently analyzed the possible association of the specific bacterial group with T2D using 42 human studies and summarized that the genera of *Blautia*, *Fusobacterium*, and *Ruminococcus* were positively associated with T2D, whereas the genera of *Akkermansia*, *Bacteroides*, *Bifidobacterium*, *Faecalibacterium*, and *Roseburia* were inversely associated with T2D. Moreover, Mobini et al. (2017) conducted a randomized, double-blind, placebo-controlled trial involving 46 Swedish patients (age 65 ± 6 years) with T2D to examine whether a 12-week administration of *L. reuteri* DSM 17938 (10^{10} CFU/day, $n = 14$) influenced the glycemic marker (HbA1c), insulin sensitivity, lipid metabolism, and fecal microbiota composition. The results showed that the supplementation of *L. reuteri* DSM 17938 only improved insulin sensitivity and did not affect microbiota composition, glycemic control, and adiposity. Larger randomized controlled trials are thus warranted to replicate the beneficial effects of probiotics on glycemic control, insulin sensitivity, lipid markers, SCFAs, and gut microbiota profiles in older adults (aged 65 years above) with T2D.

10.5 Conclusions

Despite probiotics interventions have shown promising potential in promoting healthy aging and treating age-related diseases via modulation of gut microbiota, several important issues remain controversial. To date, clinical studies supporting the health claims of probiotics tend to focus on young and middle-aged adults with age-related diseases. However, due to age-related differences in microbiota composition, the beneficial effects of probiotics observed in the younger populations should not be generalizable to older adults (> 65 years). In addition to chronological age, a growing body of evidence suggests that the efficacy of probiotics is also highly dependent on the strain, disease, dose, and length of treatment. Hence, more randomized controlled trials on elderly populations are needed to provide solid evidence about the potential benefits, safety, and efficacy of probiotics in promoting healthy aging and treating age-related diseases. Recent advances in imaging and sequencing tools can also be applied to uncover the molecular and cellular mechanisms underlying the beneficial effects of probiotics and to promote the future development of probiotic supplements and/or beverages for aging populations.

References

Abdulrahman, H., Fletcher, P. C., Bullmore, E., & Morcom, A. M. (2017). Dopamine and memory dedifferentiation in aging. *NeuroImage, 153*, 211–220.

Arseneault-Bréard, J., Rondeau, I., Gilbert, K., Girard, S. A., Tompkins, T. A., Godbout, R. , et al. (2012). Combination of *Lactobacillus helveticus* R0052 and *Bifidobacterium longum*

R0175 reduces post-myocardial infarction. *The British Journal of Nutrition*, *107*(12), 1793–1799.

Bajaj, J. S., Ahluwalia, V., Steinberg, J. L., Hobgood, S., Boling, P. A., Godschalk, M. , et al. (2016). Elderly patients have an altered gut-brain axis regardless of the presence of cirrhosis. *Scientific Reports*, *6*, 38481.

Barengolts, E., Smith, E. D., Reutrakul, S., Tonucci, L., & Anothaisintawee, T. (2019). The effect of probiotic yogurt on glycemic control in type 2 diabetes or obesity: A meta-analysis of nine randomized controlled trials. *Nutrients*, *11*(3)671.

Bartosch, S., Woodmansey, E. J., Paterson, J. C., McMurdo, M. E., & Macfarlane, G. T. (2005). Microbiological effects of consuming a symbiotic containing *Bifidobacterium bifidum*, *Bifidobacterium lactis*, and oligofructose in elderly persons, determined by real-time polymerase chain reaction and counting of viable bacteria. *Clinical Infectious Diseases*, *40*(1), 28–37.

Beaudry, K. M., & Devries, M. C. (2019). Nutritional strategies to combat type 2 diabetes in aging adults: the importance of protein. *Frontiers in Nutrition*, *6*, 138.

Benjamin, E. J., Muntner, P., Alonso, A., Bittencourt, M. S., Callaway, C. W., Carson, A. P. , et al. (2019). Heart disease and stroke statistics-2019 update: A report from the American Heart Association. *Circulation*, *139*, e56–e528.

Biagi, E., Nylund, L., Candela, M., Ostan, R., Bucci, L., Pini, E. , et al. (2010). Through ageing, and beyond: gut microbiota and inflammatory status in seniors and centenarians. *PLoS One*, *5*(5)e10667.

Britton, R. A., Irwin, R., Quach, D., Schaefer, L., Zhang, J., Lee, T. , et al. (2014). Probiotic *L. reuteri* treatment prevents bone loss in a menopausal ovariectomized mouse model. *Journal of Cellular Physiology*, *229*(11), 1822–1830.

Cattaneo, A., Cattane, N., Galluzzi, S., Provasi, S., Lopizzo, N., Festari, C. , et al. (2017). Association of brain amyloidosis with pro-inflammatory gut bacterial taxa and peripheral inflammation markers in cognitively impaired elderly. *Neurobiology of Aging*, *49*, 60–68.

Cavallini, D. C. U., Bedani, R., Bomdespacho, L. Q., Vendramini, R. C., & Rossi, E. A. (2009). Effects of probiotic bacteria, isoflavones and simvastatin on lipid profile and atherosclerosis in cholesterol-fed rabbits: A randomized double-blind study. *Lipids in Health and Disease*, *8*, 1.

Cenci, S., Weitzmann, M. N., Roggia, C., Namba, N., Novack, D., Woodring, J. , et al. (2000). Estrogen deficiency induces bone loss by enhancing T-cell production of TNF-alpha. *The Journal of Clinical Investigation*, *106*(10), 1229–1237.

Chan, Y. K., Brar, M. S., Kirjavainen, P. V., Chen, Y., Peng, J., Li, D. , et al. (2016). High fat diet induced atherosclerosis is accompanied with low colonic bacterial diversity and altered abundances that correlates with plaque size, plasma A-FABP and cholesterol: A pilot study of high fat diet and its intervention with *Lactobacillus rhamnosus* GG (LGG) or telmisartan in ApoE-/- mice. *BMC Microbiology*, *16*(1), 264.

Chen, L. H., Huang, S. Y., Huang, K. C., Hsu, C. C., Yang, K. C., Li, L. A. , et al. (2019). *Lactobacillus paracasei* PS23 decelerated age-related muscle loss by ensuring mitochondrial function in SAMP8 mice. *Aging*, *11*(2), 756–770.

Chen, L., Liu, W., Li, Y., Luo, S., Liu, Q., Zhong, Y. , et al. (2013). *Lactobacillus acidophilus* ATCC 4356 attenuates the atherosclerotic progression through modulation of oxidative stress and inflammatory process. *International Immunopharmacology*, *17*(1), 108–115.

Chan, Y. K., El-Nezami, H., Chen, Y., Kinnunen, K., & Kirjavainen, P. V. (2016). Probiotic mixture VSL#3 reduce high fat diet induced vascular inflammation and atherosclerosis in ApoE$^{(-/-)}$ mice. *AMB Express*, *6*(1), 61.

Chen, J., Ou, Y., Hu, S., Shao, L. W., & Liu, Y. (2017). Metformin extends *C. elegans* lifespan through lysosomal pathway. *eLife*, *6*, e31268.

Chiang, S., & Pan, T. (2011). Antiosteoporotic effects of *Lactobacillus*-fermented soy skim milk on bone mineral density and the microstructure of femoral bone in ovariectomized mice. *Journal of Agricultural and Food Chemistry*, *59*(14), 7734–7742.

Chowdhury, R., Guitant-Masip, M., Bunzeck, N., Dolan, R. J., & Düzel, E. (2012). Dopamine modulates episodic memory persistence in old age. *Journal of Neuroscience, 32*(41), 14193–14204.

Claesson, M. J., Cusack, S., O'Sullivan, O., Greene-Diniz, R., de Weerd, H., Flannery, E. , et al. (2011). Composition, variability, and temporal stability of the intestinal microbiota of the elderly. *Proceeding of the National Academy of Sciences (USA), 108*(Suppl. 1), 4586–4591.

Collino, S., Montoliu, I., Martin, F. P. J., Scherer, M., Mari, D., Salvioli, S. , et al. (2013). Metabolic signatures of extreme longevity in Northern Italian centenarians reveal a complex remodeling of lipids, amino acids, and gut microbiota metabolism. *PLoS One, 8*(8)e56564.

Collins, F. L., Irwin, R., Bierhalter, H., Schepper, J., Britton, R. A., Parameswaran, N. , et al. (2016). *Lactobacillus reuteri* 6475 increases bone density in intact females only under an inflammatory setting. *PLoS One, 11*(4)e0153180.

Collins, F. L., Rios-Arce, N. D., Schepper, J. D., Jones, D., Schaefer, L., Britton, R. A. , et al. (2019). Beneficial effects of *Lactobacillus reuteri* 6475 on bone mineral density in male mice is dependent on lymphocytes. *Scientific Reports, 9*, 14708.

Corpuz, H. M., Ichikawa, S., Arimura, M., Mihara, T., Kumagai, T., Mitani, T. , et al. (2018). Long-term diet supplementation with *Lactobacillus paracasei* K71 prevents age-related cognitive decline in senescence-accelerated mouse prone 8. *Nutrients, 10*(6), 762. https://doi.org/10.3390/nu10060762.

Cox, L. M., Yamanishi, S., Sohn, J., Alekseyenko, A. V., Leung, J. M., Cho, I. , et al. (2014). Altering the intestinal microbiota during a critical developmental window has lasting metabolic consequences. *Cell, 158*(4), 705–721.

Dang, F., Jiang, Y., Pan, R., Zhou, Y., Wu, S., Wang, R. , et al. (2018). Administration of *Lactobacillus paracasei* ameliorates type 2 diabetes in mice. *Food & Function, 9*(7), 3630–3639.

Danilo, C. A., Constantopoulos, E., McKee, L. A., Chen, H., Regan, J. A., Lipovka, Y. , et al. (2017). *Bifidobacterium animalis* subsp. *lactis* 420 mitigates the pathological impact of myocardial infarction in the mouse. *Beneficial Microbes, 8*(2), 257–269.

Ding, R. X., Goh, W. R., Wu, R. N., Yue, X. Q., Luo, X., Khine, W. W. T. , et al. (2019). Revisit gut microbiota and its impact on human health and disease. *Journal of Food and Drug Analysis, 27*(3), 623–631.

Distrutti, E., O'Reilly, J. A., McDonald, C., Cipriani, S., Renga, B., Lynch, M. A. , et al. (2014). Modulation of intestinal microbiota by the probiotic VSL#3 reset brain gene expression and ameliorates the age-related deficit in LTP. *PLoS One, 9*(9)e106503.

Dong, H., Rowland, I., Thomas, L. V., & Yaqoob, P. (2013). Immunomodulatory effects of a probiotic drink containing *Lactobacillus casei* Shirota in healthy older volunteers. *European Journal of Nutrition, 52*, 1853–1863.

El Aidy, S., van Baarlen, P., Derrien, M., Lindenbergh-Kortleve, D. J., Hooiveld, G., Levenez, F. , et al. (2012). Temporal and spatial interplay of microbiota and intestinal mucosa drive establishment of immune homeostasis in conventionalized mice. *Mucosal Immunology, 5*(5), 567–579.

Eloe-Fadrosh, E. A., Brady, A., Crabtree, J., Drabek, E. F., Ma, B., Mahurkar, A. , et al. (2015). Functional dynamics of the gut microbiome in elderly people during probiotic consumption. *MBio, 6*, . e00231-15.

Ettinger, G., Burton, J. P., Gloor, G. B., & Reid, G. (2017). *Lactobacillus rhamnosus* GR-1 attenuates induction of hypertrophy in cardiomyocytes but not through secreted protein MSP-1 (p75). *PLoS One, 12*(1)e0168622.

Everard, A., Matamoros, S., Geurts, L., Delzenne, N. M., & Cani, P. D. (2014). *Saccharomyces bouldari* administration changes gut microbiota and reduces hepatic steatosis, low-grade inflammation, and fat mass in obese and type 2 diabetic db/db mice. *MBio, 5*(3), e01011–e01014.

Fåk, F., & Bäckhed, F. (2012). *Lactobacillus reuteri* prevents diet-induced obesity, but not atherosclerosis, in a strain dependent fashion in Apoe-/- mice. *PLoS One*, *7*(10)e46837.

Farrokhian, A., Raygan, F., Saltani, A., Tajabadi-Ebrahimi, M., Sharifi, E. M., Karami, A. A., et al. (2019). The effects of synbiotic supplementation on carotid intima-media thickness, biomarkers of inflammation and oxidative stress in people with overweight, diabetes, and coronary heart disease: a randomized, double-blind, placebo-controlled trial. *Probiotics and Antimicrobial Proteins*, *11*(1), 133–142.

Fielding, R. A., Reeves, A. R., Jasuja, R., Liu, C., Barrett, B. B., & Lustgarten, M. S. (2019). Muscle strength is increased in mice that are colonized with microbiota from high-functioning older adults. *Experimental Gerontology*, *127*, 110722.

Flaxman, S. R., Bourne, R. R. A., Resnikoff, S., Ackland, P., Braithwaite, T., Cicinelli, M. V., et al. (2017). Global causes of blindness and distance vision impairment 1990-2020: a systematic review and meta-analysis. *The Lancet: Global Health*, *5*(12), 1221–1234.

Flores, R., Shi, J., Fuhrman, B., Xu, X., Veenstra, T. D., Gail, M. H., et al. (2012). Fecal microbial determinants of fecal and systematic estrogens and estrogen metabolites: a cross-sectional study. *Journal of Translational Medicine*, *10*, 253.

Frostegård, J. (2013). Immunity, atherosclerosis and cardiovascular disease. *BMC Medicine*, *11*, 117.

Fuhrman, B. J., Feigelson, H. S., Flores, R., Gail, M. H., Xu, X., Ravel, J., et al. (2014). Associations of the fecal microbiome with urine estrogens and estrogen metabolites in post-menopausal women. *The Journal of Clinical Endocrinology and Metabolism*, *99*(12), 4632–4640.

Gan, X. T., Ettinger, G., Huang, C. X., Burton, J. P., Haist, J. V., Rajapurohitam, C., et al. (2014). Probiotic administration attenuates myocardial hypertrophy and heart failure after myocardial infarction in the rat. *Circulation Heart Failure*, *7*(3), 491–499.

Gao, A. W., Bos, J. U. D., Sterken, M. G., Kammenga, J. E., Smith, R. L., & Houtkooper, R. H. (2018). Forward and reverse genetic approaches to uncover metabolic aging pathways in *Caenorhabditis elegans*. *Biochimica et Biophysica Acta (BBA) - Molecular Basis of Disease*, *1864*, 2697–2706.

Gao, H., Wen, J. J., Hu, J. L., Nie, Q. X, Chen, H. H., Xiong, T., et al. (2018). Polysaccharide from fermented *Momordica charantia* L. with *Lactobacillus plantarum* NCU116 ameliorates type 2 diabetes in rats. *Carbohydrate Polymers*, *201*, 624–633.

Gefen, T., Kim, G., Bolbolan, K., Geoly, A., Ohm, D., Oboudiyat, C., et al. (2019). Activated microglia in cortical white matter across cognitive aging trajectories. *Frontiers in Aging Neuroscience*, *11*, 94. https://doi.org/10.3389/fnagi.2019.00094.

Girard, S. A., Bah, T. M., Kaloustian, S., Lada-Moldovan, L., Rondeau, I., Tompkins, T. A., et al. (2009). *Lactobacillus helveticus* and *Bifidobacterium longum* taken in combination reduce the apoptosis propensity in the limbic system after myocardial infarction in a rat model. *The British Journal of Nutrition*, *102*(10), 1420–1425.

Gladyshey, V. N. (2016). Aging: progressive decline in fitness due to the rising deleteriome adjusted by genetic, environmental, and stochastic processes. *Aging Cell*, *15*(4), 594–602.

González-Burgos, I., & Feria-Velasco, A. (2008). Serotonin/dopamine interaction in memory formation. *Progress in Brain Research*, *172*, 603–623.

Govindaraju, T., Sahle, B. W., McCaffrey, T. A., McNeil, J. J., & Owen, A. J. (2018). Dietary patterns and quality of life in older adults: a systematic review. *Nutrients*, *10*(8), 971. https://doi.org/10.3390/nu10080971.

Grompone, G., Martorell, P., Llopis, S., González, N., Genovés, S., Mulet, A. P., et al. (2012). Anti-inflammatory *Lactobacillus rhamnosus* CNCM I-3690 strain protects against oxidative stress and increases lifespan in *Caenorhabditis elegans*. *PLoS One*, *7*(12)e52493.

Guillemard, E., Tondu, F., Lacoin, F., & Schrezenmeir, J. (2010). Consumption of a fermented dairy product containing the probiotic *Lactobacillus casei* DN-114001 reduces the duration of respiratory infections in the elderly in a randomized controlled trial. *The British Journal of Nutrition, 103*(1), 58–68.

Gunung, M., Li, Z., You, H., Rodrigues, R., Jump, D. B., Morgun, A. , et al. (2020). Role of gut microbiota in type 2 diabetes pathophysiology. *eBioMedicine, 51*, 102590.

Guss, J. D., Horsfield, M. W., Fontenele, F. F., Sandoval, T. N., Luna, M., Apporval, F. , et al. (2017). Alterations to the gut microbiome impair bone strength and tissue material properties. *Journal of Bone and Mineral Research, 32*(6), 1343–1353.

Guzon-Illescas, O., Perez, F. E., Crespi, V. N., Quiruirós, D. F. J., Peña, M., Alonso-Blas, C. , et al. (2019). Mortality after osteoporotic hip fractures: incidence, trends, and associated factors. *Journal of Orthopaedic Surgery and Research, 14*, 203.

Han, B., Sivaramakrishnan, P., Lin, C. J., Neve, I. A. A., He, J., Tay, L. W. R. , et al. (2017). Microbial genetic composition tunes host longevity. *Cell, 169*(7), 1249–1262.

Hayes, C. L., Dong, J., Galipeau, H. J., Jury, J., McCarville, J., Huang, X. , et al. (2018). Commensal microbiota induces colonic barrier structure and functions that contribute to homeostasis. *Scientific Reports, 8*, 14184.

Hendijani, F., & Akbari, V. (2018). Probiotic supplementation for management of cardiovascular risk factors in adults with type II diabetes: a systematic review and meta-analysis. *Clinical Nutrition, 37*(2), 532–541.

Hibberd, P. L., Kleimola, L., Fiorino, A., Botelho, C., Haverkamp, M., Andreyeva, I. , et al. (2014). No evidence of harms of probiotic *Lactobacillus rhamnosus* GG ATCC 53103 in healthy elderly—A phase I open label study to access safety, tolerability and cytokine responses. *PLoS One, 9*(12)e113456.

Hong, Y. F., Kim, H., Kim, H. S., Park, W. J., Kim, J. Y., & Chung, D. K. (2016). *Lactobacillus acidophilus* K301 inhibits atherogenesis via induction of 24(S), 25-epoxycholesterol-mediated ABCA1 and ABCG1 production and cholesterol efflux in macrophages. *PLoS One, 11*(4)e0154302.

Hor, Y. Y., Ooi, C. H., Khoo, B. Y., Choi, S. B., Seeni, A., Shamsuddin, S. , et al. (2019). *Lactobacillus* strains alleviated aging symptoms and aging-induced metabolic disorders in aged rats. *Journal of Medicinal Food, 22*(1), 1–13.

Horai, R., Zárate-Bladés, C. R., Dillenburg-Pilla, P., Chen, J., Kielczewski, J. L., Silver, P. B. , et al. (2015). Microbiota-dependent activation of an autoreactive T cell receptor provokes autoimmunity in an immunologically privileged site. *Immunity, 43*(2), 343–353.

Huang, S. Y., Chen, L. H., Wang, M. F., Hsu, C. C., Chan, C. H., Li, J. X. , et al. (2018). *Lactobacillus paracasei* PS23 delays progression of age-related cognitive decline in senescence accelerated mouse prone 8 (SAMP8) mice. *Nutrients, 10*(7), 894. https://doi.org/10.3390/nu10070894.

Huang, Y., Wang, J., Quan, G., Wang, X., Yang, L., & Zhong, L. (2014). *Lactobacillus acidophilus* ATCC 4356 prevents atherosclerosis via inhibition of intestinal cholesterol absorption in apolipoprotein E-knockout mice. *Applied and Environmental Microbiology, 80*(24), 7496–7504.

Hurez, V., Dao, V., Liu, A., Gelfond, J., Sun, L., Bergman, M. , et al. (2015). Chronic mTOR inhibition in mice with rapamycin alters T, B, myeloid, and innate lymphoid cells and gut flora and prolongs life of immune-deficient mice. *Aging Cell, 14*(6), 945–956.

Huuskonen, J., Suuronen, T., Nuutinen, T., Kyrylenko, S., & Salminen, A. (2004). Regulation of microglial inflammatory response by sodium butyrate and short-chain fatty acids. *British Journal of Pharmacology, 141*(5), 874–880.

Inana, G., Murat, C., An, W., Yao, X., Harris, I. R., & Cao, J. (2018). RPE phagocytic function declines in age-related macular degeneration and is rescued by human umbilical tissue derived cells. *Journal of Translational Medicine, 16*, 63. https://doi.org/10.1186/s12967-018-1434-6.

Inoue, T., Kobayashi, Y., Mori, N., Sakagawa, M., Xiao, J. Z., Moritani, T. , et al. (2018). Effect of combined bifidobacteria supplementation and resistance training on cognitive function, body composition and bowel habits of healthy elderly subjects. *Beneficial Microbes, 9*(6), 843–853.

International Diabetes Federation (2019). *IDF diabetes atlas* (9th ed.). Brussels, Belgium: International Diabetes Federation.

Jafarnejad, S., Djafarian, K., Fazeli, M. R., Yekaninejad, M. S., Rostamian, A., & Keshavarz, S. A. (2017). Effects of a multispecies probiotic supplement on bone health in osteopenic postmenopausal women: A randomized, double-blind, controlled trial. *Journal of the American College of Nutrition, 36*(7), 497–506.

Johnson, S. C., Rabinovitch, P. S., & Kaeberlein, M. (2013). mTOR is a key modulator of ageing and age-related disease. *Nature, 493*(7432), 338–345.

Kaeberlein, M. (2017). Translational geroscience: a new paradigm for 21st century medicine. *Translational Medicine of Aging, 1*, 1–4.

Karlsson, C., Ahrné, S., Molin, G., Berggren, A., Palmquist, I., Fredrikson, G. N. , et al. (2010). Probiotic therapy to men with incipient arteriosclerosis initiates increased bacterial diversity in colon: A randomized controlled trial. *Atherosclerosis, 208*(1), 228–233.

Khosla, S., & Pacifici, R. (2013). Estrogen deficiency, postmenopausal osteoporosis, and age-related bone loss. In *Osteoporosis: Fourth edition* (pp. 1113–1136). Elsevier Inc. https://doi.org/10.1016/B978-0-12-415853-5.00046-7.

Kiefte-de Jong, J. C., Mathers, J. C., & Franco, O. H. (2014). Nutrition and healthy aging: the key ingredients. *The Proceeding of the Nutrition Society, 73*(2), 249–259.

Kim, J. G., Lee, E., Kim, S. H., Whang, K. Y., Oh, S., & Imm, J. Y. (2009). Effects of a *Lactobacillus casei* 393 fermented milk product on bone metabolism in ovariectomized rats. *International Dairy Journal, 19*(11), 690–695.

King, C. H., Desai, H., Sylvetsky, A. C., LoTempio, J., Ayanyan, S., Carrier, J. , et al. (2019). Baseline human gut microbiota profile in healthy people and standard reporting template. *PLoS One, 14*(9)e0206484.

Kiousi, D. E., Karapetsas, A., Karolidou, K., Panayiotidis, M. I., Pappa, A., & Galanis, A. (2019). Probiotics in extraintestinal diseases: current trends and new directions. *Nutrients, 11*(4), 788. https://doi.org/10.3390/nu11040788.

Kruger, M. C., Fear, A., Chua, W. H., Plimmer, G. G., & Schollum, L. M. (2009). The effect of *Lactobacillus rhamnosus* HN001 on mineral absorption and bone health in growing male and ovariectomized female rats. *Dairy Science and Technology, 89*, 219–231.

Lambert, M. N. T., Thorup, A. C., Hansen, E. S. S., & Jeppesen, P. B. (2017). Combined red clover isoflavones and probiotics potenly reduce menopausal vasomotor symptoms. *PLoS One, 12*(6)e0176590.

Lambeth, S. M., Carson, T., Lowe, J., Ramaraj, T., Leff, J. W., Luo, L. , et al. (2015). Composition, diversity and abundance of gut microbiome in prediabetes and type 2 diabetes. *Journal of Diabetes and Obesity, 2*(3), 1–7.

Lefevre, M., Racedo, S. M., Ripert, G., Housez, B., Cazaubiel, M., Maudet, C. , et al. (2015). Probiotic strain *Bacillus subtilis* CU1 stimulates immune system of elderly during common infectious disease period: a randomized, double-blind placebo-controlled study. *Immunity & Aging, 12*, 24. https://doi.org/10.1186/s12979-015-0051-y.

Leulier, F., MacNeil, L. T., Lee, W., Rawis, J. F., Cani, P. D., Schwarzer, M. , et al. (2017). Integrative physiology: at the crossroads of nutrition, microbiota, animal physiology and human health. *Cell Metabolism, 25*(3), 522–534.

Li, C., Ding, Q., Nie, S. P., Zhang, Y. S., Xiong, T., & Xie, M. Y. (2014). Carrot juice fermented with *Lactobacillus plantarum* NCU116 ameliorates type 2 diabetes in rats. *Journal of Agricultural and Food Chemistry, 62*(49), 11884–11891.

Li, C., Huang, Q., Yang, R., Dai, Y., Zeng, J., & Wang, Q. (2019). Gut microbiota composition and bone mineral loss - epidemiologic evidence from individuals in Wuhan, China. *Osteoporosis International, 30*(5), 1003–1013.

Li, X., Wang, N., Yin, B., Fang, D., Jiang, T., Fang, S. , et al. (2016). Effects of *Lactobacillus plantarum* CCFM0236 on hyperglycaemia and insulin resistance in high-fat and streptozotocin-induced type 2 diabetic mice. *Journal of Applied Microbiology, 121*(6), 1727–1736.

Logsdon, A. F., Erickson, M. A., Rhea, E. M., Salameh, T. S., & Banks, W. A. (2018). Gut reactions: how the blood-brain barrier connects the microbiome and the brain. *Experimental Biology and Medicine, 243*(2), 159–165.

London, L. E. E., Kumar, A. H. S., Wall, R., Casey, P. G., O'Sullivan, O., Shanahan, F. , et al. (2014). Exopolysaccharide-producing probiotic lactobacilli reduce serum cholesterol and modify enteric microbiota in ApoE-deficient mice. *The Journal of Nutrition, 144*(12), 1956–1962.

López-Otín, C., Blasco, M. A., Patridge, L., Serrano, M., & Kroemer, G. (2013). The hallmarks of aging. *Cell, 153*(6), 1194–1217.

Lynn, H., Kwok, T., Wong, S. Y., Woo, J., & Leung, P. C. (2006). Angiotensin converting enzyme inhibitor use is associated with higher bone mineral density in elderly Chinese. *Bone, 38*(4), 584–588.

Malik, M., Suboc, T. M., Tvagi, S., Salzman, N., Wang, J., Ying, R. , et al. (2018). *Lactobacillus plantarum* 299v supplementation improves vascular endothelial function and reduced inflammatory biomarkers in men with stable coronary artery disease. *Circulation Research, 123*(9), 1091–1102.

Mangelsdorf, D. J., Thummel, C., Beato, M., Herrlich, P., Schütz, G., Umesono, K. , et al. (1995). The nuclear receptor superfamily: the second decade. *Cell, 83*(6), 835–839.

Martin-Montalvo, A., Mercken, W. M., Mitchell, S. J., Palacios, H. H., Mote, P. L., Scheibye-Knudsen, M. , et al. (2013). Metformin improves healthspan and lifespan in mice. *Nature Communications, 4*, 2192. https://doi.org/10.1038/ncomms3192.

McCabe, L. R., Irwin, R., Scharfer, L., & Britton, R. A. (2013). Probiotic use decreases intestinal inflammation and increases bone density in healthy male but not female mice. *Journal of Cellular Physiology, 228*(8), 1793–1798.

Miller, L. E., Lehtoranta, L., & Lehtinen, M. J. (2019). Short-term probiotic supplementation enhances cellular immune function in healthy elderly: systematic review and meta-analysis of controlled studies. *Nutrition Research, 64*, 1–8.

Miraghajani, M., Zaghian, N., Dehkohneh, A., Mirlohi, M., & Ghiasvand, R. (2019). Probiotic soy milk consumption and renal function among type 2 diabetic patients with nephropathy: a randomized control clinical trial. *Probiotics and Antimicrobial Proteins, 11*(1), 124–132.

Mizoguchi, T., Kasahara, K., Yamashita, T., Sasaki, N., Yodoi, K., Matsumoto, T. , et al. (2017). Oral administration of the lactic acid bacterium *Pediococcus acidilactici* attenuates atherosclerosis in mice by inducing tolerogenic dendritic cells. *Heart and Vessels, 32*(6), 768–776.

Mobini, R., Tremaroli, V., Ståhlman, M., Karlsson, F., Levin, M., Ljungberg, M. , et al. (2017). Metabolic effects of *Lactobacillus reuteri* DSM 17938 in patients with type 2 diabetes: A randomized controlled trial. *Diabetes, Obesity and Metabolism, 19*(4), 579–589.

Mohseni, S., Bayani, S., Bahmani, F., Tajabadi-Ebrahimi, M., Bayani, M. A., Jafari, P. , et al. (2018). The beneficial effects of probiotic administration on wound healing and metabolic status in patients with diabetic foot ulcer: A randomized, double-blind, placebo-controlled trial. *Diabetes/Metabolism Research and Reviews. 34*(3)https://doi.org/10.1002/dmrr.2970.

Moludi, J., Alizadeh, M., Davari, M., Golmohammadi, A., & Maleki, V. (2019). The efficacy and safety of probiotic intervention in attenuating cardiac remodeling following myocardial infraction: Literature review and study protocol for a randomized, double-blinded, placebo- controlled trial. *Contemporary Clinical Trials Communications, 15*, 100364.

Montazeri-Najafabady, N., Ghasemi, Y., Dabbaghmanesh, M. H., Talezadeh, P., Koohpeyma, F., & Gholami, A. (2019). Supportive role of probiotic strains in protecting rats from ovariectomy-induced cortical bone loss. *Probiotics and Antimicrobial Proteins, 11* (4), 1145–1154.

Morita, Y., Jounai, K., Sakamoto, A., Tomita, Y., Sugihara, Y., Suzuki, H. , et al. (2018). Long-term intake of *Lactobacillus paracasei* KW3110 prevents age-related chronic inflammation and retinal cell loss in physiologically aged mice. *Aging, 10*(10), 2723–2740.

Morita, Y., Miwa, Y., Jounai, K., Fujiwara, D., Kurihara, T., & Kanauchi, O. (2018). *Lactobacillus paracasei* KW3110 prevents blue light-induced inflammation and degeneration in the retina. *Nutrients, 10*(12)e1991.

Moro-Garcia, M. A., Alonso-Arias, R., Baltadjieva, M., Fernández, B. C., Fernández, B. M. A., Díaz, R. E. , et al. (2013). Oral supplementation with *Lactobacillus delbrueckii* subsp. *bulgaricus* 8481 enhances systematic immunity in elderly subjects. *Age (Dordrecht, Netherlands), 35*(4), 1311–1326.

Narva, M., Collin, M., Lamberg-Allartdt, C., Kärkkäinen, M., Poussa, T., Vapaatalo, H. , et al. (2004). Effects of long-term intervention with *Lactobacillus helveticus*-fermented milk on bone mineral density and bone mineral content in growing rats. *Annals of Nutrition and Metabolism, 48*, 228–234.

Narva, M., Nevala, R., Poussa, T., & Korpela, R. (2004). The effect of *Lactobacillus helveticus* fermented milk on acute changes in calcium metabolism in postmenopausal women. *European Journal of Nutrition, 43*(2), 61–68.

Ni, Y., Yang, X., Zheng, L., Wang, Z., Wu, L., Jiang, J. , et al. (2019). *Lactobacillus* and *Bifidobacterium* improves physiological function and cognitive ability in aged mice by the regulation of gut microbiota. *Molecular Nutrition & Food Research, 63*(22)e1900603.

Nilsson, A. G., Sundh, D., Bäckhed, F , & Lorentzon, M. (2018). *Lactobacillus reuteri* reduces bone loss in older women with low bone mineral density: A randomized, placebo-controlled, double-blind, clinical trial. *Journal of Internal Medicine, 284*(3), 303–317.

Odamaki, T., Kato, K., Sugahara, H., Hashikura, N., Takahashi, S., Xiao, J. , et al. (2016). Age-related changes in gut microbiota composition from newborn to centenarian: a cross-sectional study. *BMC Microbiology, 16*, 90. https://doi.org/10.1186/s12866-016-0708-5.

Ohlsson, C., Engdahi, C., Fåk, F., Andersson, A., Windahl, S. H., Farman, H. H. , et al. (2014). Probiotics protect mice from ovariectomy-induced cortical bone loss. *PLoS One, 9*, e92368.

O'Toole, P. W., & Claesson, M. J. (2010). Gut microbiota: changes throughout the lifespan from infancy to elderly. *International Dairy Journal, 20*(4), 281–291.

Ovadya, Y., Landsberger, T., Leins, H., Vadai, E., Gal, H., Biran, A. , et al. (2018). Impaired immune surveillance accelerates accumulation of senescent cells and aging. *Nature Communications, 9*, 5435.

Park, M. R., Ryu, S., Maburutse, B. E., Oh, N. S., Kim, S. H., Oh, S. , et al. (2018). Probiotic *Lactobacillus fermentum* strain JDFM216 stimulates the longevity and immune response of *Caenorhabditis elegans* through a nuclear hormone receptor. *Scientific Reports, 8*, e7441.

Parvaneh, K., Ebrahimi, M., Sabran, M. R., Karimi, G., Hwei, A. N. M., Abdul-Majeed, S. , et al. (2015). Probiotics (*Bifidobacterium longum*) increase bone mass density and upregulate *Sparc* and *Bmp-2* genes in rats with bone loss resulting from ovariectomy. *BioMed Research International, 2015*, 897639.

Parvaneh, M., Karimi, G., Jamaluddin, R., Ng, M. H., Zuritati, I., & Muhammad, S. I. (2018). *Lactobacillus helveticus* (ATCC 27558) upregulates Runx2 and Bmp2 and modulates bone mineral density in ovariectomy-induced bone loss rats. *Clinical Interventions in Aging, 13*, 1555–1564.

Plovier, H., Everard, A., Druart, C., Depommier, C., Van, H., Geurts, M. , et al. (2017) A purified membrane protein from *Akkermansia muciniphila* or the pasteurized bacterium improves metabolism in obese and diabetic mice. *Nature Medicine, 23*, 107–113.

Psichas, A., Sleeth, M. L., Murphy, K. G., Brooks, L., Bewick, G. A., Hanyaloglu, A. C. , et al. (2015). The short chain fatty acid propionate stimulates GLP-1 and PYY secretion via free fatty acid receptor 2 in rodents. *International Journal of Obesity, 39*, 424–429.

Pu, F., Guo, Y., Li, M., Zhu, H., Wang, S., Shen, X. , et al. (2017). Yogurt supplemented with probiotics can protect the healthy elderly from respiratory infections: A randomized controlled open-trial label. *Clinical Interventions in Aging*, *12*, 1223–1231.

Qiu, L., Tao, X., Xiong, H., Yu, J., & Wei, H. (2018). *Lactobacillus plantarum* ZDY04 exhibits a strain-specific property by lowering TMAO via the modulation of gut microbiota in mice. *Food & Function*, *9*(8), 4299–4309.

Qu, L., Ren, J., Huang, L., Pang, B., Liu, X., Liu, X. , et al. (2018). Antidiabetic effects of *Lactobacillus casei* fermented yogurt through reshaping gut microbiota structure in type 2 diabetic rats. *Journal of Agricultural and Food Chemistry*, *66*(48), 12696–12705.

Quach, D., Parameswaran, N., McCabe, L., & Britton, R. A. (2019). Characterising how probiotic *Lactobacillus reuteri* 6475 and lactobacillic acid mediate suppression of osteoclast differentiation. *Bone Reports*, *11*, 100227.

Rampelli, S., Candela, M., Turroni, S., Biagi, E., Collino, S., Franceschi, C. , et al. (2013). Functional metagenomic profiling of intestinal microbiome in extreme ageing. *Aging (Albany NY)*, *5*(12), 902–912.

Reigstad, C. S., Salmonson, C. E., Rainey, J. F., Szurszewski, J. H., Linden, D. R., Sonnenburg, J. L. , et al. (2015). Gut microbes promote colonic serotonin production through an effect of short-chain fatty acids on enterochromaffin cells. *The FASEB Journal*, *29*(4), 1395–1403.

Rinninella, E., Mele, M. C., Merendino, N., Cintoni, M., Anselmi, G., Caporossi, A. , et al. (2018). The role of diet, micronutrients and the gut microbiota in age-related macular degeneration: new perspectives from the gut-retina axis. *Nutrients*, *10*(11), 1677. https://doi.org/10.3390/nu10111677.

Romo-Araiza, A., Gutiérrez-Salmeán, G., Galván, E. J., Hernández-Frausto, M., Herrera-López, G., Romo-Parra, H. , et al. (2018). Probiotics and prebiotics as a therapeutic strategy to improve memory in a model of middle-aged rats. *Frontiers in Aging Neuroscience*, *10*, 146. https://doi.org/10.3389/fnagi.2018.00416.

Sadeghzadeh, J., Vakili, A., Sameni, H. R., Shadnoush, M., Bandegi, A. R., & Zahedi, K. M. (2017). The effect of oral consumption of probiotics in prevention of heart injury in a rat myocardial infarction model: a histopathological, hemodynamic and biochemical evaluation. *Iranian Biomedical Journal*, *21*(3), 174–181.

Salmon, A. B. (2015). About-face on the metabolic side effects of rapamycin. *Oncotarget*, *6*(5), 2585–2586.

Sampson, T. R., & Mazmanian, S. K. (2016). Control of brain development, function, and behavior by the microbiome. *Cell Host & Microbe*, *17*(5), 565–576.

Sanborn, V., Azcarate-Peril, M. A., Updegraff, J., Manderino, L. M., & Gunstad, J. (2018). A randomized clinical trial examining the impact of LGG probiotic supplementation on psychological status in middle-aged and older adults. *Contemporary Clinical Trials Communications*, *12*, 192–197.

Sanders, M. E., Merenstein, D. J., Reid, G., Gibson, G. R., & Rastall, R. A. (2019). Probiotics and prebiotics in intestinal health and disease: from biology to the clinic. *Nature Reviews Gastroenterology & Hepatology*, *15*, 605–616.

Sasaki-Adams, D. M., & Kelley, A. E. (2001). Serotonin-dopamine interactions in the control of conditioned reinforcement and motor behavior. *Neuropsychopharmacology*, *25*, 440–452.

Schepper, J. D., Collins, F. L., Rios-Arce, N. D., Raehtz, S., Schaefer, L., Gardinier, J. D. , et al. (2019). Probiotic *Lactobacillus reuteri* prevents postantibiotic bone loss by reducing intestinal dysbiosis and preventing barrier disruption. *Journal of Bone and Mineral Research*, *34*(4), 681–698.

Schlender, L., Martinez, Y. V., Adeniji, C., Reeves, D., Faller, B., Sommerauer, C. , et al. (2017). Efficacy and safety of metformin in the management of type 2 diabetes mellitus in older adults: a systematic review for the development of recommendations to reduce potentially inappropriate prescribing. *BMC Geriatrics*, *17*(1), 227. https://doi.org/10.1186/s12877-017-0574-5.

Shida, K., Sato, T., Lizuka, R., Hoshi, R., Watanabe, O., Igarashi, T. , et al. (2017). Daily intake of fermented milk with *Lactobacillus casei* strain Shirota reduces the incidence and duration of upper respiratory tract infections in healthy middle-aged office workers. *European Journal of Nutrition*, *56*(1), 45–53.

Short, K. R., Bigelow, M. L., Kahl, J., Singh, R., Coenen-Schimke, J., Raghavakaimal, S. , et al. (2005). Decline in skeletal muscle mitochondrial function with aging in human. *Proceeding of the National Academy of Sciences (USA)*, *102*(15), 5618–5623.

Siddharth, J., Chakrabarti, A., Pannérec, A., Karaz, S., Morin-Rivron, D., Masoodi, M. , et al. (2017). Aging and sarcopenia associate with specific interaction between microbes, serum biomarkers and host physiology in rats. *Aging*, *9*(7), 1698–1714.

Sierra, F. (2016). The emergence of geroscience as an interdisciplinary approach to the enhancement of health span and life span. *Cold Spring Harbor Perspectives in Medicine*, *6* (4), a025163.

Son, G. H., Altintas, O., Kim, E. J. E., Kwon, S., & Lee, S. V. (2019). Age-dependent changes and biomarkers of aging in *Caenorhabditis elegans*. *Aging Cell*, *18*(2)e12853.

Stallone, G., Infante, B., Prisciandaro, C., & Grandaliano, G. (2019). mTOR and aging: an old fashioned dress. *International Journal of Molecular Sciences*, *20*(11), 2774. https://doi.org/10.3390/ijms20112774.

Sum, Z., Sun, X., Li, J., Li, Z., Hu, Q., Li, L. , et al. (2020). Using probiotics for type 2 diabetes mellitus intervention: advances, questions, and potential. *Critical Reviews in Food Science and Nutrition*, *60*(4), 670–683.

Takimoto, T., Hatanaka, M., Hoshino, T., Takara, T., Tanaka, K., Shimizu, A. , et al. (2018). Effect of *Bacillus subtilis* C-3102 on bone mineral density in healthy postmenopausal Japanese women: a randomized, placebo-controlled, double-blind clinical trial. *Bioscience of Microbiota, Food and Health*, *37*(4), 87–96.

Tan, P. L., Eor, J. Y., Chun, T., & Kim, S. H. (2015). Immune Modulation by Probiotics. In M. T. Liong (Ed.), *Microbiology Monographs on Beneficial Microorganisms in Medical & Health Applications* (pp. 101–130). Switzerland: Springer.

Tang, T. W. H., Chen, H. C., Chen, C. Y., Yen, C. Y. T., Lin, C. J., Prajnamitra, R. P. , et al. (2019). Loss of gut microbiota alters immune system composition and cripples postinfarction cardiac repair. *Circulation*, *139*, 647–659.

Tao, Y. W., Gu, Y. L., Mao, X. Q., Zhang, L., & Pei, Y. F. (2020). Effects of probiotics on type II diabetes mellitus: A meta-analysis. *Journal of Translational Medicine*, *18*, 30.

Tiderencel, K. A., Hutcheon, D. A., & Ziegler, J. (2020). Probiotic for the treatment of type 2 diabetes: a review of randomized controlled trial. *Diabetes/Metabolism Research and Reviews*, *36*(1)e3213.

Turnbaugh, P. J., Hamady, M., Yatsunenko, T., Cantarel, B. L., Duncan, A., Ley, R. E. , et al. (2009). A core gut microbiome in obese and lean twins. *Nature*, *457*, 480–484.

Valentini, L., Pinto, A., Bourdel-Marchasson, I., Ostan, R., Brigidi, P., Turroni, S. , et al. (2015). Impact of personalized diet and probiotic supplementation on inflammation, nutritional parameters and intestinal microbiota- The "RISTOMED project": Randomized controlled trial in healthy older people. *Clinical Nutrition*, *34*(4), 593–602.

Vogt, N. M., Kerby, R. L., Dill-McFarland, K. A., Harding, S. J., Merluzzi, A. P., Johnson, S. C. , et al. (2017). Gut microbiome alterations in Alzheimer's disease. *Scientific Reports*, *7*, 13537.

Wang, G., Li, X., Zhao, J., Zhang, H., & Chen, W. (2017). *Lactobacillus casei* CCFM419 attenuates type 2 diabetes via a gut microbiota dependent mechanism. *Food & Function*, *8*(9), 3155–3164.

Wang, Y., Dilidaxi, D., Wu, Y., Sailike, J., Sun, X., & Nabi, X. H. (2020). Composite probiotics alleviate type 2 diabetes by regulating intestinal microbiota and inducing GLP-1 secretion in db/db mice. *Biomedicine & Pharmacotherapy*, *125*, 109914.

Wang, F., Yu, R., Huang, G., Cai, D., Liang, X., Su, H. , et al. (2015). Gut microbiota community and its assembly associated with age and diet in Chinese centenarians. *Journal of Microbiology and Biotechnology, 25*(8), 1195–1204.

Woodmansey, E. J. (2007). Intestinal bacterial aging. *Journal of Applied Microbiology, 102*(5), 1178–1186.

World Health Organization (2018, February 5). *Ageing and health. Retrieved from(2018, February 5). https://www.who.int/news-room/fact-sheets/detail/ageing-and-health.*

Yamori, Y., Moriguchi, E. H., Teramoto, T., Miura, A., Fukui, Y., Honda, K. , et al. (2002). Soybean isoflavones reduce postmenopausal bone resorption in female Japanese immigrants in Brazil: A ten-week study. *Journal of the American College of Nutrition, 21*(6), 560–563.

Yang, X., Yu, D., Xue, L., Li, H., & Du, J. (2020). Probiotics modulate the microbiota-gut-brain axis and improve memory deficits in aged SAMP8 mice. *Acta Pharmaceutica Sinica B, 10*(3), 475–487.

Zeng, Z., Yuan, Q., Yu, R., Zhang, J., Ma, H., & Chen, S. (2019). Ameliorative effects of probiotic *Lactobacillus paracasei* NL41 on insulin sensitivity, oxidative stress, and beta-cell function in a type 2 diabetes mellitus rat model. *Molecular Nutrition & Food Research, 63* (22)e1900457.

Zhang, J., Motyl, K. J., Irwin, R., MacDougald, O. A., Britton, R. A., & McCabe, L. R. (2015). Loss of bone and Wnt10b expression in male type 1 diabetic mice is blocked by the probiotic *Lactobacillus reuteri. Endocrinology, 156*(9), 3169–3182.

Zhao, L., Zhao, Y., Liu, R., Zheng, X., Zhang, M., Guo, H. , et al. (2017). The transcription factor DAF-16 is essential for increased longevity in *C. elegans* exposed to *Bifidobacterium longum* BB68. *Scientific Reports, 7*, 7408.

Zhou, X., Li, J., Guo, J., Geng, B., Ji, W., Zhao, Q. , et al. (2018). Gut-dependent microbial translocation induced inflammation and cardiovascular events after ST-elevation myocardial infarction. *Microbiome, 6*(1), 66.

Zinkernagel, M. S., Zysset-Burri, D. C., Keller, I., Berger, L. E., Leichtle, A. B., Largiadèr, C. R. , et al. (2017). Association of the intestinal microbiome with the development of neovascular age-related macular degeneration. *Scientific Reports, 7*, 40826. https://doi.org/10.1038/srep40826.

CHAPTER

11

TRP channels in the gut: Effect of probiotics and phyto-nutraceuticals on gut-brain-immune axis

Sushama Mohanta[a,b] and Chandan Goswami[a,b]

[a]National Institute of Science Education and Research, School of Biological Sciences, Khurda, Odisha, India, [b]Homi Bhabha National Institute, Mumbai, India

11.1 Introduction to TRP ion channels

Transient receptor potential (TRP) channels are a group of nonselective ion channels involved in a large number of cellular and physiological functions. All TRPs have six transmembrane regions in the middle portion, flanked by N-terminal and C-terminal regions that are located on the intracellular side. Functional TRP channels are tetrameric in nature. An approximate 25-amino acid long sequence, known as the "TRP-domain" and a further smaller sequence (EWKFAR, known as the TRP-box) are conserved structural features in many TRPs. The TRP-box is located at the end of the sixth transmembrane region and the beginning of the C-terminal region (Kumar, Goswami, & Goswami, 2013; Kumar, Kumari, Majhi, & Goswami, 2015). In humans, 28 TRP channels are classified into six sub-types, i.e., canonical (TRPCs), vanilloid (TRPVs), melastatin (TRPMs), mucolipins (TRPMLs), polycystins (TRPPs), and ankyrin (TRPA1) (Goswami & Hucho, 2008). TRP channels are known to be permeable for different mono and divalent cations such as Na^+, K^+, Ca^{2+}, Mg^{2+}, Mn^{2+}, Zn^{2+}, Sr^{2+}, Ni^{2+}, Fe^{2+}, etc. but are not permeable to trivalent cations (Ramsey, Delling, & Clapham, 2006). Although TRPs are "nonselective" in nature, yet most of the TRPs are fairly selective for

Probiotic Beverages
https://doi.org/10.1016/B978-0-12-818588-9.00004-8

Ca^{2+}-ions, and activation of TRPs results in Ca^{2+}-influx. TRPs are important for Ca^{2+}-absorption from the gut and urine (Ramsey et al., 2006). Due to their "nonselective" nature, TRPs have been considered as the molecular route for cellular entry of different trace elements.

TRP channels are mainly present in the animal kingdom, ranging from lower eukaryotes to humans (Ramsey et al., 2006). TRPs are also present in several parasites, such as flatworms. The parasitic TRPs can offer specific molecular targets for specific drugs and health benefits. TRPs are also present in some fungi including yeast. TRPs are generally absent in the plant kingdom. Notably, TRP channels are completely missing in all prokaryotes. These channels are polymodal in nature and can be activated by various physical stimuli such as different temperatures, mechanical force, osmolarity, pH, UV, and IR. TRPs are known to be activated or inhibited by a series of endogenous, as well as exogenous compounds, such as different toxins, lipids, peptides, small compounds, hormones, plant products, fermented products, and also by different reactive chemicals (Ramsey et al., 2006). Among the plant products, menthol and capsaicin are exemplary. Menthol acts as an activator of TRPM8, the "cold receptor" and thus induces a "cool feeling." In contrast, "capsaicin" the active ingredient of hot chili activates TRPV1 (also known as the "capsaicin receptor" or the "hot receptor"), which induces the "burning sensation" (Ramsey et al., 2006). The list of active compounds from plant sources that act on specific TRP channels is large (Yadav, Saha, Kumar, & Goswami, 2019).

Some (but not all) TRP channels have the unique ability i.e., "thermogating" behavior, which allows activation of these channels at different temperatures (Ramsey et al., 2006). Also, several TRPs, (such as TRPV1 and others) can be activated by low pH, which makes these channels responsible for acid-induced pain in the gut (Ramsey et al., 2006). Being activated or inhibited by different small, natural compounds also makes these channels ideal targets for different physiological and pathophysiological pathways.

Reports suggest that bacterial cell wall components, such as lipopolysaccharides (LPS), other bacterial toxins, and also bacterial metabolites can act on different TRPs, making them either activated or inhibited. In many cases, nociception, acute pain in the gut, and other pathophysiological problems are due to the adverse modulation of TRP channels. In contrast, certain compounds are known for their analgesic and healing ability in the gut. Also, there are fermented products and degraded food components and other metabolites that can act on these channels and can induce health benefits. Specific fermented products show their effectiveness on these TRPs (discussed later). Proper management and regulation of TRPs, as a whole, can be beneficial for health. On the other hand, improper regulation of these same channels can induce strong inflammation and tissue damage leading to serious health hazards. Therefore, TRPs in the gut tissue can act as a bidirectional knife and hold central aspects of balance between physiological and pathophysiological states. Although some studies have been conducted to correlate probiotics and some phytochemicals with TRPs, not many in-depth studies have been conducted to understand the intricate relationship between probiotics and their metabolites on TRP channels. This review focuses on the possibilities of traditionally used foods and beverages from different ethnic groups and summarizes the effects of probiotics/probiotic-based foods and beverages that can target specific TRPs for medical and physiological benefits.

11.2 Expression of TRPs in the gut

The gut has several components such as gut epithelia, smooth muscles, blood vessels, immune cells, and innervating neurons to mention a few key components. The expression of different TRPs in different cells present in the gut has been established to a large extent (Holzer, 2011; Khalil, Alliger, Weidinger, & Engel, 2018). Both absolute and relative expression of TRPs in different cells and layers of the gut is "dynamic and plastic" in nature, i.e., these expressions change with age, physiological state, exposure to different foods, immune status of the body, etc. Overall, the expression of specific TRP channels in different cells present in the gut is of importance, ranging from detecting different signaling cues, regulation of intracellular Ca^{2+}-signaling, inflammation control, the release of different hormones, enzymes, and peptides, the release of different cytokines, absorption of Ca^{2+} and other ions, decisions for food-uptake, and addiction to certain items.

11.3 TRPs in gut epithelia

Gut epithelial cells represent "the frontline" encountering a lot of tissue damage, irritants present in food, different bacteria, and toxins, different antigens, noxious molecules, nutrients, and changes in pH and temperature. The same layers of cells are also involved in the difficult task of absorbing nutrients, different ions, and communicating with the neurons and immune cells present nearby to maintain the gut's physiology and functions. TRPs play a key role in many of the functions conducted by epithelial cells. Initially, it was assumed that TRPs were exclusively present in the peripheral neuron of higher animals. However, later studies have confirmed that TRPs are present in many non-neuronal cells and expression of at least seven different TRP channels (namely TRPV1, TRPV4, TRPV6, TRPM5, TRPM8, TRPC6, and TRPA1) has been reported in the gut epithelial cells (Alaimo & Rubert, 2019). TRPV6 is expressed in gut epithelial cells and is involved in Ca^{2+}-absorption. TRPs are also expressed in specialized cells. For example, TRPA1 is expressed in highly specialized enterochromaffin cells present in gut epithelia (Nozawa, Kawabata-Shoda, Doihara, & Ito, 2009).

11.4 TRPs as regulators of the gut-neuronal system

TRPs were initially described as advanced molecules that specifically express in "sensory neurons only" and which are capable of detecting different physical and chemical stimuli. The expression of TRPs in the central nervous system was established later. The expression of TRPs in neuronal systems correlates well with different physiological and sensory functions, such as detection of temperature, osmolarity, mechanical force, light, taste, etc. Many of these "sensory functions" by neurons are also relevant for critical gut-related functions such as detection of food, feeling of starvation and satiety, digestion of food, regulation of blood glucose levels, excretion, etc. TRPs are also involved in complex functions such as food preferences, addiction, and energy balance.

In the gut, TRPs are expressed from start-to-end (i.e., from olfactory receptors and taste buds to the upper part to the rectum). TRPs are also expressed in keratinocytes in the oronasal cavity and nearby to taste buds, resulting in the perception of the five basic tastes (i.e., sweet, bitter, sour, salty, and umami) (Roper, 2014). In olfactory neurons, TRPs play an important role in the detection of food, olfactory adaption and complex functions that are applicable even to lower organisms, such as *Drosophila*. For example, TRPM5 present in olfactory neurons is involved in sensing semi chemicals and different pheromones. Similarly, expression of different members of TRPVs (TRPV1–4), TRPMs (TRPM5, TRPM8), and TRPA1 are reported in the olfactory system and the olfactory epithelium. The presence of multiple TRPs directly in type-II and type-III taste buds and associated peripheral neurons link these channels for taste perception. For example, TRPM5 is expressed in taste receptors and provides the sensitivity of sweet as well as bitter, and umami taste. TRPA1 helps in detecting the pungent taste of mustard. TRPV1 helps in detecting the taste of hot chili. TRPV1t (a TRPV1 variant) is involved in the detection of salty taste. TRPV1-positive neurons are also present in the rectal region and colonic enteric nervous system. TRPA1 is present in epithelial cells of the colon. Using *Trpa1*$^{-/-}$ animals, it has been established that nodose and dorsal root ganglia neurons innervate three different regions of the GI tract that contain TRPA1. The expression of different TRPs in peripheral neurons innervating gut tissue has been established by several studies. Notably, the expression of individual TRPs in these neurons remains "plastic" and therefore subject to change depending on multiple factors such as age, microbiome, inflammation state, and other physiological states.

Sour taste and the presence of weak acids such as lactic and acetic acid are the signatures of probiotic beverages. PKD1L3 and PKD2L1 (sour taste cells) can detect sour tastes. Probiotic beverages such as yogurt improve digestion and the reason attributed may be due to membrane depolarization and/or action potentials in PKD2L1 in the presence of weak acids (Challis & Ma, 2016). Further, it is important to note that the action potential firing is not observed in the presence of weak acids in nonsour taste cells. The $K_{ir}2.1\,K^+$ channel is responsible for sour taste transduction and regulates the secretion of gastric juice, thereby improving digestion as well as metabolism (Gilca & Dragos, 2017).

The expressions of TRPs in neurons are linked to the functions that are controlled by the gut-brain axis, a circuit that is central to physiology and pathophysiology (discussed later). Involvement of TRPs in olfactory- and taste bud–related stimulation, as well as response in the gut, develop strong chemo-attraction behavior towards a certain food or chemo-repulsion behavior to avoid certain food. For example, TRPV3 is involved in decisions related to food uptake (Singh, Kumar, Shelkar, & Singru, 2016). Often such decisions can also be linked with food preference/addiction as well. An opposite phenomenon is also relevant for humans (i.e., people with gastric problems generally avoid spicy food). Such "avoidance" of nonsuitable food is also observed in other species and such behavior is often exploited commercially. For example, the TRPV1-induced pain signal (burning sensation in the tongue and gut) results in rodents avoiding poultry foods mixed with hot chili powder. Further, Perez-Burgos, Wang, McVey Neufeld, and Kunze (2015) depicted the role of live probiotic bacteria, *Lactobacillus reuteri* in modulating TRPV1. Such probiotic strains can be used as adjunct therapeutic agents for antinociceptive effects.

11.5 TRPs as regulators of the gut-immune system

In the last 15 years, the importance of TRP channels in the immune system has been established to a large extent especially their relevance in the gut-immune system. TRPs are an important component of mucosal immunity (Khalil et al., 2018). Some of the TRPs are involved in intracellular Ca^{2+}-influx in T-cells and macrophages, a process that is a prerequisite for immune activation.

TRPs are also involved in endocannabinoid signaling. The endocannabinoid system includes different receptors, ligands, and enzymes and is representative of mind–body-medicine. For example, cannabinoid (CB) receptors and TRPV1 have common ligands, such as *N*-arachidonoyl-dopamine

(NADA) and N-arachidonoylethanolamine (AEAs). AEA is known to play an important role in maintaining immunological health in the gut. The gut tissue is full of different immune cells recognizing and secreting a large number of inflammatory factors such as histamine, ATP, bradykinin, prostaglandins, nerve-growth factors (NGF), TNFα, IL-1β as well as H^+, different proteases and neurotransmitters such as serotonin (Alaimo & Rubert, 2019). Notably, a series of probiotic factors and natural products present in foods can modulate the TRP channel activity at the gut level, induce better gut immunity and, thus, induce health benefits (discussed in later sections).

Interestingly, some probiotic bacterial strains and prebiotics are found to modulate the elevation and decrease in the CB mRNAs in the gut, hence indirectly impacting TRPs. Administration of *Lactobacillus acidophilus* in mice showed a higher expression of CB2 mRNA in the epithelial cell of the colon. Similarly, *Enterococcus faecium* when fed to *Solea solea* could upregulate CB1 mRNA. Some prebiotics, such as oligofructose, is known to reduce the expression of CB1 mRNA (McPartland, Guy, & Di Marzo, 2014). It is pertinent to suggest that the therapeutic applications of probiotics and prebiotics requires confirmatory findings on activation or deactivation of the TRPs and simultaneously the CB receptors as antagonists and agonists in different disease conditions.

Highly Ca^{2+}-selective TRPs, namely TRPV5 and TRPV6, are expressed in T-cells. Other TRPVs, namely TRPV1–TRPV4, are endogenously expressed in T-cells (Majhi, Saha, Kumar, & Goswami, 2015). TRPC3 is endogenously present in T-cells. Application of capsaicin (an activator of TRPV1) or 4α-PDD (an activator of TRPV4) results in higher levels of intracellular Ca^{2+} in the T-cells (Majhi, Sahoo, Yadav, & Goswami, 2015). Notably, pharmacological inhibition of TRPV1, or TRPV4, results in reduction of ConA-mediated immune activation. Simultaneous inhibition of TRPV1 and TRPV4 can significantly reduce T-cell activation. Similarly, TRPA1 is also involved in T-cell activation (Sahoo, Majhi, Tiwari, & Chattopadhyay, 2019).

CD4+ T-cells isolated from wild type animals express functional TRPA1. Lack of TRPA1 aggravates colitis in *Il10*$^{-/-}$ mice. Increased infiltration of both TRPA1$^+$ and TRPV1$^+$ T-cells has been observed in inflamed colon sections of patients with active inflammatory bowel disease (IBD). *Trpm8*$^{-/-}$ mice are hypersensitive to Dextran sulfate sodium (DSS)-induced colitis, and CD11c+dendritic cells from *Trpm8*$^{-/-}$ show hyperinflammatory responses to TLR-stimulation suggesting the role of TRPM8 in gut-immune functions. Furthermore, calcitonin gene-related peptide (CGRP, an inflammatory neuropeptide) content is increased in colons from naive and DSS-treated *Trpm8*$^{-/-}$ mice. This suggests that the absence of TRPM8 results in a deficient CGRP release. Treatment of *Trpm8*$^{-/-}$ mice with CGRP reversed their hyperinflammatory phenotype. TRPM8 signaling in mucosal sensory neurons appears to be indispensable for the regulation of innate inflammatory responses via the neuropeptide CGRP.

Macrophages are important contributors to the gut immune system and protect the gut tissue from invading microbes. Diverse TRP channels express endogenously in macrophages and are involved in inflammation control and the clearance of pathogens invading gut tissue. It is important to mention that certain TRPs are present in lysosomes and regulate lysosomal pH (Yadav & Goswami, 2017). Thus, TRPs represent key molecules of the lysosome-mediated bacterial clearance process. Notably, the phagocytic activity of macrophages is largely dependent on TRPV2 functions. TRPs are also present in NK cells (a type of white blood cell) and impaired activity of TRPs is linked with the development of certain diseases.

11.6 Involvement of TRPs in gut inflammation, irritable bowel syndrome, and other gut-related disorders

In the past few years, the importance of TRP channels in gut-inflammation, irritable bowel syndrome (IBS), and other gut-related disorders have become prominent and the use of specific herbal or medicinal or probiotic products are known to help overcome these problems (Chen, Mu, Zhu, Mukherjee, & Zhang, 2020). Proper neuro-immune crosstalk is a hallmark of healthy gut physiology, which often goes wrong in many gut-related disorders, such as the development of colitis. In the gut, TRPs influence multiple aspects that are interlinked to each other and that leads to gut inflammation. First, the outermost gut epithelial cells express different TRPs at the basal level. Such expressions are subject to dynamic changes and are often increased during inflammation. This inflammation is due to the direct activation of gut cells by different noxious stimuli. Second, depending on nature, the extent of the stimulation, and the molecular target present in the peripheral neurons, the nerve ends release specific neuropeptides, neurotransmitters, and other signaling compounds that lead to more inflammation and thus nociception or vice versa (i.e., analgesic effects). Third, the gut harbors a large number of immune cells (T-cells, macrophages, NK cells). These immune cells release proinflammatory or anti-inflammatory cytokines once these TRPs are activated or inhibited. For example, activation of TRPV1 can have both a proinflammatory and anti-inflammatory impact on gut tissue, depending on the extent of activation.

Due to the involvement of TRPV1 in pain, its specific role in gastrointestinal inflammation and function has been explored (Geppetti & Trevisani, 2004). Increased expression of TRPV1 in sensory nerves has been correlated with IBS development and abdominal pain (Akbar, Yiangou, Facer, et al., 2008). TRPs are also involved in the development of colitis. For example, TRPV2 knock-out animals exhibit less intestinal inflammation and develop less colitis compared to wild type (Wt) mice at clinical, histopathological, and immunohistopathological readouts. This is due to less recruitment of macrophages in the gut. In the same context, the oral application of capsaicin or AEAs (a common ligand of TRPV1 and CB2) results in a significant increase in the number of functionally active CX3CR1hi macrophages (Mϕ) (Acharya, Penukonda, Shcheglova, et al., 2017).

Oral administration of AEA to nonobese diabetic mice protects type-1-diabetes. It may be hypothesized that some probiotics suppress TRPV1, and as a result lead to relief in abdominal pain and anti-inflammatory effects. Additionally, some probiotic bacteria and yeast administration in IBS animal models have been found to regulate IL-1 and IL-6 in serum levels (Hong, Seo, Lee, & Park, 2019).

TRPV1 activation induces NO and reactive oxygen species (ROS), and TRPV1 is involved in inflammatory signaling events, at least in short-term duration. However, there are reports suggesting that TRPV1 has an anti-inflammatory and tissue-protective role as well, mainly in the case of long-term effects. For example, *Trpv1*$^{-/-}$ animals have a higher rate of local inflammation and an accelerated onset of the systemic inflammatory response syndrome suggesting a tissue-protective role of TRPV1. Accordingly, inhibition of TRPV1 or TRPA1, prevents the transition of acute to chronic inflammation and pain in chronic pancreatitis.

Lactate is known to inhibit TRPV1. Lactate is one of the prime products of most of the lactic acid bacteria and probiotic bacteria, hence this is regarded as a prime metabolite in probiotic beverages (de la Roche, Walther, Leonow, & Leffler, 2016). The addition of capsaicin to lactic acid fermentation medium during the fermentation of curd improves the L-lactate titers in the medium (Sharma, Jain, Nair, & Ramachandran, 2013). TRPV2 activation in macrophages by LPS results in enhanced cytokine production. TRPA1 is modulated by algesic stimuli and is involved in gut mechanosensation. TRPA1 is present in human epithelial cells, macrophages, and enteric ganglia cells in the colon. The upregulation of TRPA1 mRNA is detected in inflamed samples. In *Trpa1*$^{-/-}$ animals, the disease-activity-index is higher compared to wild type animals. TRPA1 is upregulated in colitis tissue and activation of TRPA1 protects gut tissue by decreasing the expressions of several proinflammatory neuropeptides, cytokines, and chemokines. However, not all TRPs are inflammatory in nature. For example, activation of TRPM8 results in an anti-inflammation process (Ramachandran, Hyun, Zhao, & Hollenberg, 2013).

Unlike TRPV1, TRPM8 (also known as the menthol receptor) plays an anti-inflammatory role in the gut (Ramachandran et al., 2013). Application of icilin (TRPM8 activator) attenuates chemically-induced colitis in wild-type but not in *Trpm8*$^{-/-}$ mice. Icilin attenuates DSS–induced colitis and inflammatory cytokine/chemokine release. *Trpm8*$^{-/-}$ animals show elevated colonic levels of CGRP compared to wild-type animals. This suggests an anti-inflammatory role for TRPM8 activation, which is due to inhibition of neuropeptide release. This points to TRPM8 as a novel therapeutic and probiotic target for colitis and other inflammatory diseases. TRPM8 performs its protective role in the intestine by inhibiting the release of inflammatory cytokines (TNF-α, IL-1, IL-6, and MCP-1). Some probiotic beverages, such as kombucha, use menthol in their formulation and hence help to activate TRPM8 and indirectly facilitate anti-inflammatory activity in the gut.

11.7 Bacterial lipopolysaccharides and bacterial toxins and their effects on TRPs

TRPs serve as the molecular targets of several toxins produced by animals and plants (toxin-TRP combinations with the chemical nature of prey–predator relationships). Reports suggest that both bacterial cell wall components, namely LPS and/or specific bacterial toxins can act on different receptors, TRPs, and other ion channels. LPS are strong immunomodulatory factors that activate TLR4-mediated innate immunity and thus activate macrophages. Studies have suggested that selected TRPs (such as TRPA1) act as alternate and potent receptors for LPS (Meseguer, Alpizar, Luis, & Viana, 2014). LPS isolated from *Escherichia coli* activates human and mouse TRPA1 isoforms expressed in heterologous systems. Such activation is independent of TLR4 as LPS-mediated activation of peripheral neurons can also be observed in *Tlr4*$^{-/-}$ but not in *Trpa1*$^{-/-}$ animals. LPS-mediated activation of peripheral neurons can be effectively blocked by TRPA1 inhibitors and can be synergistically activated by TRPA1 activators. The effectiveness of LPS-mediated TRPA1 activation and development of acute inflammation correlates well with the LPS-derived from different bacterial species that have different levels of molecular symmetry for LPS. Indeed, LPSs with the conical shape have more effectiveness than LPS with a semi conical or a cylindrical shape suggesting the impact of different bacterial genera on this process (Meseguer et al., 2014). LPS triggers calcitonin gene–related peptide (CGRP) production and induces inflammation, which is TRPA1-dependent and TLR4-independent. Notably, TRPA1's ability to act as an LPS receptor has an evolutionary origin and is observed in lower organisms as well.

The importance of TRPV1 and TRPV4 in response to bacterial components and the induction of painful signals is significant. TRPV1 can be activated by LPS, but to a lesser extent than TRPA1 (Boonen, Alpizar, Sanchez, et al., 2018) as confirmed by using *Trpv1*$^{-/-}$ as well as double-knock-out (*Trpv1*$^{-/-}$ & *Trpa1*$^{-/-}$) animals (Ferraz, Henry, Hargreaves, &

Diogenes, 2011). Similarly, cells isolated from *Trpv4*$^{-/-}$ animals cannot detect LPS-containing bacteria in vitro and thus are inefficient in terms of bacterial clearance. Airway epithelial cells show increased Ca^{2+}-influx immediately after LPS application. This response occurs by activation of TRPV4 and in a TLR4-independent manner. This LPS-mediated Ca^{2+}-influx can be reduced by pharmacological inhibition of TRPV4 and is lost in *Trpv4*$^{-/-}$ animals. TRPV4-mediates immediate LPS-induced increases in ciliary beat frequency and production of more NO help in bacterial clearance (Alpizar, Boonen, Sanchez, et al., 2017). TRPM2 also contributes to the LPS-mediated production of NO. LPS weakly activates TRPM3 and TRPM8 to promote Ca^{2+}-influx (Boonen et al., 2018). TRPM7-mediated Ca^{2+}-influx is involved in LPS-mediated endocytosis of TLR4 and subsequent macrophage activation (Schappe, Szteyn, Stremska, & Desai, 2018). Coincidentally, probiotic strains of *Weissella* sp. were found to reduce LPS-mediated proinflammatory stress in murine macrophages and to also inhibit the generation of IL-8 by human epithelial cells (Singh, Bhatia, Singh, & Bhadada, 2018). It is important to understand the impact of probiotic strains on the TRPs, especially TRPM2, TRPM3, TRPV4, and TRPM8 in inflammation caused due to LPS.

Apart from the LPS, TRP channels also become activated by different bacterial toxins and related products (Boonen et al., 2018). Some pathogenic strains of *S. aureus* produce pain and hyperalgesia due to three classes of pore-forming toxins (PFT). The first group contains an α-hemolysin (Hla). The second group represents bicomponent leukocidins, comprised of γ-hemolysins (such as HlgAB, HlgBC) and leukocidins (LukAB, LukED, LukSF). The third group represents phenol-soluble modulins (PSMs), small amphipathic α-helical peptide toxins (PSMα1, α2, α3, α4, PSMβ1, β2, and δ-toxin) that are capable of lysing cells. Interestingly, *Trpv1*$^{-/-}$ mice show less induction of heat hyperalgesia upon *S. aureus* infection compared to *Trpv1*$^{+/+}$ or *Trpv1*$^{+/-}$ animals (Blake, Baral, Voisin, & Chiu, 2018). Bacillus colonization in the intestine inhibits the infection chances of *S. aureus*. The inhibitory property of *Bacillus* sp. is attributed to a class of lipopeptide that is secreted and counteracts against the quorum sensing of *S. aureus* (Piewngam & Otto, 2020). However, the correlation between the probiotic lipopeptides with TRPs is yet to be understood.

Another classic example is the botulinum toxin produced by *Clostridium botulinum*. Botulinum toxins modulate TRPV1 (often lowering the expression of TRPV1 in peripheral neurons), reduce hyperalgesia, and different forms of pain (Fan, Chu, Wang, et al., 2017). Some probiotic microorganisms such as S. *boulardii*, *L. acidophilus*, *L. rhamnosus LGG*, and L. *reuteri* were observed to block botulinum neurotoxin serotype A in Caco-2 cells (in vitro) (Lam, Tam, Stanker, & Cheng, 2016). The administration of such probiotic strains in the presence of botulinum toxin and its effect on the TRPs is unknown. Another group of compounds is cyclodextrins, which are produced in different bacteria. Some of these, namely methyl-β-cyclodextrin, are well known for their ability to chelate membrane cholesterol, thereby affecting many transmembrane proteins, including TRPs. Another example is sirolimus, also known as rapamycin, synthesized by *Streptomyces hygroscopicus*. Rapamycin activates the TRPML directly present in lysosomes (Zhang, Chen, Gao, & Xu, 2019).

TRPs also respond to oxidized and peroxidized lipids suggesting that TRPs act as major sensors for LPS-mediated painful signals and induce inflammation (Choi, Yoo, Lim, & Hwang, 2014). The results suggest that TRPs act as pattern-recognition receptors (PRR) that detect both pathogen-associated molecular patterns (PAMPs) and danger-associated molecular patterns (DAMPs) and induce inflammasome activation in immune cells and sensory neurons relevant to the gut and other tissues (Santoni, Cardinali, Morelli, & Amantini, 2015). Therefore, probiotic microorganisms can be very useful for the neutralization of LPS, toxins, and other metabolites produced by pathogenic bacteria (mostly foodborne pathogens such as *Salmonella*, *Shigella*, *Staphylococcus aureus*, and *Clostridium botulinum*).

11.8 TRPs as regulators of the gut-brain axis

The gut harbors a large number of microbes and this microbiome is tightly linked with the factors that determine good health or disease. Notably, gut bacteria can also influence diseases of the enteric and central nervous systems, mainly by forcing the gut to produce certain neurotransmitters and other key factors. In this context, TRP channels are involved in the gutbrain axis (discussed later). Gut microbiota influences several diseases of the central and peripheral nervous system by releasing diverse neurotransmitters and other related factors (Martin, Osadchiy, Kalani, & Mayer, 2018). Several mediators derived from intestinal microbiota can, directly and indirectly, regulate pain signaling through sensitization of pain-related receptors such as TLRs, TRPs, GABA receptors, and other ion channels. Administration of probiotics, prebiotics, and synbiotics can have a beneficial effect on visceral hypersensitivity and pain including TRPs in the pathway. Hence, modification of the gut microbiota by dietary interventions, such as fecal microbiota transplantation, can be a promising means for the management of chronic pain.

The peripheral neurons, other excitatory cells present in the gut, and the fluctuation of neurotransmitters produced by the gut form a strong gut-brain-axis. The gut-brain axis is also strongly linked with the gut immune system as well as to the gut microbiome (Martin et al., 2018). Modulation of the gut-brain-axis stands as a central point that maintains the balance between physiology and pathophysiology and therapeutic approaches towards gastrointestinal diseases (Mayer, Tillisch, & Bradesi, 2006). Blocking neuronal signaling to immune cells can be helpful in managing invasive infections of Streptococcal species. In contrast, probiotic strains (such as *Lactobacillus reuteri*) can inhibit inflammatory signals. Several ion channels are involved in this gut-brain axis and are involved in the signaling of gastrointestinal pain (Brierley, Hughes, Harrington, et al., 2010). In this context, TRPs and a few other channels play a central role in the gut-brain axis (Takahashi, Kozai, & Mori, 2012). TRPs are present in different cells, detect different gut metabolites (as well as bacterial products) resulting in direct regulation of the release of different neurotransmitters and other factors from gut cells. For example, TRPA1 activation in enterochromaffin cells results in serotonin (5-hydroxytryptamine; 5-HT) secretion affecting gastrointestinal motility and activation of the reward center (Nozawa et al., 2009).

In the gut, TRPV1 serves as a molecular target for CGRP, a molecule relevant for the gut-brain axis. TRPV1 is involved in the antinociceptive effect of ghrelin (a brain-gut hormone) in the case of IBS, which also involves opioid systems. The endocannabinoid system regulates the gut-brain axis involving TRPV1. Capsaicin-mediated stimulation of TRPV1 helps in the local production of AEA, which acts on cannabinoid btype 2 (CB2) and modulates endocannabinoid signaling (Acharya et al., 2017). Capsaicin alters the gut microbiome, and this induces transcriptional changes in the hypothalamus. Olvanil, a nonpungent TRPV1 activator, has antiemetic properties. Other TRPs are also involved in the regulation of the gut-brain axis. For example, TRPM8 positive sensory nerves regulate colitogenic responses by innate immune cells by regulating CGRP release (de Jong et al., 2015). The gut-brain axis plays roles that affect complex behaviors such as addiction. Even complex behaviors, such as sex-deprivation or increased uptake of ethanol, can be linked with TRPA1, as observed in *Drosophila*. In the gut, TRPA1 is involved in the regulation of serotonin release upon activation by active components present in the food such as allyl isothiocyanate (AITC) and cinnamaldehyde. Notably, not all TRP functions involve the peripheral or central nervous system. In contrast, there are specific functions that are independent of the gut-brain axis yet involve TRPs. For example, TRPV4 is involved in the regulation of gastrointestinal motility by directly affecting smooth muscle cells. This is achieved by controlling macrophages without the involvement of the enteric nervous system. However, more detailed studies are still needed to explore the role of TRPs in the gut-brain axis.

11.9 Evolution of gut function and TRPs

The microbiome present in the gut correlates well with food availability for digestion and, thus, has a strong impact on animal evolution. It is suggested that the gut (multicellular organ and function) may have originated ~900 million years ago (interestingly, at the same time some ancient TRPs evolved). Approximately, 600 million years ago, single cells perceived the need to be in association with other cells in order to handle larger and more complex food resulting in the formation of a multicellular organization of the gut, and a "division of labor" was initiated. Gut epithelial cells have "sensory functions" that are conserved from the first multicellular animals to the complex gut of humans.

TRP channel functions are intimately linked with food selection, food options, development of different germ-layers, evolution of digestive systems, enzyme secretion, even prey–predator relationships, all collectively contributing to gut functions and, thus, species evolution. The importance of TRPs in gut evolution can be largely linked with biological functions such as sensory input against certain signaling cues, development of the gut as a tissue, ability of the gut in absorption of monovalent and divalent cations (and also trace minerals), ability of the gut to respond to different temperatures, pH, osmolality, mechanical pressure, maintenance of body temperature, the ability of different cells to release different factors (such as enzymes, peptides, transmitters, hormones, etc.) as Ca^{2+}-dependent exocytosis events and decisions for food-uptake and energy balance. Most of the TRPVs evolved in vertebrates approximately 440 million years ago (Sardar, Kumar, Bhandari, & Goswami, 2012; Kumari, Kumar, Sardar, & Goswami, 2015). The ability of TRPV1 to respond to endocannabinoid signaling is highly relevant gut physiology as TRPV1 overlaps with CB receptors. TRPA1 evolved ~900 million years ago and is present in many invertebrates and, thus, is more ancient than TRPVs (Saha, Sucharita, Majhi, & Goswami, 2019). Similarly, TRPM8 can be traced back to around 390 million years (Majhi, Saha, et al., 2015).

11.10 Variability in TRPs in the human population and choice of food/beverage selections

The choice of foods and food preferences is a complex phenomenon observed in all species. In humans, both of these properties have a strong linkage with multiple factors, such as the origin of different ethnic groups, culture, geographic location, food availability, age of the individual, lifestyle, etc. The key players involved in such a process are typically associated with complex tasks such as neurological rewards, physiological benefits, immune response, etc. This is due to the bioactive ingredients present in food and metabolites produced in the gut, which act on specific receptors and channels inducing physiological effects. The microbiome present in the gut can affect health either positively or negatively. Antibiotic-induced changes in the gut microbiome can adversely affect gut endocannabinoidome signaling, hippocampal neuroglial reorganization, and depression. Such negative aspects can be overcome by applying probiotic species such as *Lactobacillus casei* DG (LCDG) (Guida, Turco, Iannotta, & Maione, 2018). In such a context, TRPs (and other channels) are instrumental for these above-mentioned functions.

Genome-sequencing has indicated that in human populations, the TRPs have a large number of variants globally, which represent mainly point mutations, isotypes, splice variants, etc. (Ghosh, Kaur, Kumar, & Goswami, 2016; Majhi, Saha, et al., 2015). At present, these global variances have not been classified into different groups, but such a large number of variants may have importance in different sensory behaviors and other responses against different stimuli. As a proof-of-concept, it has been reported that TRPM8 polymorphisms increase the risk of IBS. It is a common observation that the choice of certain foods or beverages, and specific products are variable depending on the region, local environment, and ecological niche. Accordingly, the use of different plant-based spices and fermented products varies in different countries, environments, and ethnic groups. For example, both consumption of hot chili (containing capsaicin/capsaicinoids) and tolerance to high doses of capsaicin occurs more in tropical countries. Accordingly, the consumption of alcoholic beverages is higher in temperate countries and the use of foods with more fermented spices is common in countries with high-environmental temperatures. Similarly, the consumption of alcohol is higher in colder regions and Scandinavian countries.

11.11 Food supplements and their effects on TRPs

At present, a number of small compounds are known that act on single or even multiple TRPs. In general, these compounds represent different small compounds, lipid molecules, and also vitamins. Most of these compounds are available in plant products and act as channel activators. Several plant products induce health benefits through TRPs and not all of these compounds are discussed here (Yadav et al., 2019). It is worth mentioning that there are several phytochemicals and active compounds that act on diverse ion channels including TRPs. However, as an example, the health benefits of capsaicin are briefly discussed below.

While excess capsaicin may cause tissue inflammation and tissue damage, a mild dose of dietary capsaicin can provide immense health benefits as suggested by several studies. For example, capsaicin reduces overall obesity by increasing body metabolism and overall body glucose regulation. TRPV1 activation by capsaicin also enhances insulin secretion and sensitization in diabetic mice. Activation of TRPV1 by capsaicin in the gut can help to reduce obesity-induced insulin resistance hepatic steatosis. Oral capsaicin enhances a discreet population of macrophages and confers protection from autoimmune diabetes. Long-term diets with capsaicin attenuate experimental autoimmune neuritis. Capsaicin reduces the expression of proinflammatory cytokines and enhances anti-inflammatory cytokines in the sciatic nerve. Capsaicin reduces demyelination and infiltration of immune cells (T-cells and macrophages) in the areas of injured nerves. As a result, oral capsaicin treatment can induce regulatory macrophages in the small intestine and provide health benefits. Capsaicin also helps in M1-M2 macrophage polarization, which helps in the protection of dopaminergic neurons against LPS-challenges and it induces T-cell activation (Majhi, Sahoo, et al., 2015). Some traditional lactic acid fermented foods and beverages contain capsaicin, as chili is used as a condiment in their formulation. For example, *pazhaya sadham* (fermented rice beverage) and *koozh* (fermented millet porridge) that are the ethnic fermented beverages of Tamil Nadu, contain a mild level of capsaicin (Antony, Ilango, Chelliah, Ramakrishnan, & Ravichandran, 2020) that may help modulate the optimum activity of TRPV1.

11.12 Different probiotic factors that can target TRPs in the gut

The use of probiotics is an age-old custom and well adapted to certain health benefits. Some probiotics are known to reduce gut-pain significantly and to provide multiple health benefits. The use of probiotics remains a common practice recommended by physicians and followed by many, yet the actual chemistry and biology behind their use remain underexplored. While most of the probiotics work on ROS- and NOS-mediated pathways, the actual molecular targets and small components present in the probiotics are not well characterized. However, some studies provide a strong "proof-of-concept" that probiotics act on TRP channels and provide health benefits. For example, a high dose of capsaicin-induced gut pain can be reduced by the application of a strain *Lactobacillus reuteri* (DSM 17938) (Perez-Burgos et al., 2015). Even its conditioned medium reduces the capsaicin-induced pain in a dose-dependent manner suggesting that the soluble product of the DSM strain is involved in this effect. This strain blocks the capsaicin-evoked Ca^{2+}-rise and capsaicin-induced currents in primary DRG neurons. Another *Lactobacillus* strain fails to do this, suggesting that the effect of the particular

DSM strain on TRPV1 is highly specific. The effect of the DSM strain is valid only in the case of live *Lactobacillus reuteri*. Dead cells fail to prevent the capsaicin-induced currents. The specificity of DSM is also confirmed by using *Trpv1*$^{-/-}$ animals. It is suggested that live *Lactobacillus reuteri* sheds some products such as micro vesicles (~150 nm in size) that contain many of the surface and other bacterial components contained in the parent bacteria. These micro-vesicles may diffuse through the tissues and finally stimulate the peripheral neurons present in the gut.

Another example is 10-oxo-12(Z)-octadecenoic acid, a linoleic acid metabolite produced by lactic acid bacteria in the gut, which affects TRPV1 (Kim, Furuzono, Yamakuni, & Goto, 2017). The dietary presence of KetoA enhances energy expenditure and protects animals from diet-induced obesity. This effect is more prominent in wild-type and not in *Trpv1*$^{-/-}$ animals suggesting the involvement of TRPV1 in this process. Indeed, KetoA activates TRPV1, as observed by Ca^{2+}-imaging experiments and whole-cell patch-clamp measurements. KetoA-mediated activation of TRPV1 enhances noradrenaline turnover in adipose tissues. KetoA also up-regulates factors that regulate brown adipocyte functions, such as uncoupling protein 1 (UCP1) in white adipose tissue (WAT). By using obese and diabetic model KK-Ay mice, it was shown that KetoA intake manages obesity-associated metabolic disorders. In *Trpv1*$^{-/-}$ mice, neither the KetoA-induced antiobesity effect nor UCP1 up-regulation was observed. This suggests that the antiobesity effect of KetoA is caused by TRPV1 activation–mediated browning in white adipose tissue. As KetoA is produced in the gut, it could, therefore, be involved in the regulation of host energy metabolism effectively. The gut bacterium *Akkermansia muciniphila* has certain health benefits. An increase in the population of *Akkermansia muciniphila* shows an antiobesity effect of capsaicin in animals fed with a high fat diet (Shen, Shen, Zhao, & Le, 2017).

TRPA1 also serves as a molecular target for several probiotic factors. Several myrosinase activating bacteria (mainly *Enterobacter* sp.) are used in the preparation of Thai fermented cabbage. These hydrolyze the glucosinolates (GSLs) present in fresh cabbage and produce isothiocyanates, nitriles, thiocyanates, etc. A prominent bioactive product in this fermented food is AITC (TRPA1 activator), which has several health benefits such as chemoprevention, anti-inflammatory, antioxidant, and immunomodulatory activity. AITC is also produced by GSL-metabolizing bacteria (Luang-In, Deeseenthum, Udomwong, & Gregori, 2018). Cinnamaldehyde present in several cinnamon beverages can activate TRPA1 at micromolar concentrations and exert health benefits (Helal, Tagliazucchi, Verzelloni, & Conte, 2014). Polyphenol compounds (such as epigallocatechin gallate) present in green tea and fermented tea activate TRPA1.

Not only bacterial but also fungal fermented products are known to act on TRP channels. For example, onydecalins (fungal polyketides produced by fungal fermentation) show antihistoplasma activity and also block TRP activity and in the future, this area will be of additional interest. A classic example of a fermented product is ethanol, which acts directly on several TRP channels. While the list of fermented products that act on TRPs and other channels is certainly very large, Table 11.1 briefly summarizes some key TRP channels that are subject to probiotic factor–mediated activation or inhibition.

TABLE 11.1 Examples of fermented metabolite products affecting TRP channels

Name of the channel	Fermented metabolites	Source of fermented metabolite	Strains involved
TRPV1	Ethanol, Furanmethanol, H_2S, low pH, Lysophophatidic acid, Short chain fatty acids (SCFA), NO, H_2O_2	Kefir, Kombucha, wine, soya sauce	*Kluyveromyces marxianus*, *Saccharomyces cerevisiae*, *Saccharomyces unisporus*, *Acetobacter*, *Gluconobacter*
TRPA1	AITC, cinnamaldehyde, acetaldehyde, H_2S, lysophophatidic acid, flavonoids, formaldehyde, polyphenols, CO_2	Sauerkraut, Kombucha, cinnamon beverages, carbonated beverages, kefir, wine	*Enterobacter xiangfangensis*, *Enterococcus casseliflavus*, *Streptococcus thermophilus*, *Lactobacillus*, *Lactococcus*
TRPM8	Ethanol, SCFA	Kefir, kombucha, beer, cheese	*Escherichia coli*, *Acetobacter aceti*, *Propionibacterium*, *Bifidobacteria*, *Saccharomyces cerevisiae*
TRPC	H_2S, flavonoids, NO, H_2O_2, low pH	Wine, kombucha	*Bifidobacterium*, *Saccharomyces cerevisiae*
TRPM2	H_2O_2, AMP	Kefir	*Bifidobacterium bifidum*, *Lactobacillus* sp.
TRPV3 TRPV4	NO	Sauerkraut Kimchi	*Enterococcus faecalis*, *Enterobacteriaceae* *Lactobacillus* sp.
TRPM7, TRPM4	ATP, AMP, ADP	Carbohydrate fermentation, beer, wine, cheese, yogurt	*Streptococcus*, *Lactobacillus*, *Saccharomyces cerevisiae*

11.13 Prospects and conclusions

TRPs were discovered in the 1980s and subsequently established as molecular targets of different physical and chemical stimuli. At present, several studies have confirmed the expression of different TRPs in diverse cells comprising the gut tissues. The function of these cells and the impact of TRPs in the gut-brain axis and gut-immune axis have been established. In such cross-talk, TRPs appear to have a wide range of effects, as these channels can function as taste receptors as well as key molecules responsible for painful tissue damage (Holzer, 2011). It is well established that gut microbiota can regulate pain in the peripheral and central nervous system, and they can induce several health benefits. Targeting gut microbiota by diet and pharmabiotic intervention represents new therapeutic strategies for the management of chronic pain. While pathogenic bacteria and their components such as LPS can induce health damage, it has been established that friendly microbial components and products, such as probiotic foods and beverages, can induce several health benefits that go beyond gut-related problems such as depression, reproductive failure, cardiac issues, etc., which involve different TRPs. Therefore, proper diets and managing the gut microbiome by targeting TRPs can bring immense health benefits, which are not only restricted to the gut, but also in the central nervous system and systemic immune response. However, further studies in this direction and public awareness are still needed.

Acknowledgment

SM and CG acknowledge the intramural financial support from National Institute of Science Education and Research, DAE, Govt. of India. The authors thank all of the laboratory members for critical comments on this manuscript. CG serves as a DAAD research ambassador.

References

Acharya, N., Penukonda, S., Shcheglova, T., & Srivastava, P. K. (2017). Endocannabinoid system acts as a regulator of immune homeostasis In the gut. *Proceedings of the National Academy of Sciences of the United States of America, 114*(19), 5005–5010. https://doi.org/10.1073/pnas.1612177114.

Akbar, A., Yiangou, Y., Facer, P., & Ghosh, S. (2008). Increased capsaicin receptor TRPV1-expressing sensory Fibres In irritable bowel syndrome and their correlation with abdominal pain. *Gut, 57*(7), 923–929. https://doi.org/10.1136/gut.2007.138982.

Alaimo, A., & Rubert, J. (2019). The pivotal role of TRP channels in homeostasis and diseases throughout the gastrointestinal tract. *International Journal of Molecular Sciences, 20*(21), 5277. https://doi.org/10.3390/ijms20215277.

Alpizar, Y. A., Boonen, B., Sanchez, A., & Talaver, K. (2017). TRPV4 activation triggers protective responses to bacterial lipopolysaccharides in airway epithelial cells. *Nature Communications, 8*, 1059 1–13 (2017). https://doi.org/10.1038/s41467-017-01201-3.

Antony, U., Ilango, S., Chelliah, R., Ramakrishnan, S. R., & Ravichandran, K. (2020). Ethnic fermented foods and beverages of Tamil Nadu. In J. P. Tamang (Ed.), *Ethnic fermented foods and beverages of India: Science history and culture* (pp. 539–560). Singapore: Springer.

Blake, K. J., Baral, P., Voisin, T., & Chiu, I. M. (2018). *Staphylococcus aureus* produces pain through pore-forming toxins and neuronal TRPV1 that is silenced by QX-314. *Nature Communications, 9,* 37 1–15(2018). https://doi.org/10.1038/s41467-017-02448-6.

Boonen, B., Alpizar, Y. A., Sanchez, A., & Talavera, K. (2018). Differential effects of lipopolysaccharide on mouse sensory TRP channels. *Cell Calcium, 73,* 72–81. https://doi.org/10.1016/j.ceca.2018.04.

Brierley, S. M., Hughes, P. A., Harrington, A. M., & Blackshaw, L. A. (2010). Identifying the ion channels responsible for signaling gastro-intestinal based pain. *Pharmaceuticals (Basel), 3*(9), 2768–2798. https://doi.org/10.3390/ph3092768.

Challis, R. C., & Ma, M. (2016). Sour taste finds closure in a potassium channel. *Proceedings of the National Academy of Sciences of the United States of America, 113*(2), 246–247.

Chen, Y., Mu, J., Zhu, M., Mukherjee, A., & Zhang, H. (2020). Transient receptor potential channels and inflammatory bowel disease. *Frontiers in Immunology, 11,* 180. https://doi.org/10.3389/fimmu.2020.00180.

Choi, S. I., Yoo, S., Lim, J. Y., & Hwang, S. W. (2014). Are sensory TRP channels biological alarms for lipid peroxidation? *International Journal of Molecular Sciences, 15*(9), 16430–16457. https://doi.org/10.3390/ijms150916430.

de Jong, P. R., Takahashi, N., Peiris, M., Bertin, S., Lee, J., Gareau, M. G., … Raz, E. (2015). TRPM8 on mucosal sensory nerves regulates colitogenic responses by innate immune cells via CGRP. *Mucosal Immunology, 8*(3), 491–504. https://doi.org/10.1038/mi.2014.82.

de la Roche, J., Walther, I., Leonow, W., & Leffler, A. (2016). Lactate is a potent inhibitor of the capsaicin receptor TRPV1. *Scientific Reports. 6,* 36740https://doi.org/10.1038/srep36740.

Fan, C., Chu, X., Wang, L., & Li, T. (2017). Botulinum toxin type a reduces TRPV1 expression in the dorsal root ganglion In rats with adjuvant-arthritis pain. *Toxicon, 133,* 116–122. https://doi.org/10.1016/j.toxicon.2017.05.001.

Ferraz, C. C., Henry, M. A., Hargreaves, K. M., & Diogenes, A. (2011). Lipopolysaccharide from *Porphyromonas gingivalis* sensitizes capsaicin-sensitive nociceptors. *Journal of Endodontia, 37*(1), 45–48. https://doi.org/10.1016/j.joen.2007.07.001.

Geppetti, P., & Trevisani, M. (2004). Activation and sensitisation of the vanilloid receptor: Role in gastrointestinal inflammation and function. *British Journal of Pharmacology, 141* (8), 1313–1320. https://doi.org/10.1038/sj.bjp.0705768.

Ghosh, A., Kaur, N., Kumar, A., & Goswami, C. (2016). Why individual thermo sensation and pain perception varies? Clue of disruptive mutations in TRPVs from 2504 human genome data. *Channels (Austin, Tex), 10*(5), 339–345. https://doi.org/10.1080/19336950.2016.1162365.

Gilca, M., & Dragos, D. (2017). Extraoral taste receptor discovery: new light on ayurvedic pharmacology. *Evidence-based Complementary and Alternative Medicine,*5435831 30 pages (2017). https://doi.org/10.1155/2017/5435831.

Goswami, C., & Hucho, T. (2008). Submembraneous microtubule cytoskeleton: Biochemical and functional interplay of TRP channels with the cytoskeleton. *The FEBS Journal, 275*(19), 4684–4699. https://doi.org/10.1111/j.1742-4658.2008.06617.x.

Guida, F., Turco, F., Iannotta, M., & Maione, S. (2018). Antibiotic-induced microbiota perturbation causes gut endocannabinoidome changes, hippocampal neuroglial reorganization and depression In mice. *Brain, Behavior, and Immunity, 67,* 230–245. https://doi.org/10.1016/j.bbi.2017.09.001.

Helal, A., Tagliazucchi, D., Verzelloni, E., & Conte, A. (2014). Bioaccessibility of polyphenols and cinnamaldehyde in cinnamon beverages subjected to in vitro gastro-pancreatic digestion. *Journal of Functional Foods, 7,* 506–516. https://doi.org/10.1016/j.jff.2014.01.005.

Holzer, P. (2011). TRP channels in the digestive system. *Current Pharmaceutical Biotechnology, 12*(1), 24–34. https://doi.org/10.2174/138920111793937862.

Hong, K. B., Seo, H., Lee, J. S., & Park, Y. (2019). Effects of probiotic supplementation on post-infectious irritable bowel syndrome in rodent model. *BMC Complementary and Alternative Medicine*. *19*(1)195https://doi.org/10.1186/s12906-019-2610-9.

Khalil, M., Alliger, K., Weidinger, C., & Engel, M. A. (2018). Functional role of transient receptor potential channels in immune cells and epithelia. *Frontiers in Immunology*, *9*, 174. https://doi.org/10.3389/fimmu.2018.00174.

Kim, M., Furuzono, T., Yamakuni, K., & Goto, T. (2017). 10-oxo-12(Z)-Octadecenoic acid, a linoleic acid metabolite produced by gut lactic acid bacteria, enhances energy metabolism by activation of TRPV1. *The FASEB Journal*, *31*(11), 5036–5048. https://doi.org/10.1096/fj.201700151R.

Kumar, A., Goswami, L., & Goswami, C. (2013). Importance of TRP channels in pain: Implications for stress. *Frontiers in Bioscience (Scholar Edition)*, *5*, 19–38. https://doi.org/10.2741/s356.

Kumar, A., Kumari, S., Majhi, R. K., & Goswami, C. (2015). Regulation of TRP channels by steroids: Implications in physiology and diseases. *General and Comparative Endocrinology*, *220*, 23–32. https://doi.org/10.1016/j.ygcen.2014.10.004.

Kumari, S., Kumar, A., Sardar, P., & Goswami, C. (2015). Influence of membrane cholesterol in the molecular evolution and functional regulation of TRPV4. *Biochemical and Biophysical Research Communications*, *456*(1), 312–319. https://doi.org/10.1016/j.bbrc.2014.11.077.

Lam, T. I., Tam, C. C., Stanker, L. H., & Cheng, L. W. (2016). Probiotic microorganisms inhibit epithelial cell internalization of botulinum neurotoxin serotype A. *Toxins*, *8*(12), 377. https://doi.org/10.3390/toxins8120377.

Luang-In, V., Deeseenthum, S., Udomwong, P., & Gregori, M. (2018). Formation of sulforaphane and iberin products from thai cabbage fermented by myrosinase-positive bacteria. *Molecules*, *23*(4), 955. https://doi.org/10.3390/molecules23040955.

Majhi, R. K., Saha, S., Kumar, A., & Goswami, C. (2015). Expression of temperature-sensitive ion channel TRPM8 in sperm cells correlates with vertebrate evolution. *PeerJ*, *3*, e1310. https://doi.org/10.7717/peerj.1310.

Majhi, R. K., Sahoo, S. S., Yadav, M., & Goswami, C. (2015). Functional expression of TRPV channels in T cells and their implications in immune regulation. *The FEBS Journal*, *282*(14), 2661–2681. https://doi.org/10.1111/febs.13306.

Martin, C. R., Osadchiy, V., Kalani, A., & Mayer, E. A. (2018). The brain-gut-microbiome axis. *Cellular and Molecular Gastroenterology and Hepatology*, *6*(2), 133–148. https://doi.org/10.1016/j.jcmgh.2018.04.003.

Mayer, E. A., Tillisch, K., & Bradesi, S. (2006). Modulation of the brain-gut axis as a therapeutic approach in gastrointestinal disease. *Alimentary Pharmacology & Therapeutics*, *24* (6), 919–933. https://doi.org/10.1111/j.1365-2036.2006.03078.x.

McPartland, J. M., Guy, G. W., & Di Marzo, V. (2014). Care and feeding of the endocannabinoid system: A systematic review of potential clinical interventions that upregulate the endocannabinoid system. *PLoS One*, *9*(3), e89566. https://doi.org/10.1371/journal.pone.0089566.

Meseguer, V., Alpizar, Y. A., Luis, E., & Viana, F. (2014). TRPA1 channels mediate acute neurogenic inflammation and pain produced by bacterial endotoxins. *Nature Communications*, *5*, 3125. https://doi.org/10.1038/ncomms4125.

Nozawa, K., Kawabata-Shoda, E., Doihara, H., & Ito, H. (2009). TRPA1 regulates gastrointestinal motility through serotonin release from enterochromaffin cells. *Proceedings of the National Academy of Sciences of the United States of America*, *106*, 3408–3413. https://doi.org/10.1073/pnas.0805323106.

Perez-Burgos, A., Wang, L., McVey Neufeld, K. A., & Kunze, W. A. (2015). The TRPV1 channel in rodents is a major target for Antinociceptive effect of the probiotic *Lactobacillus reuteri* DSM 17938. *The Journal of Physiology*, *593*(17), 3943–3957. https://doi.org/10.1113/JP270229.

Piewngam, P., & Otto, M. (2020). Probiotics to prevent *Staphylococcus aureus* disease? *Gut Microbes*, *11*(1), 94–101.

Ramachandran, R., Hyun, E., Zhao, L., & Hollenberg, M. D. (2013). TRPM8 activation attenuates inflammatory responses in mouse models of colitis. *Proceedings of the National Academy of Sciences of the United States of America*, *110*(18), 7476–7481. https://doi.org/10.1073/pnas.1217431110.

Ramsey, I. S., Delling, M., & Clapham, D. E. (2006). An introduction to TRP channels. *Annual Review of Physiology*, *68*, 619–647. https://doi.org/10.1146/annurev.physiol.68.040204.100431.

Roper, S. D. (2014). TRPs in taste and chemesthesis. *Handbook of Experimental Pharmacology*, *223*, 827–871. https://doi.org/10.1007/978-3-319-05161-1_5.

Saha, S., Sucharita, S., Majhi, R. K., & Goswami, C. (2019). TRPA1 is selected as a semi-conserved channel during vertebrate evolution due to its involvement in spermatogenesis. *Biochemical and Biophysical Research Communications*, *512*(2), 295–302. https://doi.org/10.1016/j.bbrc.2019.02.121.

Sahoo, S. S., Majhi, R. K., Tiwari, A., & Chattopadhyay, S. (2019). Transient receptor potential Ankyrin1 channel is endogenously expressed in T cells and is involved In immune functions. *Bioscience Reports*. *39*(9)https://doi.org/10.1042/BSR20191437. BSR20191437.

Santoni, G., Cardinali, C., Morelli, M. B., & Amantini, C. (2015). Danger- and pathogen-associated molecular patterns recognition by pattern-recognition receptors and ion Channels of the transient receptor potential family triggers the inflammasome activation in immune cells and sensory neurons. *Journal of Neuroinflammation*, *12*, 21. https://doi.org/10.1186/s12974-015-0239-2.

Sardar, P., Kumar, A., Bhandari, A., & Goswami, C. (2012). Conservation of tubulin-binding sequences in TRPV1 throughout evolution. *PLoS One*, *7*(4), e31448. https://doi.org/10.1371/journal.pone.0031448.

Schappe, M. S., Szteyn, K., Stremska, M. E., & Desai, N. B. (2018). Chanzyme TRPM7 mediates the Ca^{2+} influx essential for lipopolysaccharide-induced toll-like receptor 4 endocytosis and macrophage activation. *Immunity*, *48*(1), 59–74. e5(2018). https://doi.org/10.1016/j.immuni.2017.11.026.

Sharma, S., Jain, S., Nair, G. N., & Ramachandran, S. (2013). Capsicum annuum enhances L-lactate production by *Lactobacillus acidophilus*: Implication in curd formation. *Journal of Dairy Science*, *96*(7), 4142–4148.

Shen, W., Shen, M., Zhao, X., & Le, S. (2017). Anti-obesity effect of capsaicin in mice fed with high-fat diet is associated with an increase in population of the gut bacterium *Akkermansia muciniphila*. *Frontiers in Microbiology*, *8*, 272. https://doi.org/10.3389/fmicb.2017.00272.

Singh, S., Bhatia, R., Singh, A., & Bhadada, S. K. (2018). Probiotic attributes and prevention of LPS-induced pro-inflammatory stress in RAW264. 7 macrophages and human intestinal epithelial cell line (Caco-2) by newly isolated *Weissella cibaria* strains. *Food & Function*, *9*(2), 1254–1264.

Singh, U., Kumar, S., Shelkar, G. P., & Singru, S. P. (2016). Transient receptor potential vanilloid 3 (TRPV3) in the ventral tegmental area of rat: Role in modulation of the mesolimbic-dopamine reward pathway. *Neuropharmacology*, *110*(Pt A), 198–210. https://doi.org/10.1016/j.neuropharm.2016.04.012.

Takahashi, N., Kozai, D., & Mori, Y. (2012). TRP channels: Sensors and transducers of gasotransmitter signals. *Frontiers in Physiology*, *3*, 324. https://doi.org/10.3389/fphys.2012.00324.

Yadav, M., & Goswami, C. (2017). TRPV3 mutants causing Olmsted syndrome induce impaired cell adhesion and nonfunctional lysosomes. *Channels (Austin, Tex)*, *11*(3), 196–208. https://doi.org/10.1080/19336950.2016.1249076.

Yadav, M., Saha, S., Kumar, A., & Goswami, C. (2019). Plant and natural products as modulators of TRP channels. *Biological Research & Reviews*, 1–13.

Zhang, X., Chen, W., Gao, Q., & Xu, H. (2019). Rapamycin directly activates lysosomal mucolipin TRP channels independent of mTOR. *PLoS Biology*. *17*(5)e3000252https://doi.org/10.1371/journal.pbio.3000252.

CHAPTER

12

Application of genomics, transcriptomics, and proteomics in probiotic research

Susrita Sahoo[a], *Soumya R. Mahapatra*[a], *Namrata Misra*[a,b], *and Mrutyunjay Suar*[a,b]

[a]School of Biotechnology, Kalinga Institute of Industrial Technology (KIIT), Deemed to be University, Bhubaneswar, India; [b]KIIT-Technology Business Incubator (KIIT-TBI), Kalinga Institute of Industrial Technology (KIIT), Deemed to be University, Bhubaneswar, India

12.1 Overview

Over the past few years, probiotics have been widely explored owing to their advantageous effects on human health and their benefits in the production of fermented products, especially probiotic beverages (Khaneghah et al., 2020; Million, Lagier, Yahav, & Paul, 2013; Sidhu & Alkandari, 2020; Tannock, 1998). The entire genome sequence data of several bacterial genomes provides a platform for the application of an omics approach to understanding the detailed functional analysis of target genes and enzymes for the development of potentially engineered strains (Aggarwal, Breedon, Davis, Hwang, & Chang, 2020; Barra, Danino, & Garrido, 2020). These multidimensional omics platforms, specifically genomics, transcriptomics, and proteomics, also help to elucidate the complex structure-function relationships of microorganisms (Fig. 12.1). Moreover, comparative genomics has escalated our understanding of microbial metabolism by providing valuable insights into genomic structure, gene function, location, and underlying several metabolic and biological pathways responsible for particular biological phenomena.

To further accelerate experimental studies, various bioinformatic databases and web servers have been recently developed that systematically

https://doi.org/10.1016/B978-0-12-818588-9.00009-7

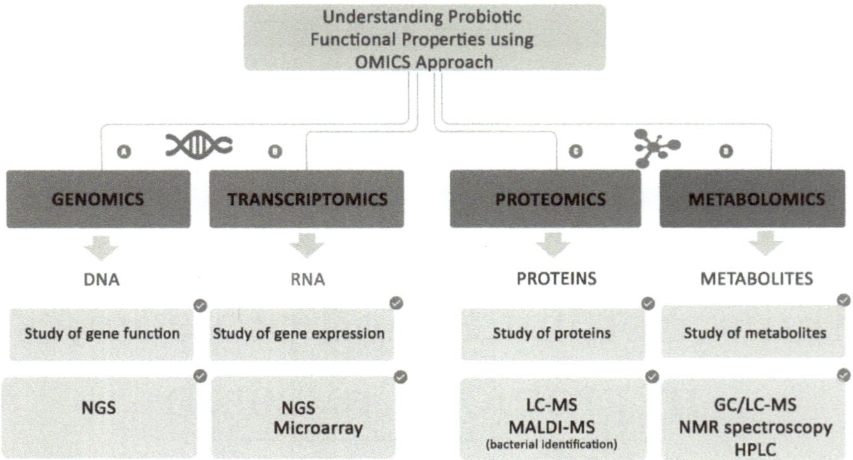

FIG. 12.1 Schematics representation of the application of "Omics" approaches to study probiotic functional properties. *Modified from Day, R. L., Harper, A. J., Woods, R. M., Davies, O. G., & Heaney, L. M. (2019). Probiotics: Current landscape and future horizons.* Future Science OA, 5*(4), FSO391.*

store various genomic and biological data pertinent to probiotic bacterial strains. These publicly available comprehensive resources can also be applied as platform tools by biologists, especially probiotic food and beverage manufacturers, for designing strategies to develop genetically engineered strains with better efficacy and probiotic properties (Yadav, Kumar, Baweja, & Shukla, 2018).

This chapter presents a comprehensive outline of the current advances in different omics approaches viz., genomics, transcriptomics, and proteomics applications in the field of probiotics, followed by a series of bioinformatics resources available for understanding the physiology and functionality of probiotics. The recent application of these approaches provides comprehensive knowledge on the precise interactions between probiotics bacterial species and the host, including their relationship with the gut microflora.

12.2 OMICS-approaches to study probiotics and beneficial effects on the host

Owing to the significant beneficial effects of probiotic food and beverages (Alraefaei, Taibi, & Comelli, 2020), as shown in Fig. 12.2, the genome sequences of several promising probiotic strains are currently available, laying out the framework for further application of omics approaches, namely genomics, transcriptomics, and proteomics for probiotics. This

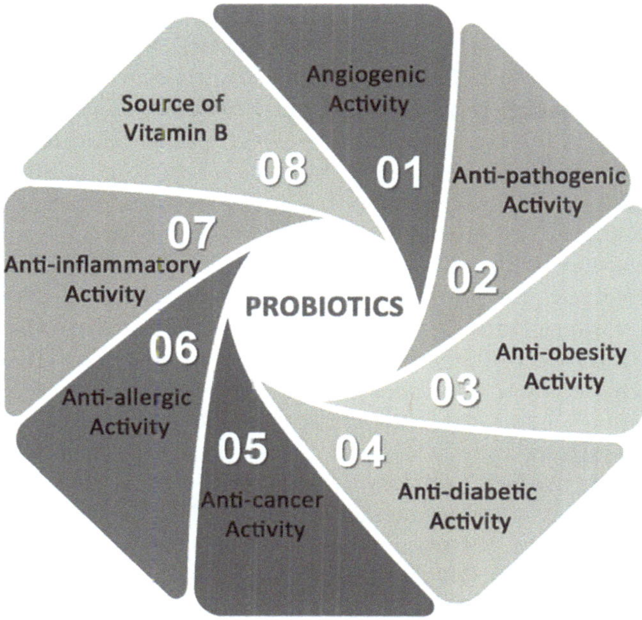

FIG. 12.2 Benefits of probiotics in a wide range of disease conditions. *Modified from Kerry, R. G., Patra, J. K., Gouda, S., Park, Y., Shin, H. S., & Das, G. (2018). Benefaction of probiotics for human health: A review.* Journal of Food and Drug Analysis, 26*(3), 927–939.*

section describes the recent implementation of omics approaches to understand the functional role of probiotics and their mechanism of action.

12.2.1 Genomics

The genome-scale study of probiotic bacteria, also known as "probiogenomics," provides insights into the phylogenomic evolution of diverse bacterial species and a molecular-level understanding of their beneficial effects on health (Ventura et al., 2009). Over the past few years, advanced research on probiotics and the availability of genomics data has significantly improved our understanding of the functionality of different probiotic organisms, particularly the species belonging to the genus *Lactobacillus* and of some *Bifidobacterium* species (Suez, Zmora, & Elinav, 2020). Moreover, this complete genomic information has also improved our knowledge of the mechanisms for adaptation of lactobacilli and bifidobacteria to the human gut environment and interactions with the host.

Sequencing of lactic acid bacteria (LAB) and comparative genomics between its close ancestor, *Bacillus*, has revealed that evolutionary loss of ancestral genes, approximately 600 to 1,200 genes of its overall genetic repertoire, has resulted in an evolution in *Lactobacillus* (Makarova & Koonin, 2007). A major segment of these lost genes includes the key biosynthetic enzymes that are generally involved in sporulation (Makarova & Koonin, 2007). In 2020, details about 220 whole-genome sequencing projects on *Lactobacillus* are now publicly available at Genome, NCBI (https://www.ncbi.nlm.nih.gov/genome/). The genus *Lactobacillus* consists of a diverse clade of LAB belonging to the Firmicutes phylum, which is mostly Gram-positive, nonmotile, catalase-negative, acid-tolerant, anaerobic/microaerophilic, nonspore forming, and low in guanine-cytosine (GC) content (Hammes & Vogel, 1995). Previous studies have shown that LAB are ecologically niche-specific; for example *L. delbrueckii* subsp. *Bulgaricus*, and *L. helveticus* are generally found in dairy products, while *L. acidophilus* and *L. gasseri* are present widely in humans and animal gastrointestinal tracts (GITs) and species such as *L. brevis, L. pentosus, L. plantarum*, and *L. paracasei* can be found in a variety of niches. Furthermore, it is observed that LAB have small-sized genomes (average genome size of 2 Mb, with a coding capacity of 2,000 genes) in comparison to other related bacteria, due to the genome reduction process resulting in the maintenance of a few important genes that are required for niche-specific survival (Makarova et al., 2006).

Health-promoting effects of *Lactobacilli* on humans have generated increasing interest in the investigation of their genomic and molecular features. Among all LAB, the genomic size of *Lactobacillus* is the largest and the most diverse, ranging from 1.23 Mb (*L. sanfranciscensis*) to 4.91 Mb (*L. parakefiri*) (Sun et al., 2015). The *Lactobacillus* pan-genome has nearly 14,000 proteins, while its core genome contains 383 orthologs. Nearly 100 out of 383 genes are organized in operon-like clusters, also found to be conserved in a small number of other related Gram-positive bacteria (Kant, Blom, Palva, Siezen, & de Vos, 2011; Smokvina et al., 2013).

L. plantarum WCFS1 was the first *Lactobacillus* strain sequenced (Kleerebezem et al., 2003), followed shortly by the sequencing of *L. johnsonii NC533* (Pridmore et al., 2004) and *L. acidophilus NCFM* (Altermann et al., 2005). The genomic data shed light on various genomic features, for instance, adaptation islands of strain *WCFS1* belonging to *L. plantarum*, scarcity of basic metabolic pathways in *L. johnsonii strain NC553*, and distinctive structures known as potential autonomous units (PAU) in *L. acidophilus NCFM*. The majority of the LAB have relatively small genome sizes, however, *L. plantarum* holds a larger genome, obtained due to horizontal gene transfer (Kleerebezem et al., 2003), with a size of approximately 3.24 Mb, a protein count of 2968, and a 44.5% GC content. The core genome of *L. plantarum* is comprised of 1425 genes

(Evanovich, de Souza Mendonça Mattos, & Guerreiro, 2019). More significantly are three gene clusters, which play a vital role in the interaction with the environment, such as the clusters responsible for producing exopolysaccharides (responsible for antioxidant and antitumor activity) and a nonribosomal derived hybrid peptide-polyketide (a natural product with pharmaceutical applications). These clusters were generally obtained in an evolutionary action because of their GC profile; thereby, it is proposed that adaptations are essential for survival in a particular niche (Siezen et al., 2010). Strain JDM1 of *L. plantarum* is a commercially used probiotic strain, especially in China, which appears to have lost 100 kb as compared to strain *WCFS1*; the loss of genes is associated with sugar metabolism and transport (Zhang et al., 2009). *L. delbrueckii* consists of two industrially important subspecies viz., *bulgaricus* (1.8 Mb), globally used in the manufacture of probiotic yogurt and subspecies *lactis* (2 Mb), primarily utilized in the production of cheese (El Kafsi et al., 2014). Apart from being a crucial starter for the manufacture of long-ripened Italian and Swiss-type cheeses, strains *of L. helveticus* are also used to ferment meat and plant materials, including their probiotic activity in the GIT and urogenital tract of both animals and humans (Strahinic et al., 2013; Taverniti & Guglielmetti, 2012; Broadbent et al., 2011; Giraffa, 2014). The genome sizes of *Lactobacilli* vary from 1.87 to 2.38 Mbp with an average 37% GC content. Widely utilized in various dairy products as probiotics and also as a flavor contributing strain in yogurt, cheese, and sweet acidophilus milk, strains of *L. acidophilus* are part of a larger group comprising several species such as *L. amylovorus, L. acidophilus, L. gallinarum, L. crispatus, L. gasseri, L. johnsonii, and L. gasseri* (Berger et al., 2007; Buriti, Da Rocha, & Saad, 2005; Ejtahed et al., 2011; Ong, Henriksson, & Shah, 2007; Ramachandran, Lacher, Pfeiler, & Elkins, 2013). The strain *L. acidophilus NCFM* was the first *L. acidophilus* to be sequenced (Altermann et al., 2005). Currently, 16 different strains of *L. acidophilus* have been sequenced with genomes size varying between 1.25 and 2.05 Mbp, and approximately 35% GC content. Even though both the biochemical and phenotypic characterization of strains exhibit a certain level of variation, genotypic studies reveal minimal diversity within the genomes of these species (Bull et al., 2014; Ramachandran et al., 2013; Stahl & Barrangou, 2013). However, the genome analysis of *L. johnsonii FI9785* shows its role as a competitive exclusion agent against pathogens in poultry (Wegmann et al., 2009).

L. rhamnosus ATCC53103 and *GG* are probiotic strains that have been commercially used for many years in several beverages and foods (Kankainen et al., 2009; Morita et al., 2009). *L. rhamnosus* genomes have a comparatively high number of proteins compared to other sequenced intestinal lactobacilli and are particularly required for the metabolism and transport of carbohydrates and amino acids, and for defense mechanisms.

Additionally, *L. rhamnosus* contains proteins, encoded by a three-gene cluster and with conserved W x L domains, useful for attachment to the peptidoglycan on cell surfaces (Brinster, Furlan, & Serror, 2007; Siezen et al., 2006). These gene clusters are uniquely found in a few plant-associated Gram-positive bacteria; however, none are reported in intestinal lactobacilli (Siezen et al., 2006). Most importantly, the *L. rhamnosus GG* strain has a spaCBA gene cluster, which encodes for three unique secreted pilin proteins with conserved LPXTG sequence as peptidoglycan anchors, and these are completely absent in *L. rhamnosus LC705* (Kankainen et al., 2009). Notably, SpaA is a crucial scaffolding protein on which the minor pili proteins, namely SpaB and SpaC are attached. However, utilizing the insertional inactivation of the spaC protein, a reduced SpaC protein was generated, and this occurred in cells with significant decreased binding to human mucus (Kankainen et al., 2009). This suggests that the presence of SpaC-containing pili may elucidate the prolonged tenacity of the *L. rhamnosus GG* strain in the GIT than the *LC705* strain (Kankainen et al., 2009) and also could be an important factor for increased health beneficial effects of probiotic strains belonging to *L. rhamnosus*.

Several bioinformatic analyses of the sequenced genomes between the *Lactobacilli* and milk or plant isolates have illustrated distinct differences crucial for niche adaptation. For example, genomes of milk-adapted *L. helveticus* and *L. bulgaricus* (Callanan et al., 2008; Makarova et al., 2006) comprise an array of genes responsible for the metabolism of milk-derived sugars and a few additional carbohydrates (Ventura et al., 2009). A coherent indication of adaptation to the human GIT environment is exhibited through augmentation of putative mucus-binding enzymes that are known to be involved in the breakdown of carbohydrate molecules (Boekhorst, Wels, Kleerebezem, & Siezen, 2006; Siezen et al., 2006). Moreover, distinct adaptation to the human GIT is shown clearly by the presence of a bile salt hydrolase (BSH) enzyme coded by every sequenced intestinal *Lactobacilli* (Lambert, 2008).

Furthermore, various *Lactobacillus* strains are widely known for their potential to produce B-group vitamins, for example, *L. plantarum* strain *LZ95* produces riboflavin and *L. reuteri ZJ03* supplements vitamin B12 content in soy-yogurt (Capozzi, Russo, Dueñas, López, & Spano, 2012; Gu, Zhang, Song, Li, & Zhu, 2015; Li, Zhou, & Gu, 2016). Moreover, it was noted that *L. plantarum strain* WCSF1 is capable of producing a substantial quantity of folate, but not riboflavin (Kleerebezem et al., 2003; LeBlanc et al., 2011; Wegkamp et al., 2010), unlike LAB strain *L. plantarum* LZ227 isolated from cow milk, which showed the ability to produce both riboflavin and folate. Studies have confirmed that strains that lack *rib* genes or with partial *rib* structural genes are impotent in terms of the production of riboflavin (Kleerebezem et al., 2003). An absolute functional *rib* operon includes genes *ribA* (3, 4-dihydroxy-2-butanone

4-phosphate synthase), *ribB* (riboflavin synthase with alpha subunit), *ribG* (deaminase and reductase, riboflavin specific), and *ribH* (a riboflavin synthase with beta subunit). These genes, which are typically found in LAB strain LZ227, are responsible for the synthesis of riboflavin in probiotic strains.

Members belonging to genus *Bifidobacterium* are immotile, Gram-positive, anaerobic bacteria. They include strikingly less phylogenetic and genomic variations (Ventura et al., 2007). Originally, these were isolated from the fecal matter of newborns, and, to date, approximately 50 species have been isolated from animals, humans, and insects (Favier, Vaughan, De Vos, & Akkermans, 2002; Tissier, 1900). *Bifidobacteria* are one of the well-known commensal bacteria, which originated in the human colon and dominate the evolving microbiome in breast-fed newborns (Klaenhammer et al., 2002).

Since the sequencing of the first bacterial genome, exponential advancements in sequencing and annotation have resulted in over a thousand publicly available probiotic microorganism genomes being sequenced (Table 12.1).

The first Bifidobacteria colonizer, *B. longum subsp. infantis* was isolated from a newborn, and it has the largest genome at 2.83 Mb (Sela et al., 2008). The *B. longum* subsp. genome encompasses comprehensive pathways for the production of essential vitamins and a specific gene cluster, with a size of 43 kb, for digestion of human milk oligosaccharides (HMO). However, subsequently, the total numbers of *Bifidobacterium* were observed to decline progressively with the age of the host, while others became more dominant. Another commonly found *Bifidobacteria* species in the GI tract is *Bifidobacterium animalis* subsp. lactis with a genome size of only 1.9 Mb, which is widely used as a probiotic in North America and Europe. This bacterium is devoid of human milk oligosaccharide cluster, as post-weaned organisms do not entail this functionality. However, a fructooligosaccharide (fos) gene cluster is present to produce the enzymes necessary for the breakdown and utilization of health-promoting fructooligosaccharides. Moreover, *B. animalis* subsp. *lactis* AD011, derived from a fecal sample of a healthy breast-fed infant, has increased immunomodulatory activity (Kim et al., 2008). Its genome encodes more glycosylases responsible for degrading plant- or milk-derived oligosaccharides, and the fos gene cluster for processing of fructooligosaccharides (Kim et al., 2009a, 2009b). The *B. animalis* subsp. *lactis* DSM10140 and B1-04 strains differ only by 4 indels and 47 single nucleotide polymorphisms (SNPs) (Barrangou et al., 2009a, 2009b).

Comparative genomic analysis is useful to assign a potential function to uncharacterized genes sharing sequence similarity with functionally annotated genes. Approximately, 60% of the genes of *B. thetaiotaomicron*, 70% of *B. longum*, and 70% of *L. plantarum*, have been assigned putative

TABLE 12.1 Details on whole-genome sequenced potential probiotics bacteria

Species	Strain	Accession	Isolation source	Reference
Bifidobacterium adolescentis	ATCC 15703	NC_008618	Human feces	Ramirez-Farias et al. (2008)
Bifidobacterium animalis subsp. *lactis*	AD011	NC_011835	Human infant feces	Kim et al. (2009a, 2009b)
Bifidobacterium animalis subsp. *lactis*	ATCC SD5219	NC_012814	Human infant feces	Barrangou et al. (2009a, 2009b)
Bifidobacterium animalis subsp. *lactis*	DSM 10140	NC_012815	Swiss yoghurt	Barrangou et al. (2009a, 2009b)
Bifidobacterium breve	UCC203			Leahy, Higgins, Fitzgerald, and Van Sinderen (2005)
Bifidobacterium longum	NCC2705	NC_004307	Human infant feces	Schell et al. (2002)
Bifidobacterium longum	DJO10A	NC_010816	Human adolescent feces	Lee et al. (2008)
Bifidobacterium longum subsp. *infantis*	ATCC 15697	NC_011593	Human infant feces	Sela et al. (2008)
Propionibacterium freundenreichii	ATCC9614		Swiss cheese	Altermann et al. (2005)
Lactobacillus acidophilus	NCFM	NC_006814	Human intestine	Makarova et al. (2006)
Lactobacillus casei	ATCC 334	NC_008526	Emmental cheese	Aleksandrzak-Piekarczyk, Koryszewska-Bagińska, and Bardowski (2013)
Lactobacillus delbrueckii subsp. *bulgaricus*	ATCC BAA-365	NC_008529	French starter culture	Makarova et al. (2006)
Lactobacillus delbrueckii subsp. *bulgaricus*	ATCC 11842	NC_008054	Bulgarian yoghurt	Van de Guchte et al. (2006)
Lactobacillus fermentum	IFO 3956	NC_010610	Japanese fermented plant	Morita et al. (2008)

TABLE 12.1 Details on whole-genome sequenced potential probiotics bacteria—cont'd

Species	Strain	Accession	Isolation source	Reference
Lactobacillus gasseri	ATCC 33323	NC_008530	Human intestine	Makarova et al. (2006)
Lactobacillus helveticus	DPC 4571	NC_010080	Swiss cheese	Callanan et al. (2008)
Lactobacillus johnsonii	NCC533	NC_005362	Human intestine	Pridmore et al. (2004)
Lactobacillus johnsonii	FI9785	FN298497	Poultry	Wegmann et al. (2009)
Lactobacillus plantarum	WCFS1	NC_004567	Human saliva	Kleerebezem et al. (2003)
Lactobacillus plantarum	JDM1	NC_012984		Zhang et al. (2009)
Lactobacillus reuteri	F275, JCM1112	NC_010609	Human adult intestine	Morita et al. (2008)
Lactobacillus rhamnosus	GG	NC_013198	Human feces	Kankainen et al. (2009)
Lactobacillus rhamnosus	ATCC53103	AP011548	Human intestine	Morita et al. (2009)
Lactobacillus salivarius	UCC118	NC_007929	Human small intestine	Claesson et al. (2006)
Leuconostoc citreum	KM20	NC_010471	Korean fermented vegetables	Kim, Choi, and Ji (2008)

function, showing the need to identify and annotate the functions of the uncharacterized hypothetical genes and the encoded proteins. In addition to expanding the knowledge about intestinal microbiota composition and activity, various culture-independent metagenomic studies were performed in order to unravel genes and their functions in a specific digestive environment. Metagenomic approaches have helped to predict the community structure of the microbiota, by revealing the wide microbial diversity and subsequently, identifying various enterotypes of the human gut microbiome. With the advancement of metagenomic approaches, the understanding of the structure and diversity of the gut microbial community and their genetic composition have been substantially improved. Thereby, the integration of genomics and microbiome studies can provide valuable insights about the probiotic mechanisms of action and factors influencing its efficiency, thus further facilitating the development of improved engineered probiotic strains.

12.2.2 Transcriptomics

A transcriptome is usually defined as the initial product of genome expression, while the genome is defined as the collection of all DNA present in the nucleus and the mitochondria. Comprehensive transcriptional profiling of bacterial species, in their native environment, helps in understanding the underpinning molecular functions that regulate the interaction between probiotics and humans, or with other microbes found in the GIT. Several reports have discussed the genome transcriptional responses to the gastrointestinal environment, such as the existence of bile salts (Alcantara & Zuniga, 2012; Koskenniemi et al., 2011; Ruiz et al., 2012; Ruiz et al., 2012; Whitehead, Versalovic, Roos, & Britton, 2008), milk from different sources (Turroni et al., 2011), the effect of growth in various oligosaccharides (Barrangou et al., 2006; Gilad et al., 2010), showing a series of molecular approaches that probiotics could utilize to control the GIT conditions. Moreover, transcriptomics has also been reported to be useful for the establishment of novel molecular toolboxes for further metabolic level analyses of probiotic organisms. For instance, a transcriptomic study showed the existence of a bile-inducible efflux transporter, in different bifidobacterial species, which plays a vital role in bile tolerance (Ruiz, Zomer, O'Connell-Motherway, van Sinderen, & Margolles, 2012; Gueimonde, Garrigues, van Sinderen, de los Reyes-Gavilán, & Margolles, 2009; Ruiz, O'Connell-Motherway, et al., 2012). Likewise, a combination of transcriptomes belonging to *L. plantarum* under diverse ecological circumstances has identified gene-regulatory networks with important functions in fermentation (Bron et al., 2012).

Complete genome transcriptomic reports belonging to several probiotics and their intervention in the GIT channel of animal models, instead of in vitro laboratory circumstances, have advanced our understanding of the probiotic lifestyle in the GIT environment by identifying important housekeeping genes, including some essential colonization factors (Denou et al., 2008; Foroni et al., 2011; Marco et al., 2009; O'Connell-Motherway et al., 2011). Likewise, another study on the differentiation of the *L. plantarum* transcriptome between mouse and human intestines, surprisingly showed convergence in the gut adaption reaction to both of the hosts (Marco et al., 2010). Also, a comparative transcriptomics analysis between various strains belonging to the phylum Bifidobacterium, in the intestine of a mouse model with fecal cultures, revealed an array of genes involved in the production of sugar transporters and glycosidases in vivo (Ishikawa et al., 2011). Further, transcriptomic studies will be essential to obtain a comprehensive picture of downstream reactions of the host and pathways triggered in response to probiotics that might assist in the identification and molecular assistance of probiotic effects.

For example, studies performed on responses of the human GIT to *L. plantarum* WCFS1 reported effects on immune modulation, lipid metabolism, cellular growth, and cell-cell signaling on the GIT, which were regulated at the transcriptional level, confirming the significance of transcriptomic profiles in deciphering molecular information from complex samples (Leimena et al., 2012; McNulty et al., 2011; Troost et al., 2008; Van Baarlen et al., 2011).

12.2.3 Proteomics

The word "Proteome" is widely defined as "complete protein complements of a cell or subcellular fraction of a microorganism in a defined growth phase under a definite physiological condition" (Gorg, Boguth, Obermaier, & Weiss, 1998; Aebersold & Mann, 2003; Di Cagno, De Angelis, Calasso, & Gobbetti, 2011). Several studies have corroborated that proteomics is a useful platform for characterizing different probiotic bacterial strains as the method can determine the global variation in the synthesis of proteins as a response to different microbial environments (Aires et al., 2010; Sánchez, Ruiz, de los Reyes-Gavilán, & Margolles, 2008). Specifically, two-dimensional gel electrophoresis (2-DE) is a method used for generating maps in reference to probiotic species, permitting both inter-strain and interspecies distinction. For example, it has been used to understand the molecular mechanism involving the response of bile salt in some vital LAB strains such as *L. rhamnosus GG, L. plantarum* 299V, and *L. delbrueckii subsp. lactis* 200; as well as responses to acidic pH in *B. animalis, B. longum, L. casei,* and *L. reuteri* (Burns et al., 2010; Koskenniemi et al., 2011). Furthermore, this method is used to decipher the relationship between distinct strains in coculture media (Ruiz et al., 2009) and for the identification of molecules engaged in the interaction of probiotics with the host environment, such as the identification of target extracellular proteins and surface-associated proteins (Izquierdo et al., 2009; Kelly et al., 2005; Sanchez et al., 2007; Sánchez et al., 2008). Furthermore, various earlier reports have indicated that it is useful in analyzing bacterial responses to different physiological stresses, such as findings on the response of *B. longum* BBMN68 to an oxidative stress environment (Xiao et al., 2011) and the *L. reuteri* response to selenium exploitation for nutraceutical perseverance (Lamberti et al., 2011; Mangiapane et al., 2011). Additionally, it is also utilized to identify various metabolic regulatory pathways that allow probiotics to grow with changeable carbon sources (Liu et al., 2011).

As 2-DE is used to identify specific types of protein, other novel techniques have been developed to analyze the complete probiotic proteome (Beck et al., 2009; Koponen et al., 2012; Koskenniemi et al., 2009; Laakso et al., 2011; Wu et al., 2012; Yuan et al., 2008). Differential staining techniques, based on fluorescent probes, have been widely utilized to illustrate the specific proteins expressed at low-level pH and also to detect the proteins involved in post-translational modification (Koponen et al., 2012; Wu et al., 2012). However, the biggest challenge of this technique is that it sometimes fails to predict proteins that are highly hydrophobic or are generally expressed at extremely minimal levels (Sánchez et al., 2008). To overcome this problem, different molecular labeling methods and numerous gel free–based methods are used, which include protease breakdown and solubilization of substances extracted from bacteria, followed by bifurcation complex liquid chromatography systems (Coute, Hernandez, Appel, Sanchez, & Margolles, 2007; Ruiz, Sánchez, de los Reyes-Gavilán, Gueimonde, & Margolles, 2009; Vitali et al., 2007; Vitali, Wasinger, Brigidi, & Guilhaus, 2005).

Considering the host gut-proteome as a fundamental element for maintaining the mutualistic relationship between host-to-microbiota, metaproteomics, a complementary approach to metagenomics, is crucial to identify and address the function encoded by the gut microbes. Metaproteomic studies are focused on the large-scale characterization of proteins from environmental microbiota, like the human gut (Petriz & Franco, 2017) and to characterize differential protein profiles under altered physiological conditions (Lee, Chin, Neoh, & Jamal, 2017; Li et al., 2011). Importantly, metaproteomics approaches have the potential to critically explore microbial functionality, which could further assist in an understanding of the underlying pathophysiology and devise strategies in disease prevention and management for improved human health.

Recently, in-silico analysis of putative hypothetical protein sequences has become an integral part of proteomics research. Several bioinformatics tools are available such as SignalP (www.cbs.dtu.dk/services/SignalP-3.0/) for predicting presence of N-terminal signal peptides, and Transmembrane Helices Hidden Markov Models (TMHMM) (http://www.cbs.dtu.dk/services/TMHMM/) for identifying hydrophobic transmembrane regions. Additionally, bioinformatics tools such as Pfam (https://pfam.xfam.org/) and Structural Classification of Proteins (SCOP) database (http://scop.mrc-lmb.cam.ac.uk/) are used to identify and study the sequence-function relationship of conserved consensus sequences, particularly found on surface proteins such as sugar-binding, mucus-binding, fibronectin-binding, and collagen-binding domains, which have been shown to play an integral role in the interaction between host and probiotic bacterial species.

12.3 Probiotic focused bioinformatics databases

To further accelerate the omics studies, various bioinformatics databases have been recently developed that systematically provide genomic functional details of the microorganisms, usage surveillance, evaluation of the labeling and safety information, and other essential nutritional details pertinent to probiotics. These publicly available comprehensive resources can be useful in further experimental research on probiotics.

A number of bioinformatics databases have been developed to facilitate advanced research in probiotics. For example, PROBIO is a comprehensive repository of information on all probiotics reported to date (Tao et al., 2017). It provides in-depth knowledge about various functions of the probiotic and its functional classes (that are assigned by the International Classification of Disease [ICD] codes), taxonomic lineages, both commercial and growth phase, and also provides hyperlinks to the entire genome sequence data available at the National Center for Biotechnology Information (NCBI) (Coordinators, 2017) and the Microbial Genome Database (MGD) (Uchiyama, Mihara, Nishide, & Chiba, 2015). Additionally, the PROBIO database in March of 2020 (http://bidd2.nus.edu.sg/probio/homepage.htm) included information on 167 clinical trials, 448 commercialized, and 382 literature reports on probiotics. The rich data available at PROBIO is useful for deciphering the molecular mechanisms of the probiotic bacterial species and also for the identification of novel probiotic strains.

Likewise, the Probiotics Database (PBDB) is freely available at http://lzubiodrugs.com and provides complete nutritional details and other important biological information on 1730 known probiotics present in fermented food and beverages (Zhao et al., 2019).

12.4 Future application of omics in development of engineered probiotics strains

Numerous omics and bioinformatics approaches have paved novel research roadmaps for in-depth exploration of probiotics aimed at improving human health. The traditional approach of identification of novel probiotics that starts with constructing a strain library using a culturomics approach is an extremely laborious and time-consuming process (Lagier et al., 2016). However, by application of multidisciplinary omics strategies, identification of target biomolecules and strains becomes easier and faster and these can be further validated by experimental studies.

In addition to elucidating the importance of a healthy microbiota to host health, it is essential to have a clear understanding of the contributions of the varied constituents of the community. The application of multi-omics approaches will certainly be useful in this regard by providing more in-depth knowledge of the complex structure-function relationships of the microbial communities. Recently, by employing the various omics methods, vital microorganisms have been genetically modified into so-called "genomic tape recorders" that have the potential of observing events and storing the information to be further analyzed at a later time (Farzadfard & Lu, 2014). Even though this technology is still not widely studied in the probiotics field, it could be used to construct engineered strains that can track the ecological changes inside the GIT.

Furthermore, it has been reported that the marginal differences in the gene content between genetically homologous probiotic strains could be a major reason for significant variations in phenotypes (Zeevi et al., 2019). For example, in the *Bifidobacterium* genus, the genetic differences between

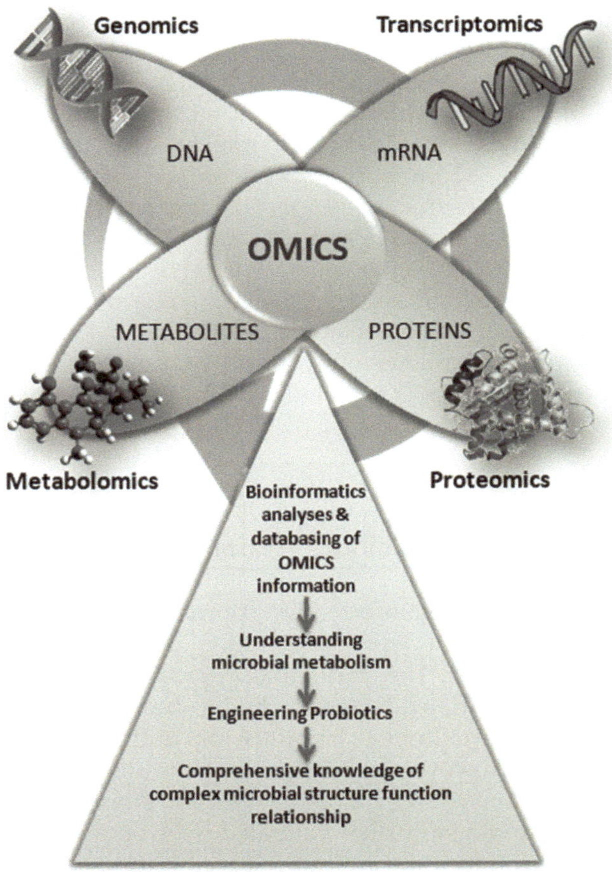

FIG. 12.3 Schematic representation of the application of OMICS approach in probiotics research.

various strains of the same species underlie variations in their carbohydrate utilization profiles (Arboleya et al., 2018). In this regard, bioinformatics techniques and the application of various computational tools and databases can play a major role in pinpointing the target genes responsible for conferring probiotic traits in an organism and to assist in the detailed studies of the structure-function relationships of the encoded enzymes (Fig. 12.3). These insights will certainly act as a framework for further laboratory experiments to develop genetically engineered probiotic strains with optimum properties for industrial applications.

References

Aebersold, R., & Mann, M. (2003). Mass spectrometry-based proteomics. *Nature, 422*, 198–207.

Aggarwal, N., Breedon, A. M. E., Davis, C. M., Hwang, I. Y., & Chang, M. W. (2020). Engineering probiotics for therapeutic applications: Recent examples and translational outlook. *Current Opinion in Biotechnology, 65*, 171–179.

Aires, J., Anglade, P., Baraige, F., Zagorec, M., Champomier-Verges, M. C., & Butel, M. J. (2010). Proteomic comparison of the cytosolic proteins of three *Bifidobacterium longum* human isolates and *B. longum* NCC2705. *BMC Microbiology, 10*, 29. https://doi.org/10.1186/1471-2180-10-29.

Alcantara, C., & Zuniga, M. (2012). Proteomic and transcriptomic analysis of the response to bile stress of *Lactobacillus casei* BL23. *Microbiology, 158*, 1206–1218.

Aleksandrzak-Piekarczyk, T., Koryszewska-Bagińska, A., & Bardowski, J. (2013). Genome sequence of the probiotic strain *Lactobacillus rhamnosus* (formerly *Lactobacillus casei*) LOCK900. *Genome Announcements, 1*(4). e00640-13.

Alraefaei, A., Taibi, A., & Comelli, E. M. (2020). Probiotic supplements–basic concepts of the gut microbiome and the role of probiotics to sustain health. P. A. Spagnuolo (Ed.), *Vol. 23. Nutraceuticals and human health: The food-to-supplement paradigm* (pp. 185–203). Royal Society of Chemistry.

Altermann, E., Russell, W. M., Azcarate-Peril, M. A., Barrangou, R., Buck, B. L., McAuliffe, O., et al. (2005). Complete genome sequence of the probiotic lactic acid bacterium *Lactobacillus acidophilus* NCFM. *Proceedings of the National Academy of Sciences of the United States of America, 102*(11), 3906–3912.

Arboleya, S., Bottacini, F., O'Connell-Motherway, M., Ryan, C. A., Ross, R. P., Van Sinderen, D., et al. (2018). Gene-trait matching across the *Bifidobacterium longum* pan-genome reveals considerable diversity in carbohydrate catabolism among human infant strains. *BMC Genomics, 19*(1), 33. https://doi.org/10.1186/s12864-017-4388-9.

Barra, M., Danino, T., & Garrido, D. (2020). Engineered probiotics for detection and treatment of inflammatory intestinal diseases. *Frontiers in Bioengineering and Biotechnology, 8*, 265.

Barrangou, R., Azcarate-Peril, M. A., Duong, T., Conners, S. B., Kelly, R. M., & Klaenhammer, T. R. (2006). Global analysis of carbohydrate utilization by *Lactobacillus acidophilus* using cDNA microarrays. *Proceedings of the National Academy of Sciences of the United States of America, 103*, 3816–3821.

Barrangou, R., Briczinski, E. P., Traeger, L. L., Loquasto, J. R., Richards, M., Horvath, P., et al. (2009a). Comparison of the complete genome sequences of *Bifidobacterium animalis* subsp. lactis DSM 10140 and Bl-04. *Journal of Bacteriology, 191*(13), 4144–4151.

Barrangou, R., Briczinski, E. P., Traeger, L. L., Loquasto, J. R., Richards, M., Horvath, P., et al. (2009b). Comparison of the complete genome sequences of *Bifidobacterium animalis subsp. lactis* DSM 10140 and Bl-04. *Journal of Bacteriology, 191*, 4144–4151.

Beck, H. C., Madsen, S. M., Glenting, J., Petersen, J., Israelsen, H., Norrelykke, M. R., et al. (2009). Proteomic analysis of cell surface-associated proteins from probiotic *Lactobacillus plantarum*. *FEMS Microbiology Letters, 297*, 61–66.

Berger, B., Pridmore, R. D., Barretto, C., Delmas-Julien, F., Schreiber, K., Arigoni, F., et al. (2007). Similarity and differences in the *Lactobacillus acidophilus* group identified by polyphasic analysis and comparative genomics. *Journal of Bacteriology, 189*(4), 1311–1321.

Boekhorst, J., Wels, M., Kleerebezem, M., & Siezen, R. J. (2006). The predicted secretome of *Lactobacillus plantarum* WCFS1 sheds light on interactions with its environment. *Microbiology, 152*, 3175–3183.

Brinster, S., Furlan, S., & Serror, P. (2007). C-terminal WxL domain mediates cell wall binding in *Enterococcus faecalis* and other gram-positive bacteria. *Journal of Bacteriology, 189*, 1244–1253.

Broadbent, J. R., Cai, H., Larsen, R. L., Hughes, J. E., Welker, D. L., De Carvalho, V. G., et al. (2011). Genetic diversity in proteolytic enzymes and amino acid metabolism among *Lactobacillus helveticus* strains. *Journal of Dairy Science, 94*(9), 4313–4328.

Bron, P. A., Wels, M., Bongers, R. S., van Bokhorst-van de Veen, H., Wiersma, A., Overmars, L., et al. (2012). Transcriptomes reveal genetic signatures underlying physiological variations imposed by different fermentation conditions in *Lactobacillus plantarum*. *PLoS One, 7*, e38720.

Bull, M. J., Jolley, K. A., Bray, J. E., Aerts, M., Vandamme, P., Maiden, M. C., et al. (2014). The domestication of the probiotic bacterium *Lactobacillus acidophilus*. *Scientific Reports, 4*, 7202.

Buriti, F. C., Da Rocha, J. S., & Saad, S. M. (2005). Incorporation of *Lactobacillus acidophilus* in Minas fresh cheese and its implications for textural and sensorial properties during storage. *International Dairy Journal, 15*(12), 1279–1288.

Burns, P., Sánchez, B., Vinderola, G., Ruas-Madiedo, P., Ruiz, L., Margolles, A., et al. (2010). Inside the adaptation process of *Lactobacillus delbrueckii subsp. lactis* to bile. *International Journal of Food Microbiology, 142*, 132–141.

Callanan, M., Kaleta, P., O'Callaghan, J., O'Sullivan, O., Jordan, K., McAuliffe, O., et al. (2008). Genome sequence of *Lactobacillus helveticus*, an organism distinguished by selective gene loss and insertion sequence element expansion. *Journal of Bacteriology, 190*(2), 727–735.

Capozzi, V., Russo, P., Dueñas, M. T., López, P., & Spano, G. (2012). Lactic acid bacteria producing B-group vitamins: a great potential for functional cereals products. *Applied Microbiology and Biotechnology, 96*(6), 1383–1394.

Claesson, M. J., Li, Y., Leahy, S., Canchaya, C., van Pijkeren, J. P., Cerdeño-Tárraga, A. M., et al. (2006). Multireplicon genome architecture of *Lactobacillus salivarius*. *Proceedings of the National Academy of Sciences of the United States of America, 103*(17), 6718–6723.

Coordinators, N. R. (2017). Database resources of the national center for biotechnology information. *Nucleic Acids Research, 45*(Database issue), D12.

Coute, Y., Hernandez, C., Appel, R. D., Sanchez, J. C., & Margolles, A. (2007). Labeling of *Bifidobacterium longum* cells with C-13-substituted leucine for quantitative proteomic analyses. *Applied and Environmental Microbiology, 73*, 5653–5656.

Denou, E., Pridmore, R. D., Berger, B., Panoff, J. M., Arigoni, F., & Brussow, H. (2008). Identification of genes associated with the long-gut-persistence phenotype of the probiotic *Lactobacillus johnsonii* strain NCC533 using a combination of genomics and transcriptome analysis. *Journal of Bacteriology, 190*, 3161–3168.

Di Cagno, R., De Angelis, M., Calasso, M., & Gobbetti, M. (2011). Proteomics of the bacterial cross-talk by quorum sensing. *Journal of Proteomics, 74*, 19–34.

Ejtahed, H. S., Mohtadi-Nia, J., Homayouni-Rad, A., Niafar, M., Asghari-Jafarabadi, M., Mofid, V., et al. (2011). Effect of probiotic yogurt containing *Lactobacillus acidophilus* and *Bifidobacterium lactis* on lipid profile in individuals with type 2 diabetes mellitus. *Journal of Dairy Science, 94*(7), 3288–3294.

El Kafsi, H., Binesse, J., Loux, V., Buratti, J., Boudebbouze, S., Dervyn, R., et al. (2014). Genome sequence of *Lactobacillus delbrueckii* subsp. *lactis* CNRZ327, a dairy bacterium with anti-inflammatory properties. *Genome Announcements, 2*(4), e00328-14.

Evanovich, E., de Souza Mendonça Mattos, P. J., & Guerreiro, J. F. (2019). Comparative genomic analysis of *Lactobacillus plantarum:* An overview. *International Journal of Genomics, 2019*, 4973214. https://doi.org/10.1155/2019/4973214.

Farzadfard, F., & Lu, T. K. (2014). Genomically encoded analog memory with precise in vivo DNA writing in living cell populations. *Science, 346*(6211), 1256272.

Favier, C. F., Vaughan, E. E., De Vos, W. M., & Akkermans, A. D. (2002). Molecular monitoring of succession of bacterial communities in human neonates. *Applied and Environmental Microbiology, 68*(1), 219–226.

Foroni, E., Serafini, F., Amidani, D., Turroni, F., He, F., Bottacini, F., et al. (2011). Genetic analysis and morphological identification of pilus-like structures in members of the genus *Bifidobacterium. Microbial Cell Factories, 10,* S16. https://doi.org/10.1186/1475-2859-10-S1-S16.

Gilad, O., Jacobsen, S., Stuer-Lauridsen, B., Pedersen, M. B., Garrigues, C., & Svensson, B. (2010). Combined transcriptome and proteome analysis of *Bifidobacterium animalis subsp. lactis* BB-12 grown on xylo-oligosaccharides and a model of their utilization. *Applied and Environmental Microbiology, 76*, 7285–7291.

Giraffa, G. (2014). *Lactobacillus helveticus*: importance in food and health. *Frontiers in Microbiology, 5*, 338. https://doi.org/10.3389/fmicb.2014.00338.

Gorg, A., Boguth, G., Obermaier, C., & Weiss, W. (1998). Two-dimensional electrophoresis of proteins in an immobilized pH 4–12 gradient. *Electrophoresis, 19*, 1516–1519.

Gu, Q., Zhang, C., Song, D., Li, P., & Zhu, X. (2015). Enhancing vitamin B12 content in soy-yogurt by *Lactobacillus reuteri. International Journal of Food Microbiology, 206*, 56–59.

Gueimonde, M., Garrigues, C., van Sinderen, D., de los Reyes-Gavilán, C. G., & Margolles, A. (2009). Bile-inducible efflux transporter from *Bifidobacterium longum* NCC2705, conferring bile resistance. *Applied and Environmental Microbiology, 75*, 3153–3160.

Hammes, W. P., & Vogel, R. F. (1995). The genus lactobacillus. B. J. B. Wood, & W. H. Holzapfel (Eds.), *Vol. 2. The genera of lactic acid bacteria* (pp. 19–54). Boston, MA: Springer.

Ishikawa, E., Shima, T., Sudam, K., Shirasawa, Y., Sato, T., & Umesaki, Y. (2011). Comparison of *Bifidobacterium breve* strain Yakult transcriptomes in germ-free mice with those in fecal cultures. *Journal of Bioscience and Bioengineering, 112*, 451–457.

Izquierdo, E., Horvatovich, P., Marchioni, E., Aoude-Werner, D., Sanz, Y., & Ennahar, S. (2009). 2-DE and MS analysis of key proteins in the adhesion of *Lactobacillus plantarum*, a first step toward early selection of probiotics based on bacterial biomarkers. *Electrophoresis, 30*, 949–956.

Kankainen, M., Paulin, L., Tynkkynen, S., von Ossowski, I., Reunanen, J., Partanen, P., et al. (2009). Comparative genomic analysis of *Lactobacillus rhamnosus* GG reveals pili containing a human-mucus binding protein. *Proceedings of the National Academy of Sciences of the United States of America, 106*, 17193–17198.

Kant, R., Blom, J., Palva, A., Siezen, R. J., & de Vos, W. M. (2011). Comparative genomics of lactobacillus. *Microbial Biotechnology, 4*(3), 323–332.

Kelly, P., Maguire, P. B., Bennett, M., Fitzgerald, D. J., Edwards, R. J., Thiede, B., et al. (2005). Correlation of probiotic *Lactobacillus salivarius* growth phase with its cell wall associated proteome. *FEMS Microbiology Letters, 252*, 153–159.

Khaneghah, A. M., Abhari, K., Eş, I., Soares, M. B., Oliveira, R. B., Hosseini, H., et al. (2020). Interactions between probiotics and pathogenic microorganisms in hosts and foods: A review. *Trends in Food Science & Technology, 95*, 205–218.

Kim, J. Y., Choi, Y. O., & Ji, G. E. (2008). Effect of oral probiotics (*Bifidobacterium lactis* AD011 and *Lactobacillus acidophilus* AD031) administration on ovalbumin-induced food allergy mouse model. *Journal of Microbiology and Biotechnology, 18*, 1393–1400.

Kim, J. F., Jeong, H., Lee, J. S., Choi, S. H., Ha, M., Hur, C. G., et al. (2008). Complete genome sequence of *Leuconostoc citreum* KM20. *Journal of Bacteriology, 190*(8), 3093–3094.

Kim, J. F., Jeong, H., Yu, D. S., Choi, S. H., Hur, C. G., Park, M. S., et al. (2009a). Genome sequence of the probiotic bacterium *Bifidobacterium animalis* subsp. lactis AD011. *Journal of Bacteriology, 191*(2), 678–679.

Kim, J. F., Jeong, H., Yu, D. S., Choi, S. H., Hur, C. G., Park, M. S., et al. (2009b). Genome sequence of the probiotic bacterium *Bifidobacterium animalis subsp. lactis* AD011. *Journal of Bacteriology, 191*, 678–679.

Klaenhammer, T., Altermann, E., Arigoni, F., Bolotin, A., Breidt, F., Broadbent, J., et al. (2002). Discovering lactic acid bacteria by genomics. In R. J. Siezen, J. Kok, T. Abee, & G. Schasfsma (Eds.), *Lactic acid bacteria: Genetics, metabolism and applications* (pp. 29–58). Dordrecht: Springer.

Kleerebezem, M., Boekhorst, J., van Kranenburg, R., Molenaar, D., Kuipers, O. P., Leer, R., et al. (2003). Complete genome sequence of *Lactobacillus plantarum* WCFS1. *Proceedings of the National Academy of Sciences of the United States of America, 100*(4), 1990–1995.

Koponen, J., Laakso, K., Koskenniemi, K., Kankainen, M., Savijoki, K., Nyman, T. A., et al. (2012). Effect of acid stress on protein expression and phosphorylation in *Lactobacillus rhamnosus* GG. *Journal of Proteomics, 75*, 1357–1374.

Koskenniemi, K., Koponen, J., Kankainen, M., Savijoki, K., Tynkkynen, S., de Vos, W. M., et al. (2009). Proteome analysis of *Lactobacillus rhamnosus* GG using 2-D DIGE and mass spectrometry shows differential protein production in laboratory and industrial type growth media. *Journal of Proteome Research, 8*, 4993–5007.

Koskenniemi, K., Laakso, K., Koponen, J., Kankainen, M., Greco, D., Auvinen, P., et al. (2011). Proteomics and transcriptomics characterization of bile stress response in probiotic *Lactobacillus rhamnosus* GG. *Molecular & Cellular Proteomics. 10*, https://doi.org/10.1074/mcp.M110.002741. M110.002741.

Laakso, K., Koskenniemi, K., Koponen, J., Kankainen, M., Surakka, A., Salusjarvi, T., et al. (2011). Growth phase-associated changes in the proteome and transcriptome of *Lactobacillus rhamnosus* GG in industrial-type whey medium. *Microbial Biotechnology, 4*, 746–766.

Lagier, J. C., Khelaifia, S., Alou, M. T., Ndongo, S., Dione, N., Hugon, P., et al. (2016). Culture of previously uncultured members of the human gut microbiota by culturomics. *Nature Microbiology, 1*(12), 1–8.

Lambert, J. M. (2008). *Bile salt hydrolase in* Lactobacillus plantarum*: Functional analysis and delivery to the intestinal tract of the host.* (Dissertation)Wageningen University.(2008). *https://library.wur.nl/WebQuery/wurpubs/365433.*

Lamberti, C., Mangiapane, E., Pessione, A., Mazzoli, R., Giunta, C., & Pessione, E. (2011). Proteomic characterization of a selenium-metabolizing probiotic *Lactobacillus reuteri* Lb2 BM for nutraceutical applications. *Proteomics, 11*, 2212–2221.

Leahy, S. C., Higgins, D. G., Fitzgerald, G. F., & Van Sinderen, D. (2005). Getting better with bifidobacteria. *Journal of Applied Microbiology, 98*(6), 1303–1315.

LeBlanc, J. G., Laiño, J. E., del Valle, M. J., Vannini, V. V., van Sinderen, D., Taranto, M. P., et al. (2011). B-Group vitamin production by lactic acid bacteria–current knowledge and potential applications. *Journal of Applied Microbiology, 111*(6), 1297–1309.

Lee, P. Y., Chin, S. F., Neoh, H. M., & Jamal, R. (2017). Metaproteomic analysis of human gut microbiota: where are we heading? *Journal of Biomedical Science, 24*(1), 36.

Lee, J. H., Karamychev, V. N., Kozyavkin, S. A., Mills, D., Pavlov, A. R., Pavlova, N. V., et al. (2008). Comparative genomic analysis of the gut bacterium *Bifidobacterium longum* reveals loci susceptible to deletion during pure culture growth. *BMC Genomics*, *9*(1), 247.

Leimena, M. M., Wels, M., Bongers, R. S., Smid, E. J., Zoetendal, E. G., & Kleerebezem, M. (2012). Comparative analysis of *Lactobacillus plantarum* WCFS1 transcriptomes by using DNA microarray and next-generation sequencing technologies. *Applied and Environmental Microbiology*, *78*, 4141–4148.

Li, X., LeBlanc, J., Truong, A., Vuthoori, R., Chen, S. S., Lustgarten, J. L., et al. (2011). A metaproteomic approach to study human-microbial ecosystems at the mucosal luminal interface. *PLoS One*, *6*(11).

Li, P., Zhou, Q., & Gu, Q. (2016). Complete genome sequence of *Lactobacillus plantarum* LZ227, a potential probiotic strain producing B-group vitamins. *Journal of Biotechnology*, *234*, 66–70.

Liu, D. W., Wang, S. A., Xu, B., Guo, Y. H., Zhao, J. L., Liu, W., et al. (2011). Proteomics analysis of *Bifidobacterium longum* NCC2705 growing on glucose, fructose, mannose, xylose, ribose, and galactose. *Proteomics*, *11*, 2628–2638.

Makarova, K. S., & Koonin, E. V. (2007) Evolutionary genomics of lactic acid bacteria. *Journal of Bacteriology*, *189*(4), 1199–1208.

Makarova, K., Slesarev, A., Wolf, Y., Sorokin, A., Mirkin, B., Koonin, E., et al. (2006). Comparative genomics of the lactic acid bacteria. *Proceedings of the National Academy of Sciences of the United States of America*, *103*(42), 15611–15616.

Mangiapane, E., Lamberti, C., Galano, E., Pessione, A., Giunta, C., Amoresano, A., et al. (2011). Physiological changes induced by selenium in a probiotic *Lactobacillus reuteri* strain: A proteomic study. *The FEBS Journal*, *278*, S432.

Marco, M. L., de Vires, M. C., Wels, M., Molenaar, D., Mangell, P., Ahrne, S., et al. (2010). Convergence in probiotic *Lactobacillus* gut-adaptive responses in humans and mice. *The ISME Journal*, *4*, 1481–1484.

Marco, M. L., Peters, T. H. F., Bongers, R. S., Molenaar, D., van Hemert, S., Sonnenburg, J. L., et al. (2009). Lifestyle of *Lactobacillus plantarum* in the mouse cecum. *Environmental Microbiology*, *11*, 2747–2757.

McNulty, N. P., Yatsunenko, T., Hsiao, A., Faith, J. J., Muegge, B. D., Goodman, A. L., et al. (2011). The impact of a consortium of fermented milk strains on the gut microbiome of gnotobiotic mice and monozygotic twins. *Science Translational Medicine*, *3*, 106ra106.

Million, M., Lagier, J. C., Yahav, D., & Paul, M. (2013). Gut bacterial microbiota and obesity. *Clinical Microbiology and Infection*, *19*(4), 305–313.

Morita, H., Toh, H., Fukuda, S., Horikawa, H., Oshima, K., Suzuki, T., et al. (2008). Comparative genome analysis of *Lactobacillus reuteri* and *Lactobacillus fermentum* reveal a genomic island for reuterin and cobalamin production. *DNA Research*, *15*(3), 151–161.

Morita, H., Toh, H., Oshima, K., Murakami, M., Taylor, T. D., Igimi, S., et al. (2009). Complete genome sequence of probiotic *Lactobacillus rhamnosus* ATCC 53103. *Journal of Bacteriology*, *191*(24), 7630–7631.

O'Connell-Motherway, M., Zomer, A., Leahy, S. C., Reunanen, J., Bottacini, F., Claesson, M. J., et al. (2011). Functional genome analysis of *Bifidobacterium breve* UCC2003 reveals type IVb tight adherence (tad) pili as an essential and conserved host colonization factor. *Proceedings of the National Academy of Sciences of the United States of America*, *108*, 11217–11222.

Ong, L., Henriksson, A., & Shah, N. P. (2007). Proteolytic pattern and organic acid profiles of probiotic Cheddar cheese as influenced by probiotic strains of *Lactobacillus acidophilus*, *Lb. paracasei*, *Lb. casei* or *Bifidobacterium* sp. *International Dairy Journal*, *17*(1), 67–78.

Petriz, B. A., & Franco, O. L. (2017). Metaproteomics as a complementary approach to gut microbiota in health and disease. *Frontiers in Chemistry*, *5*, 4.

Pridmore, R. D., Berger, B., Desiere, F., Vilanova, D., Barretto, C., Pittet, A. C., et al. (2004). The genome sequence of the probiotic intestinal bacterium *Lactobacillus johnsonii* NCC 533.

Proceedings of the National Academy of Sciences of the United States of America, 101(8), 2512–2517.

Ramachandran, P., Lacher, D. W., Pfeiler, E. A., & Elkins, C. A. (2013). Development of a tiered multilocus sequence typing scheme for members of the *Lactobacillus acidophilus* complex. *Applied and Environmental Microbiology, 79*(23), 7220–7228.

Ramirez-Farias, C., Slezak, K., Fuller, Z., Duncan, A., Holtrop, G., & Louis, P. (2008). Effect of inulin on the human gut microbiota: stimulation of *Bifidobacterium adolescentis* and *Faecalibacterium prausnitzii*. *British Journal of Nutrition, 101*(4), 541–550.

Ruiz, L., Álvarez-Martín, P., Mayo, B., de los Reyes-Gavilán, C. G., Gueimonde, M., & Margolles, A. (2012). Controlled gene expression in bifidobacteria by use of a bile-responsive element. *Applied and Environmental Microbiology, 6*, 307–318.

Ruiz, L., Coute, Y., Sánchez, B., de los Reyes-Gavilán, C. G., Sanchez, J. C., & Margolles, A. (2009). The cell-envelope proteome of *Bifidobacterium longum* in an in vitro bile environment. *Microbiology, 155*, 957–967.

Ruiz, L., O'Connell-Motherway, M., Zomer, A., de los Reyes-Gavilán, C. G., Margolles, A., & van Sinderen, D. (2012). A bile-inducible membrane protein mediates bifidobacteria bile resistance. *Microbial Biotechnology, 5*, 523–535.

Ruiz, L., Sánchez, B., de los Reyes-Gavilán, C. G., Gueimonde, M., & Margolles, A. (2009). Coculture of *Bifidobacterium longum* and *Bifidobacterium breve* alters their protein expression profiles and enzymatic activities. *International Journal of Food Microbiology, 133*, 148–153.

Ruiz, L., Zomer, A., O'Connell-Motherway, M., van Sinderen, D., & Margolles, A. (2012). Discovering novel bile protection systems in *Bifidobacterium breve* UCC2003 through functional genomics. *Applied and Environmental Microbiology, 78*, 1123–1131.

Sanchez, B., Champomier-Verges, M. C., Collado, M. D., Anglade, P., Baraige, F., Sanz, Y., et al. (2007). Low-pH adaptation and the acid tolerance response of *Bifidobactetium longum* biotype longum. *Applied and Environmental Microbiology, 73*, 6450–6459.

Sánchez, B., Ruiz, L., de los Reyes-Gavilán, C. G., & Margolles, A. (2008). Proteomics of stress response in *Bifidobacterium*. *Frontiers in Bioscience, 13*, 6905–6919.

Schell, M. A., Karmirantzou, M., Snel, B., Vilanova, D., Berger, B., Pessi, G., et al. (2002). The genome sequence of *Bifidobacterium longum* reflects its adaptation to the human gastrointestinal tract. *Proceedings of the National Academy of Sciences of the United States of America, 99* (22), 14422–14427.

Sela, D. A., Chapman, J., Adeuya, A., Kim, J. H., Chen, F., Whitehead, T. R., et al. (2008). The genome sequence of *Bifidobacterium longum subsp. infantis* reveals adaptations for milk utilization within the infant microbiome. *Proceedings of the National Academy of Sciences of the United States of America, 105*, 18964–18969.

Sidhu, J. S., & Alkandari, D. (2020). Overview of probiotics in cancer prevention and therapy. In *Functional foods in cancer prevention and therapy* (pp. 261–282). Academic Press.

Siezen, R., Boekhorst, J., Muscariello, L., Molenaar, D., Renckens, B., & Kleerebezem, M. (2006). *Lactobacillus plantarum* gene clusters encoding putative cell-surface protein complexes for carbohydrate utilization are conserved in specific gram-positive bacteria. *BMC Genomics, 7*, 126. https://doi.org/10.1186/1471-2164-7-126.

Siezen, R. J., Tzeneva, V. A., Castioni, A., Wels, M., Phan, H. T., Rademaker, J. L., et al. (2010). Phenotypic and genomic diversity of *Lactobacillus plantarum* strains isolated from various environmental niches. *Environmental Microbiology, 12*(3), 758–773.

Smokvina, T., Wels, M., Polka, J., Chervaux, C., Brisse, S., Boekhorst, J., et al. (2013). *Lactobacillus paracasei* comparative genomics: towards species pan-genome definition and exploitation of diversity. *PLoS One, 8*(7)e68731.

Stahl, B., & Barrangou, R. (2013). Complete genome sequence of probiotic strain *Lactobacillus acidophilus* La-14. *Genome Announcements, 1*(3). e00376-13.

Strahinic, I., Lozo, J., Terzic-Vidojevic, A., Fira, D., Kojic, M., Golic, N., et al. (2013). Technological and probiotic potential of BGRA43 a natural isolate *of Lactobacillus helveticus*. *Frontiers in Microbiology*, *4*, 2. https://doi.org/10.3389/fmicb.2013.00002.

Suez, J., Zmora, N., & Elinav, E. (2020). Probiotics in the next-generation sequencing era. *Gut Microbes*, *11*(1), 77–93.

Sun, Z., Harris, H. M., McCann, A., Guo, C., Argimón, S., Zhang, W., et al. (2015). Expanding the biotechnology potential of lactobacilli through comparative genomics of 213 strains and associated genera. *Nature Communications*, *6*(1), 1–13.

Tannock, G. W. (1998). Studies of the intestinal microflora: a prerequisite for the development of probiotics. *International Dairy Journal*, *8*(5-6), 527–533.

Tao, L., Wang, B., Zhong, Y., Pow, S. H., Zeng, X., Qin, C., et al. (2017). Database and bioinformatics studies of probiotics. *Journal of Agricultural and Food Chemistry*, *65*(35), 7599–7606.

Taverniti, V., & Guglielmetti, S. (2012) Health-promoting properties of *Lactobacillus helveticus*. *Frontiers in Microbiology*, *3*, 392. https://doi.org/10.3389/fmicb.2012.00392.

Tissier, H. (1900). *Recherchers sur la flora intestinale normale et pathologique du nourisson*. Paris, France: University of Paris.

Troost, F. J., van Baarlen, P., Lindsey, P., Kodde, A., de Vos, W. M., Kleerebezem, M., et al. (2008). Identification of the transcriptional response of human intestinal mucosa to *Lactobacillus plantarum* WCFS1 in vivo. *BMC Genomics*, *9*, 374. https://doi.org/10.1186/1471-2164-9-374.

Turroni, F., Foroni, E., Serafini, F., Viappiani, A., Montanini, B., Bottacini, F., et al. (2011). Ability of *Bifidobacterium breve* to grow on different types of milk: Exploring the metabolism of milk through genome analysis. *Applied and Environmental Microbiology*, *77*, 7408–7417.

Uchiyama, I., Mihara, M., Nishide, H., & Chiba, H. (2015). MBGD update 2015: microbial genome database for flexible ortholog analysis utilizing a diverse set of genomic data. *Nucleic Acids Research*, *43*(D1), D270–D276.

Van Baarlen, P., Troost, F., van der Meer, C., Hooiveld, G., Boekschoten, M., Brummer, R. J. M., et al. (2011). Human mucosal in vivo transcriptome responses to three lactobacilli indicate how probiotics may modulate human cellular pathways. *Proceedings of the National Academy of Sciences of the United States of America*, *108*, 4562–4569.

Van de Guchte, M., Penaud, S., Grimaldi, C., Barbe, V., Bryson, K., Nicolas, P., et al. (2006). The complete genome sequence of *Lactobacillus bulgaricus* reveals extensive and ongoing reductive evolution. *Proceedings of the National Academy of Sciences of the United States of America*, *103*(24), 9274–9279.

Ventura, M., Canchaya, C., Tauch, A., Chandra, G., Fitzgerald, G. F., Chater, K. F., et al. (2007). Genomics of Actinobacteria: Tracing the evolutionary history of an ancient phylum. *Microbiology and Molecular Biology Reviews*, *71*(3), 495–548.

Ventura, M., O'Flaherty, S., Claesson, M. J., Turroni, F., Klaenhammer, T. R., van Sinderen, D., et al. (2009). Genome-scale analysis of health-promoting bacteria: Probiogenomics. *Nature Reviews Microbiology*, *7*, 61–71.

Vitali, B., Turroni, S., Dal Piaz, F., Candela, M., Wasinger, V., & Brigidi, P. (2007). Genetic and proteomic characterization of rifaximin resistance in *Bifidobacterium infantis* BI07. *Research in Microbiology*, *158*, 355–362.

Vitali, B., Wasinger, V., Brigidi, P., & Guilhaus, M. (2005). A proteomic view of *Bifidobacterium infantis* generated by multi-dimensional chromatography coupled with tandem mass spectrometry. *Proteomics*, *5*, 1859–1867.

Wegkamp, A., Mars, A. E., Faijes, M., Molenaar, D., de Vos, R. C., Klaus, S. M., et al. (2010). Physiological responses to folate overproduction in *Lactobacillus plantarum* WCFS1. *Microbial Cell Factories*, *9*(1), 100. https://doi.org/10.1186/1475-2859-9-100.

Wegmann, U., Overweg, K., Horn, N., Goesmann, A., Narbad, A., Gasson, M. J., et al. (2009). The complete genome sequence of *Lactobacillus johnsonii* FI9785, a competitive exclusion agent against pathogens in poultry. *Journal of Bacteriology*, *191*, 7142–7143.

Whitehead, K., Versalovic, J., Roos, S., & Britton, R. A. (2008). Genomic and genetic characterization of the bile stress response of probiotic *Lactobacillus reuteri* ATCC 55730. *Applied and Environmental Microbiology, 74*, 1812–1819.

Wu, C. D., Zhang, J., Chen, W., Wang, M., Du, G. C., & Chen, J. (2012). A combined physiological and proteomic approach to reveal lactic-acid-induced alterations in *Lactobacillus casei* Zhang and its mutant with enhanced lactic acid tolerance. *Applied Microbiology and Biotechnology, 93*, 707–722.

Xiao, M., Xu, P., Zhao, J. Y., Wang, Z., Zuo, F. L., Zhang, J. W., et al. (2011). Oxidative stress-related responses of *Bifidobacterium longum* subsp. longum BBMN68 at the proteomic level after exposure to oxygen. *Microbiology, 157*, 1573–1588.

Yadav, R., Kumar, V., Baweja, M., & Shukla, P. (2018). Gene editing and genetic engineering approaches for advanced probiotics: A review. *Critical Reviews in Food Science and Nutrition, 58*(10), 1735–1746.

Yuan, J., Wang, B., Sun, Z. K., Bo, X., Yuan, X., He, X., et al. (2008). Analysis of host inducing proteome changes in *Bifidobacterium longum* NCC2705 grown in vivo. *Journal of Proteome Research, 7*, 375–385.

Zeevi, D., Korem, T., Godneva, A., Bar, N., Kurilshikov, A., Lotan-Pompan, M., et al. (2019). Structural variation in the gut microbiome associates with host health. *Nature, 568*(7750), 43–48.

Zhang, Z. Y., Liu, C., Zhu, Y. Z., Zhong, Y., Zhu, Y. Q., Zheng, H. J., et al. (2009). Complete genome sequence of *Lactobacillus plantarum* JDM1. *Journal of Bacteriology, 191*(15), 5020–5021.

Zhao, W., Liu, Y., Latta, M., Ma, W., Wu, Z., & Chen, P. (2019). Probiotics database: a potential source of fermented foods. *International Journal of Food Properties, 22*(1), 198–217.

PART IV

Production and quality

CHAPTER

13

Starter cultures for probiotic beverages: A comparative study of traditional and modern approaches

Nasim Khorshidian[a], Mojtaba Yousefi[a], Neda Mollakhalili Meybodi[b], and Amir M. Mortazavian[c]

[a]Food Safety Research Center (Salt), Semnan University of Medical Sciences, Semnan, Iran; [b]Department of Food Sciences and Technology, School of Public Health, Shahid Sadoughi University of Medical Sciences, Yazd, Iran; [c]Department of Food Science and Technology, National Nutrition and Food Technology Research Institute, Faculty of Nutrition Sciences, Food Science and Technology, Shahid Beheshti University of Medical Sciences, Tehran, Iran

13.1 Introduction

Fermentation is an old process of food preservation that has some additional advantages, including the improvement of nutritional status and sensory characteristics of food products, as well as the reduction of toxic and antinutritional factors (Ashaolu, 2019; Chilton, Burton, & Reid, 2015). There are many beneficial effects associated with the consumption of fermented food products including lowering blood cholesterol, prevention of diabetes, obesity, osteoporosis, cancers, allergies, and improvement of the immune system (Şanlier, Gökcen, & Sezgin, 2019).

In many traditional fermented foods and beverages, fermentation would be initiated spontaneously due to the presence of suitable microflora within the food matrix. However, nowadays, most food fermentations are

Probiotic Beverages
https://doi.org/10.1016/B978-0-12-818588-9.00018-8

performed on a large scale and through inoculation of desired and well-adapted microorganisms named as starter cultures (Vinicius De Melo Pereira et al., 2019). The main microorganisms involved in the fermentation of these matrices include lactic acid bacteria (LAB), yeasts, and molds that conduct alcoholic, lactic, and malolactic fermentation and generate diverse principal and secondary metabolites (Ashaolu, 2019).

Among fermented food products, fermented dairy and nondairy beverages comprise a major part of the human diet (Kandylis, Pissaridi, Bekatorou, Kanellaki, & Koutinas, 2016). Furthermore, increased attention has been paid to developing various functional beverages due to easier distribution and storage, to providing various sizes, shapes, and appearance, as well as ease of use and enhanced delivering sources for various functional ingredients, such as probiotics (Corbo, Bevilacqua, Petruzzi, Casanova, & Sinigaglia, 2014). Many LAB and yeast species exert probiotic activity and there are numerous studies reporting on the isolation of probiotic microorganisms from traditional fermented foods and beverages (Kandasamy, Kavitake, & Shetty, 2018, Yousefi Asli, Khorshidian, Mohammad Mortazavian, & Hosseini, 2017). Probiotic LABs and yeasts are extensively incorporated into dairy and nondairy beverages due to their health-promoting properties (Khorshidian, Yousefi Asli, Hosseini, Shadnoush, & Mortazavian, 2016) as well as being utilized as starter cultures (Gupta & Abu-Ghannam, 2012; Mohammadi et al., 2017). The ability of probiotics to use the various substrates is strain-specific and this should be considered in the formulation of probiotic fermented beverages (Sridharan & Das, 2019). In recent years, there has been an increasing tendency toward the development of new starter cultures through the isolation of naturally occurring strains and the improvement of some strains by biotechnological techniques to achieve the desired favorable characteristics (Johansen, 2018).

13.2 Starter cultures

Fermentation is initiated in three main ways. The oldest method for the production of fermented foods used the indigenous inhabitant microorganisms in the raw material. In this case, the presence of the correct microorganisms and suitable conditions for their growth are essential factors for a successful fermentation (Shrivastava & Ananthanarayan, 2015). Despite providing these conditions, there is no guarantee that a fermented product with the desired quality characteristics will be produced. Another method is "back-slopping," which involves inoculation of the raw material with a previously-fermented substrate. This helps decrease fermentation time and is more predictable (Johansen, 2018). However, because of the high microbial load in back-slopping and the difficulty in inoculating a reproducible number of cells, this strategy has been gradually replaced by the use of starter cultures (Vinicius De Melo Pereira et al., 2019).

Starter cultures have an important role in fermented food production as final product characteristics such as sensorial and safety properties are affected by the starter cultures. They generally consist of bacteria, yeasts, molds, and their combination among which, lactic acid bacteria (LAB) and yeasts are the most extensively used microorganisms. It has been reported that at least 195 species of bacteria and 69 species of yeasts and molds are used in food fermentation (Kandasamy et al., 2018).

Based on the incubation and manufacturing temperatures under which starter cultures are used, they are classified as mesophilic or thermophilic. Mesophilic cultures grow and produce lactic acid at moderate temperatures (about 30°C), with thermophilic cultures operating at higher temperatures (about 42°C) (Altieri, Ciuffreda, Di Maggio, & Sinigaglia, 2017). However, the most common way to classify starter cultures is based on the complexity of the culture and the way it reproduces. Mostly, starter cultures are derived from natural starters that contain an undefined mixture of different strains and/or species. Sometimes, commercial mixed-strain starters (MSS), which are obtained from the best natural starters, are reproduced under controlled conditions for the specific type of products. Natural starter cultures and commercial MSS, due to their long history, are called traditional starters. On the other hand, defined strain starters (DSS) generally consist of only a small number of selected strains, providing more control on the composition and properties of the cultures (Altieri et al., 2017; Parente & Cogan, 2004). Traditional cultures can be composed of many strains of various bacterial species; sometimes yeasts and molds are also involved in the development of various properties of the final products (Broome, Powell, & Limsowtin, 2002). Traditional starter cultures have been utilized for particular or traditional products and their industrial usage is limited. Fig. 13.1 illustrates starter culture types and their characteristics.

According to Corbo, Racioppo, Monacis, and Speranza (2017), the main reason manufacturers use commercial starters is fear of product failure, but it should be noted that the use of commercial starters hinders the possibility of developing unique products. To prevent the production of products with flattening sensory properties and lacking typical desired characteristics, the use of "typical" microbial starters isolated from fermented foods that are the most adapted to the particular intrinsic ecology of the food matrix and exhibit desirable technological and hygienic properties has been suggested (Corbo et al., 2017). However, due to the use of defined strains and/or species ratio in defined strain starters and their high reproducible performance and high phage resistance, defined strain starters have now mostly replaced the traditional starters for industrial-scale production (Carminati et al., 2010).

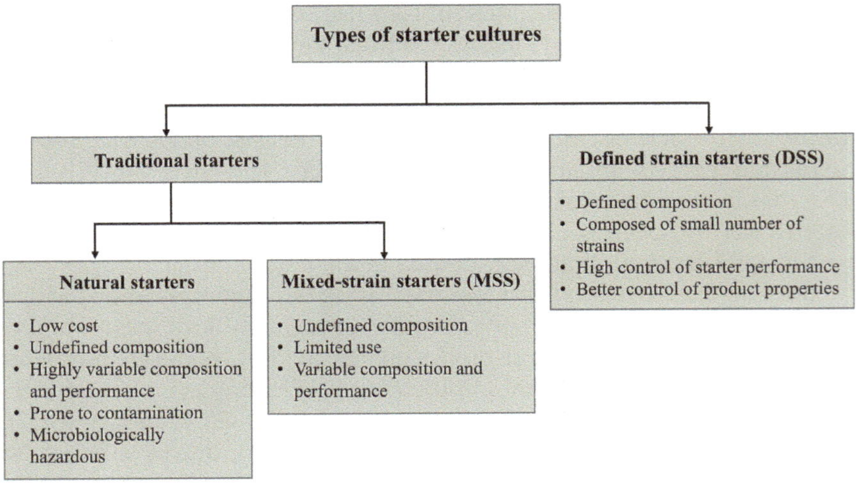

FIG. 13.1 Different types of starter cultures and their characteristics.

13.2.1 Selection criteria for starter cultures

It is crucial to consider some important criteria in the selection of starter cultures for fermented foods and beverages since the final quality characteristics of the product are modulated by the metabolic activity of the strains. It has been emphasized by the Food and Drug Administration (FDA) and the European Food Safety Authority (EFSA) that microbial species intended for use in fermented food products should belong to the group known as "generally recognized as safe" (GRAS) and with specified taxonomy (Ashaolu, 2019). Starter cultures should be capable of utilizing a wide spectrum of substrates, grow rapidly, as well as be resistant to stress conditions during fermentation such as osmotic stress, accumulation of organic acids and alcohol, increases in temperature, and decreases in pH (Parsons & Rock, 2013).

Sensory acceptability is of paramount importance in the development of fermented foods and beverages (Granato, Branco, Cruz, Faria, & Shah, 2010). Starter cultures using organic substrates can generate several metabolites such as organic acids, esters, and carbonyl compounds, which induce flavor and aroma in fermented products. Thus, the employment of suitable microbial strains, without a negative effect on sensory characteristics, should be considered (Peyer, Zannini, & Arendt, 2016). Fermented food products are easily contaminated with fungi, which can impose technological and health implications. It has been reported that some strains of *Lactobacillus*, *Leuconostoc*, and *Pediococcus* possess antifungal activities through the production of various metabolites (organic acids, hydrogen peroxide, carbon dioxide, diacetyl, and bacteriocins) and can be used as

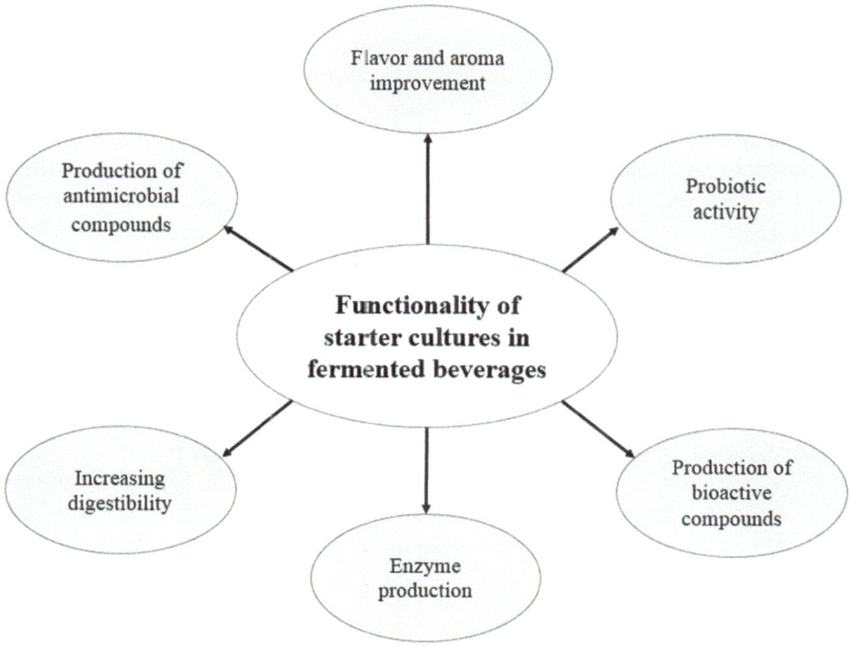

FIG. 13.2 The functionality of starter cultures in fermented beverages.

bioprotective cultures in some fermented food products (Ben Said, Gaudreau, Dallaire, Tessier, & Fliss, 2019; Sadiq et al., 2019).

It has been expressed that some microbial strains, especially LABs and yeasts, can promote the nutritional and health quality of fermented food products via the production of vitamins (folate, riboflavin, vitamin K), conjugated linolenic (CLNA) and linoleic acid (CLA), antihypertensive peptides, carotenoids, phenolic compounds, phytase, and proteases (Melini, Melini, Luziatelli, Ficca, & Ruzzi, 2019). Incorporation of these strains into fermented food products can be a promising tool for the development of foods with healthful effects and higher acceptance by consumers. The functionality of starter cultures in fermented beverages is illustrated in Fig. 13.2.

13.3 Bacteria as starter cultures in probiotic beverages

The most widely used bacteria as starter cultures in beverages are lactic acid bacteria. They are a large group of bacteria belonging to the genera *Bifidobacterium*, *Enterococcus*, *Lactobacillus*, *Leuconostoc*, *Lactococcus*, *Propionibacterium*, *Pediococcus*, *Streptccoccus*, *Tetragenococcus*, *Vagococcus*, and

Weissella (Kavitake, Kandasamy, Devi, & Shetty, 2018). They are gram-positive, noncore forming, rod- or cocci-shaped bacteria that metabolize sugars and generate lactic acid (Bintsis, 2018). LABs exert various functionalities in fermented foods including contributions to flavor and texture via metabolic pathways, production of bioactive compounds, and the bio-preservation of foods (Wedajo, 2015). There are numerous indigenous fermented beverages produced in different parts of the world where LAB play a significant role in fermentation and product development. Some LAB and yeast cultures present probiotic activity and have been commercialized as starter cultures in global markets including, *Lactobacillus acidophilus* NCFM, *Lactobacillus rhamnosus* HN001 (DR20), and *Bifidobacterium lactis* HN019 (DR10) (Danisco, USA), *Lactobacillus casei* strain Shirota and *Bifidobacterium breve* strain (Yakult, Japan), *Lactobacillus fermentum* VRI003 (PCC) (Probiomics, Australia), *L. rhamnosus* R0011 (Institut Rosell, Canada), *Streptococcus oralis* KJ3 (Oragenics, Inc., USA), and *Saccharomyces cerevisiae* and *boulardii*) (Biocodex USA) (Tamang, Shin, Jung, & Chae, 2016). Table 13.1 represents some selected publications regarding cereal, fruit, and vegetable–based probiotic beverages.

TABLE 13.1 Selected publications on probiotic cereal, fruit and vegetable–based beverages.

Beverage type	Probiotic strain	Remark	Reference
Cereal-based			
Maize	*L. paracasei* BGP1, *L. casei* BGP93, *L. rhamnosus* LRB, *L. acidophilus* PRO	Beverages fermented by L. *acidophilus* or *L. rhamnosus* were well accepted by trained and untrained panels and suitable for commercial production of probiotic maize-based beverages	Nyanzi, Jooste, Abu, and Beukes (2010)
Beverages containing malt, barley and their mixtures	*L. plantarum* and *L. acidophilus*	The growth of probiotic bacteria increased in the presence of malt and significant amounts of lactic acid were produced The bacterial cell counts were above probiotic levels	Rathore, Salmerón, and Pandiella (2012)

TABLE 13.1 Selected publications on probiotic cereal, fruit and vegetable–based beverages—cont'd

Beverage type	Probiotic strain	Remark	Reference
Oat flour and barley malt	*L. acidophilus* NCIMB 8821, *L. plantarum* NCIMB 8826 *L. reuteri* NCIMB 11951	The cell viability was 10^8 cfu/mL and pH values were in the range of 3.3 to 3.7 The beverage containing *L. plantarum* and malt obtained the highest acceptability and level of acetaldehyde	Salmerón, Thomas, and Pandiella (2015)
Sprouted wheat, barley, pearl millet, and green gram (mung bean) along with oatmeal and soymilk	*L. acidophilus* NCDC14	Acidity and pH in different probiotic drink samples were in the acidity range of 0.45 to 1.02% and pH 4.11 to 4.49, respectively with higher in green gram-based drinks Regarding good sensory acceptability scores (>7) and probiotic counts, wheat, barley and green gram at 6 g, while pearl millet at a 4 g level with 50:50 mL of soymilk and distilled water can be considered suitable for the development of probiotic drinks	Mridula and Sharma (2015)
Rice	*L plantarum* L7	The highest concentrations of lactic acid (4.95 mg/g), acetic acid (0.36 mg/g), and succinic acid (0.37 mg/g) were obtained on the 4th, 5th, and 3rd days of fermentation, respectively. The cell population was 8.32 log cfu/mL at the end of fermentation	Giri, Sen, Saha, Sukumaran, and Park (2018)

Continued

TABLE 13.1 Selected publications on probiotic cereal, fruit and vegetable–based beverages—cont'd

Beverage type	Probiotic strain	Remark	Reference
Fruit and vegetable–based			
Litchi juice	*L. casei*	A beverage with good overall acceptance was produced. Total phenolics and antioxidant capacity were retained. Viability of bacteria after 4 weeks of storage was 8 log cfu/mL	Zheng et al. (2014)
Peach juice	*L. plantarum* DSMZ 20179, *L. delbrueckii* DSMZ 15996, *L. casei* DSMZ 20011	*L. delbrueckii* grew well in peach juice, reached nearly 10×10^9 cfu/mL, after 48 h of fermentation and was capable of sugar consumption, pH decreases and production of lactic acid during fermentation After four weeks of cold storage at 4 °C, the viable cell counts of L. *delbrueckii* were 1.72×10^7 cfu/mL in fermented peach juice	Pakbin, Razavi, Mahmoudi, and Gajarbeygi (2014)
Cashew apple juice	*L. casei* NRRL B-442	The optimum conditions for probiotic cashew apple juice production were an initial pH 6.4, fermentation temperature of 30°C, inoculation level of 7.48 Log cfu/mL (*L. casei*) and a 16 h fermentation process Viable cell counts were higher than 8 Log cfu/mL throughout the storage period (42 days)	Pereira, Maciel, and Rodrigues (2011)

TABLE 13.1 Selected publications on probiotic cereal, fruit and vegetable–based beverages—cont'd

Beverage type	Probiotic strain	Remark	Reference
Coconut water	*L. plantarum*	This beverage contained the desired cell population of *L. plantarum*. The addition of sucrose and artificial coconut flavor to the fermented beverage led to greater acceptability of the product	Prado et al. (2015)
Pomegranate juice	*L. bulgaricus* and L. *plantarum*	Inoculation of juice with 10% bacteria and a fermentation of 7h resulted in a beverage containing 10^9 cfu/mL probiotic bacteria	Thakur and Sharma (2017)
Pomegranate juice	*L. plantarum* (NRRLB-227), *L. casei* (NRRL B-1922) *L. bulgaricus* (CFFCB0043) and L. *salivarius* (NRRL B-1949)	*L. casei* had a better growth profile and higher biomass density at 37°C at pH around 3.5–4	Mustafa et al. (2019)
Tomato juice	*L. acidophilus* LA39, *L. plantarum* C3, *L. casei* A4 *L. delbrueckii* D7	The survival of the four lactobacillus strains in fermented tomato juice with low pH varied between 10^6 and 10^8 cfu mL^{-1}, with the highest viability shown by *L. acidophilus* and *L. delbrueckii* during 30 days storage at 4°C	Yoon, Woodams, and Hang (2004)
Cabbage juice	*L. plantarum* C3 *L. casei* A4 *L. delbrueckii* D7	Bacteria grew well on cabbage juice and reached about 10^9 cfu/mL after 48h of fermentation. After 4 weeks of cold storage, the viable cell counts of L. *plantarum* and	Yoon, Woodams, and Hang (2006)

Continued

TABLE 13.1 Selected publications on probiotic cereal, fruit and vegetable–based beverages—cont'd

Beverage type	Probiotic strain	Remark	Reference
		L. delbrueckii were 4.1×10^7 and 4.5×10^5 cfu/mL, respectively. *L. casei* did not survive at the low pH and lost cell viability completely after 2 weeks of the cold storage	
Beet juice	*L. plantarum* *L. acidophilus* *L. casei* *L. delbrueckii*	*L. acidophilus* and *L. plantarum* showed the ability to reduce pH from 6.3 to 4.5 after 2 h of fermentation at 30°C. *L. acidophilus* had less stability during storage compared to *L. plantarum*, *L. casei*, and *L. delbrueckii*, which showed viabilities ranging between 10^6 cfu/mL and 10^8 cfu/mL during 4 weeks of storage at 4°C	Yoon, Woodams, and Hang (2005)

Depending on the metabolic pathway employed, the LAB can be classified into two groups: homo-fermentative LAB use the Embden-Meyerhof pathway, ferment hexoses via glycolysis, and generate lactic acid as the main product; hetero-fermentative LAB use the pentose phosphate or the phosphoketolase pathway for hexose fermentation and produce carbon dioxide and ethanol, in addition to lactic acid (Prückler et al., 2015). Malolactic fermentation is a secondary fermentation performed by LAB in wine, where L-malic acid is converted to L-lactic acid and CO_2, leading to acidity reduction in wines and ciders (Liu, 2002). Other compounds, which are secondary metabolites, such as higher alcohols, polyols, esters, organic acids, ketones, short-chain fatty acids, and aldehydes, are produced at various levels.

LABs are potential sources of diverse enzymes that are excreted into the food matrix or that can be extracted and employed during fermentation. LAB strains with amylolytic enzymes can convert starch into lactic acid. They can be utilized in cereal-based fermented beverages (Blandino, Al-Aseeri, Pandiella, Cantero, & Webb, 2003). LABs with proteolytic activity can excrete bioactive peptides during the production of fermented milk-based beverages (Elfahri, Vasiljevic, Yeager, & Donkor, 2016). LAB glycosidases and esterases can contribute to the development of aroma precursors and fruity aroma and flavor compounds (Bergsveinson, Kajala, & Ziola, 2017). The enzymes in LAB responsible for the production of multiple metabolites in fermented beverages are summarized in Table 13.2.

TABLE 13.2 Enzymes in LAB and yeast species used as starter cultures in fermented beverages.

Enzyme	LAB species	Fermented Beverage	Reference
Malolactic	*L. plantarum* PCS 26	Apple juice	Dimitrovski, Velickova, Langerholc, and Winkelhausen (2015)
		Jerusalem artichoke juice	Dimitrovski, Velickova, Dimitrovska, Langerholc, and Winkelhausen (2016)
	L. plantarum (DSM 16365, DSM 20174, DSM 10492, DSM 100813) and *Oenococcus oeni*	Black chokeberry and sea buckthorn juices	Markkinen, Laaksonen, Nahku, Kuldjärv, and Yang (2019)
Proteolytic and peptidolytic	*L. casei* strains	Fermented milk	Li et al. (2017)
	L. helveticus strains	Fermented milk	Elfahri et al. (2016)
	K. marxianus YMP45 and *S. cerevisiae* YAM14	Chhurpi	Rai, Kumari, Sanjukta, and Sahoo (2016)
	K. marxianus	Fermented milk	Li, Sadiq, Liu, Chen, and He (2015)
Glycosidase	*L. acidophilus* DSMZ 20079 and *L. plantarum* DSMZ 20174	Pomegranate juice	Mousavi et al. (2013)
Polysaccharide-degrading	*L. plantarum* (NCIMB 8826) and *L. acidophilus* (NCIMB 8821)	Barley-malt	Rathore et al. (2012)
Esterase	*L. acidophilus* F-46	Fermented dandelion (*Taraxacum officinale*) beverage	Kim and Baik (2015)

13.4 Yeasts as starter cultures in beverages

Yeasts are eukaryotic microorganisms frequently found in fermented foods and beverages (Rai, Pandey, & Sahoo, 2018). They are involved in alcohol production, generation and utilization of organic acids, improvement of flavor, aroma, and texture, increase of nutritive value by the production of vitamins and bioactive peptides, and reduction of antinutritional factors and toxins (Chaves-López et al., 2014; Rai, Sanjukta, & Jeyaram, 2017). They play an important role in food fermentation through the production of enzymes (e.g., amylase, cellulase, β-glucosidase, invertase, lipase, pectinase, protease, phytase) that favor various biochemical processes. Yeasts are a rich source of β-glucosidase, which converts bound polyphenols to their free form and increases their bioavailability in fermented foods and beverages (Gaensly, Agustini, Da Silva, Picheth, & Bonfim, 2015) (Table 13.2). They participate in the fermentation of various beverages such as amasi, kefir, kumis, boza, kvass, salgam, togwa, kombucha, and many others (Baschali, Tsakalidou, Kyriacou, Karavasiloglou, & Matalas, 2017).

The most frequently used yeast in food and beverage fermentation is *Saccharomyces cerevisiae*. It is the main yeast involved in the production of alcoholic beverages such as wine and beer. It also produces carbonyl compounds, esters, sulfur lactones, and organic acids during fermentation and these secondary metabolites affect flavor (Jayaram et al., 2013). *S. cerevisiae* transforms fermentable sugars (glucose, sucrose, fructose, and maltose) to pyruvate through glycolysis, which is decarboxylated into acetaldehyde and then converted to ethanol (Walker & Stewart, 2016).

It has been reported that some yeast species have probiotic properties including *S. cerevisiae, Kluyveromyces marxianus, Kluyveromyces lactis, Debaromyces hansenii, Saccharomyces boulardii, Torulaspora delbrueckii, Candida krusei, Yarrowia lipolytica, Pichia fermentans,* and *Pichia kudriavzevii* (Rai et al., 2018).

Yeasts can cooperate with other microorganisms in the production of fermented foods and beverages. They can decrease the growth of unfavorable microorganisms by producing inhibitory compounds and they can also produce vitamins, amino acids, and free sugars that lead to the enhancement of LAB growth, while the LAB can reduce the pH of a medium and provide a suitable environment for yeast growth (Aidoo, Rob Nout, & Sarkar, 2006; Chen, Aorigele, Wang, Simujide, & Yang, 2015).

13.5 Coculture/mixed culture application in probiotic beverages

A mixed culture is defined as the combination of two or more microorganisms that belong to the same group or from different microbial groups (e.g., bacteria and yeast, bacteria and fungi, fungi and yeast, and other combinations) (Hesseltine, 1991). Although using single-strain cultures is common in the production of some products, for other products the utilization of mixed cultures has multiple advantages including higher yield, better sensory characteristics, and the bulk production of favorable metabolites. With the mixed culture, there is a metabolic activity, the exchange of the generated metabolites and signals, prevention or augmentation of the growth of other microorganisms, and better utilization of substrates within the matrix cab occur (Adebo et al., 2018). In the case of probiotic cultures, it can take a long time to reach the desired low pH values in a fermentation, which is not acceptable from an industrial viewpoint due to the decrease in output and the increased chance of microbial contamination. This problem can be addressed through the application of mixed cultures (Do Amaral Santos, Da Silva Libeck, & Schwan, 2014).

Application of the co-culture of yeast and LAB has been reported for the production of some functional milk products enriched in antihypertensive peptides (Rai et al., 2017). Yeasts have also been utilized for the viability enhancement of probiotic LAB (Liu & Tsao, 2009). Some examples of mixed culture applications in fermented beverages are summarized in Table 13.3.

TABLE 13.3 Selected studies on the application of mixed cultures in fermented beverages.

Beverage	Mixed culture	Remarks	Reference
Soy beverage	*S. thermophilus* and *L. helveticus*	The ability of L. *helveticus* to bio-convert isoflavones decreased	Champagne, Tompkins, Buckley, and Green-Johnson (2010)
Goat beverage	*L. lactis* and *L. lactis* subsp. *Cremoris* along with *Saccharomyces fragilis*	The mixed culture used shortened fermentation time in addition to the production of a high quality goat beverage	Agata and Jan (2012)
Apricot juice	Lactobacillus and bifidobacterium strains	Higher cell yield, antioxidant activity and acetic acid levels were reported	Bujna, Farkas, Tran, Sao Dam, and Nguyen (2018)
Durian juice	*Williopsis saturnus* and *L. casei*	The yeast increased probiotic viability and improved the aroma profile by producing volatile compounds	Lu, Putra, and Liu (2018)

Continued

TABLE 13.3 Selected studies on the application of mixed cultures in fermented beverages.—cont'd

Beverage	Mixed culture	Remarks	Reference
Beer	*L. paracasei* L26 and *S. cerevisiae* S-04	Probiotic bacteria were stable and capable of producing lactic acid in addition to the excellent metabolic activity of the yeast	Chan, Chua, Toh, and Liu (2019)
Maize-based beverages	*S. cerevisiae* CCMA 0731, *S. cerevisiae* CCMA 0732 and L. *paracasei* LBC-81	Viability of strains was higher than 6 log cfu/mL. Various volatile compounds such as acids, alcohols, aldehydes, esters, and ketones were present in the beverages	Menezes, Ramos, Dias, and Schwan (2018)
Beverages based on cassava and rice	*L. plantarum* CCMA 0743, *T. delbrueckii* CCMA 0235 and commercial L. *acidophilus* LAC-04	Co-culture of LAB strains with *T. delbrueckii* can improve the product digestibility, LAB growth, and antioxidant activity with acceptable sensory properties	Freire, Ramos, Da Costa Souza, Cardoso, and Schwan (2017)
Fermented soy milk	*S. boulardii* and LAB	Aglycones, isoflavones, and antioxidant activity increased	Rekha and Vijayalakshmi (2008)
Fermented milk	*P. kudriavzevii* KL84A and *L. plantarum* LAT3	ACE-inhibitory properties increased in the beverage	Chaves-López et al. (2012)

13.6 Bioactive compounds in beverages produced by starter cultures

It has been reported that starter cultures are capable of releasing nutritive and bioactive compounds into beverages thereby enhancing the health-promoting properties of these products. In this context, attempts have been made to use starter cultures as cell factories, for the industrial production of these metabolites in a pure form, or to promote their synthesis in situ in fermented foods (Melini et al., 2019; Torino, Font De Valdez, & Mozzi, 2015).

Some LAB species can produce B-group vitamins; a promising strategy for the bio-fortification of foods (Leblanc et al., 2011). Exopolysaccharides (EPS) are long-chain polysaccharides synthesized by LAB. They consist of repeating units of sugars (glucose, galactose, mannose, fructose, and rhamnose) or sugar derivatives and noncarbohydrate constituents and are divided into different categories depending on the composition and mechanism of production (Ibarburu et al., 2015; Llamas-Arriba et al., 2018). They are known to influence the physicochemical (viscosity, stability, and water holding capacity) and sensory characteristics of the final product, alongside offering the bacteria protection toward environmental conditions (Torino et al., 2015). The technological features of EPS are linked with interactions with water as well as gel formation (Ripari, 2019). In dairy-based and cereal-based fermented beverages, EPS plays an important role in the sensory properties of the final product (Torino et al., 2015).

Conjugated linoleic acid (CLA) is a term attributed to the positional and geometric isomers of linoleic acid with conjugated double bonds. It exerts several biological activities such as anticarcinogenic, antidiabetic, anti-inflammatory, anti-obesity, and antioxidant (Hur, Kim, Bahk, & Park, 2017; Yang et al., 2015, 2017). Milk and dairy products are one of the main sources of CLA in the human diet and fermentation is considered to be one of the most important natural ways of increasing CLA levels in food products (Blasi & Cossignani, 2019). It has been reported that besides rumen bacteria, strains of *Bifidobacterium*, *Enterococcus*, *Lactobacillus*, *Lactococcus*, *Propionibacterium*, and *Streptococcus* have the capability for CLA production, due to the presence of the linoleate isomerase enzyme (Blasi & Cossignani, 2019). Factors affecting CLA production include the bacterial strain, level of linoleic acid, the fermentation media, as well as the fermentation conditions (Yang et al., 2017). For example, CLA was produced by nine potential probiotic LAB strains isolated from kefir in de Man, Rogosa, and Sharpe (MRS) broth with supplementation of sunflower seed oil (Vieira et al., 2017). Dahiya and Puniya (2017) isolated CLA producing lactobacilli from dairy products and screening results in MRS broth indicated that *L. plantarum*, *L. gasseri*, *L. fermentum*, and *L. salivarius* were all capable of CLA production and the highest level of CLA was generated by L. *plantarum* HIF15 in skim milk. In a study conducted by Colakoglu and Gursoy (2011), an adjunct culture (*L. reuteri* ATCC 55739 or *L. lactis* subsp. *lactis* IO-1), along with conventional starter cultures, were used to produce a yogurt drink with an increased CLA level.

The compound γ-aminobutyric acid (GABA) is produced by various LAB species. For example, in mature coconut water by *L. plantarum* DW12 (Kantachote, Ratanaburee, Hayisama-Ae, Sukhoom, & Nunkaew, 2017), in fermented milk by L. *plantarum* PU11 (Nejati et al., 2013), in Korean Bokbunja wine by *S. cerevisiae* (Song & Baik, 2014) and fermented black soybean milk by *L. brevis* FPA 3709 (Ko, Lin, & Tsai, 2013).

Generation of bioactive peptides, such as the angiotensin-I-converting enzyme (ACE) inhibitory peptide during milk whey fermentation by

Lactobacillus helveticus (Narva, Halleen, Väänänen, & Korpela, 2004) and *L. casei* (Li et al., 2017), has been reported. Augmentation of antioxidant activity during fermentation have been observed in different food matrices, such as fermented milk prepared by *Pedicoccus pentosaceus* (Balakrishnan & Agrawal, 2014), apple juice fermented with *L. plantarum* ATCC 14917 (Li et al., 2019), a millet-based beverage (Raabadi) with *L. plantarum* RYPR1 (Yadav, Puniya, & Shukla, 2016), and a grape beverage fermented with *L. plantarum*, *L. rhamnosus*, and *L. casei* (Khanniri, Sohrabvandi, Mortazavian, Khorshidian, & Malganji, 2018). Table 13.4 represents some selected publications on fermented beverages and the bioactive compounds within them produced during fermentation.

TABLE 13.4 Selected publications on fermented beverages containing bioactive compounds.

Type of bioactive compound	Type of beverage	Microorganisms	Reference
EPS (extracellular polymeric substances)	Kefir	*Lactobacillus kefiranofaciens*	Prado et al. (2015)
	Pulque	*Leuconostoc citreum* *Leuconostoc kimchii*	Escalante et al. (2008)
	Ogi	*L. plantarum* YO 175	Adesulu-Dahunsi, Jeyaram, Sanni, and Banwo (2018)
	Boza	*L. citreum* (E55) and L. *lactis* (A47)	Heperkan, Daskaya-Dikmen, and Bayram (2014)
	Quinoa-based fermented beverage	*L. plantarum* Q823, *L. casei* Q11, and *L. lactis* ARH74	Ludena Urquizo et al. (2017)
Vitamin B			
Riboflavin	Kefir-like cereal-based beverages	*L. plantarum* M5MA1-B2 + kefir starters	Yépez et al. (2019)
Folic acid	Rice-based fermented beverage	*L. fermentum* KKL1	Ghosh et al. (2015)
B12	Mature coconut water	*L. plantarum* DW12	Kantachote et al. (2017)

TABLE 13.4 Selected publications on fermented beverages containing bioactive compounds—cont'd

Type of bioactive compound	Type of beverage	Microorganisms	Reference
CLA (conjugated linoleic acid)			
	Fermented soy milk	*L. plantarum* P1201	Lee et al. (2018)
	Dahi	*L. acidophilus* and *L. casei*	Yadav, Jain, and Sinha (2007)
	Fermented milk	*B. animalis* subsp. *Lactis*	Moghadam et al. (2019)
	Fermented milk	*L. rhamnosus* + yogurt culture	Xu, Boylston, and Glatz (2006)
GABA (γ-aminobutyric acid)			
	Grape must beverage	*L. plantarum* DSM19463	Di Cagno et al. (2010)
	Raspberry juice	*L. brevis* GABA100	Kim, Lee, Ji, Lee, and Hwang (2009)
	Red seaweed beverage	*L. plantarum* DW12	Ratanaburee, Kantachote, Charernjiratrakul, Penjamras, and Chaiyasut (2011)
Selenium	Beer	*S. cerevisiae* and *Saccharomyces uvarum*	Sánchez-Martínez et al. (2012)
Bioactive peptides			
	Fermented soy milk	*L. plantarum* C2	Singh and Vij (2018)
	Sprouted quinoa yogurt beverages	*L. casei*	Obaroakpo et al. (2019)

13.7 Immobilization technology for starter cultures

In recent years, there has been rising interest in the use of immobilized cells as an alternative to conventional free cells in food fermentations. Cell immobilization presents numerous advantages, such as increasing fermentation productivity and cell stability, the possibility of continuous processing, and decreasing the costs of recovery and downstream processing (Kourkoutas, Bekatorou, Banat, Marchant, & Koutinas, 2004). Immobilization methods can be categorized into entrapment within a porous matrix, adsorption on a solid carrier, self-aggregation by flocculation, and covalent binding. Carriers for food production must be nontoxic and stable during processing, and high loading capacity is desirable (Mitropoulou, Nedovic, Goyal, & Kourkoutas, 2013).

Encapsulation is a process that entraps the active substances in a wall material and protects it from environmental conditions. It has been used extensively for the entrapment of probiotic cells by a variety of polymers and different materials (Kavitake et al., 2018). Biopolymers such as alginate, carrageenan, starch, xanthan, gelatin, cellulose, milk, and whey proteins have been used as coating materials for the encapsulation of probiotic cells (Kosseva, 2011).

Altieri et al. (2019) immobilized *S. cerevisiae* W13 on apple pieces and used it for cider production. It was observed that apple pieces as the carrier could be used 10 times and the yeast had similar performance in terms of ethanol production as free yeast cells. The fermentation efficiency of thermally dried immobilized kefir co-culture on casein was investigated by Dimitrellou et al. (2008). The results showed that immobilization of the kefir culture maintained cell viability fermentation activity for 1 year.

Another example is the use of immobilized technology for the fermentation of cornelian cherry juice. Mantzourani et al. (2018) used *L. plantarum* ATTC14917 in free or immobilized form for the fermentation of cornelian cherry juice at 30°C for 24h followed by storage at 4°C for 28days. Analysis of residual sugar and organic acids revealed that sugar content was reduced by 62% in the case of free cells and 66% in immobilized cells at the 4th week of storage. Lactic acid content increased during storage reaching the maximum level of 97.8 and 148.5mg/100mL at the 4th week of storage in free and immobilized cells, respectively. The total phenolic content of the fermented cornelian cherry juice with immobilized cells was recorded in higher levels (214–264mg GAE/100mL) for all of the cold storage times compared to the fermented juice with free cells (165–199mg GAE/100mL) and the nonfermented juice (135–169mg GAE/100mL). Immobilized cells retained their viability at higher levels (9.95 log cfu/mL at the 4th week) compared to free cells (7.36 log cfu/mL at the 4th week). In a later study by Mantzourani et al. (2019), cornelian cherry juice was fermented with L. *paracasei* K5 in free form or immobilized in wheat bran at 30°C for 24h and then kept for 28days at 4°C. The results of the chemical analysis showed that immobilization of the bacteria increased the fermentation activity of *L. paracasei* K5.

13.8 Conclusions

Production of fermented dairy and nondairy beverages has future potential for the development of more functional foods. Probiotic food products are one of the largest functional food markets, and comprehensive research is being conducted in designing probiotic beverages. Several lactobacilli and bifidobacteria species have been utilized as starter cultures in fermented beverages, which have improved the quality and healthful characteristics, as well as the sensory properties of the beverages. There is still a need to explore potential new starter cultures with better-defined characteristics, which can be isolated from different sources as well as new fermentable substrates for the production of novel probiotic beverages. Furthermore, technological challenges, including the stability and viability of probiotics and their sensory characteristics should be considered in the development of these products. The optimization of fermentation technology, proper selection of probiotic strains and substrates, with respect to safety, fermentative activity, organoleptic properties, nutritiveness, degree of bioactivity, and compatibility between the probiotics is of the greatest importance in the development of probiotic beverages.

References

Adebo, O. A., Njobeh, P. B., Adeboye, A. S., Adebiyi, J. A., Sobowale, S. S., Ogundele, O. M., et al. (2018). Advances in fermentation technology for novel food products. In S. Panda, & P. Shetty (Eds.), *Innovations in technologies for fermented food and beverage industries* (pp. 71–87). UK: Springer.

Adesulu-Dahunsi, A. T., Jeyaram, K., Sanni, A. I., & Banwo, K. (2018). Production of exopolysaccharide by strains of *Lactobacillus plantarum* YO175 and OF101 isolated from traditional fermented cereal beverage. *PeerJ*, *6*, e5326.

Agata, L., & Jan, P. (2012). Production of fermented goat beverage using a mixed starter culture of lactic acid bacteria and yeasts. *Engineering in Life Sciences*, *12*, 486–493.

Aidoo, K. E., Rob Nout, M., & Sarkar, P. K. (2006). Occurrence and function of yeasts in Asian indigenous fermented foods. *FEMS Yeast Research*, *6*, 30–39.

Altieri, C., Campaniello, D., Speranza, B., Sinigaglia, M., Corbo, M. R., & Bevilacqua, A. (2019). Immobilization of *Saccharomyces cerevisiae* on apple pieces to produce cider. *Fermentation*, *5*, 1–9.

Altieri, C., Ciuffreda, E., Di Maggio, B., & Sinigaglia, M. (2017). Lactic acid bacteria as starter cultures. In B. Speranza, A. Bevilacqua, M. R. Corbo, & M. Sinigaglia (Eds.), *Starter cultures in food production* (pp. 1–15). UK: John Wiley& Sons.

Ashaolu, T. J. (2019). A review on selection of fermentative microorganisms for functional foods and beverages: The production and future perspectives. *International Journal of Food Science & Technology*, *54*, 2511–2519.

Balakrishnan, G., & Agrawal, R. (2014). Antioxidant activity and fatty acid profile of fermented milk prepared by *Pediococcus pentosaceus*. *Journal of Food Science and Technology*, *51*, 4138–4142.

Baschali, A., Tsakalidou, E., Kyriacou, A., Karavasiloglou, N., & Matalas, A.-L. (2017). Traditional low-alcoholic and non-alcoholic fermented beverages consumed in European countries: a neglected food group. *Nutrition Research Reviews*, *30*, 1–24.

Ben Said, L., Gaudreau, H., Dallaire, L., Tessier, M., & Fliss, I. (2019). Bioprotective culture: A new generation of food additives for the preservation of food quality and safety. *Industrial Biotechnology*, *15*, 138–147.

Bergsveinson, J., Kajala, I., & Ziola, B. (2017). Next-generation sequencing approaches for improvement of lactic acid bacteria-fermented plant-based beverages. *AIMS Microbiology*, *3*, 8–24.

Bintsis, T. (2018). Lactic acid bacteria as starter cultures: An update in their metabolism and genetics. *AIMS Microbiology, 4*, 665–684.

Blandino, A., Al-Aseeri, M., Pandiella, S., Cantero, D., & Webb, C. (2003). Cereal-based fermented foods and beverages. *Food Research International, 36*, 527–543.

Blasi, F., & Cossignani, L. (2019). Fermentation as a strategy to increase conjugated linoleic acid in dairy products. *Large Animal Review, 25*, 101–104.

Broome, M., Powell, I., & Limsowtin, G. (2002). Cheese starter cultures: Specific properties. *Encyclopaedia of dairy science* (pp. 269–275). Vol. 1(pp. 269–275). ·Academic Press, UK.

Bujna, E., Farkas, N. A., Tran, A. M., Sao Dam, & Nguyen, Q. D. (2018). Lactic acid fermentation of apricot juice by mono- and mixed cultures of probiotic *Lactobacillus* and *Bifidobacterium* strains. *Food Science and Biotechnology, 27*(2), 547–554.

Carminati, D., Giraffa, G., Quiberoni, A., Binetti, A., Suárez, V., & Reinheimer, J. (2010). Advances and trends in starter cultures for dairy fermentations. In F. Mozzi, R. Raya, & G. Vignolo (Eds.), *Biotechnology of lactic acid bacteria: Novel applications* (pp. 177–192). UK: John Wiley& Sons.

Champagne, C. P., Tompkins, T. A., Buckley, N. D., & Green-Johnson, J. M. (2010). Effect of fermentation by pure and mixed cultures of *Streptococcus thermophilus* and *Lactobacillus helveticus* on isoflavone and B-vitamin content of a fermented soy beverage. *Food Microbiology, 27*, 968–972.

Chan, M. Z. A., Chua, J. Y., Toh, M., & Liu, S.-Q. (2019). Survival of probiotic strain *Lactobacillus paracasei* L26 during co-fermentation with *S. cerevisiae* for the development of a novel beer beverage. *Food Microbiology, 82*, 541–550.

Chaves-López, C., Serio, A., Paparella, A., Martuscelli, M., Corsetti, A., Tofalo, R. , et al. (2014). Impact of microbial cultures on proteolysis and release of bioactive peptides in fermented milk. *Food Microbiology, 42*, 117–121.

Chaves-López, C., Tofalo, R., Serio, A., Paparella, A., Sacchetti, G., & Suzzi, G. (2012). Yeasts from Colombian kumis as source of peptides with angiotensin I converting enzyme (ACE) inhibitory activity in milk. *International Journal of Food Microbiology, 159*, 39–46.

Chen, Y., Aorigele, C., Wang, C., Simujide, H., & Yang, S. (2015). Screening and extracting mycocin secreted by yeast isolated from koumiss and their antibacterial effect. *Journal of Food and Nutrition Research, 3*, 52–56.

Chilton, S., Burton, J., & Reid, G. (2015). Inclusion of fermented foods in food guides around the world. *Nutrients, 7*, 390–404.

Colakoglu, H., & Gursoy, O. (2011). Effect of lactic adjunct cultures on conjugated linoleic acid (CLA) concentration of yoghurt drink. *Journal of Food, Agriculture and Environment, 9*, 60–64.

Corbo, M. R., Bevilacqua, A., Petruzzi, L., Casanova, F. P., & Sinigaglia, M. (2014). Functional beverages: The emerging side of functional foods: Commercial trends, research, and health implications. *Comprehensive Reviews in Food Science and Food Safety, 13*, 1192–1206.

Corbo, M. R., Racioppo, A., Monacis, N., & Speranza, B. (2017). Commercial starters or autochtonous strains? That is the question. In B. Speranza, A. Bevilacqua, M. R. Corbo, & M. Sinigaglia (Eds.), *Starter cultures in food production* (pp. 174–198). UK: John Wiley& Sons.

Dahiya, D. K., & Puniya, A. K. (2017). Isolation, molecular characterization and screening of indigenous lactobacilli for their abilities to produce bioactive conjugated linoleic acid (CLA). *Journal of Food Science and Technology, 54*, 792–801.

Di Cagno, R., Mazzacane, F., Rizzello, C. G., De Angelis, M., Giuliani, G., Meloni, M. , et al. (2010). Synthesis of γ-aminobutyric acid (GABA) by *Lactobacillus plantarum* DSM19463: Functional grape must beverage and dermatological applications. *Applied Microbiology and Biotechnology, 86*, 731–741.

Dimitrellou, D., Tsaousi, K., Kourkoutas, Y., Panas, P., Kanellaki, M., & Koutinas, A. A. (2008). Fermentation efficiency of thermally dried immobilized kefir on casein as starter culture. *Process Biochemistry, 43*, 1323–1329.

Dimitrovski, D., Velickova, E., Dimitrovska, M., Langerholc, T., & Winkelhausen, E. (2016). Synbiotic functional drink from Jerusalem artichoke juice fermented by probiotic *Lactobacillus plantarum* PCS26. *Journal of Food Science and Technology, 53*, 766–774.

Dimitrovski, D., Velickova, E., Langerholc, T., & Winkelhausen, E. (2015). Apple juice as a medium for fermentation by the probiotic *Lactobacillus plantarum* PCS 26 strain. *Annals of Microbiology, 65*, 2161–2170.

Do Amaral Santos, C. C. A., Da Silva Libeck, B., & Schwan, R. F. (2014). Co-culture fermentation of peanut-soy milk for the development of a novel functional beverage. *International Journal of Food Microbiology, 186*, 32–41.

Elfahri, K., Vasiljevic, T., Yeager, T., & Donkor, O. (2016). Anti-colon cancer and antioxidant activities of bovine skim milk fermented by selected *Lactobacillus helveticus* strains. *Journal of Dairy Science, 99*, 31–40.

Escalante, A., Giles-Gómez, M., Hernández, G., Córdova-Aguilar, M. S., López-Munguía, A., Gosset, G. , et al. (2008). Analysis of bacterial community during the fermentation of pulque, a traditional Mexican alcoholic beverage, using a polyphasic approach. *International Journal of Food Microbiology, 124*, 126–134.

Freire, A. L., Ramos, C. L., Da Costa Souza, P. N., Cardoso, M. G. B., & Schwan, R. F. (2017). Nondairy beverage produced by controlled fermentation with potential probiotic starter cultures of lactic acid bacteria and yeast. *International Journal of Food Microbiology, 248*, 39–46.

Gaensly, F., Agustini, B. C., Da Silva, G. A., Picheth, G., & Bonfim, T. M. B. (2015). Autochthonous yeasts with β-glucosidase activity increase resveratrol concentration during the alcoholic fermentation of *Vitis labrusca* grape must. *Journal of Functional Foods, 19*, 288–295.

Ghosh, K., Ray, M., Adak, A., Halder, S. K., Das, A., Jana, A. , et al. (2015). Role of probiotic *Lactobacillus fermentum* KKL1 in the preparation of a rice based fermented beverage. *Bioresource Technology, 188*, 161–168.

Giri, S. S., Sen, S. S., Saha, S., Sukumaran, V., & Park, S. C. (2018). Use of a potential probiotic, *Lactobacillus plantarum* L7, for the preparation of a rice-based fermented beverage. *Frontiers in Microbiology, 9*, 1–11.

Granato, D., Branco, G. F., Cruz, A. G., Faria, J. D. A. F., & Shah, N. P. (2010). Probiotic dairy products as functional foods. *Comprehensive Reviews in Food Science and Food Safety, 9*, 455–470.

Gupta, S., & Abu-Ghannam, N. (2012). Probiotic fermentation of plant based products: Possibilities and opportunities. *Critical Reviews in Food Science and Nutrition, 52*, 183–199.

Heperkan, D., Daskaya-Dikmen, C., & Bayram, B. (2014). Evaluation of lactic acid bacterial strains of boza for their exopolysaccharide and enzyme production as a potential adjunct culture. *Process Biochemistry, 49*, 1587–1594.

Hesseltine, C. W. (1991). Mixed-culture fermentations: An introduction to oriental food fermentations. In G. Zeikus, & E. A. Johnson (Eds.), *Mixed cultures in biotechnology* (pp. 1–16). New York: McGraw Hill.

Hur, S. J., Kim, H. S., Bahk, Y. Y., & Park, Y. (2017). Overview of conjugated linoleic acid formation and accumulation in animal products. *Livestock Science, 195*, 105–111.

Ibarburu, I., Puertas, A. I., Berregi, I., Rodríguez-Carvajal, M. A., Prieto, A., & Dueñas, M. T. (2015). Production and partial characterization of exopolysaccharides produced by two *Lactobacillus suebicus* strains isolated from cider. *International Journal of Food Microbiology, 214*, 54–62.

Jayaram, V. B., Cuyvers, S., Lagrain, B., Verstrepen, K. J., Delcour, J. A., & Courtin, C. M. (2013). Mapping of *Saccharomyces cerevisiae* metabolites in fermenting wheat straight-dough reveals succinic acid as pH-determining factor. *Food Chemistry, 136*, 301–308.

Johansen, E. (2018). Use of natural selection and evolution to develop new starter cultures for fermented foods. *Annual Review of Food Science and Technology, 9*, 411–428.

Kandasamy, S., Kavitake, D., & Shetty, P. H. (2018). Lactic acid bacteria and yeasts as starter cultures for fermented foods and their role in commercialization of fermented foods. In S. Panda, & P. Shetty (Eds.), *Innovations in technologies for fermented food and beverage industries* (pp. 25–52). UK: Springer.

Kandylis, P., Pissaridi, K., Bekatorou, A., Kanellaki, M., & Koutinas, A. A. (2016). Dairy and non-dairy probiotic beverages. *Current Opinion in Food Science*, *7*, 58–63.

Kantachote, D., Ratanaburee, A., Hayisama-Ae, W., Sukhoom, A., & Nunkaew, T. (2017). The use of potential probiotic *Lactobacillus plantarum* DW12 for producing a novel functional beverage from mature coconut water. *Journal of Functional Foods*, *32*, 401–408.

Kavitake, D., Kandasamy, S., Devi, P. B., & Shetty, P. H. (2018). Recent developments on encapsulation of lactic acid bacteria as potential starter culture in fermented foods–A review. *Food Bioscience*, *21*, 34–44.

Khanniri, E., Sohrabvandi, S., Mortazavian, A. M., Khorshidian, N., & Malganji, S. (2018). Effect of fermentation, cold storage and carbonation on the antioxidant activity of probiotic grape beverage. *Current Nutrition & Food Science*, *14*, 335–340.

Khorshidian, N., Yousefi Asli, M., Hosseini, H., Shadnoush, M., & Mortazavian, A. M. (2016). Potential anticarcinogenic effects of lactic acid bacteria and probiotics in detoxification of process-induced food toxicants. *Iranian Journal of Cancer Prevention*, *9*, 1–13.

Kim, J.-H., & Baik, S.-H. (2015). Preparation and characterization of fermented dandelion (*Taraxacum officinale*) beverage using *Lactobacillus acidophilus* F46 having cinnamoyl esterase activity. *Food Science and Biotechnology*, *24*, 583–593.

Kim, J. Y., Lee, M. Y., Ji, G. E., Lee, Y. S., & Hwang, K. T. (2009). Production of γ-aminobutyric acid in black raspberry juice during fermentation by *Lactobacillus brevis* GABA100. *International Journal of Food Microbiology*, *130*, 12–16.

Ko, C. Y., Lin, H.-T. V., & Tsai, G. J. (2013). Gamma-aminobutyric acid production in black soybean milk by *Lactobacillus brevis* FPA 3709 and the antidepressant effect of the fermented product on a forced swimming rat model. *Process Biochemistry*, *48*, 559–568.

Kosseva, M. R. (2011). Immobilization of microbial cells in food fermentation processes. *Food and Bioprocess Technology*, *4*, 1089–1118.

Kourkoutas, Y., Bekatorou, A., Banat, I. M., Marchant, R., & Koutinas, A. (2004). Immobilization technologies and support materials suitable in alcohol beverages production: A review. *Food Microbiology*, *21*, 377–397.

Leblanc, J., Laiño, J. E., Del Valle, M. J., Vannini, V. V., Van Sinderen, D., Taranto, M. P. , et al. (2011). B-group vitamin production by lactic acid bacteria–current knowledge and potential applications. *Journal of Applied Microbiology*, *111*, 1297–1309.

Lee, J. H., Kim, B., Hwang, C. E., Haque, M. A., Kim, S. C., Lee, C. S. , et al. (2018). Changes in conjugated linoleic acid and isoflavone contents from fermented soymilks using *Lactobacillus plantarum* P1201 and screening for their digestive enzyme inhibition and antioxidant properties. *Journal of Functional Foods*, *43*, 17–28.

Li, C., Kwok, L.-Y., Mi, Z., Bala, J., Xue, J., Yang, J., et al. (2017). Characterization of the angiotensin-converting enzyme inhibitory activity of fermented milks produced with *Lactobacillus casei*. *Journal of Dairy Science*, *100*, 9495–9507.

Li, Y., Sadiq, F. A., Liu, T., Chen, J., & He, G. (2015). Purification and identification of novel peptides with inhibitory effect against angiotensin I-converting enzyme and optimization of process conditions in milk fermented with the yeast *Kluyveromyces marxianus*. *Journal of Functional Foods*, *16*, 278–288.

Li, Z., Teng, J., Lyu, Y., Hu, X., Zhao, Y., & Wang, M. (2019). Enhanced antioxidant activity for apple juice fermented with *Lactobacillus plantarum* ATCC14917. *Molecules*, *24*, 1–12.

Liu, S.-Q. (2002). Malolactic fermentation in wine–beyond deacidification. *Journal of Applied Microbiology*, *92*, 589–601.

Liu, S.-Q., & Tsao, M. (2009). Enhancement of survival of probiotic and non-probiotic lactic acid bacteria by yeasts in fermented milk under non-refrigerated conditions. *International Journal of Food Microbiology*, *135*, 34–38.

Llamas-Arriba, M. G., Pérez-Ramos, A., Puertas, A. I., López, P., Prieto, A., & Dueñas, M. T. (2018). Characterization of *Pediococcus ethanolidurans* CUPV141: a β-D-glucan-and heteropolysaccharide-producing bacterium. *Frontiers in Microbiology, 9*, 1–15.

Lu, Y., Putra, S. D., & Liu, S.-Q. (2018). A novel non-dairy beverage from durian pulp fermented with selected probiotics and yeast. *International Journal of Food Microbiology, 265*, 1–8.

Ludena Urquizo, F. E., García Torres, S. M., Tolonen, T., Jaakkola, M., Pena-Niebuhr, M. G., Von Wright, A. , et al. (2017). Development of a fermented quinoa-based beverage. *Food Science & Nutrition, 5*, 602–608.

Mantzourani, I., Nouska, C., Terpou, A., Alexopoulos, A., Bezirtzoglou, E., Panayiotidis, M. , et al. (2018). Production of a novel functional fruit beverage consisting of Cornelian cherry juice and probiotic bacteria. *Antioxidants, 7*, 1–10.

Mantzourani, I., Terpou, A., Alexopoulos, A., Bezirtzoglou, E., Bekatorou, A., & Plessas, S. (2019). Production of a potentially synbiotic fermented Cornelian cherry (*Cornus mas* L.) beverage using *Lactobacillus paracasei* K5 immobilized on wheat bran. *Biocatalysis and Agricultural Biotechnology, 17*, 347–351.

Markkinen, N., Laaksonen, O., Nahku, R., Kuldjärv, R., & Yang, B. (2019). Impact of lactic acid fermentation on acids, sugars, and phenolic compounds in black chokeberry and sea buckthorn juices. *Food Chemistry, 286*, 204–215.

Melini, F., Melini, V., Luziatelli, F., Ficca. A. G., & Ruzzi, M. (2019). Health-promoting components in fermented foods: An up-to-date systematic review. *Nutrients, 11*, 1–24.

Menezes, A. G. T., Ramos, C. L., Dias, D. R., & Schwan, R. F. (2018). Combination of probiotic yeast and lactic acid bacteria as starter culture to produce maize-based beverages. *Food Research International, 111*, 187–197.

Mitropoulou, G., Nedovic, V., Goyal, A., & Kourkoutas, Y. (2013). Immobilization technologies in probiotic food production. *Journal of Nutrition and Metabolism, 2013*, 1–16.

Moghadam, B. E., Keivaninahr, F., Nazemi, A., Fouladi, M., Mokarram, R. R., & Benis, K. Z. (2019). Optimization of conjugated linoleic acid production by *Bifidobacterium animalis* subsp. Lactis and its application in fermented milk. *LWT-Food Science and Technology, 108*, 344–352.

Mohammadi, R., Yousefi, M., Sarlak, Z., Shah, N. P., Mortazavian, A. M., Sadeghi, E. , et al. (2017). Influence of commercial culture composition and cow milk to soy milk ratio on the biochemical, microbiological, and sensory characteristics of a probiotic fermented composite drink. *Food Science and Biotechnology, 26*, 749–757.

Mousavi, Z. E., Mousavi, S. M., Razavi, S. H., Hadinejad, M., Emam-Djomeh, Z., & Mirzapour, M. (2013). Effect of fermentation of pomegranate juice by *Lactobacillus plantarum* and *Lactobacillus acidophilus* on the antioxidant activity and metabolism of sugars, organic acids and phenolic compounds. *Food Biotechnology, 27*, 1–13.

Mridula, D., & Sharma, M. (2015). Development of non-dairy probiotic drink utilizing sprouted cereals, legume and soymilk. *LWT-Food Science and Technology, 62*, 482–487.

Mustafa, S. M., Chua, L. S., El-Enshasy, H. A., Abd Majid, F. A., Hanapi, S. Z., & Abdul Malik, R. (2019). Effect of temperature and pH on the probiotication of *Punica granatum* juice using *Lactobacillus* species. *Journal of Food Biochemistry, 43*, e12805.

Narva, M., Halleen, J., Väänänen, K., & Korpela, R. (2004). Effects of *Lactobacillus helveticus* fermented milk on bone cells in vitro. *Life Sciences, 75*, 1727–1734.

Nejati, F., Rizzello, C. G., Di Cagno, R., Sheikh-Zeinoddin, M., Diviccaro, A., Minervini, F. , et al. (2013). Manufacture of a functional fermented milk enriched of angiotensin-I converting enzyme (ACE)-inhibitory peptides and γ-amino butyric acid (GABA). *LWT- Food Science and Technology, 51*, 183–189.

Nyanzi, R., Jooste, P. J., Abu, J. O., & Beukes, E. M. (2010). Consumer acceptability of a synbiotic version of the maize beverage mageu. *Development Southern Africa, 27*, 447–463.

Obaroakpo, J. U., Liu, L., Zhang, S., Lu, J., Pang, X., & Lv, J. (2019). α-Glucosidase and ACE dual inhibitory protein hydrolysates and peptide fractions of sprouted quinoa yoghurt beverages inoculated with *Lactobacillus casei*. *Food Chemistry, 299*, 124985.

Pakbin, B., Razavi, S. H., Mahmoudi, R., & Gajarbeygi, P. (2014). Producing probiotic peach juice. *Biotechnology and Health Sciences*, *1*(3)e24683.

Parente, E., & Cogan, T. (2004). Starter cultures: General aspects. In P. Fox, P. McSweeny, T. Cogan, & T. Guinee (Eds.), *Cheese: Chemistry, physics and microbiology* (pp. 123–148). UK: Academic Press.

Parsons, J. B., & Rock, C. O. (2013). Bacterial lipids: Metabolism and membrane homeostasis. *Progress in Lipid Research*, *52*, 249–276.

Pereira, A. L. F., Maciel, T. C., & Rodrigues, S. (2011). Probiotic beverage from cashew apple juice fermented with *Lactobacillus casei*. *Food Research International*, *44*, 1276–1283.

Peyer, L. C., Zannini, E., & Arendt, E. K. (2016). Lactic acid bacteria as sensory biomodulators for fermented cereal-based beverages. *Trends in Food Science & Technology*, *54*, 17–25.

Prado, M. R., Blandón, L. M., Vandenberghe, L. P., Rodrigues, C., Castro, G. R., Thomaz-Soccol, V. , et al. (2015). Milk kefir: Composition, microbial cultures, biological activities, and related products. *Frontiers in Microbiology*, *6*, 1–10.

Prado, F. C., Lindner, J. D. D., Inaba, J., Thomaz-Soccol, V., Brar, S. K., & Soccol, C. R. (2015). Development and evaluation of a fermented coconut water beverage with potential health benefits. *Journal of Functional Foods*, *12*, 489–497.

Prückler, M., Lorenz, C., Endo, A., Kraler, M., Dürrschmid, K., Hendriks, K. , et al. (2015). Comparison of homo- and heterofermentative lactic acid bacteria for implementation of fermented wheat bran in bread. *Food Microbiology*, *49*, 211–219.

Rai, A. K., Kumari, R., Sanjukta, S., & Sahoo, D. (2016). Production of bioactive protein hydrolysate using the yeasts isolated from soft chhurpi. *Bioresource Technology*, *219*, 239–245.

Rai, A. K., Pandey, A., & Sahoo, D. (2018). Biotechnological potential of yeasts in functional food industry. *Trends in Food Science & Technology*, *83*, 129–137.

Rai, A. K., Sanjukta, S., & Jeyaram, K. (2017). Production of angiotensin I converting enzyme inhibitory (ACE-I) peptides during milk fermentation and their role in reducing hypertension. *Critical Reviews in Food Science and Nutrition*, *57*, 2789–2800.

Ratanaburee, A., Kantachote, D., Charernjiratrakul, W., Penjamras, P., & Chaiyasut, C. (2011). Enhancement of γ-aminobutyric acid in a fermented red seaweed beverage by starter culture *Lactobacillus plantarum* DW12. *Electronic Journal of Biotechnology*, *14*, 1–14.

Rathore, S., Salmerón, I., & Pandiella, S. S. (2012). Production of potentially probiotic beverages using single and mixed cereal substrates fermented with lactic acid bacteria cultures. *Food Microbiology*, *30*, 239–244.

Rekha, C., & Vijayalakshmi, G. (2008). Biomolecules and nutritional quality of soymilk fermented with probiotic yeast and bacteria. *Applied Biochemistry and Biotechnology*, *151*, 452–463.

Ripari, V. (2019). Techno-functional role of exopolysaccharides in cereal-based, yogurt-like beverages. *Beverages*, *5*, 1–13.

Sadiq, F. A., Yan, B., Tian, F., Zhao, J., Zhang, H., & Chen, W. (2019). Lactic acid bacteria as antifungal and anti-mycotoxigenic agents: A comprehensive review. *Comprehensive Reviews in Food Science and Food Safety*, *18*, 1403–1436.

Salmerón, I., Thomas, K., & Pandiella, S. S. (2015). Effect of potentially probiotic lactic acid bacteria on the physicochemical composition and acceptance of fermented cereal beverages. *Journal of Functional Foods*, *15*, 106–115.

Sánchez-Martínez, M., Da Silva, E. G. P., Pérez-Corona, T., Cámara, C., Ferreira, S. L., & Madrid, Y. (2012). Selenite biotransformation during brewing. Evaluation by HPLC–ICP-MS. *Talanta*, *88*, 272–276.

Şanlier, N., Gökcen, B. B., & Sezgin, A. C. (2019). Health benefits of fermented foods. *Critical Reviews in Food Science and Nutrition*, *59*, 506–527.

Shrivastava, N., & Ananthanarayan, L. (2015). Use of the backslopping method for accelerated and nutritionally enriched idli fermentation. *Journal of the Science of Food and Agriculture*, *95*, 2081–2087.

Singh, B. P., & Vij, S. (2018). In vitro stability of bioactive peptides derived from fermented soy milk against heat treatment, pH and gastrointestinal enzymes. *LWT, 91*, 303–307.

Song, N. E., & Baik, S. H. (2014). Identification and characterization of high GABA and low biogenic amine producing indigenous yeasts isolated from Korean traditional fermented Bokbunja (*Rubus coreanus* Miquel) wine. *Journal of Biotechnology, 185*, S83.

Sridharan, S., & Das, K. M. S. (2019). A study on suitable non dairy food matrix for probiotic bacteria–A systematic review. *Current Research in Nutrition and Food Science Journal, 7*, 5–16.

Tamang, J. P., Shin, D.-H., Jung, S.-J., & Chae, S.-W. (2016). Functional properties of microorganisms in fermented foods. *Frontiers in Microbiology, 7*, 1–13.

Thakur, M., & Sharma, R. (2017). Development of probiotic pomegranate beverage and its physico-chemical and microbial characterization. *International Journal of Pure & Applied Bioscience, 5*, 35–41.

Torino, M. I., Font De Valdez, G., & Mozzi, F. (2015). Biopolymers from lactic acid bacteria. Novel applications in foods and beverages. *Frontiers in Microbiology, 6*, 834. https://doi.org/10.3389/fmicb.2015.00834.

Vieira, C. P., Cabral, C. C., Da Costa Lima, B. R., Paschoalin, V. M. F., Leandro, K. C., & Conte-Junior, C. A. (2017). *Lactococcus lactis* ssp. Cremoris MRS47, a potential probiotic strain isolated from kefir grains, increases cis-9, trans-11-CLA and PUFA contents in fermented milk. *Journal of Functional Foods, 31*, 172–178.

Vinicius De Melo Pereira, G., De Carvalho Neto, D. P., Junqueira, A. C. D. O., Karp, S. G., Letti, L. A., Magalhães Júnior, A. I. , et al. (2019). A review of selection criteria for starter culture development in the food fermentation industry. *Food Reviews International*, 1–33. https://doi.org/10.1080/87559129.2019.1630636.

Walker, G. M., & Stewart, G. G. (2016). *Saccharomyces cerevisiae* in the production of fermented beverages. *Beverages, 2*, 1–12.

Wedajo, B. (2015). Lactic acid bacteria: Benefits, selection criteria and probiotic potential in fermented food. *Journal of Probiotics & Health, 3*, 1–9.

Xu, S., Boylston, T. D., & Glatz, B. A. (2006). Effect of inoculation level of *Lactobacillus rhamnosus* and yogurt cultures on conjugated linoleic acid content and quality attributes of fermented milk products. *Journal of Food Science, 71*, 275–280.

Yadav, H., Jain, S., & Sinha, P. (2007). Production of free fatty acids and conjugated linoleic acid in probiotic dahi containing *Lactobacillus acidophilus* and *Lactobacillus casei* during fermentation and storage. *International Dairy Journal, 17*, 1006–1010.

Yadav, R., Puniya, A. K., & Shukla, P. (2016). Probiotic properties of *Lactobacillus plantarum* RYPR1 from an indigenous fermented beverage Raabadi. *Frontiers in Microbiology, 7*, 1–9.

Yang, B., Chen, H., Stanton, C., Ross, R. P., Zhang, H., Chen, Y. Q. , et al. (2015). Review of the roles of conjugated linoleic acid in health and disease. *Journal of Functional Foods, 15*, 314–325.

Yang, B., Gao, H., Stanton, C., Ross, R. P., Zhang, H., Chen, Y. Q. , et al. (2017). Bacterial conjugated linoleic acid production and their applications. *Progress in Lipid Research, 68*, 26–36.

Yépez, A., Russo, P., Spano, G., Khomenko, I., Biasioli, F., Capozzi, V. , et al. (2019). In situ riboflavin fortification of different kefir-like cereal-based beverages using selected Andean LAB strains. *Food Microbiology, 77*, 61–68.

Yoon, K. Y., Woodams, E. E., & Hang, Y. D. (2004). Probiotication of tomato juice by lactic acid bacteria. *Journal of Microbiology (Seoul, Korea), 42*, 315–318.

Yoon, K. Y., Woodams, E. E., & Hang, Y. D. (2005). Fermentation of beet juice by beneficial lactic acid bacteria. *LWT- Food Science and Technology, 38*, 73–75.

Yoon, K. Y., Woodams, E. E., & Hang, Y. D. (2006). Production of probiotic cabbage juice by lactic acid bacteria. *Bioresource Technology, 97*, 1427–1430.

Yousefi Asli, M., Khorshidian, N., Mohammad Mortazavian, A., & Hosseini, H. (2017). A review on the impact of herbal extracts and essential oils on viability of probiotics in fermented milks. *Current Nutrition & Food Science, 13*, 6–15.

Zheng, X., Yu, Y., Xiao, G., Xu, Y., Wu, J., Tang, D. , et al. (2014). Comparing product stability of probiotic beverages using litchi juice treated by high hydrostatic pressure and heat as substrates. *Innovative Food Science & Emerging Technologies, 23*, 61–67.

PART V

Technologies and legalities

CHAPTER

14

Kefir, kombucha, and sour beers

Lopamudra Sahu[a] *and Sandeep K. Panda*[b]

[a]Department of Botany, Utkal University, Bhubaneswar, India, [b]School of Biotechnology, KIIT University, Bhubaneswar, India

14.1 Introduction

Fermentation is an ancient food processing technique that has been used for the preservation of food since time immemorial (Behera & Panda, 2020). Common fermented foods include yogurts, sausages, vinegars, vegetable pickles, fermented milks, cheeses, vegetable protein/amino acid/peptide sauces, alcoholic foods/beverages, leavened and sourdough breads. Milk and cultured dairy products are one of the oldest fermented products. Fermented dairy products containing probiotics are of interest due to their curative and protective attributes (Sahu & Panda, 2018). *Lactobacillus* and *Bifidobacterium* are the prime bacterial genera in these probiotic products, while others such as *Pediococcus, Enterococcus,* and *Lactobacillus* are also prevalent (Sahu, Panda, Paramithiotis, Zdolec, & Ray, 2016). Lactic acid bacteria (LAB), as probiotics, have shown therapeutic effects in diseases such as rheumatoid arthritis and cancer (Furuya, Shimizu, & Kawamori, 2011; Marco, Pavan, & Kleerebezem, 2006). Lately, there has been a strong focus on functional foods with probiotic microorganisms and health-promoting organic ingredients. Fermented probiotic beverages are gaining in popularity because modern-day consumers are more health-conscious and inclined towards organic and natural foods, with some consumers preferring functional nonalcoholic beverages over alcoholic beverages. The global trends and preferences of consumers have attracted innovation and diversification of functional food production. This has given an impetus to the manufacturers to expand their markets in the production of nonalcoholic beverages, especially the probiotic beverages that have a cultural background.

Some of the beverages currently of great interest to modern consumers include kefir, kombucha, and sour beer. Kefir and kombucha, as probiotic

Probiotic Beverages
https://doi.org/10.1016/B978-0-12-818588-9.00008-5

beverages, are described in detail later in this chapter. Also highlighted is the manufacture and increasing popularity of sour beers.

14.2 Brief background of kefir, kombucha, and sour beer

Kefir is prepared from the fermentation of kefir grains, both traditional and commercially available ones, with varieties of raw milk (cow, goat, buffalo, camel, sheep), water, coconut/soy milk, vegetable juices, etc. (Behera, Panda, Kayitesi, & Mulaba-Bafubiandi, 2016). Kefir grains are constituted of a consortium of microorganisms that accumulate on a complex proteinaceous and polysaccharide substrate, which include LAB (*Lactobacillus paracasei, L. kefiri, L. buchneri*, etc.), acetic acid bacteria, and yeast (namely *Saccharomyces cerevisiae* and *Kluyveromyces lactis)* (Fig. 14.1).

Though the kefir produced from milk is the main familiar indigenous fermented beverage, an alternative kefir drink has also been prepared by replacing milk with water enriched with sugar (John & Deeseenthum, 2015). Cocoa, juices of specific fruits, yam, sesame, and bean extracts are also used as a source of nutrients for the replacement of milk in the preparation of kefir (Corona et al., 2016; da Costa, de Alencar, & dos Santos Leandro, 2018; Puerari, Magalhaes, & Schwan, 2012; Randazzo et al., 2016).

Sharifi, Moringa, and Mortazavi (2017) reviewed the potential of kefir as a dietary probiotic for cancer prevention and treatment and the involvement of the kefir complex in the synthesis of anticancer bioactive components. The large amounts of good bacteria in kefir aid in digestion and it

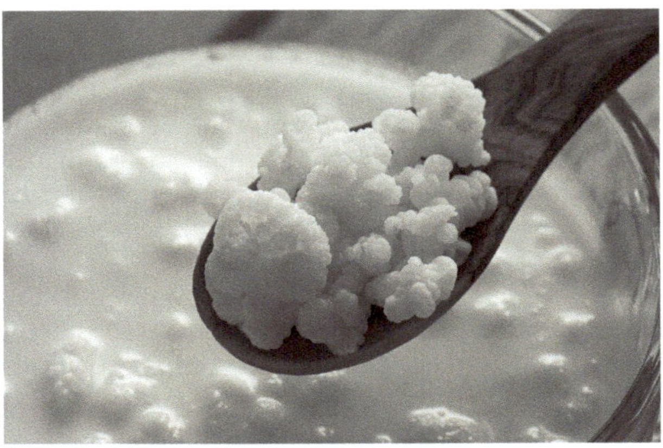

FIG. 14.1 Kefir grains used for the fermentation of kefir.

contains a wider nutrient content than yogurt. It has become an alternative and highly beneficial beverage for lactose-intolerant populations, another driving factor for its market size growth. In the modern era of the food industry, kefir is finding wide use as probiotic content in the production of frozen desserts, dips, and sauces, and consumption of kefir as a digestive supplement has been of importance for the growth of the kefir market. Though the production and consumption of kefir are high in Europe, it is also predicted to grow at a positive rate in other parts of Asia Pacific and North American regions in the near future.

Kombucha was a traditionally home-brewed beverage that has recently been repositioned into a classy and nutrient-rich fermented product, with gut-friendly probiotics. Kombucha is prepared by the fermentation of sweetened tea using a conglomerate of microorganisms (e.g., *Acetobacter* spp., *Gluconobacter oxydans*, *Bacterium gluconicum*) and yeast (e.g., *Schizosaccharomyces* spp., *Saccharomyces* spp., *Candida* spp., or *Pichia* spp. etc.) for 10–14days. The market value of bottled kombucha is on the rise, and it is becoming a popular beverage in the United States. Kombucha drinks, because of their fizzy taste and unique flavors, have outpaced similar beverages available in the market in terms of popularity. Kombucha tea marketability is boosted because of the incorporation of innovative styles and flavors that appease and attract consumers. Cutting-edge brewing techniques, along with usage of superior quality raw materials, have resulted in the premiumization of kombucha tea, resulting in some consumers being diverted from mainstream beers.

Although technically a beer, sour beer is being marketed as the "hottest cold drink!" In a market obsessed with innovative, obscure, and complex beers, this funky beer has created a niche for itself. Traditionally produced and consumed in Belgium, this beer has now gained tremendous popularity throughout the world. The degree and character of tartness are key attributes. The desired flavor of sour beers may require several months, or even years, of aging. Various assortments of sour flavors are achieved by utilizing several bacteria such as *Lactobacilli*, *Acetobacter*, and *Pediococci*, as well as yeast (*Dekkera/Brettanomyces*) singly or in a consortium. Lactic and acetic acids are primarily responsible for the sourness in most sour beers. The beers are brewed purposely with selected microorganisms to obtain those sour, acidic, and tart flavors due to the use of wild yeast and/or bacterial strains. Some sour styles are also characterized by an additional salty flavor. Sour beers can vary widely in flavor and intensity. The acidity level in the beer imparts sourness to the beer, and it is because of bacteria such as *Lactobacillus* and *Pediococcus*, which as part of the brewing process, create lactic acid and acetic acid. Table 14.1 depicts some of the health benefit claims of kefir, kombucha, and sour beers.

TABLE 14.1 Some beneficial health claims of kefir, kombucha, and sour beer from different studies.

Probiotic beverage	Health claims	References
Kefir	Anti-microbial activity Anti-bacterial effect	Bourrie, Willing, and Cotter (2016) John and Deeseenthum (2015)
	Anti-hypertensive effect	Rosa et al. (2017) Friques et al. (2015)
	Reduction in cholesterol and Hypocholesterolemic effects	Rosa et al. (2017) Bourrie et al. (2016) Klippel et al. (2016)
	Reduces lactose intolerance	Rosa et al. (2017)
	Anti-inflammatory effect	Prado et al. (2016)
	Anti-carcinogenic effects	Rafie, Hamedani, Ghiasvand, and Miraghajani (2015) Sharifi et al. (2017) Alshaar et al. (2017)
	Improves insulin resistance Relieves hyperglycemia, insulin resistance, and hyperlipidemia, and improves intracellular metabolic imbalance and glycemic control in diabetes mellitus	Ostadrahimi et al. (2015) Pereira, Pimenta, and Porto (2016)
	Anti-allergic effects	Nielsen, Gurakan, and Unlu (2014)
	Increases calcium absorption rates, reduces parathyroid (PTH) level and bone resorption	Rizzoli and Biver (2017)
Kombucha	Anti-oxidant properties	Aidoo (2015)
	Anti-hyperglycemic activity	Dias and Shenoy (2016)
	Hypoglycemic activity	Lobo and Shenoy (2015a)
	Anti-hyperlipidemic activity	Lobo and Shenoy (2015a, 2015b) Lobo, Sagar, and Shenoy (2017)
	Anti-carcinogenic effects, cell proliferation, and increased detoxification	Dufresne and Farnworth (2000) Jayabalan, Malbasa, Loncar, Vitas, and Sathishkumar (2014)

TABLE 14.1 Some beneficial health claims of kefir, kombucha, and sour beer from different studies.—cont'd

Probiotic beverage	Health claims	References
	Anti-microbial activity	Bhattacharya et al. (2016) Al-Kalifawi (2014) Santos Jr., Batista, Rodrigues, Filho, and Lima (2009)
	Hepatoprotective	Dias and Shenoy (2016)
	Prevention against foot and mouth disease	Fu, Wu, Lv, He, and Jiang (2015)
	Anti-fungal activity Prevention/treatment of Malassezia infections	Yuniarto, Anggadiredja, and Aqidah (2016) Battikh, Chaieb, Bakhrouf, and Ammar (2013) Mahmoudi et al. (2016)
Sour beer	Vitamin B synthesis	Katina et al. (2007)
	Non-allergic	

14.3 Preparation technology

14.3.1 Processing of kefir

Kefir is produced both traditionally and commercially for industrial purposes. Mostly cow's milk is preferred; other raw materials such as goat and sheep milk are also used. Nondairy sources (rice, soy, peanut, walnut) can replace the milk of cow, sheep, and goat for kefir production (Wyk, 2019). Traditional kefir production is carried out by the inoculation of kefir grains into milk. Fresh milk is thermally treated for sterilization and further kefir grains (containing microorganisms) at a dose of 2%–10% are added to the sterilized milk at 20–25°C. Fermentation is conducted for 18–24h and the inoculants (kefir grains) are sieved out and stored under cold conditions for subsequent applications (Otles & Cagindi, 2003).

Commercial kefir production is carried out using different methods, but the overall standard procedure is usually similar to that of the traditional type. Microbial and biochemical control methods are adapted for the processing of fresh milk prior to homogenization and thermal treatment at 90–95°C for up to 10min. The temperature of the milk is reduced to ambient temperature, usually, 18–24°C and fermentation is initiated with the inoculation of kefir grains at 2%–8%. Fermentation is allowed for 18–24h followed by bottling, maturation, and storage (4°C) (Otles & Cagindi, 2003). Currently, lyophilized microorganisms are preferred by commercial kefir manufacturers to avoid any chance of interference by unwanted microorganisms (Hertzler & Clancy, 2003).

Several methods are adapted for the storage of kefir grains. The common methods are the application of lyophilization, freeze and vacuum drying, as well as storage at low temperatures. The grains can remain viable (microbiologically active) over 7–8months if stored at −20°C (Nogay, 2019). However, activity is higher (12–18months) in the dry form.

14.3.2 Manufacturing kombucha

Black tea/green tea and white sugar (5, 7.5, 10, 15, and 20g/L) are the preferred substrates for the preparation of kombucha. The Kombucha pellicle is a smooth disc with a hard, even, viscous mass of yeast and bacteria (Fig. 14.2).

It is placed in a container, and to it, cold-black tea with sugar is added. It usually requires about 8–12days, to complete the first fraction of the kombucha; a portion of it is taken out for use and extra tea is filled into the jar. The matured kombucha pellicle is thick, around 1cm, and can generate a measurable amount of the probiotic drink on a daily basis. Time to time, the peeling of segments of the pellicle/SCOBY is performed to initiate fresh cultures.

Other methods include the bottling of kombucha for storage and consumption after a time interval. The process is similar to the former one and

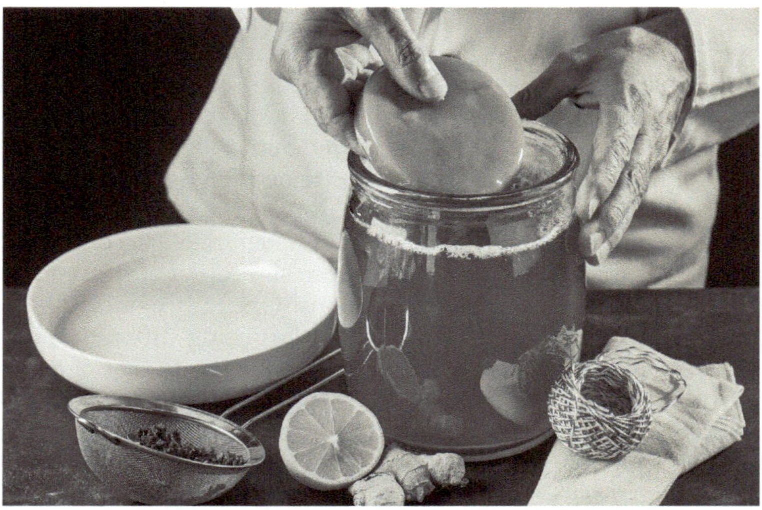

FIG. 14.2 Kombucha with pellicle and glass container.

a large glass jar is used instead. Fermentation is carried out for 7–8 days at 22–30°C in a closed jar, shielded with a paper towel/coffee filter held with strings. To start a new batch, one portion of kombucha is transferred to a container (glass) and stored under cold conditions, whereas the other portion is applied to initiate a fresh fermentation. After every batch of Kombucha fermentation, there is a formation of a new deposit on the top of the earlier culture. The components permeate and fermentation takes place, the carbohydrate (sugar) is metabolized using various enzymes to produce vitamins, minerals, and organic acids, thus converting a sugar-rich black tea into a healthy, flavorful, probiotic drink. The end product is mildly alcoholic (0.5%–1%), carbonated, and is a slightly acidic product in terms of organoleptic attributes, similar to the flavor of a light vinegar. After the completion of fermentation, the beverage is subjected to straining, bottling, sealing using a hygienic cap, and refrigeration. Kombucha pellicles must be handled with care to prevent contamination by harmful bacteria and molds.

14.3.3 Sour beer fermentation

The common process of beer production encompasses malting and brewing. Malting entails the artificially induced germination of a crop by steeping and germination followed by kilning to create malt colors and aromas. The brewing process encompasses wort preparation that includes mashing and boiling, fermentation, maturation, and filtration and/or stabilization.

Sour beer is a special type of beer historically produced using indigenous methods. The fermentation of sour beer involves not only a specific strain of yeast but also other microorganisms to obtain the distinctive flavor of the beer (Thompson Witrick, Duncan, Hurley, & O'Keefe, 2017). The other microorganisms involved in the typical sour and tart flavor of the beer include bacteria such as LAB, *Pediococcus,* and among the yeast *Brettanomyces*. The use of the probiotic lactobacilli, *Lactobacillus paracasei* L26, as a starter culture for lambic beer production is an innovative way of utilizing this live probiotic microbe for extra health beneficial properties, whereas standard sour beers use wild, as well as commercial LAB for wort acidification (Alcine, Chua, Toh, & Liu, 2019).

Souring of beer is accomplished either by kettle souring or by a mixed culture fermentation. In kettle souring, fermentation of the wort with microorganisms is carried out for 24–48 h, followed by boiling with hops and then an alcoholic fermentation with brewer's yeast. In contrast in a mixed culture fermentation, the LAB is inoculated into the fermentation medium during the primary fermentation, along with brewer's yeast or during the secondary fermentation (aging) by using souring microorganisms in the barrel.

Heterolactic fermenting yeasts, other than *S. cerevisiae*, are used for primary souring of the wort, and souring occurs during primary fermentation without the role of LAB. The yeast strains *Lachancea fermentati*, *Hanseniaspora vineae*, *Wickerhamomyces anomalus*, and *Schizosaccharomyces japonicus* have shown exceptional attenuation and medium-to-high flocculation (Osburn et al., 2018). Lambic beer, which is one of the most common beers of Belgium, is exposed to wild yeast and native bacteria during the progress of the fermentation. *Pediococcus*, *Acetobacter*, LAB, *Brettanomyces*, and *Saccharomyces* species are the microorganisms involved in the fermentation of lambic beer, and their use adds to the distinctive features of this beer.

14.4 Microbial dynamics in kefir, kombucha, and sour beer during the course of fermentation

During fermentation, microbial consortia and the production of metabolites influence the quality and efficacy of the fermented product for human consumption. Although microbiological and molecular techniques are adapted to identify the microorganisms for the period of the fermentation process, with the advent of modern high-throughput sequencing methods, it has become easier to detect the microorganisms at different stages of fermentation, along with their metabolites.

14.4.1 Kefir

Culturing methods have been the traditional way to study the microbial diversity of kefir, in which different LAB species have been found to be the dominant bacteria in the beverage and the kefir grain. Of late, advanced sequencing techniques have been employed to study the microbial diversity and dynamics in different kefir grains and it was observed that *Lactobacillus*, among bacteria, and *Ascomycota* among fungi, are the dominating genera (Marsh, O'Sullivan, Hill, Ross, & Cotter, 2013; Nalbantoglu et al., 2014). In contrast, *Lactobacillus*, *Lactococcus*, *Acetobacter*, and *Leuconostoc* among bacteria and *Kazachstania*, *Kluyveromyces*, *Naumovozyma*, and *Saccharomyces* among fungi were found to control the microbiota of kefir milk (Garofalo et al., 2015; Korsak et al., 2015). Walsh et al. (2016) carried out a detailed analysis based on metagenomics and metabolomics to study the gene content and microbial diversity/population from kefir of three different regions, during a 24h fermentation. Their studies divulged that *Lactobacillus kefiranofaciens* was governing the initial period of fermentation; however, in the latter stages, *Leuconostoc mesenteroides* dominated the medium. This progression was confirmed by the presence of the genes engaged in the synthesis of aromatic amino acids in L. *mesenteroides* but absent from *L. kefiranofaciens*.

Furthermore, the dominance of the microorganisms in the fermentation medium of kefir is understood from the corresponding volatile compounds and their respective pathways. For example, acetic acid generation is linked with *Acetobacter* spp., lactic acid is connected with LAB, and esters with *Saccharomyces* spp. Hence, ester and ketone production can be enhanced by inoculation of *L. kefiranofaciens*, acetic acid, and 2,3-butanedione generation can be influenced positively by *L. mesenteroides*, thereby supporting the fundamental relationship between microbial taxa and flavors. Studies examined the specific genera and species of microorganisms with different volatile compounds, and it was revealed that the microbes in kefir had the essential genes for the generation of these compounds. Recently, Nogay (2019) reviewed the details of the microbial characteristics of kefir.

14.4.2 Kombucha

During the fermentation of kombucha, the yeasts and bacteria utilize substrates in numerous ways, which also corresponds to various metabolites. As yeasts break down (enzymatic) sucrose into glucose and fructose and generate ethanol through the glycolytic pathway, glucose is utilized by acetic acid bacteria (AAB) for the production of gluconic acid and ethanol is utilized for the generation of acetic acid. The pH of kombucha falls with the generation of organic acids during the fermentation period. Marsh, O'Sullivan, Hill, Ross, and Cotter (2014) used high-ended amplicon sequencing methods on the DNAs acquired from the pellicles, which were obtained from five different regions and the analogous kombucha at two particular time intervals of fermentation. Their studies revealed that *Gluconacetobacter* spp. were the predominant bacteria present, while *Acetobacter* was detected in trace populations. A significant *Lactobacillus* populace was also found to be prevalent in the latter part of the fermentation. *Zygosaccharomyces, Dekkera,* and *Kazachstania* were the three genera of yeast populations found. Though *Zygosaccharomyces* dominated the fermented beverage, many additional genera were observed in the pellicles.

In contrast, a study carried out by Chakravorty et al. (2016), using next-generation sequencing, showed that the genus *Candida* was the prominent microbe in the system, while *Saccharomyces* was observed in very low proportions up to 14 days, but *Zygosaccharomyces* was not observed in their process as in earlier studies by Marsh et al. (2014).

The other important yeast genera that were dominant were *Lachancea* and *Kluyveromyces*. The authors studied the bacterial community by combining a low-resolution Terminal restriction fragment length polymorphism (T-RFLP) analysis followed by a high-resolution throughput screening (HTS) analysis, which revealed a major prokaryotic genus as *Komagataeibacter* with respect to *Acetobacter* and *Gluconacetobacter*. A study was carried out by Coton et al. (2017) on the microbial ecology of kombucha fermentation using green/black tea by microbial and metabarcoding processes. They reported that *Acetobacteraceae* spp. were the dominant followed by *Lactobacteriaceae*, whereas *Dekkera* spp., *Hanseniaspora* spp. and *Zygosaccharomyces* spp. were common among the yeasts during fermentation. However, the species diversity fell over the fermentation period (8 days). *Gluconacetobacter europaeus, G. oxydans, G. saccharivorans,* and *Acetobacter peroxydans* were the overriding species of AAB.

Several groups of microorganisms maintain symbiotic relationships during the fermentation of kombucha. The microbial dynamics in kombucha fermentation is complex, leading to a series of biochemical reactions. As sucrose is the source of sugar, yeasts act on it through their periplasmic invertase enzyme and hydrolyze it into glucose and fructose. Some acetic acid bacteria produce gluconic acid and glucuronic acid through the fermentation of glucose. Yeasts also produce ethanol from glucose and the ethanol can be subsequently oxidized by acetic acid bacteria for the production of acetic acid. Simultaneously, acetic acid affects the production of ethanol by yeasts. In the complex symbiotic microbial relationship, the prime microbial metabolites of kombucha are ethanol, glycerol, D-saccharic acid, organic acids such as lactic acid, oxalic acid, malic acid, etc. (Laureys, Britton, & Clippeleer, 2020).

14.4.3 Sour beers

The traditional method of fermentation of lambic beer encompasses four phases (Enterobacteriaceae phase, main fermentation phase, acidification phase, and maturation phase). The *Enterobacteriaceae* phase fermentation continues for 30–40 days. The prominent microbes in this phase are *Enterobacter* spp., *Klebsiella* spp., *Escherichia coli, Hafnia alvei,* cycloheximide-resistant yeasts *Hanseniaspora uvarum* and *Saccharomyces dairensis,* as well as *Saccharomyces uvarum*. This phase is followed by the main fermentation for a period of 3–4 months and is distinguished by the presence of *S. cerevisiae, S. bayanus/pastorianus,* and *S. uvarum*. Subsequent fermentation (acidification phase) continues for 4 to 8 months and is dominated by *Pediococcus* spp. along with *Lactobacillus* spp., and

Brettanomyces spp. The last maturation phase begins 10 months from the initiation of fermentation, during which the fermentation medium is gradually attenuated and a fall in the population of LAB is observed. However, it is important to note that AAB were isolated throughout the entire fermentation process (Spitaels et al., 2015).

De Roos, Vandamme, and De Vuyst (2018) explained the changes in the microbial species and the formation of the metabolic biochemicals all through the different phases of fermentation of lambic beer. The authors observed malolactic fermentation by *Pediococcus damnosus*, uptake of acetoin by *Dekkera* spp., metabolism of maltooligosaccharides simultaneously, possibly by the yeasts, and a shortened enterobacterial phase despite lactic acid generation for acidification of wort, were some of the newest fermentation characteristics. Though the microorganisms as described above are almost similar in the craft beer fermentations, researchers have identified various novel species of micro-organisms based on their genomic studies by using sophisticated techniques along with the culture-based ones (Panda, 2019).

Hi-C sequencing was applied for the assemblage of draft genome sequences from sour beer microbial diversity and *D. bruxellensis*, *P. kudriavzevii*, and *S. cerevisiae* and interspecies-hybrid yeast of *Pichia* composed of *P. membranifaciens* and an unknown interrelated species. *Acetobacter pomorum* and another *Acetobacter* species, and LAB, *Pediococcus damnosus* and a novel *Lactobacillus* species were observed (Heil et al., 2017). Osburn et al. (2018) further suggested the exclusion of LAB for souring in beer fermentation and instead proposed heterofermentative yeast for lactic acid production during primary fermentation. Five yeast species (*Hanseniaspora vineae, Lachancea fermentati, Lachancea thermotolerans, Schizosaccharomyces japonicus, and Wickerhamomyces anomalus*) out of the 300 strains selected could produce lactic acid, ethanol, and carbon dioxide efficiently by using a sugar substrate through heterolactic fermentation. A large-scale and bacteria-free brewing process with the four strains exhibited the efficiency of the yeasts; they were very attenuative, yielded a substantial amount of lactic acid, and produced pleasurable aromatic and flavored compounds.

In the fermentation of sour beer, both alcoholic (through yeast) and lactic acid (mostly through selected bacteria) fermentation are conducted. Counting and monitoring the growth of microorganisms, namely yeast and bacteria, are important during the course of the fermentation. Although a yeast count can be conducted by hemocytometer and image cytometers, an appropriate bacterial count in sour beer is a constraint. However, the traditional bacterial fermentation is followed by the fall of pH or rise in the acidity, and the counting of bacteria can be conducted by colony counts on agar plates.

14.5 Health-promoting potentials of kefir, kombucha, and sour beer

Kefir, a fermented milk beverage, is produced by cocultures (LAB, AAB, and yeast), which are enveloped by kefiran (an exopolysaccharide, a glucogalactan). A novel bioactive compound i.e. a polysaccharide EPS_DN1 secreted by *Lactobacillus kefiranofaciens* isolated from kefir may be a potential natural antibiotic (Jeong et al., 2017). Atalar (2018) used cold-pressed hazelnut milk to manufacture a functional kefir beverage that was known to have more health-beneficial potential than cow's milk samples because of its bioactive nature and lipid profile. The addition of hazelnut milk was also reported to improve the structural properties of kefir samples. Novel bioactive peptides with antihypertensive effects and the potential of inhibiting ACE activity in vivo were identified from bovine milk fermented using two dissimilar proteomic methods (matrix-assisted laser desorption ionization- time-of-fiight [MALDI-TOF] and Shotgun Proteomics) (Amorim et al., 2019). Such discovery on novel milk-derived bioactive peptides in kefir may signal avenues and directions to the dairy-based manufacturers to expand and promote the products with new health claims and special functional characteristics.

Kombucha drink is a carbonated acidic beverage with a tinge of sweetness due to the various metabolites and organic biochemical compounds generated by the co-culture of bacteria and yeast. Chandrakala, Lobo, and Dias (2019) reviewed the bioactive compounds of kombucha and its health benefits. The presence of many antioxidants, vitamins (B1, B2, B6, B12, C), amino acids, enzymes, polyphenols, and flavonoids and their effects on health have been assessed. Jayabalan and Waisundara (2019) reviewed the functional aspects of kombucha tea and the metabolites associated with it. A study by Villarreal-Soto et al. (2019) reported that the bioactive compounds from the extracts of fermented black tea with the kombucha conglomerate could be enhanced by using two types (geometrically different) of vessels followed by repeated extractions with solvents of escalating polarity. Forty-seven compounds were identified by GC-MS and their study revealed that fermentation kinetics were enhanced and the final anti-inflammatory and antiproliferative properties were improved with an elevated surface/height (s/h) ratio.

Similarly, in sour beer, LAB provide a bioprotective property against food spoilage and pathogens during the brewing process (Rouse & van Sinderen, 2008). This unique beer utilizes lactic acid bacteria, namely *Pediococcus* sp. and *Lactobacillus* spp. The biocontrol activity of the bacteria is due to the production of several antimicrobial compounds during their metabolic activities. The production of lactic acid, bacteriocin, cyclic dipeptides, and some unknown metabolites and proteins inhibit the proliferation of undesirable bacteria and fungi in the fermentation medium.

Probiotic bacteria in beer are also known to synthesize health-promoting metabolites, functional biochemicals, and most commonly vitamin B in the fermentation medium (Katina et al., 2007). Researchers are engaged in developing sour beers with live probiotic lactic acid bacteria for delivering these beneficial probiotic microorganisms to consumers through a popular alcoholic beverage in order to overcome the disadvantages of dairy-based probiotic beverages (i.e., lactose intolerance, allergy, and cholesterol content).

14.6 Current market status, consumers' preference and future of kefir, kombucha, and sour beer

A recent research report estimated that the worth of the global kefir business was USD 1.57 billion in 2017 (Global Kefir Market, 2018) and is projected to escalate to USD 2.89 billion by 2024 at a compound annual growth rate (CAGR) of 6.1% (during 2019 to 2024) (Market Research Future, 2020). Based on the type of product, the market for kefir is segmented as organic, Greek, frozen, and low-fat kefir.

Organic kefir is gaining popularity across different regions and this segment represented a significant market stake in 2017. The increasing inclination for organic food, paired with increasing nutrition-conscious consumers among the global population, is anticipated to fuel the growth of the organic kefir products in the years to come. The second important segment is the Greek kefir. The other segments such as low-fat kefir and frozen kefir are expected to grow at a considerable CAGR during 2017–2024. Companies operating in the kefir market are competing for market share. The major commercial manufacturers of kefir are Lifeway Foods Inc., Fresh Made, Inc., Hain Celestial Group, and Wallaby Yogurt Company, Danone SA, Nourish Kefir, and Kenmare Living Foods.

Similarly, the popularity and advantage of kombucha over other beverages is due to its twin benefits of being a flavorful drink, as well as having functional properties. The growing awareness among the consumers about the health advantages of organic products and products manufactured using organic constituents has caused an upsurge in the sales of organic food and beverages. Kombucha, being mostly an organic and highly energizing beverage, with its healthy and nutritive properties, is giving a significant boost to market sales in the beverage industry (Future Market Insights, 2018). In 2016, beverage giant PepsiCo acquired KeVita, a popular functional probiotic and kombucha manufacturer owing to the growing demand for kombucha in the market. There was a rise of 37.4% in the sales of kombucha and other fermented beverages in 2018 (Watson, 2018) and it is the most popular among the functional low alcoholic fermented beverages on the market (Nielsen Insights, 2018).

The North American region is predicted to rise at a CAGR of 15.2% during the predicted time and to reach a market value of US$ 2089.6 million by 2027, followed by Europe, which has accounted for a market share of 34.0% in 2018. According to the Future Market Insights Report (2018), the kombucha market is expected to witness a lucrative growth, CAGR of 18.5% in the APEJ (Asia-Pacific region except Japan) region over the forecast period (Future Market Insights, 2018). In 2014, North America held a large stake in the global market for kombucha sales and the highest contributor was the U.S. It is expected that for developing countries, such as China and India, in the near future there would be an increase in the demand for kombucha and innovative variants such as health and energy drinks.

In Germany and Japan, there is projected to be decent growth of the kombucha market in comparison to India and other Asia-Pacific countries. Some of the leading producers of kombucha based in the US are Millennium Products, Inc., Reed's, Inc., The Hain Celestial Group Revive Kombucha, Kosmic Kombucha, Cell - Nique Corporation, Buchi Kombucha, GT's Kombucha, Townshend's Tea Company, Humm Kombucha LLC, Nesalla Kombucha, Live Soda Kombucha, and Kombucha Wonder Drink, while Red Bull GmbH is from Austria. These companies are engaged in many new approaches such as market surveys, mergers, acquisitions, online sales approaches, and partnerships with other firms to expand their business territory (Grand View Research, 2018; Transparency Market Research, 2014).

It is predicted that the craft beer sales will reach USD 107.85 billion by 2024, with a CAGR of 14.1% during 2019–2024. There is also a demand for low-alcoholic/nonalcoholic beverages among the health-conscious consumers, which has triggered the production of low alcoholic content beers with improved taste and flavors. The market among Asian consumers is also expected to increase with the rising popularity of craft beers in the continent. Even in the UK, the demand for low-alcohol drinks by volume has soared in supermarkets. One additional motivating factor is that the low-alcohol beers are often less costly to buy and produce compared to their higher alcoholic counterparts (often due to alcohol taxes).

14.7 Blending of beverages and the market purview!

Fusion beverages are taking over the traditional beverage categories and have given dimensions to innovative products, which have attracted consumers worldwide. Researchers are more focused on studying the effect of blending beverages with ingredients that would provide more health benefits than the traditional ones. Sun, Li, and Chen (2015) studied kombucha mixed with wheatgrass, which has superior and more stable antioxidant properties over the traditional kombucha formula and could be recommended for consumption as a novel beverage. Manufacturers are also experimenting with multiple ingredients such as berries, herbs, spices and condiments, coffee, and adding these flavors to attract consumers. For example, in the preparation of Buchi Kombucha, various ingredients are combined in the recipe such as organic apple juice, freshly pressed organic ginger, lime juice, etc. In 2018, the Starbucks Corporation produced kombucha in six different flavors under its brand "Evolution Juice." The Canadian kombucha company, Rise Kombucha, for the first time has ventured into the markets of the United States (Transparency Market Research, 2014).

The increasing preference for organic food and beverages coupled with rising numbers of health conscious customers is expected to fuel the growth of the organic kefir segment in the years to come. The second important segment is the Greek kefir. Based on the application, the kefir market is categorized into dips and dressings, drinks and smoothies, dairy products, and dietary supplements. Based on the flavor, the market for kefir is classified into regular and flavored. Regular kefir is widely preferred by consumers, owing to its health benefits and nutritional importance. Flavored kefir is anticipated to register considerable growth in the future. This future growth is attributed to changing consumer preferences and the high demand for diverse dairy products (Global Kefir Market, 2018).

Though the idea of sour beer at first does not appear very appealing, sour beer's complexity of flavors has gained popularity among stylish beer and wine consumers. Fruit concentrates are also blended with sour beer for special flavors. Lost styles and flavored craft beers have been renewed in the United States, Australia, New Zealand, Canada, Japan, and Scandinavia and regions of Europe are leading the market and offering substitutes to traditional lagers. High sales of craft beer over traditional beers in the local and international markets are due to an increased distribution network while offering exciting new flavors and tastes to the consumers as well as good tasting low alcohol by volume (ABV) beers.

14.8 Advances in technology and future perspectives

Technological advancement has triggered the large-scale production of fermented beverages to meet the demand of consumers. Proteomics and genomics approaches have been proven to be powerful tools to study the complex bacteria-yeast interactions and their functions in food fermentations. Bechtner, Xu, Behr, Ludwig, and Vogel (2019) validated comparative proteomics for the exploration of interrelationship involving LAB and yeast to forecast metabolic exchanges in water kefir. Apple-vinegar-based kefir was produced, and the bioactivity of the kefir particles was estimated by applying a Biospeckle Laser (Viana, Magalhaaes-Guedesa, Braga Jr., Diasc, & Schwan, 2017). Novel technology (use of immobilized kefir particles) eliminated the employment of centrifugal separators that require higher energy and investment. The use of immobilized-cell biomass (kefir grains) provided a microbial consortium. Wyk (2019) has recently reviewed the microbial and biochemical aspects of kefir beverages and kefir grains. The developments in OMIC-methods (high throughput techniques such as genomics, metagenomics, metabolomics, metaproteomics, next-generation sequencing) to accomplish an appropriate culture and technology are discussed.

Soy-whey, a byproduct generated during the manufacture of tofu and soy protein, can be transformed into an innovative beverage by the application of a kombucha microbial consortia (Tu, Tang, Azi, Hu, & Dong, 2019). This is an intelligent conversion of waste into a palatable beverage. Holistic integration of meta-omic tools combined with the present-day artificial intelligence (AI) can bring new insights into predicting an ideal kefir culture towards efficient production of kefir drinks. Coupling of metabarcoding and culture-dependent approaches can provide an outline about the diversity of microorganisms, and microbes that are recalcitrant for culturing, and their possible roles in the processing of kombucha (Coton et al., 2017).

As craft beers are often unpasteurized and unfiltered, they are potential vehicles for delivering health benefits. For example, probiotic bacteria (*Lactobacillus paracasei L26)* were co-fermented with *S. cerevisiae* for the development of a sour beer (Alcine et al., 2019). Capece et al. (2018) studied the effect of the integration of *S. cerevisiae* var. *boulardii* (Sb) (probiotic) along with *S. cerevisiae* for beer fermentation. Such an introduction of traits was observed to enhance the antioxidant potential and phenolic content of beer, thereby increasing the health benefits of these low alcoholic or alcohol-free beers.

14.9 Conclusions

This chapter has examined three important probiotic beverages with an indigenous origin, currently accepted as a modern drink with several health-promoting potentials. The transformation of microbial technologies in recent years has enabled food manufacturers and technocrats to refine and fine-tune the process of producing kefir, kombucha, and sour beer. This chapter has also detailed the microorganisms involved in the fermentation of these beverages and the metabolites produced during the process. In the future, some of these technologies will be helpful in the revival of other indigenous probiotic beverages that are currently limited to particular regions of the globe, making them available to a wider consumer audience.

References

Aidoo, E. (2015). *Studies on the cytotoxicity and antioxidant activity of tea Kombucha* (Doctoral dissertation). University of Ghana.

Alcine, C. M. Z., Chua, J. Y., Toh, M., & Liu, S. Q. (2019). Survival of probiotic strain *Lactobacillus paracasei* L26 during co-fermentation with *S. cerevisiae* for the development of a novel beer beverage. *Food Microbiology, 82*, 541–550.

Al-Kalifawi, E. J. (2014). Study the antimicrobial effect of Kombucha tea on bacteria isolated from diabetic foot ulcer. *Journal of Biotechnology Research Center, 8*(4), 27–32. Special edition.

Alshaar, I. A., Aloklah, B., Al-Deen, R. B., Aljamali, M., Alkadry, R., & Albiski, F. (2017). *In vitro* anticancer properties of kefir and kefir products produced by a novel method in Syria. *International Journal of Pharmaceutical Science Invention, 6*(5), 1–6.

Amorim, F. G., Coitinho, L. B., Dias, A. T., Friques, A. G. F., Monteiro, B. L., Rezende, L. C. D., et al. (2019). Identification of new bioactive peptides from kefir milk through proteopeptidomics: Bioprospection of antihypertensive molecules. *Food Chemistry, 282*, 109–119.

Atalar, I. (2018). Functional kefir production from high pressure homogenized hazelnut milk. *LWT Food Science and Technology*. https://doi.org/10.1016/j.lwt.2019.03.013.

Battikh, H., Chaieb, K., Bakhrouf, A., & Ammar, E. (2013). Antibacterial and antifungal activities of black and green kombucha teas. *Journal of Food Biochemistry, 37*(2), 231–236.

Bechtner, J., Xu, D., Behr, J., Ludwig, C., & Vogel, R. F. (2019). Proteomic analysis of *Lactobacillus nagelii* in the presence of *Saccharomyces cerevisiae* isolated from water kefir and comparison with *Lactobacillus hordei*. *Frontiers in Microbiology, 2019*. https://doi.org/10.3389/fmicb.2019.00325.

Behera, S. S., & Panda, S. K. (2020). Ethnic and industrial probiotic foods and beverages: Efficacy and acceptance. *Current Opinion in Food Science, 32*, 29–36.

Behera, S. K., Panda, S. K., Kayitesi, E., & Mulaba-Bafubiandi, A. F. (2016). Kefir & Koumiss: Origin, health benefits & current status. In R. C. Ray, & D. Montet (Eds.), *Fermented foods: Part 2. Technological interventions* (pp. 401–417). Boca Raton: CRC Press.

Bhattacharya, D., Bhattacharya, S., Patra, M. M., Chakravorty, S., Sarkar, S., Chakraborty, W., et al. (2016). Antibacterial activity of polyphenolic fraction of kombucha against enteric bacterial pathogens. *Current Microbiology, 73*(6), 885–896.

Bourrie, B. C. T., Willing, B. P., & Cotter, P. D. (2016). The microbiota and health promoting characteristics of the fermented beverage kefir. *Frontiers in Microbiology, 7*, 647.

Capece, A., Romaniello, R., Pietrafesa, A., Siesto, G., Pietrafesa, R., Zambuto, M., et al. (2018). Use of *Saccharomyces cerevisiae* var. *boulardii* in co-fermentations with *S. cerevisiae* for the production of craft beers with potential healthy value-added. *International Journal of Food Microbiology, 284*, 22–30.

Chakravorty, S., Bhattacharya, S., Chatzinotas, A., Chakraborty, W., Bhattacharya, D., & Gachhui, R. (2016). Kombucha tea fermentation: Microbial and biochemical dynamics. *International Journal of Food Microbiology, 220*, 63–72.

Chandrakala, S. K., Lobo, R. O., & Dias, F. O. (2019). Kombucha (bio-tea): An elixir for life? *Nutrients in Beverages, 12*, 591–616.

Corona, O., Randazzo, W., Alessandro, M., Guarcello, R., Nicola, F., Erten, H., et al. (2016). Characterization of kefir-like beverages produced from vegetable juices. *Journal of Food Science and Technology, 66*, 572–581.

Coton, M., Pawtowski, A., Taminiau, B., Burgaud, G., Deniel, F., Coulloumme-Labarthe, L., et al. (2017). Unraveling microbial ecology of industrial-scale kombucha fermentations by metabarcoding and culture-based methods. *FEMS Microbiology Ecology, 93*. https://doi.org/10.1093/femsec/fix048.fix048.

da Costa, M. R., de Alencar, E. R., & dos Santos Leandro, E. (2018). Characterization of the kefir beverage produced from yam (*Colocasia esculenta* L.), sesame seed (*Sesamum indicum* L.) and bean (*Phaseolus vulgaris* L.) extracts. *Journal of Food Science and Technology, 55*, 4851–4858. https://doi.org/10.1007/s13197-018-3419-0.

De Roos, J., Vandamme, P., & De Vuyst, L. (2018). Wort substrate consumption and metabolite production during lambic beer fermentation and maturation explain the successive growth of specific bacterial and yeast species. *Frontiers in Microbiology, 9*, 2763. https://doi.org/10.3389/fmicb.2018.02763.

Dias, F. O., & Shenoy, C. K. (2016). Protective effect of Kombucha on diabetic nephropathy in Streptozotocin—Induced diabetic rats. *International Journal of Science and Research, 5*(3), 945–948.

Dufresne, C., & Farnworth, E. (2000). Tea, Kombucha, and health: A review. *Food Research International, 33*(6), 409–421.

Friques, A. G., Arpini, C. M., Kalil, I. C., Gava, A. L., Leal, M. A., Porto, M. L., et al. (2015). Chronic administration of the probiotic kefir improves the endothelial function in spontaneously hypertensive rats. *Journal of Translational Medicine, 13*, 390. https://doi.org/10.1186/s12967-015-0759-7.

Fu, N., Wu, J., Lv, L., He, J., & Jiang, S. (2015). Anti-foot-and-mouth disease virus effects of Chinese herbal kombucha in vivo. *Brazilian Journal of Microbiology, 46*(4), 1245–1255.

Furuya, H., Shimizu, Y., & Kawamori, T. (2011). Sphingolipids in cancer. *Cancer Metastasis Reviews, 30*(3–4), 567–576.

Future Market Insights (FMI). (2018). *Kombucha market*. REP-GB-7815, 175 p https://www.futuremarketinsights.com/reports/kombucha-market.

Garofalo, C., Osimani, A., Milanovic, V., Aquilanti, L., De Filippis, F., Stellato, G., et al. (2015). Bacteria and yeast microbiota in milk kefir grains from different Italian regions. *Food Microbiology, 49*, 123–133.

Global Kefir Market. (2018). https://www.zionmarketresearch.com/report/kefir-market.

Grand View Research. (2018). *Kombucha market size, share & trends analysis report by flavor (original, flavored), by distribution channel (supermarkets, health stores, online stores), by region, and segment forecasts, 2018–2025*. 99p https://www.grandviewresearch.com/industry-analysis/kombucha-market.

Heil, C. S., Burton, J. N., Liachko, I., Friedrich, A., Hanson, N. A., Morris, C. L., et al. (2017). Identification of a novel interspecific hybrid yeast from a metagenomic spontaneously inoculated beer sample using Hi-C. *Yeast, 35*(1), 71–84. https://doi.org/10.1002/yea.3280.

Hertzler, S. R., & Clancy, S. M. (2003). Kefir improves lactose digestion and tolerance in adults with lactose maldigestion. *Journal of the American Dietetic Association, 103*, 582–587.

Jayabalan, R., Malbasa, R. V., Loncar, E. S., Vitas, J. S., & Sathishkumar, M. (2014). A review on kombucha tea-microbiology, composition, fermentation, beneficial effects, toxicity, and tea fungus. *Comprehensive Reviews in Food Science and Food Safety, 13*(4), 538–550.

Jayabalan, R., & Waisundara, V. Y. (2019). Kombucha as a functional beverage. In A. M. Grumezescu, & A. M. Holban (Eds.), *Vol. 11. Functional and medicinal beverages* (pp. 413–446). Cambridge: Academic Press (Chapter 12).

Jeong, D., Kim, D.-H., Kang, I.-B., Kim, H., Song, K.-Y., Kim, H.-S., et al. (2017). Characterization and antibacterial activity of a novel exopolysaccharide produced by *Lactobacillus kefiranofaciens* DN1 isolated from kefir. *Food Control, 78*, 436–442.

John, S. M. J., & Deeseenthum, S. (2015). Properties and benefits of kefir—A review. *Journal of Science and Technology, 37*, 275–282.

Katina, K., Liukkonen, K. H., Kaukovirta-Norja, A., Adlercreutz, H., Heinonen, S. M., Lampi, A.-M., et al. (2007). Fermentation-induced changes in the nutritional value of native or germinated rye. *Journal of Cereal Science*, *46*(3), 348–355.

Klippel, B. F., Duemke, L. B., Leal, M. A., Friques, A. G., Dantas, E. M., Dalvi, R. F., et al. (2016). Effects of kefir on the cardiac autonomic tones and baroreflex sensitivity in spontaneously hypertensive rats. *Frontiers in Physiology*, *7*, 211. https://doi.org/10.3389/fphys.2016.00211.

Korsak, N., Taminiau, B., Leclercq, M., Nezer, C., Crevecoeur, S., Ferauche, C., et al. (2015). Evaluation of the microbiota of kefir samples using metagenetic analysis targeting the 16S and 26S ribosomal DNA fragments. *Journal of Dairy Science*, *98*, 3684–3689.

Laureys, D., Britton, S., & Clippeleer, J. D. (2020). Kombucha tea fermentation: A review. *Journal of the American Society of Brewing Chemists*, *78*(3), 165–174.

Lobo, R. O., Sagar, B. K. C., & Shenoy, C. K. (2017). Bio-tea prevents membrane destabilization during isoproterenol-induced myocardial injury. *Journal of Microscopy Ultrastructure*, *5*, 146–154.

Lobo, R. O., & Shenoy, C. K. (2015a). Evaluation of Kombucha consumption against myocardial infarction. *International Journal of Science and Research*, *4*(6), 237–238.

Lobo, R. O., & Shenoy, C. K. (2015b). Myocardial potency of bio-tea against isoproterenol induced myocardial damage in rats. *Journal of Food Science and Technology*, *52*(7), 4491–4498.

Mahmoudi, E., Saeidi, M., Marashi, M. A., Moafi, A., Mahmoodi, V., & Zeinolabedini Zamani, M. (2016). In vitro activity of kombucha tea ethyl acetate fraction against *Malassezia* species isolated from seborrhoeic dermatitis. *Current Medical Mycology*, *2*(4), 30–36.

Marco, M. L., Pavan, S., & Kleerebezem, M. (2006). Towards understanding molecular modes of probiotic action. *Current Opinion in Biotechnology*, *17*(2), 204–210.

Market Research Future. (July 2020). *Global kefir market research report*. https://www.marketresearchfuture.com/reports/kefir-market-4367.

Marsh, A. J., O'Sullivan, O., Hill, C., Ross, R. P., & Cotter, P. D. (2013). Sequencing- based analysis of the bacterial and fungal composition of kefir grains and milks from multiple sources. *PLoS One*, *8*. https //doi.org/10.1371/journal.pone.0069371.

Marsh, A. J., O'Sullivan, O., Hill, C., Ross, R. P., & Cotter, P. D. (2014). Sequence-based analysis of the bacterial and fungal compositions of multiple kombucha (tea fungus) samples. *Food Microbiology*, *38*, 171–178.

Nalbantoglu, U., Cakar, A., Dogan, H., Abaci, N., Ustek, D., Sayood, K., et al. (2014). Metagenomic analysis of the microbial community in kefir grains. *Food Microbiology*, *41*, 42–51. https://doi.org/10.1016/j.fm.2014.01.014.

Nielsen, B., Gurakan, G. C., & Unlu, G. (2014). Kefir: A multifaceted fermented dairy product. *Probiotics and Antimicrobial Proteins*, *6*, 123–135.

Nielsen Insights. (2018). *No signs of fizzing out: America's love of sparkling water remains strong through August. (CPG, FMCG & Retail 08-24-2018)*. https://www.nielsen.com/us/en/insights/news/2018/no-signs-of-fizzing-out-americas-love-of-sparkling-water-remains-strong.html (Accessed 24 January 2020).

Nogay, N. H. (2019). Kefir beverage and its effects on health. In A. M. Grumezescu, & A. M. Holban (Eds.), *Milk-based beverages* (pp. 273–296). Cambridge: Woodhead Publishing.

Osburn, K., Amaral, J., Metcalf, S. R., Nickens, D. M., Rogers, C. M., Sausen, C., et al. (2018). Primary souring: A novel bacteria-free method for sour beer production. *Food Microbiology*, *70*, 76–84.

Ostadrahimi, A., Taghizadeh, A., Mobasseri, M., Farrin, N., Payahoo, L., Gheshlaghi, Z. B., et al. (2015). Effect of probiotic fermented milk (kefir) on glycemic control and lipid profile in type 2 diabetic patients: A randomized double-blind placebo-controlled clinical trial. *Iranian Journal of Public Health*, *44*, 228–237.

Otles, S., & Cagindi, O. (2003). Kefir: A probiotic dairy-composition, nutritional and therapeutic aspects. *Pakistan Journal of Nutrition, 2*, 54–59.

Panda, S. K. (2019). *Technology for wine and beer production from Ipomoea batatas*. Boca Raton: CRC Press.

Pereira, T. M. C., Pimenta, F. S., & Porto, M. L. (2016). Coadjuvants in the diabetic complications: Nutraceuticals and drugs with pleiotropic effects. *International Journal of Molecular Sciences, 17*. https://doi.org/10.3390/ijms17081273/.

Prado, M. R. M., Boller, C., Zibetti, R. G. M., de Souza, D., Pedroso, L. L., & Soccol, C. R. (2016). Anti-inflammatory and angiogenic activity of polysaccharide extract obtained from Tibetan kefir. *Microvascular Research, 108*, 29–33.

Puerari, C., Magalhaes, K. T., & Schwan, R. F. (2012). New cocoa pulp-based kefir beverages: Microbiological, chemical composition and sensory analysis. *Food Research International, 48*, 634–640.

Rafie, N., Hamedani, S. G., Ghiasvand, R., & Miraghajani, M. (2015). Kefir and cancer: A systematic review of literatures. *Archives of Iranian Medicine, 18*(12), 852–857.

Randazzo, W., Corona, O., Guarcello, R., Francesca, N., Germana, M. A., Erten, H., et al. (2016). Development of new non-dairy beverages from Mediterranean fruit juices fermented with water kefir microorganisms. *Food Microbiology, 54*, 40–51.

Rizzoli, R., & Biver, E. (2017). Effects of fermented milk products on bone. *Calcified Tissue International, 102*(4), 489–500. https://doi.org/10.1007/s00223-017-0317-9.

Rosa, D. D., Dias, M. M., Grzeskowiak, Ł. M., Reis, S. A., Conceiçao, L. L., & Maria do Carmo, G.P. (2017). Milk kefir: Nutritional, microbiological and health benefits. *Nutrition Research Reviews, 30*, 82–96.

Rouse, S., & van Sinderen, D. (2008). Bioprotective potential of lactic acid bacteria in malting and brewing. *Journal of Food Protection, 71*(8), 1724–1733.

Sahu, L., & Panda, S. K. (2018). Innovative technologies and implications in fermented food and beverage industries: An overview. In S. K. Panda, & P. H. C. Shetty (Eds.), *Innovations in technologies for fermented food and beverage industries* (pp. 1–23). Switzerland: Springer.

Sahu, L., Panda, S. K., Paramithiotis, S., Zdolec, N., & Ray, R. C. (2016). Biogenic amines in fermented foods: Overview. In D. Montet, & R. C. Ray (Eds.), *Fermented foods, Part I: Biochemistry and biotechnology* (pp. 318–332). Boca Raton: CRC Press.

Santos, R. J., Jr., Batista, R. A., Rodrigues, S. A., Filho, L. U. X., & Lima, A. S. (2009). Antimicrobial activity of broth fermented with Kombucha colonies. *Journal of Microbial and Biochemical Technology, 1*(1), 72–78.

Sharifi, M., Moringa, A., & Mortazavi, D. (2017). Kefir: A powerful probiotic with anticancer properties. *Medical Oncology, 34*(11), 183. https://doi.org/10.1007/s12032-017-1044-9.

Spitaels, F., Wieme, A. D., Janssens, M., Aerts, M., Van Landschoot, A., De Vuyst, L., et al. (2015). The microbial diversity of an industrially produced lambic beer shares members of a traditionally produced one and reveals a core microbiota for lambic beer fermentation. *Food Microbiology, 49*, 23–32. https://doi.org/10.1016/j.fm.2015.01.008.

Sun, T. Y., Li, J. S., & Chen, C. (2015). Effects of blending wheatgrass juice on enhancing phenolic compounds and antioxidant activities of traditional kombucha beverage. *Journal of Food and Drug Analysis, 23*, 709–718.

Thompson Witrick, K., Duncan, S., Hurley, K., & O'Keefe, S. F. (2017). Acid and volatiles of commercially-available lambic beers. *Beverages, 3*(4), 51. https://doi.org/10.3390/beverages3040051.

Transparency Market Research. (2014). *Kombucha market - global industry analysis, size, share, growth, trends and forecast 2016–2023*. https://www.transparencymarketresearch.com/kombucha-market.html.

Tu, C., Tang, S., Azi, F., Hu, W., & Dong, M. (2019). Use of kombucha consortium to transform soy whey into a novel functional beverage. *Journal of Functional Foods, 52*, 81–89.

Viana, R. O., Magalhaaes-Guedesa, K. T., Braga, R. A., Jr., Diasc, D. R., & Schwan, R. F. (2017). Fermentation process for production of apple-based kefir vinegar: Microbiological, chemical and sensory analysis. *Brazilian Journal of Microbiology, 48*, 592–601.

Villarreal-Soto, S. A., Beauforta, S., Bouajilaa, J., Soucharda, J. P., Renard, T., Rollan, S., et al. (2019). Impact of fermentation conditions on the production of bioactive compounds with anticancer, anti-inflammatory and antioxidant properties in kombucha tea extracts. *Process Biochemistry, 83*, 44–54.

Walsh, A. M., Crispie, F., Kilcawley, K., O'Sullivan, O., O'Sullivan, M. G., Claesson, M. J., et al. (2016). Microbial succession and flavor production in the fermented dairy beverage kefir. *Msystems, 1*(5). https://doi.org/10.1128/msystems.00052-16. e00052-16.

Watson, E. (2018). *Fermentation on fire: US retail sales of kombucha and other fermented beverages surged 37.4% in 2017*. https://www.foodnavigator-usa.com/Article/2018/02/13/Fermentation-on-fire-US-retail-sales-of-kombucha-and-other-fermented-beverages-surged-37.4-in-2017# (Accessed 24 January 2020).

Wyk, J. V. (2019). Kefir: The champagne of fermented beverages. In A. M. Grumezescu, & A. M. Holban (Eds.), *Fermented beverages* (pp. 473–527). Cambridge: Woodhead Publishing.

Yuniarto, A., Anggadiredja, K., & Aqidah, R. A. N. (2016). Antifungal activity of kombucha tea against human pathogenic fungi. *Asian Journal of Pharmaceutical and Clinical Research, 9*(5), 253–255. https://doi.org/10.22159/ajpcr.2016.v9i5.13432.

CHAPTER

15

Probiotic lactobacillus strains for enhanced health benefits (genetic engineering and microencapsulation)

Gargi Dey[a], Didier Montet[b], and Phillippe Thonart[c]

[a]School of Biotechnology, KIIT University, Bhubaneswar, India, [b]UMR95 QualiSud Cirad Université of Montpellier, Montpellier, France, [c]Walloon Center for Industrial Biology, Microbial Technology Unit, University of Liège, Gembloux, Belgium

15.1 Introduction

The spread of food-borne pathogens and emerging low grade inflammation and related co-morbidities are prevailing health concerns. Several conventional and nonconventional strategies have evolved over the past decade to address these concerns. Among these, the popular one that is being explored widely is in the application of probiotic formulations. A survey of the current market shows an impressive list of both dairy and nondairy probiotic food formats fortified with different strains of lactobacillus. There is immense scope for improvement in this field. One of the most recent developments in this field is that of bioengineered probiotic strains designed to possess properties to prevent or alleviate specific pathogens and inflammatory conditions. There is the possibility of acquiring tailor-made probiotic strains through the application of genetic engineering techniques. This chapter focuses on various strategies that can be used to design recombinant probiotic strains and the wide range of infection and disease conditions where these strains may be applied as effective therapeutic solutions. Considering the complexity of the intestinal

https://doi.org/10.1016/B978-0-12-818588-9.00015-2

environment, many more beneficial effects may be harnessed by way of influencing the composition and activities of the gut microbiota. For instance, the performance of the probiotic strains can definitely be enhanced further, be it for production of antiinfectives, toxin neutralization, enhancement of anti-inflammatory responses, as oral vaccines, or for antitumor potential.

15.2 Current global probiotic products

The probiotic market is expected to reach 76.8 billion USD by 2024 (MarketWatch Press Release, 2019). Initially, when probiotic products emerged in the market, dairy products were the main food formats and vehicles. With each passing year, this segment of the market has witnessed a number of innovations, especially from the production point of view. Most of the advances have been in the selection of probiotic cultures and in technological improvements for the preservation and survival of probiotic cultures during storage periods. However, the most dramatic innovations that the global market has seen have been in the development of numerous nondairy probiotic products. Emerging evidence has confirmed that gut healthy products may be developed from synergistic formulations of plant carbohydrates and phenolics. This rationale has been widely adapted by food companies, which now offer a wide range of probiotic products based on fruit, vegetable, and cereal food formats. The current non-dairy commercial products that are being marketed globally are summarized in Table 15.1.

15.3 Emerging techniques for future probiotics

There are still several bottlenecks and gaps in the current technology and new nondairy food formats pose their own set of challenges, necessitating standardization of each type of formulation and technological upgrades. Furthermore, health will continue to be at the forefront of novel product development. To date, conventional probiotic strains have been applied for prevention of diseases.

Fortunately, to sustain the global demand for more innovation, there have been continuous efforts to meet these demands. Research has focused on emerging techniques for designing genetically engineered lactobacillus strains with health benefits and disease reduction potentials. In parallel, techniques such as microencapsulation are being fine-tuned to achieve technological advancements in product development platforms.

TABLE 15.1 Current global non-dairy probiotic products based on *Lactobacillus* strains.

Sl no	Brand name	Food format	Probiotic strain	Country
1.	Biola	Fruit juice	*Lb. rhamnosus*	Norway
2.	Danone-Proviva	Fruit drink	*Lb. plantarum*	Sweden
3.	Bravo Easy kit for fruit juice	Fruit juice	*Lb. salivarius* *Lb. acidophilus* *Lb. casei, Lb. rhamnosus, Lactococcus lactis, Bifidobacterium*	Switzerland
4.	Body Ecology Passion Fruit Biotic	Passion fruit	*Lb. acidophilus* *Lb. delbrueckii*	USA
5.	Garden of Life RAW organic Kids Probiotic	Raw organic fruits and vegetable blend	*Lb. gasseri, Lb. plantarum, Lb. casei, Lb. acidophilus, B. lactis*	USA
6.	Good Belly	Fruit juice drink	*Lb. plantarum 299v*	USA
7.	ProbiBravo Friscus	Fruit drink	*Lb. plantarum, Lb. paracasei*	Sweden
8.	Healthy Life Probiotic Juice	Fruit juice	*Lb. plantarum, Lb. paracasei*	Australia
9.	Oasis, health Break Probiotic juice	Fruit juice	*Lb. rhamnosus*	Canada
10.	Rela, Biogaia	Fruit juice	*Lb. reuteri*	Sweden
11.	Valio Bioprofit	Fruit juice	*Lb. rhamnosus*	Finland
12.	Macrolife, Macrogreens Superfood Bars	Cereal Bars	*Lb. acidophilus* *Lb. rhamnosus* *Lb. bulgaricus* *B. longus* *B. breve*	USA
13.	Yog Active Probiotic cereals	Cereals	*Lb. acidophilus*	Germany
14.	Daiya	Coconut cream and Pea protein	*Lb. plantarum* *Lb. casei*	Canada
15.	Rainbow Light Probiolicious Gummies	Berry Flavored	*Lb. sporogenes*	USA
16.	ProDenta	Chewing gum	*Lb. reuteri* Prodentis	Sweden
17.	CocoBiotic	Organic grains and Wild Crafted coconuts	*Lb. acidophilus* *Lb. delbrueckii*	Australia

From Dey, G. (2018). Non dairy probiotic foods: Innovations and market trends, In: S. Panda & P.H. Shetty (Eds.), Innovations in technologies for fermented food and beverages industries *(pp. 19–174). Springer.*

In the next sections of this chapter, the recent aspects of genetic engineering and microencapsulation techniques applied in this field are discussed. This chapter also includes an in-depth discussion on the diverse range of new probiotic strains that have been designed to target different disease conditions.

15.3.1 Genetic engineering techniques for designing novel probiotic strains

The discovery of several genetic tools for the engineering of probiotic strains has provided a deeper understanding of the host microbiota interactions and the underlying mechanisms, thereby facilitating the engineering of strain variants with tailored functionalities (Shigemori & Shimosato, 2017; Yadav, Kumar, Baweja, & Shukla, 2018). Clustered Regularly Interspaced Short Palindromic Repeats (CRISPR) is one such technology that has accelerated the evolution of gene editing across the globe (Barrangou & Notebaart, 2019). CRISPR and its associated Cas proteins are comprised of adaptive immune systems against foreign nucleic acid, such as phages and plasmids (Hidalgo-Cantabrana, O'Flaherty, & Barrangou, 2017). They are a part of the prokaryotic defense system and are present in several bacterial species and in most archaeal species. Apart from the potential role as a genome editing tool in eukaryotes, several studies have also established the use of CRISPR-Cas9 systems in the genetic engineering of bacterial species, especially food-based starter cultures (Bravo & Landete, 2017). The CRISPR-Cas systems provide several advantages over phages and plasmids (Bikard & Barrangou, 2017; Flora & Welcker, 2017).

Currently, the CRISPR-Cas system is classified into three distinct types and ten subtypes for each of which signature genes have been identified. Typically, the Type I CRISPR mechanism contains the Cas3 gene with distinct helicase and DNase activities. The Type II CRISPR-Cas systems include the 'HNH'-type system and Cas9 that is required for gene silencing. The Type III CRISPR-Cas systems contain polymerase and RAMP modules, which can be further divided into subtypes III-A (Mtube or CASS6) and III-B (polymerase-RAMP module).

Among the three systems, Type II CRISPR-Cas is one of the most extensively studied systems owing to the programmable, precise, portable, and efficient Cas9 nuclease (Hidalgo-Cantabrana, Goh, & Barrangou, 2019). The Cas9 endonuclease can potentiate DNA binding and cleavage through an engineered single guide RNA (sgRNA) sequence. Therefore, utilizing the sequence-specific targeting of nucleic acid via RNA-guided CRISPR-associated (Cas) effector protein has provided an exciting platform for remodeling the defense machinery into programmable genome editing tools. For example, the Cas9 endonuclease from Streptococcus pyogenes (SpyCas9) Class 2 Type II CRISPR-Cas system can be transferred with a target-specific chimeric sgRNA for accurate cleavage of DNA (Jinek et al., 2012). CRISPR-based technologies have been used to edit several bacterial genomes, such as Escherichia coli, Streptococcus pneumoniae, *Clostridium sp.*, *Streptomyces sp.*, and probiotic *Lactobacillus* species (Goh & Barrangou, 2019). More specifically, in the case of lactobacilli, the endogenous Types I and II CRISPR-Cas systems can be used, as well as the heterologous expression of Types II and V systems can be utilized in strains that do not possess a functional CRISPR-Cas system (Goh & Barrangou, 2019). Also, the plasticity of bacterial genomes, along with the CRISPR-Cas systems, has become an important tool to improve the characteristics of probiotic strains through genome manipulation (Dy, Pitman, & Fineran, 2013). The presence of the CRISPR-Cas system in lactic acid bacteria (LAB) provides novel opportunities to specifically engineer these endogenous systems for various applications, including the delivery of self-targeting templates on plasmids for genotype alteration, which includes mutations, deletions, or insertions, by co-delivering recombination templates (Hidalgo-Cantabrana et al., 2017). It is also important to note that due to the ubiquitous nature of phages and mobile genetic elements in the native niches of lactobacillus species, the elements of the CRISPR-Cas systems are mostly found in the genus where the CRISPR repeats were detected (in 60% of the 1262 lactobacillus genomes). It has also been found that spacers in several species match to phages and plasmids. Analyzing the distribution of the complete CRISPR-Cas systems in lactobacilli showed an over representation of Type II (subtype A) systems, followed by Type I (subtype E) and III systems. However, Types IV, V, and VI CRISPR-cas systems were not detected in lactobacilli (Crawley, Henriksen, Stout, Brandt, & Barrangou, 2018). Although some species possess the Type II systems, others encode the Type I systems and notably Lactobacillus fermentum and *Lactobacillus salivarius* possess all three systems (Goh & Barrangou, 2019). It is important to note that the CRISPR-Cas systems are universal among strains of *Lactobacillus jensenii* and *Lactobacillus mucosae*, whereas all *Lactobacillus acidophilus* strains have degenerated CRISPR loci, with only remnants of CRISPR arrays present in the genome. The Type II systems in lactobacilli provide for the exploitation of novel Cas9 proteins that have properties distinct from the canonical SpyCas9, SthCas9, SauCas9, or NmeCas9 for CRISPR editing with expanded PAM specificities. Certain examples of the utilization if endogenous Types I and II systems and heterologous Types II and V systems for engineering of probiotic lactobacilli as living therapeutics have been taken into account in this chapter. CRISPR-Cas systems in lactobacilli are considered to be able to facilitate the engineering of probiotics to enhance the inherent properties of the strains for improved therapeutic functionality. It is important for a probiotic strain to be able to withstand diverse environments for optimum functionality in the host environment (Capozzi, Arena, Russo, Spano, & Fiocco, 2015). For instance, overexpression of groESL, a native molecular chaperone or a heterologous expression of a listerial betaine uptake system, was demonstrated by Lactobacillus paracasei and *Bifidobacterium breve* to improve stress tolerance including temperature, oxidative, and osmotic stress (Corcoran, Stanton, Fitzgerald, & Ross, 2008). Another important factor that promotes stress tolerance in probiotics is the potential to synthesize glycogen, exopolysaccharide (EPS) production, expression of cell surface adhesins, and enhanced expression of exporter systems for bile detoxification (Caggianiello, Kleerebezem, & Spano, 2016; Hosseini Nezhad, Hussain, & Britz, 2015). All of these factors can be modulated to potentiate functionality of probiotics under in vivo conditions (Sleator & Hill, 2008). The human gut microbiota modulates the bioactivities of glycosylated phytochemicals, thereby affecting host physiology and the composition of the gut microbiota (Hernandez-Hernandez, 2019). Therefore, introduction of these sugar catabolic genes, via the CRISPR-based gene knock-in technology, can be considered as a promising approach for enhanced utilization of such complex oligosaccharides. In a study by Goh, Lee, and Hutkins (2007), the authors induced a FosE operon into a non-FOS fermenting strain (Lactobacillus rhamnosus GG), thereby enabling the strain to metabolize FOS, inulin, sucrose, and levan. Therefore by integrating the CRISPR-Cas systems, one could introduce new probabilities for genome enhancement of probiotics to improve host health along with enhancing the functional attributes of existing characteristics. *Streptococcus thermophilus*, due to its native CRISPR-Cas systems, has been used extensively as a screening tool for the selection of specific genotypes occurring in a heterologous population (Hao, Cui, & Qu, 2018; Lander, 2016).

Also, this system has been used to modulate important characteristics enhancing the starter culture phenotype, for instance EPS production (Xiong et al., 2019). A single nucleotide mutation can be introduced into polymerase epsC using the CRISPR-Cas system, along with a plasmid carrying a targeting guide RNA, and a donor template sequence containing the mutation that results in the production of a different EPS with altered properties (Hidalgo-Cantabrana et al., 2015). Several CRISPR-Cas systems have been identified in other LAB strains, such as *Lactococcus lactis* and *Bifidobacterium*, which can be exploited to enhance probiotic traits so as to improve industrial manufacturing techniques, human health, and immune modulation (Briner et al., 2015; Ichikawa et al., 2017; Millen et al., 2019). The CRISPR-Cas systems can also be used to enhance the bile salt hydrolase activity of probiotics by replacing the original promoter of bshA with a highly efficient pgm promoter, enhancing bshA transcription and boosting bshA activity (Ruiz, Margolles, & Sánchez, 2013; Yang et al., 2019).

The cell surface of probiotic organisms is an important factor as it initiates molecular interactions between the bacteria and host cells (Kim et al., 2010). By targeting the fibronectin-binding proteins (Fbp), mucin-binding proteins (Mub), collagen-binding proteins (Cbp) via the CRISPR-Cas systems can be used to enhance host colonization and gut retention properties of probiotics or even to modulate the host immune response (Johnson et al., 2016). Also, the application of the CRISPR-Cas systems can be used for rational designing of vaccines and aid in precise genome engineering for targeted delivery (Klotz & Barrangou, 2018). This can be applied to design vaccines for mucosal delivery to sexually transmitted diseases, selectively target antibiotic resistance genes, and screen the loss of antibiotic resistance genes.

Specifically in food, the CRISPR-Cas systems can also be used to selectively remove spoilage bacteria by utilizing CRISPR-based antimicrobials and allowing for the alteration of complex ecological niche composition, while in parallel, improving human health. Overall, this technique can be used to enhance and modulate the functionality of probiotic strains and aid in developing the next generation of food cultures with novel traits.

15.3.2 Applications of genetically engineered probiotic organisms for improved health benefits

Genetically, engineered probiotics can have a pivotal role in nutrition, therapeutics and in health industries. In recent years, genetically modified probiotics have been designed for efficient and site-specific delivery of gene therapy vectors, drugs, for the synthesis of physiologically active metabolites, as well as for diagnostic aids. Modern tools of synthetic biology and genetic engineering facilitate the construction of genetic circuits and precise fine-tuning of transgenic expressions.

15.3.2.1 Genetically modified probiotic strains targeting inflammatory bowel disease and irritable bowel syndrome

Several irritable bowel syndrome (IBS) susceptible genes have linked the pathogenesis of IBD to the gut mucosal homeostasis, innate and adaptive immunity, and stress response (Loddo & Romano, 2015; Zhao & Burisch, 2019). A balanced interplay between the pro-inflammatory markers (tumor necrosis factor, TNF-α, IL-1β) and the anti-inflammatory markers (IL-10, TGF-β) is known to play a crucial role in controlling inflammatory responses in patients with IBD. Various studies in the past have shown the efficacy of monoclonal antibodies against TNF-α in the maintenance of remission in patients suffering from ulcerative colitis (UC) and Crohn's disease (CD) (Crowe et al., 2018; Nedelkopoulou,

Vadamalayan, Vergani, & Mieli-Vergani, 2017). Although the anti-TNF-α antibodies have limited side effects, the immunogenic property can lead to allergic responses, autoimmune diseases, or primary resistance to the anti-TNF-α antibodies (Murdaca, Colombo, & Puppo, 2009; Protic, Schoepfer, Yawalkar, Vavricka, & Seibold, 2016). Considering that at least some of these adverse effects would be prevented by changing the path of the drug delivery from parenteral to enteral, in addition to avoiding the risk of antibody degradation during digestion, Simčič, Berlec, Stopinšek, and Štrukelj (2019) developed a recombinant *L. lactis* that could bind to TNF-α. The recombinant *L. lactis,* being a non-adherent strain, would not just be excreted along with TNF-α. The authors suggested that more than 85% of the binding capacity could be retained when incubated under simulated gastric conditions. They evaluated the TNF-α binding capacity of the genetically engineered *L. lactis* bearing TNF-α affibodies and their role in down-regulating the immune response in IBD subjects ex vivo. Recombinant *L. lactis* at a concentration of 1×10^9 and 1×10^8 CFU/mL, could bind to TNF-α by 22.6% and 18.4%, respectively ($p < 0.05$). The genetically modified *L. lactis* in cultures of inflamed intestinal tissues from IBD patients significantly increased the expression of IL-10 and downregulated the expression of TNF-α and IL-1β in comparison to the sterile culture. They reported that the genetically engineered *L. lactis* containing TNF-α affibodies bound to TNF-α by $62.8 \pm 11.9\%$ ($p = 0.026$) relative to the control in mucosal tissues from 11 IBD patients. Overall, *L. lactis* could therefore constitute a promising alternative approach for treating IBD.

IBS is characterized by chronic abdominal pain and intestinal dysfunction, which has been associated with psychological stress, increased gut permeability, altered gut motility, and more recently, the presence of a low grade inflammation of the gut mucosa. Several authors have reported on the potential of probiotic strains in the secretion of the anti-inflammatory cytokine, IL-10, as a therapy in the treatment of gastrointestinal inflammation (Wadwa et al., 2016; Yanaba et al., 2011). In research conducted by Martín et al. (2014), genetically modified *L. lactis* was observed to secrete IL-10 under a stress-inducible controlled expression system and its efficacy was tested in a dinitrobenzenesulfonic acid-induced chronic inflammatory model in mice. They reported that oral administration of the genetically engineered *L. lactis* secreting IL-10 gave significantly higher protection in terms of gut permeability and activation of immune functions. Surprisingly, it was reported that the wild-type *L. lactis* strain failed to decrease the intestinal hyperpermeability significantly ($P > 0.05$). This study suggests the possibility for the use of an IL-10-producing strain to treat inflammation mediated colitis in patients suffering from functional disorders such as IBS.

Nitric oxide (NO) is another important biomarker in patients with IBD (Soufli, Toumi, Rafa, & Touil-Boukoffa, 2016). The levels of NO produced by intestinal epithelial cells is 100 fold higher in patients with IBD, compared to healthy subjects (Baranipour et al., 2018). NO is also produced by macrophages as an antimicrobial agent (Krausz et al., 2015; Kutty, Ho, & Kumar, 2017); however, most bacteria have evolved over time to develop a resistance to NO exposure (Privett, Broadnax, Bauman, Riccio, & Schoenfisch, 2012). In this context, McKay et al., 2018 developed a genetically engineered probiotic E. coli that selectively synthesizes a model biotherapeutic, a granulocyte macrophage-colony stimulating factor (GM-CSF). The authors reported that GM-CSF has the ability to restore the gut mucosal barrier function via interactions with epithelial cells and also to act as an agonist against pathogenic strains. They reported on the ability of this genetically engineered probiotic strain to accumulate at sites with elevated NO concentrations and that it could secrete GM-CSF, which was biologically active. Further, in an *in vitro* CD model, the authors also demonstrated activation of the probiotic strain in the presence of NO, with an increased expression of GM-CSF in response to basal NO secretion. Overall, this study suggests interesting concepts that can be utilized to develop "smart" probiotic strains for the treatment of IBD, by incorporating therapeutic genes.

In another study by Del Carmen et al. (2014), a genetically modified probiotic strain of S. thermophilus CRL 807 produced anti-oxidant enzymes, which reduced the severity of inflammation in a trinitrobenzenesulfonic acid (TNBS)-induced colitis model. S. thermophilus CRL 807 was transformed with plasmid harboring genes encoding catalase (CAT) and superoxide dismutase (SOD). With the genetically modified probiotic strain, there was a significant reduction in histological scores, weight loss, and lower liver microbial translocation. The genetically modified strain could also regulate cytokine production by increasing the expression of the anti-inflammatory cytokine IL-10 and decreasing the expression of the pro-inflammatory cytokine IL-17 in the gut of TNBS treated mice. Overall, this study suggests there is a clinical use for genetically modified (GM) probiotics. Genetically, engineered S. thermophilus CRL 807 was developed through the introduction of a gene expressing an anti-oxidant enzyme, showed enhanced anti-inflammatory activities, and the authors suggest its usefulness as a novel therapeutic target for IBD.

The oxidative stress in host cells are counteracted by a series of complex anti-oxidant mechanisms involving several enzymatic and non-enzymatic components, such as SOD, CAT, glutathione peroxidase (GSH-Px), glutathione reductase (GR), glutathione-s-transferase (GST), vitamin E, vitamin C, and melatonin (Pereira, Grácio, Teixeira, & Magro, 2015; Zhang & Tsao, 2016). However, during excessive oxidant-generating conditions, the normal antioxidant mechanism may be insufficient. Several researchers have depicted the role of reactive oxygen metabolites in mediating intestinal damage in IBD, thereby disrupting epithelial integrity and initiating the inflammatory pathways (Pavlick et al., 2002; Zuo et al., 2017). In this context, Han et al., 2006 studied the efficacy of live recombinant SOD producing probiotic strains (*L. lactis* and *L. plantarum*) in improving TNBS induced experimental colitis in rats. A significant reduction in microscopic and macroscopic damage, myeloperoxidase (MPO) activity, and attenuation of nitrotyrosine was mediated by the wild type *L. lactis* strain and the genetically engineered *Lb. lactis* and *Lb. plantarum* strain, but not wild-type *Lb. plantarum* strain. Overall, the efficiency of the recombinant SOD-producing LAB in enhancing the anti-inflammatory potential of the probiotic strains in experimental colitis was shown, which could potentially be used as a novel therapeutic target in the treatment of IBD.

Another study investigated the therapeutic ability of a recombinant *Lactobacillus gasseri* producing manganese (Mn) SOD from S. thermophilus to reduce the symptoms of experimental colitis in IL-10 deficient mice (Carroll et al., 2007). Mn SOD is an isoform of SOD found in humans, which is known to have protective effects in IBD. The results of this study showed that *Lb. gasseri* expressing MnSOD could significantly reduce inflammation in IL-10 deficient mice compared to untreated mice. It also showed that MnSOD producing *Lb. gasseri* could retain normal numbers of goblet cells and the crypt architecture in the colitis mice model. The study demonstrated the role of MnSOD in enhancing the anti-inflammatory properties of *Lb. gasseri* for colitis.

Leblanc and co-workers (LeBlanc et al., 2011) studied the anti-inflammatory effects of genetically engineered *Lb. casei* BL23 producing catalase (CAT) and SOD in a TNBS-induced colitis model. It was revealed that the mice administered with the genetically modified CAT and SOD producing *Lb. casei* BL23 recovered faster in terms of initial weight loss, increased intestinal enzymatic activity, and downregulation of intestinal inflammation compared to the mice treated with the wild-type probiotic strain or the untreated animals. Mice that were treated with the CAT or SOD producing strains showed lower microbial counts in the liver compared to the TNBS treated group, elucidating the role of CAT+ and SOD+ *Lb. casei* BL23 in attenuating TNBS induced damage in a mice model of colitis.

Genetically modified probiotics for production of anti-inflammatory compounds

In another study, *L. lactis* was genetically modified to produce murine TNF neutralizing nanobodies, as therapeutic proteins against inflammatory markers in dextran sulfate sodium (DSS)-induced chronic colitis (Vandenbroucke et al., 2010). Administration of an anti-mTNF nanobody secreting *L. lactis* was shown to significantly reduce inflammation in colitis-induced mice. The nanobody secreting *L. lactis* was also efficient in downregulating signs of enterocolitis in IL-10 deficient mice and specificity of the nanobodies was reported. The *L. lactis* producing anti-m TNF nanobodies did not induce a systemic immune intervention in IL-10 deficient mice in comparison to the systemic anti-TNF therapy. These results suggest a possible therapeutic application of this recombinant LAB strain in the treatment of IBD in humans.

IL-27, belonging to the IL-12 family, is reported to play an important role in immune suppression (Zwirner & Ziblat, 2017). It has the ability to antagonize Th17 development, induce anti-inflammatory cytokine IL-10 production, inhibit IL-6 induced T-cell proliferation, and promote T-regulatory cell generation. Low expression of IL-27 gene has also been reported to be associated with the early onset of IBD in humans (Hanson et al., 2014). Hanson and co-workers (Hanson et al., 2014) investigated the mucosal delivery of immunosuppressive IL-27 by a genetically modified *L. lactis* and its ability to downregulate markers of chronic enterocolitis in mice. They reported that administration of the recombinant *L. lactis* protected the murine models from T-cell transfer induced enterocolitis and mortality. The disease activity scores histological features were regulated upon recombinant *L. lactis* treatment. Also, the levels of pro-inflammatory cytokines IL-1α, IL-6, IFN-γ, and IL-23 were significantly reduced and increased expression of IL-1α was reported in mice treated with recombinant *L. lactis*. The recombinant strain was also reported to reduce the numbers of CD4+ and IL-17+ T cells in gut-associated lymphoid tissue and was effective in reducing colitis in mice by increasing the production of IL-10.

The roles of proteases and their endogenous inhibitors in the pathology of IBD have been established (Carroll & Maharshak, 2013). Intestinal tissues from IBD subjects have shown an increased proteolytic activity (Siddiqui, Majid, & Abid, 2017). This can be attributed to either an upregulation of protease expression, or a decreased expression of endogenous protease inhibitors, or both. Motta et al. (2011) reported that transgenic mice producing human Elafin, an endogenous serine protease inhibitor, could successfully protect different mice models of IBD. Therefore, in 2015 Bermúdez-Humarán et al. (2015) developed recombinant strains of *L. lactis* that could secrete two anti-inflammatory cytokines, IL-10 and TGF-β1, and a serine protease inhibitor (Elafin and Secretory Leukocyte Protease Inhibitor — SLPI) and tested efficacy in a DSS-induced mouse model of colitis. The study revealed that administration with either of the recombinant *L. lactis* secreting serine protease inhibitors, Elafin or SLPI, could attenuate intestinal inflammation and significantly reduce all clinical parameters of inflammation, including macroscopic and microscopic colonic damage scores, colon thickness, and MPO activities compared to mice treated with the wild-type strain of *L. lactis*. Interestingly, the protective effect was much lower in the case of mice treated with recombinant *L. lactis* producing IL-10 or TGF-B1. The best result was seen in case of mice treated with Elafin producing *L. lactis*, suggesting efficiency of serine protease inhibitors as anti-inflammatory agents for the treatment of IBD.

Trefoil factors belong to the class of non-mitogenic peptides that play an active role in the protection and repair of the intestinal epithelium (Remaut, Braat, Vandenbroucke, Rotteiers, & Steidler, 2006). Due to their dense structure, they are resistant to proteases. Several studies had shown the protective or healing effect of trefoil peptides in different models of intestinal inflammation; however, no reports have documented the development of trefoil-based drugs in the treatment of IBD. Moreover, orally administered TFF could be non-beneficial as it adheres to the mucus of the small intestine and is absorbed at the caecum. Therefore, in 2004, Vandenbrouchke and coworkers (Vandenbroucke et al., 2004) developed a recombinant *L. lactis* producing TFF and evaluated its ability to protect against DSS-induced colitis in a murine model. Administration of TFF-secreting *L. lactis* resulted in targeted delivery of TFF at the mucosa of the colon. They reported a significant decrease in morbidity, mortality, and enhanced healing in mice treated with the recombinant strain of *L. lactis* producing TFF. The strain also stimulated the expression of prostaglandin-endoperoxide synthase 2. Transgenic mice deficient of the IL-10 gene also showed protection against DSS-induced colitis and improvement in the inflammatory parameters upon being treated with TFF producing *L. lactis*, suggesting an opportunity for the utilization of such a recombinant strain for effective management of colitis and epithelial damage in humans.

The enzyme 15-lipoxygenase-1 (15-LOX-1) plays a pivotal role in the oxidative metabolism of arachidonic acid, thereby producing lipoxin, a potent anti-inflammatory agent. Lipoxin A_4 (LXA_4) is not just known to stimulate the phagocytosis of apoptotic leukocytes by macrophages, but also aids in inhibiting superoxide and peroxynitrite formation and expression of IL-8 (József, Zouki, Petasis, Serhan, & Filep, 2002; Sodin-Semrl, Taddeo, Tseng, Varga, & Fiore, 2000). LXA_4 has been reported to inhibit the activator protein-1 (AP-1) and nuclear factor-kB in human leukocytes. In spite of being a small potent molecule, the short half-life of lipoxin in vivo makes usage limited as an anti-inflammatory agent. In 2014, Saraiva et al. (2015) used a recombinant *L. lactis* secreting 15-LOX-1 enzyme to deliver lipoxins, at the site of inflammation in the intestines, and tested anti-inflammatory efficacy in a TNBS induced IBD model. Administration of fermented milk (by recombinant *L. lactis* producing 15-LOX-1) depicted a significant reduction in intestinal damage associated with inflammatory bowel disease. The experimental group treated with the recombinant *L. lactis* showed the least decrease in live body weight compared to the TNBS treated control and the wild type *L. lactis* treated group. The lowest macroscopic and microscopic damage scores were recorded in the mice treated with the fermented milk by the *L. lactis* strain producing 15-LOX1, suggesting potential in combating inflammation in patients with colitis with the 15-LOX 1 producing strain *L. lactis*.

Genetically engineered probiotics in the production of anti-inflammatory cytokine IL-10

Different approaches in IL-10 delivery In 2013, Del Carmen et al. (2013) developed a genetically engineered strain of *L. lactis* that secreted fibronectin-binding protein A (FnBPA+) from Staphylococcus aureus. They studied its site specific ability to deliver pValac:il-I0, using a eukaryotic DNA expression vector which contained the ORF coding for IL-I0 of Mus musculus directly inside of the eukaryotic cells. The use of *L. lactis* secreting FnBPA+ A can be attributed to its ability to act as an adhesion, or an invasion, facilitating the adhesion or internalization into the host cells. Experimental mice fed with *L. lactis* MO1363 FnBPA+ containing pValac:il-I0 were found to have significantly decreased severity of TNBS-induced colitis, compared to the *L. lactis* MG1363 FnBPA+ (Wt group) or to mice without any treatment. A significant decrease in the mean histological score was reported along with a decrease in the body weight loss in mice administered with *L. lactis* MO1363 FnBPA+ containing pValac:il-I0. Mice administered with *L. lactis* MO1363 FnBPA+ containing pValac:il-I0 also aided in a significant decrease in the IL-17+ cells and in an increase in the ratio of IL-10/L-17 producing cells in comparison to the other treatment groups, suggesting that *L. lactis* MG 1363 FnBPA+ pValac:IL-l0 was a potential candidate as a DNA-delivery agent in the treatment of IBD in humans.

Zurita-Turk et al. (2014) evaluated the therapeutic potential of two *L. lactis* strains, the invasive *L. lactis* MG1363 FnBPA + strain, and the wild-type *L. lactis* MG1363 carrying the pValac:il-10 plasmid, a eukaryotic DNA expression vector coding for IL-10, in combating experimental inflammation induced by DSS in a murine model. They found that both of the strains carrying the pValac:il-10 plasmid were capable of downregulating intestinal inflammation in experimental mice models. Both groups showed a lower disease activity index, histological activity index, and an improvement in colon length, in comparison to the DSS control group and the *L. lactis* MG1363 FnBPA + strain, and the *L. lactis* MG1363 strains devoid the pValac:il-10 plasmid. Furthermore, only the mice receiving *L. lactis* MG1363 FnBPA + pValac:il-10 showed a significant increase in IL-10 levels and the concentration of secretory immunoglobulins A (IgA), a first line of defense against mucosal compromise, absent in case of IBD compared to the other test groups. The potential of *L. lactis* MG1363 FnBPA + pValac:il-10 as a good candidate for combating intestinal inflammation was confirmed.

The *L. lactis* strain NCDO2118 has been reported to possess a novel regulated expression system, with the ability to target heterologous proteins to the cytoplasm or to the extracellular medium (Asensi et al., 2013). Another expression system, namely the xylose-inducible expression system (XIES) has been reported to be highly controlled and efficient in producing high levels of long-term targeted proteins (Miyoshi et al., 2004). Del Carmen et al. (2011) reported the anti-inflammatory effects of a milk fermented with *L. lactis* producing IL-10 using the XIES system in a TNBS-induced coltis murine model. Results revealed a significant increase in body weight and a decrease in liver microbial translocation in mice administered with recombinant *L. lactis*, Sec strain (targeted Il-10 delivery in the extracellular medium) post TNBS induction in comparison to the *L. lactis*, Cyt strain (targeted IL-10 delivery in the cytoplasm). Both recombinant strains, Cyt and Sec, were reported to be efficient in lowering histological damage scores compared to the wild type treated group or the TNBS control group. A slight increase in the IL-10-producing immune cells was observed in mice receiving milks fermented by the Cyt or Sec strains, compared to those from the TNBS and the TNBS-Wt group. The study also revealed an increase in the ratio of IL-10/IFN- γ, IL-10/IL-12, and IL-10/IL-17 in mice treated with Cyt and Sec fermented milk, compared to those from the TNBS and the TNBS-Wt groups. Overall, this study depicted the efficacy of IL-10 producing *L. lactis* in the treatment of IBD.

15.3.2.2 Genetically modified probiotic strains for other health applications

Hypertension

About 20% of the world population today is suffering from serious hypertension (Wijeratne et al., 2018). Reports suggest the association of serious hypertension with cardiovascular diseases and other disorders, such as dyslipidemia, abdominal obesity, glucose intolerance, hyperuremia, and hyperinsulinemia (Landsberg et al., 2013; Soltani, Rasheed, Kapusta, & Reisin, 2013; Wu, Gladden, Ahmed, Ahmed, & Filippatos, 2016). Angiotensin-converting enzymes (ACEs) are a dipeptidylcarboxypeptidase, which has an integral role in regulating blood pressure as a result of the renin-angiotensin system. ACE has the ability to transform the inactive peptide, angiotensin I into angiotensin II, a potent vasoconstrictor, thereby inactivating the catalytic function of bradykinin, a peptide that causes dilation of blood vessels (Tiret et al., 1994). Although synthetic ACE inhibitors are routinely used in the treatment of hypertension, they are often accompanied with side effects, such as skin rashes, difference in tastes, and coughs. An alternative strategy in the treatment of hypertension includes the development of natural ACE inhibitory peptides

(ACEIPs). One important ACEIP, belonging to the yellowfin sole frame protein (YFP) family, has been observed to significantly decrease blood pressure in hypertensive rats (Jung et al., 2006). Another study reported on the application of tuna frame protein (TFP) in reducing blood pressure in a hypertensive rat model (Lee, Qian, & Kim, 2010). Based on this information, in 2015 Yang and co-workers (Yang et al., 2015) investigated the potential of a genetically engineered Lactobacillus plantarum NC8 (producing recombinant ACEIP from YFP and TFP) and effects on regulation of hypertension. They reported that oral delivery of genetically modified *Lb. plantarum* NC8 (RLP) could significantly regulate blood pressure and that the effect lasted for approximately 10 days post treatment ($P < 0.01$). They also showed that treatment with RLP could reduce the angiotensin II and endothelin levels in the plasma, heart, and kidney of spontaneous hypertensive rats, along with a significant reduction in triglyceride levels, showing the potential of RLP in the treatment of hypertension.

Phenylketonuria

The inability to convert dietary phenylalanine to tyrosine by the hepatic enzyme phenylalanine hydroxylase (PAH), is mostly due to genetic mutations, and leads to phenylketonuria (Scriver, 2007). In the absence of active PAH, phenylalanine and its alternative metabolites, such as phenylketone, accumulate in the blood to neurotoxic levels, thereby leading to severe neurological damage, such as tremors, seizures, and even mental retardation (Dixon, MacDonald, White, & Stafford, 2015). The only effective treatment for phenylketonuria is restriction of dietary phenylalanine intake (Ahring et al., 2009). As an alternative strategy, Durrer, Allen, and Von Herbing (2017) genetically engineered Lactobacillus reuteri 100-23C, which could express a phenylalanine lyase gene from Anabaena variabilis (AvPAL). Treatment of phenylketonuria mice with recombinant Lactobacillus reuteri 100-23C resulted in a reduction of blood phenylalanine levels ($p < 0.0005$) compared to untreated controls. Furthermore fecal cultures revealed that *Lb. reuteri* 100-23C was recovered post-4 months of treatment with the recombinant strain. No immune response against AvPAL was reported during experimentation. The study provides interesting insights for the utilization of genetically engineered probiotic strains as a potential therapy for phenylketonuria.

Bacterial and viral infections

With the emergence of new pathogens, broader approaches for the development of anti-infective agents are needed and GM probiotics have the ability to deliver a combined therapy of antimicrobial property, immune-modulation, and anticancer effects (Singh, Mal, Gautam, & Mukesh, 2019).

Several strategies have been evolved for the development of anti-infective designer probiotic strains, among which the most successful ones are blocking of pathogen-receptor binding, expression of receptor-mimic structures on cell surface, and neutralization of toxins (Sleator, Gahan, & Hill, 2001).

A few lactobacilli strains have been explored for construction of designer probiotics. A recombinant *Lb. gasseri* was designed as an oral vaccine against Streptococcus pyogenes. *Lb. gasseri* was engineered to express the M6 protein (CRR 6) of Streptococcus pyogenes. Oral intervention with a recombinant *Lb. gasseri* strain in mice demonstrated protective action against a S. pyogenes challenge (Mansour & Abdelaziz, 2016). Another gram-positive bacterium, Clostridium perfringens, is the causative organism for food poisoning, necrotic enteritis, intestinal inflammation, and toxemia. As an intestinal inhabitant, this organism poses greater risks, since any changes in the gut environment, such as diet, can facilitate its proliferation, resulting in intestinal inflammation and toxemia. As an alternative to antibiotic therapy, the possibility of host immunization using designer *Lactobacillus casei* strains has been explored. The *Lb. casei* strain, ppPG-α/L casei 393, designed by Gao et al. (2019) expressed the toxoid of the C. perfringens toxin. The strain was tested as an oral vaccine against C. perfringens and with BALB/c mice, and it was observed to induce significant amounts of secretory IgA in the intestinal mucus.

The potential of *Lactobacilli* strains to synthesize specific antimicrobial metabolites has also been explored while genetically engineering the probiotics. Recently, Peng, Tabashsum, Patel, Bernhardt, and Biswas (2018) reported the efficiency of CLA producing *Lb. casei* in controlling the *Salmonella enteric* serovar *Typhimurium* (ST) and enterohaemorrhagic E. coli (EHEC). In 2019, Tabashsum, Peng, Kahan, Rahaman, and Biswas (2019) constructed a recombinant *Lb. casei,* which could overproduce conjugated linoleic acid (CLA) for the control of pathogenic *Campylobacter jejuni*.

Apart from enterobacterial infections, reported cases of gastrointestinal infection with human norovirus are also high. An alternative therapeutic strategy that has emerged is to apply engineered probiotic strains for protein delivery. A strain of *L. paracasei* was engineered for heterologous expression of the 3D8 single chain variable fragment (3D8scFv) protein, which prevents induction of murine norovirus when injected into the intestinal lumen (Hoang et al., 2015).

Similarly, the strain *Lb. brevis* DT24 was designed to express colicin E2 and this recombinant strain showed activity against uropathogenic E. coli. Currently eukaryotic probiotic strains such as S. cerevisiae are also being explored as anti-infective vaccination strategies. For example, Palma & Colleagues (Palma, Garcia-Bates, Martins, & Douradinha, 2019) have reported work on a designer yeast S. cerevisiae that overexpresses the antigen HIV-1 gag protein, with testing on dendritic cells (DC). Only

DCs matured with designer yeast cells (expressing gag proteins) were able to efficiently perform antigen presentation to CD^{8+} T cells (Trivedi, Jena, & Seshadri, 2014).

Another strain of lactobacillus, *viz.*, recombinant *Lb. acidophilus* was constructed to express the bivalent antigen espA-Tir-M (ET) against EHEC O157:H7 as a candidate vaccine. (Lin et al., 2017).

Anti-tumor activity

Immunotherapy, more specifically checkpoint inhibitors, is considered to be among the most efficacious therapies in cancer treatment. However, there has been association with certain adverse effects, such as hepatic toxicity, skin rashes, and endocrine disorders (Scotté, Ratta, & Beuzeboc, 2019). It is therefore important to design more specific delivery systems for checkpoint blockade inhibitors, with minimal side effects. Several past studies have shown application of genetically engineered bacteria that sense and respond to the inflammation, infection, and cancer (He, Yuan, Zhong, Siddikee, & Dai, 2016; Saltepe, Kehribar, Su Yirmibeşoğlu, & Şafak Şeker, 2017). Especially in cancer, it has been shown that systemic administration of bacteria can serve as efficient tumor drug delivery vehicles via their ability to selectively colonize tumors. Very recently, Gurbatri et al. (2019) genetically transformed the probiotic bacteria, Escherichia coli Nissile 1917, which had the ability to locally and controllably release programmed cell death protein-ligand 1 (PD-L1), and anti- cytotoxic T-lymphocyte associated protein-4 (CTLA-4). The optimized lysing circuit mechanism was designed such that the recombinant probiotic bacteria carrying the anti-PD-L1 nanobody could grow and colonize the necrotic tissue core, thereby lyse-releasing the anti-PD-L1 nanobody blocking the interaction of PD-1/PD-L1 in between tumor and T cells. The authors reported an enhanced efficacy of the genetically modified probiotic strain expressing anti PD-L1 nanobody in lowering tumor growth rate, compared to the plasmid based lysing variant, and its efficiency was comparable to a monoclonal antibody against PD-L1. Furthermore, a reduced tumor growth was reported and its complete clearance when administered with a combined therapy of a nanobody against CTLA-4 and the probiotically-expressed PD-L1 nanobody in a multiple syngeneic mouse model. There is hope for the successful development of an engineered probiotic system for improved delivery of checkpoint inhibitors.

For diagnostics as a biosensor

Numerous studies in the past have shown the potential of bacteria to affect tumor growth (Diop-Frimpong, Chauhan, Krane, Boucher, & Jain, 2011; Iida et al., 2013). Researchers suggest that the intravenous administration of bacteria could have the ability to selectively grow on tumors without affecting host health and function (Li et al., 2003; Yazawa, Fujimori, Amano, Kano, & Taniguchi, 2000). This behavior of bacterial cells can be attributed to the suppressed immune activity within the tumor, along with the availability of nutrients in the necrotic tumor core, thereby prompting the exploitation of such tumor-specific bacterial growth as a tool for cancer diagnosis. Various studies also suggest the use of microbes as programmable delivery vehicles or as therapeutic or diagnostic agents (Kucherenko, Topolnikova, & Soldatkin, 2019; Lubkowicz et al., 2018). Consistent with these reports, in 2015 Danino et al. (2015) developed a recombinant E. coli Nissile 1917, as a biosensor to identify biomarkers of liver metastasis in urine samples. The recombinant E. coli specifically colonized the tumor tissue in rodent models with liver metastasis and could generate a high contrast urine signal through the selective expansion in liver metastases. It also enhanced the expression of the lacZ reporter, shown to cleave a substrate that could produce small marker molecules easily detected in urine. The bioengineered E. coli was reported to be safe and did not show any adverse health effects post-12 months of oral delivery, demonstrating that the utilization and careful programming of probiotics could be used to selectively delivery synthetic gene circuits in affected tissue environments in vivo.

15.3.3 Microencapsulation techniques for improved technological benefits

Microencapsulation has become a technology of interest to increase the viability of probiotics in food products and during product storage. Storage at different temperatures has shown better results for the coated cells by a factor of between 10 and 100 (Yao et al., 2017). In addition, microencapsulation technologies also improve resistance to gastric acidity and bile salts. The physiological efficacy of probiotics at the level of gastrointestinal transit is thus improved. There are many recent reviews concerning techniques and applications (Burgain, Gaiani, Cailliez-Grimal, Jeandel, & Scher, 2013; Foerst & Santivarangkna, 2016; Haffner & Pasc, 2018; Martín, Lara-Villoslada, Ruiz, & Morales, 2015; Šipailienė & Petraitytė, 2018). Different techniques are frequently described, in particular emulsion, atomization, extrusion, coacervation, and vibratory extrusion. De Prisco and Mauriello (2016) have reviewed applications concerning food products. Polysaccharides, such as alginate, carrageenan, chitosan, starch, gelatin, and also fats and waxes, are the most utilized materials. They are allowed in food production and for nutraceuticals. All species used as probiotics (*Lactobacillus, Bifidobacterium, Saccharomyces Enterococcus*, and *Bacillus)* can be encapsulated. Liu et al. (2019) describe each technique in detail and divide the processes into two categories: those using a high-temperature process (spray drying, fluid bed drying) as opposed to those using low temperatures (mainly technical supercritical, freeze drying, extrusion, emulsion). Other characteristics deserve attention, such as particle size, or obtaining a solid product with a low water content.

For the influence of temperature, atomization is a classic example. A spray drying process atomizes the wet slurry solution at high velocity and produces dry granulated powders by injecting hot air, at temperatures between 130 and 200°C (Arepally & Goswami, 2019). This treatment allows for the dehydration of an emulsion and the production of particles of various dimensions; the viability percentage is low because it partially destroys membrane structure and cellular constituents, such as proteins, nucleic acids, and oxidizes phospholipids (Peighambardoust, Tafti, & Hesari, 2011). Note that the oxidation phenomenon is one of the elements responsible for cell mortality; therefore, some use nitrogen in the atomization process.

In order to decrease the mortality percentage, protectors of different categories can be used (simple sugars, hydrocolloids, proteins, and antioxidants). In comparison, freeze drying requires freezing (−40°C) of an emulsion of alginate beads, produced by precipitation, followed by vacuum sublimation. The viability percentage is greater than for atomization and can reach 70 to 80% depending on the protectors used. Note that these are very similar to those used in atomization. With respect to particle size, electrospraying technology can reduce particle size to plus or minus 100 μm and increase cell viability (Coghetto, Brinques, & Ayub, 2016).

The latter technology highlights the importance of the water content of the encapsulated product. At an industrial level, the producer of starters is not the one that incorporates it into the finished product. In this case, a solid formulation is much easier to use. Frozen preparations can also be found. For the encapsulated probiotic, the situation will probably be the same and research should focus on this type of product.

Parameters influencing the stability of encapsulated probiotics are very similar to probiotics: temperature, water activity, and the gas composition surrounding the powder. These elements are related to the oxidation of lipids, especially membrane phospholipids, macromolecules, especially proteins, and nucleic acids. These oxidations can be demonstrated by the determination of fatty acids, soluble proteins (Coulibaly, Amenan, Lognay, Fauconnier, & Thonart, 2009), and the products of the oxidation of nucleic acids, which are more complex to analyze.

A methodology including thermal, colloidal, and surface analyses of powder (solid-in-gaseous phase), and dispersed (solid-in-aqueous phase) samples has been developed for probiotics and Razafindralambo, Delvigne, and Blecker (2019) provide explanations for cell behavior during storage. This approach could be used to better understand the improved stability of encapsulated probiotics and how to optimize the composition of the matrix.

Regarding the applications of encapsulation, publications refer to various fields (bakery, chocolate, fruit and vegetables, dairy products) where the properties highlighted are an increase in cell viability during the process or during storage. Encapsulation is often performed with hydrocolloids. Some producers use hydrocolloids as additives during lyophilization to realize a protective coating without claiming the use.

15.3.3.1 Challenges of encapsulating probiotics

The publications cited above show the development of various probiotic encapsulation techniques and these techniques improve, in different ways, the desired characterizations and especially the survival of the probiotics in the products, without definitively solving the issue, as the most important factor is keeping the storage temperature at constant humidity (Dianawati, Lim, Ooi, & Shah, 2017). The price of encapsulated probiotics must be compatible with the costs of their incorporation into nutraceutical or food products. If the price of probiotics varies from 200 to 500 USD per kilogram at a bacterial concentration of 10 exp. 11 per gram, the price of encapsulated probiotics should be between 500 and 700 USD for the same characteristics. The difference in price must be recovered based on the stability of the preparation and the effectiveness of the preparation at the intestinal level; this is possible for *Lactobacillus* and *Bifidobacteria,* which have improved stability and resistance to acidity (Wang, Korber, Low, & Nickerson, 2015). They compete with the system of gastro-resistant capsules and resistant probiotics, such as Bacillus coagulans and *Clostridium acetobutylicum.* These microorganisms are used in the form of spores (Konuray & Erginkaya, 2018).

In order to improve the competitiveness of the encapsulation technology, various ways can be considered (Chen, Wang, Liu, & Gong, 2017). First, the encapsulation techniques proposed must absolutely use products recognized as food approved and techniques must be compatible with industrial production; this is not always the case, One limiting factor in encapsulation is the support used and the second is that the technology must often incorporate a drying process. The most frequently used supports are hydrocolloids and especially alginate combined with another component (Gandomi, Abbaszadeh, Misaghi, Bokaie, & Noori, 2016). Extrusion techniques have been patented for specific particle sizes (Vésale Pharma, 2017; Quintens et al., 2017), and the drying technology remains as freeze drying, which is an expensive technology in terms of investment and energy.

In order to reduce the cost of encapsulated probiotics, the growth of bacteria can occur in the matrix, for example in alginate, in order to reach a higher concentration. More techniques using emulsions and spray drying are being developed. Scale-up of the emulsion and atomization can be achieved relatively easily for a lower price compared to other technologies

(Dianawati et al., 2017) However, viability losses at atomization remain high. One of the challenges of encapsulation is to arrive at a technology that can be industrialized at a reasonable price. Spraying can be one track, without excluding other techniques derived from the pharmaceutical industry.

The support and the coating are not the only challenges of this technology. Too few studies have examined the consequences of the incorporation of probiotics in terms of the organoleptic properties of products. If the size of the particles is mentioned, then the other organoleptic properties are often not the subject of systematic studies, for example taste. In conclusion, the challenge of this technology remains its industrialization, not only as a nutraceutical product in a powder, but also as a consumer food product.

15.4 Conclusions

An orchestrated understanding of mechanisms of strain specific probiotics, development of techniques, such as CRISPR, and elucidation of infective pathways and the pathophysiology of diseases, have paved way for bioengineered probiotic strains. Applications of these specific genetically engineered probiotics, as a novel approach to target intestinal infections and inflammatory conditions, appear to have great potential. However, like any other genetically modified organisms, the safety of genetically engineered probiotic strains needs to be evaluated thoroughly. The risk exposure determination, risk, and safety assessment must be ensured.

References

Ahring, K., Bélanger-Quintana, A., Dokoupil, K., Ozel, H. G., Lammardo, A. M., MacDonald, A., et al. (2009). Dietary management practices in phenylketonuria across European centres. *Clinical Nutrition*, *28*(3), 231–236.

Arepally, D., & Goswami, T. K. (2019). Effect of inlet air temperature and gum arabic concentration on encapsulation of probiotics by spray drying. *LWT*, *99*, 583–593.

Asensi, G. F., de Sales, N. F. F., Dutra, F. F., Feijó, D. F., Bozza, M. T., Ulrich, R. G., et al. (2013). Oral immunization with *Lactococcus lactis* secreting attenuated recombinant *Staphylococcal* enterotoxin B induces a protective immune response in a murine model. *Microbial Cell Factories*, *12*(1), 32. https://doi.org/10.1186/1475-2859-12-32.

Baranipour, S., Kadijani, A. A., Qujeq, D., Shahrokh, S., Haghazali, M., Mirzaei, A., et al. (2018). Inducible nitric oxide synthase as a potential blood-based biomarker in inflammatory bowel diseases. *Gastroenterology and Hepatology from Bed to Bench*, *11*(Suppl 1), S124–S128.

Barrangou, R., & Notebaart, R. A. (2019). CRISPR-directed microbiome manipulation across the food supply chain. *Trends in Microbiology*, *27*(6), 489–496.

Bermúdez-Humarán, L. G., Motta, J. P., Aubry, C., Kharrat, P., Rous-Martin, L., Sallenave, J. M., et al. (2015). Serine protease inhibitors protect better than IL-10 and TGF-β anti-inflammatory cytokines against mouse colitis when delivered by recombinant *Lactococci*. *Microbial Cell Factories*, *14*(1), 26. https://doi.org/10.1186/s12934-015-0198-4.

Bikard, D., & Barrangou, R. (2017). Using CRISPR-Cas systems as antimicrobials. *Current Opinion in Microbiology*, *37*, 155–160.

Bravo, D., & Landete, J. M. (2017). Genetic engineering as a powerful tool to improve probiotic strains. *Biotechnology and Genetic Engineering Reviews*, *33*(2), 173–189.

Briner, A. E., Lugli, G. A., Milani, C., Duranti, S., Turroni, F., Gueimonde, M., et al. (2015). Occurrence and diversity of CRISPR-Cas systems in the genus *Bifidobacterium*. *PLoS One*, *10*(7), e0133661.

Burgain, J., Gaiani, C., Cailliez-Grimal, C., Jeandel, C., & Scher, J. (2013). Encapsulation of *Lactobacillus rhamnosus* GG in microparticles: Influence of casein to whey protein ratio on bacterial survival during digestion. *Innovative Food Science & Emerging Technologies*, *19*, 233–242.

Caggianiello, G., Kleerebezem, M., & Spano, G. (2016). Exopolysaccharides produced by lactic acid bacteria: From health-promoting benefits to stress tolerance mechanisms. *Applied Microbiology and Biotechnology*, *100*(9), 3877–3886.

Capozzi, V., Arena, M. P., Russo, P., Spano, G., & Fiocco, D. (2015). Stressors and food environment: Toward strategies to improve robustness and stress tolerance in probiotics. *Applied Microbiology and Biotechnology*, *98*(17), 7569–7581.

Carroll, I. M., Andrus, J. M., Bruno-Bárcena, J. M., Klaenhammer, T. R., Hassan, H. M., & Threadgill, D. S. (2007). Anti-inflammatory properties of *Lactobacillus gasseri* expressing manganese superoxide dismutase using the interleukin 10-deficient mouse model of colitis. *American Journal of Physiology. Gastrointestinal and Liver Physiology*, *293*(4), G729–G738.

Carroll, I. M., & Maharshak, N. (2013). Enteric bacterial proteases in inflammatory bowel disease-pathophysiology and clinical implications. *World journal of gastroenterology: WJG*, *19*(43), 7531–7543.

Chen, J., Wang, Q., Liu, C. M., & Gong, J. (2017). Issues deserve attention in encapsulating probiotics: Critical review of existing literature. *Critical Reviews in Food Science and Nutrition*, *57*(6), 1228–1238.

Coghetto, C. C., Brinques, G. B., & Ayub, M. A. Z. (2016). Probiotics production and alternative encapsulation methodologies to improve their viabilities under adverse environmental conditions. *International Journal of Food Sciences and Nutrition*, *67*(8), 929–943.

Corcoran, B. M., Stanton, C., Fitzgerald, G., & Ross, R. P. (2008). Life under stress: The probiotic stress response and how it may be manipulated. *Current Pharmaceutical Design*, *14*(14), 1382–1399.

Coulibaly, I., Amenan, A. Y., Lognay, G., Fauconnier, M. L., & Thonart, P. (2009). Survival of freeze-dried *Leuconostoc mesenteroides* and *Lactobacillus plantarum* related to their cellular fatty acids composition during storage. *Applied Biochemistry and Biotechnology*, *157*(1), 70–84.

Crawley, A. B., Henriksen, E. D., Stout, E., Brandt, K., & Barrangou, R. (2018). Characterizing the activity of abundant, diverse and active CRISPR-Cas systems in lactobacilli. *Scientific Reports*, *8*(1), 11544. https://doi.org/10.1038/s41598-018-29746-3.

Crowe, J. S., Roberts, K. J., Carlton, T. M., Maggiore, L., Cubitt, M. F., Clare, S., Harcourt, K., Reckless, J., MacDonald, T.T., Ray, K.P., Vossenkämper., A., & Vossenkämper, A. (2018). Preclinical development of a novel, orally-administered anti-tumour necrosis factor domain antibody for the treatment of inflammatory bowel disease. Scientific Reports, 8 (1), 4941. https://doi.org/10.1038/s41598-018-23277-7

Danino, T., Prindle, A., Kwong, G. A., Skalak, M., Li, H., Allen, K., et al. (2015). Programmable probiotics for detection of cancer in urine. *Science Translational Medicine*, *7*(289), 289ra84.

De Prisco, A., & Mauriello, G. (2016). Probiotication of foods: A focus on microencapsulation tool. *Trends in Food Science & Technology*, *48*, 27–39.

Del Carmen, S., de LeBlanc, A. D. M., Martin, R., Chain, F., Langella, P., Bermúdez-Humarán, L. G.,et al. (2014). Genetically engineered immunomodulatory *Streptococcus thermophilus* strains producing antioxidant enzymes exhibit enhanced anti-inflammatory activities. *Applied and Environmental Microbiology*, *80*(3), 869–877.

Del Carmen, S., De Leblanc, A. D. M., Perdigon, G., Pereira, V. B., Miyoshi, A., Azevedo, V., et al. (2011). Evaluation of the anti-inflammatory effect of milk fermented by a strain of IL-10-producing *Lactococcus lactis* using a murine model of Crohn's disease. *Journal of Molecular Microbiology and Biotechnology*, *21*(3–4), 138–146.

Del Carmen, S., Zurita-Turk, M., Lima, F. A., Dos Santos, J. C., Leclercq, S. Y., Chatel, J. M., et al. (2013). A novel interleukin-10 DNA mucosal delivery system attenuates intestinal inflammation in a mouse model. *European Journal of Inflammation*, *11*(3), 641–654.

Dianawati, D., Lim, S. F., Ooi, Y. B. H., & Shah, N. P. (2017). Effect of type of protein-based microcapsules and storage at various ambient temperatures on the survival and heat tolerance of spray dried *Lactobacillus acidophilus*. *Journal of Food Science*, *82*(9), 2134–2141.

Diop-Frimpong, B., Chauhan, V. P., Krane, S., Boucher, Y., & Jain, R. K. (2011). Losartan inhibits collagen I synthesis and improves the distribution and efficacy of nanotherapeutics in tumors. *Proceedings of the National Academy of Sciences*, *108*(7), 2909–2914.

Dixon, M., MacDonald, A., White, F., & Stafford, J. (2015). Disorders of amino acid metabolism, organic acidaemias and urea cycle disorders. *Clinical Paediatric Dietetics. 381*, https://doi.org/10.1002/9781118915349.ch17.

Durrer, K. E., Allen, M. S., & Von Herbing, I. H. (2017). Genetically engineered probiotic for the treatment of phenylketonuria (PKU); assessment of a novel treatment in vitro and in the PAHenu2 mouse model of PKU. *PLoS One*, *12*(5)e0176286.

Dy, R. L., Pitman, A. R., & Fineran, P. C. (2013). Chromosomal targeting by CRISPR-Cas systems can contribute to genome plasticity in bacteria. *Mobile Genetic Elements*, *3*(5)e1003454.

Flora, A., & Welcker, J. (2017). CRISPR genome engineering: Advantages and limitations. *Rodent Research Models, 22*. https://www.taconic.com/taconic-insights/model-generation-solutions/crispr-genome-engineering-advantages-limitations.html.

Foerst, P., & Santivarangkna, C. (2016). *Advances in probiotic technology.* Boca Raton: CRC Press.

Gandomi, H., Abbaszadeh, S., Misaghi, A., Bokaie, S., & Noori, N. (2016). Effect of chitosan-alginate encapsulation with inulin on survival of *Lactobacillus rhamnosus* GG during apple juice storage and under simulated gastrointestinal conditions. *LWT- Food Science and Technology*, *69*, 365–371.

Gao, X., Ma, Y., Wang, Z., Bai, J., Jia, S., Feng, B., et al. (2019). Oral immunization of mice with a probiotic *Lactobacillus casei* constitutively expressing the α-toxoid induces protective immunity against *Clostridium perfringens* α-toxin. *Virulence*, *10*(1), 166–179.

Goh, Y. J., & Barrangou, R. (2019). Harnessing CRISPR-Cas systems for precision engineering of designer probiotic lactobacilli. *Current Opinion in Biotechnology*, *56*, 163–171.

Goh, Y. J., Lee, J. H., & Hutkins, R. W. (2007). Functional analysis of the fructooligosaccharide utilization operon in *Lactobacillus paracasei* 1195. *Applied and Environmental Microbiology*, *73*(18), 5716–5724.

Gurbatri, C., Coker, C., Hinchliffe, T. E., Lia, I., Castro, S., Treuting, P. M., et al. (2019). Engineered probiotics for local tumor delivery of checkpoint blockade nanobodies. *Science Translational Medicine*, *12*(530), eaax0876. https://doi.org/10.1126/scitranslmed.aax0876.

Haffner, F. B., & Pasc, A. (2018). Freeze-dried alginate-silica microparticles as carriers of probiotic bacteria in apple juice and beer. *LWT*, *91*, 175–179.

Han, W., Mercenier, A., Ait-Belgnaoui, A., Pavan, S., Lamine, F., van Swam, I. I., et al. (2006). Improvement of an experimental colitis in rats by lactic acid bacteria producing superoxide dismutase. *Inflammatory Bowel Diseases*, *12*(11), 1044–1052.

Hanson, M. L., Hixon, J. A., Li, W., Felber, B. K., Anver, M. R., Stewart, C. A., et al. (2014). Oral delivery of IL-27 recombinant bacteria attenuates immune colitis in mice. *Gastroenterology*, *146*(1), 210–221.

Hao, M., Cui, Y., & Qu, X. (2018). Analysis of CRISPR-Cas system in *Streptococcus thermophilus* and its application. *Frontiers in Microbiology, 9*, 257. https://doi.org/10.3389/fmicb.2018.00257.

He, W., Yuan, S., Zhong, W. H., Siddikee, M. A., & Dai, C. C. (2016). Application of genetically engineered microbial whole-cell biosensors for combined chemosensing. *Applied Microbiology and Biotechnology, 100*(3), 1109–1119.

Hernandez-Hernandez, O. (2019). *In vitro* gastrointestinal models for prebiotic carbohydrates: A critical review. *Current Pharmaceutical Design, 25*(32), 3478–3483.

Hidalgo-Cantabrana, C., Goh, Y. J., & Barrangou, R. (2019). Characterization and repurposing of type I and type II CRISPR–Cas systems in bacteria. *Journal of Molecular Biology, 431*(1), 21–33.

Hidalgo-Cantabrana, C., O'Flaherty, S., & Barrangou, R. (2017). CRISPR-based engineering of next-generation lactic acid bacteria. *Current Opinion in Microbiology, 37*, 79–87.

Hidalgo-Cantabrana, C., Sánchez, B., Álvarez-Martín, P., López, P., Martínez-Álvarez, N., Delley, M., et al. (2015). A single mutation in the gene responsible for the mucoid phenotype of *Bifidobacterium animalis* subsp. *lactis* confers surface and functional characteristics. *Applied and Environmental Microbiology, 81*(23), 7960–7968.

Hoang, P. M., Cho, S., Kim, K. E., Byun, S. J., Lee, T. K., & Lee, S. (2015). Development of *Lactobacillus paracasei* harboring nucleic acid-hydrolyzing 3D8 scFv as a preventive probiotic against murine norovirus infection. *Applied Microbiology and Biotechnology, 99*(6), 2793–2803.

Hosseini Nezhad, M., Hussain, M. A., & Britz, M. L. (2015). Stress responses in probiotic *Lactobacillus casei. Critical Reviews in Food Science and Nutrition, 55*(6), 740–749.

Ichikawa, H. T., Cooper, J. C., Lo, L., Potter, J., Terns, R. M., & Terns, M. P. (2017). Programmable type III-A CRISPR-Cas DNA targeting modules. *PLoS One, 12*(4), e0176221.

Iida, N., Dzutsev, A., Stewart, C. A., Smith, L., Bouladoux, N., Weingarten, R. A., et al. (2013). Commensal bacteria control cancer response to therapy by modulating the tumor microenvironment. *Science, 342*(6161), 967–970.

Jinek, M., Chylinski, K., Fonfara, I., Hauer, M., Doudna, J. A., & Charpentier, E. (2012). A programmable dual-RNA–guided DNA endonuclease in adaptive bacterial immunity. *Science, 337*(6096), 816–821.

Johnson, B. R., Hymes, J., Sanozky-Dawes, R., Henriksen, E. D., Barrangou, R., & Klaenhammer, T. R. (2016). Conserved S-layer-associated proteins revealed by exoproteomic survey of S-layer-forming lactobacilli. *Applied and Environmental Microbiology, 82*(1), 134–145.

József, L., Zouki, C., Petasis, N. A., Serhan, C. N., & Filep, J. G. (2002). Lipoxin A4 and aspirin-triggered 15-epi-lipoxin A4 inhibit peroxynitrite formation, NF-κB and AP-1 activation, and IL-8 gene expression in human leukocytes. *Proceedings of the National Academy of Sciences, 99*(20), 13266–13271.

Jung, W. K., Mendis, E., Je, J. Y., Park, P. J., Son, B. W., Kim, H. C., et al. (2006). Angiotensin I-converting enzyme inhibitory peptide from yellowfin sole (*Limanda aspera*) frame protein and its antihypertensive effect in spontaneously hypertensive rats. *Food Chemistry, 94*(1), 26–32.

Kim, M., Ashida, H., Ogawa, M., Yoshikawa, Y., Mimuro, H., & Sasakawa, C. (2010). Bacterial interactions with the host epithelium. *Cell Host & Microbe, 8*(1), 20–35.

Klotz, C., & Barrangou, R. (2018). Engineering components of the *Lactobacillus* S-layer for biotherapeutic applications. *Frontiers in Microbiology, 9*. https://doi.org/10.3389/fmicb.2018.02264.

Konuray, G., & Erginkaya, Z. (2018). Potential use of *Bacillus coagulans* in the food industry. *Foods, 7*(6), 92. https://doi.org/10.3390/foods7060092.

Krausz, A. E., Adler, B. L., Cabral, V., Navati, M., Doerner, J., Charafeddine, R. A., et al. (2015). Curcumin-encapsulated nanoparticles as innovative antimicrobial and wound healing agent. *Nanomedicine: Nanotechnology, Biology and Medicine, 11*(1), 195–206.

Kucherenko, I. S., Topolnikova, Y. V., & Soldatkin, O. O. (2019). Advances in the biosensors for lactate and pyruvate detection for medical applications: A review. *TrAC Trends in Analytical Chemistry*, *110*, 160–172.

Kutty, S. K., Ho, K. K. K., & Kumar, N. (2017). Nitric oxide donors as antimicrobial agents. In *Nitric oxide donors* (pp. 169–189). Academic Press.

Lander, E. S. (2016). The heroes of CRISPR. *Cell*, *164*(1–2), 18–28.

Landsberg, L., Aronne, L. J., Beilin, L. J., Burke, V., Igel, L. I., Lloyd-Jones, D., et al. (2013). Obesity-related hypertension: Pathogenesis, cardiovascular risk, and treatment: A position paper of the Obesity Society and the American Society of Hypertension. *The Journal of Clinical Hypertension*, *15*(1), 14–33.

LeBlanc, J. G., Del Carmen, S., Miyoshi, A., Azevedo, V., Sesma, F., Langella, P., et al. (2011). Use of superoxide dismutase and catalase producing lactic acid bacteria in TNBS induced Crohn's disease in mice. *Journal of Biotechnology*, *151*(3), 287–293.

Lee, S. H., Qian, Z. J., & Kim, S. K. (2010). A novel angiotensin I converting enzyme inhibitory peptide from tuna frame protein hydrolysate and its antihypertensive effect in spontaneously hypertensive rats. *Food Chemistry*, *118*(1), 96–102.

Li, X., Fu, G. F., Fan, Y. R., Liu, W. H., Liu, X. J., Wang, J. J., et al. (2003). *Bifidobacterium adolescentis* as a delivery system of endostatin for cancer gene therapy: Selective inhibitor of angiogenesis and hypoxic tumor growth. *Cancer Gene Therapy*, *10*(2), 105–111.

Lin, R., Zhang, Y., Long, B., Li, Y., Wu, Y., Duan, S., et al. (2017). Oral immunization with recombinant *Lactobacillus acidophilus* expressing esp A-Tir-M confers protection against enterohemorrhagic *Escherichia coli* O157: H7 challenge in mice. *Frontiers in Microbiology*, *8*, 417. https://doi.org/10.3389/fmicb.2017.00417.

Liu, H., Cui, S. W., Chen, M., Li, Y., Liang, R., Xu, F., et al. (2019). Protective approaches and mechanisms of microencapsulation to the survival of probiotic bacteria during processing, storage and gastrointestinal digestion: A review. *Critical Reviews in Food Science and Nutrition*, *59*(17), 2863–2878.

Loddo, I., & Romano, C. (2015). Inflammatory bowel disease: Genetics, epigenetics, and pathogenesis. *Frontiers in Immunology*, *6*, 551. https://doi.org/10.3389/fimmu.2015.00551.

Lubkowicz, D., Ho, C. L., Hwang, I. Y., Yew, W. S., Lee, Y. S., & Chang, M. W. (2018). Reprogramming probiotic *Lactobacillus reuteri* as a biosensor for *Staphylococcus aureus* derived AIP-I detection. *ACS Synthetic Biology*, *7*(5), 1229–1237.

Mansour, M. M., & Abdelaziz, S. A. (2016). Oral immunization of mice with engineered Lactobacillus gasseri NM713 strain expressing Streptococcus pyogenes M6 antigen. *Microbiology and Immunology*, *60*, 527–532. https://doi.org/10.1111/1348-0421.12397.

MarketWatch Press Release. (2019). *Probiotics market 2019 global industry trends, share, size, demand, growth opportunities, industry revenue, future and business analysis by forecast – 2024. June 4.* https://www.marketwatch.com/press-release/probiotics-market-2019-global-industry-trends-share-size-demand-growth-opportunities-industry-revenue-future-and-business-analysis-by-forecast-2024-2019-06-04.

Martín, M. J., Lara-Villoslada, F., Ruiz, M. A., & Morales, M. E. (2015). Microencapsulation of bacteria: A review of different technologies and their impact on the probiotic effects. *Innovative Food Science & Emerging Technologies*, *27*, 15–25.

Martín, R., Martín, R., Chain, F., Chain, F., Miquel, S., Miquel, S., et al. (2014). Effects in the use of a genetically engineered strain of *Lactococcus lactis* delivering in situ IL-10 as a therapy to treat low-grade colon inflammation. *Human Vaccines & Immunotherapeutics*, *10*(6), 1611–1621.

McKay, R., Ghodasra, M., Schardt, J., Quan, D., Pottash, A. E., Shang, W., et al. (2018). A platform of genetically engineered bacteria as vehicles for localized delivery of therapeutics: Toward applications for Crohn's disease. *Bioengineering & Translational Medicine*, *3*(3), 209–221.

Millen, A. M., Samson, J. E., Tremblay, D. M., Magadán, A. H., Rousseau, G. M., Moineau, S., et al. (2019). *Lactococcus lactis* type III-A CRISPR-Cas system cleaves bacteriophage RNA. *RNA Biology*, *16*(4), 461–468.
Miyoshi, A., Jamet, E., Commissaire, J., Renault, P., Langella, P., & Azevedo, V. (2004). A xylose-inducible expression system for *Lactococcus lactis*. *FEMS Microbiology Letters*, *239*(2), 205–212.
Motta, J. P., Magne, L., Descamps, D., Rolland, C., Squarzoni-Dale, C., Rousset, P., et al. (2011). Modifying the protease, antiprotease pattern by elafin overexpression protects mice from colitis. *Gastroenterology*, *140*(4), 1272–1282.
Murdaca, G., Colombo, B. M., & Puppo, F. (2009). Anti-TNF-α inhibitors: A new therapeutic approach for inflammatory immune-mediated diseases: An update upon efficacy and adverse events. *International Journal of Immunopathology and Pharmacology*, 557–565. https://doi.org/10.1177/039463200902200301.
Nedelkopoulou, N., Vadamalayan, B., Vergani, D., & Mieli-Vergani, G. (2017). Anti-TNF a treatment in children and adolescents with combined inflammatory bowel disease and autoimmune liver disease. *Journal of Pediatric Gastroenterology and Nutrition*, *66*(1), 100–105.
Palma, M. L., Garcia-Bates, T. M., Martins, F. S., & Douradinha, B. (2019). Genetically engineered probiotic *Saccharomyces cerevisiae* strains mature human dendritic cells and stimulate gag-specific memory CD8+ T cells ex vivo. *Applied Microbiology and Biotechnology*, *103*(13), 5183–5192.
Pavlick, K. P., Laroux, F. S., Fuseler, J., Wolf, R. E., Gray, L., Hoffman, J., et al. (2002). Role of reactive metabolites of oxygen and nitrogen in inflammatory bowel disease. *Free Radical Biology and Medicine*, *33*(3), 311–322.
Peighambardoust, S. H., Tafti, A. G., & Hesari, J. (2011). Application of spray drying for preservation of lactic acid starter cultures: A review. *Trends in Food Science & Technology*, *22*(5), 215–224.
Peng, M., Tabashsum, Z., Patel, P., Bernhardt, C., & Biswas, D. (2018). Linoleic acids overproducing Lactobacillus casei limits growth, survival, and virulence of *Salmonella Typhimurium* and Enterohaemorrhagic *Escherichia coli*. *Frontiers in Microbiology*, *9*, 1–14. https://doi.org/10.3389/fmicb.2018.02663.
Pereira, C., Grácio, D., Teixeira, J. P., & Magro, F. (2015). Oxidative stress and DNA damage: Implications in inflammatory bowel disease. *Inflammatory Bowel Diseases*, *21*(10), 2403–2417.
Privett, B. J., Broadnax, A. D., Bauman, S. J., Riccio, D. A., & Schoenfisch, M. H. (2012). Examination of bacterial resistance to exogenous nitric oxide. *Nitric Oxide*, *26*(3), 169–173.
Protic, M., Schoepfer, A., Yawalkar, N., Vavricka, S., & Seibold, F. (2016). Development of psoriasis in IBD patients under TNF-antagonist therapy is associated neither with anti-TNF-antagonist antibodies nor trough levels. *Scandinavian Journal of Gastroenterology*, *51*(12), 1482–1488.
Quintens, J. H. H., De Jeude, J. L. V. L., Brandau, T., Strohm, H., Schwinn, J., & Vesale Pharma SA and Brace Gmbh. (2017). *Microencapsulated probiotic substance and process of manufacture*. U.S. Patent 9,554,590.
Razafindralambo, H., Delvigne, F., & Blecker, C. (2019). Physico-chemical approach for characterizing probiotics at the solid and dispersed states. *Food Research International*, *116*, 897–904.
Remaut, E., Braat, H., Vandenbroucke, K., Rotteiers, P., & Steidler, L. (2006). Clinical potential of *Lactococcus lactis* mediated delivery of human interleukin-10 and trefoil factors. *Bioscience and Microflora*, *25*(3), 81–97.
Ruiz, L., Margolles, A., & Sánchez, B. (2013). Bile resistance mechanisms in *Lactobacillus* and *Bifidobacterium*. *Frontiers in Microbiology*, *4*, 396. https://doi.org/10.3389/fmicb.2013.00396.
Saltepe, B., Kehribar, E. S., Su Yirmibeşoğlu, S. S., & Şafak Şeker, U. O. (2017). Cellular biosensors with engineered genetic circuits. *ACS Sensors*, *3*(1), 13–26.

Saraiva, T. D. L., Morais, K., Pereira, B., de Azevedo, V., Rocha, C., Prosperi, C., et al. (2015). Milk fermented with a 15-lipoxygenase-1-producing *Lactococcus lactis* alleviates symptoms of colitis in a murine model. *Current Pharmaceutical Biotechnology*, *16*(5), 424–429.

Scotté, F., Ratta, R., & Beuzeboc, P. (2019). Side effects of immunotherapy: A constant challenge for oncologists. *Current Opinion in Oncology*, *31*(4), 280–285.

Scriver, C. R. (2007). The PAH gene, phenylketonuria, and a paradigm shift. *Human Mutation*, *28*(9), 831–845.

Shigemori, S., & Shimosato, T. (2017). Applications of genetically modified immunobiotics with high immunoregulatory capacity for treatment of inflammatory bowel diseases. *Frontiers in Immunology*, *8*, 22. https://doi.org/10.3389/fimmu.2017.00022.

Siddiqui, I., Majid, H., & Abid, S. (2017). Update on clinical and research application of fecal biomarkers for gastrointestinal diseases. *World Journal of Gastrointestinal Pharmacology and Therapeutics*, *8*(1), 39–46.

Simčič, S., Berlec, A., Stopinšek, S., & Štrukelj, B. (2019). Engineered and wild-type *L. lactis* promote anti-inflammatory cytokine signalling in inflammatory bowel disease patient's mucosa. *World Journal of Microbiology and Biotechnology*, *35*(3), 45. https://doi.org/10.1007/s11274-019-2615-z.

Singh, B., Mal, G., Gautam, S. K., & Mukesh, M. (2019). Designer probiotics: The next-gen high efficiency biotherapeutics. In *Advances in animal biotechnology* (pp. 71–79). Cham: Springer.

Šipailienė, A., & Petraitytė, S. (2018). Encapsulation of probiotics: Proper selection of the probiotic strain and the influence of encapsulation technology and materials on the viability of encapsulated microorganisms. *Probiotics and Antimicrobial Proteins*, *10*(1), 1–10.

Sleator, R. D., Gahan, C. G., & Hill, C. (2001). Identification and disruption of the proBA locus in *Listeria monocytogenes*: Role of proline biosynthesis in salt tolerance and murine infection. *Applied and Environmental Microbiology*, *67*(6), 2571–2577.

Sleator, R. D., & Hill, C. (2008). New frontiers in probiotic research. *Letters in Applied Microbiology*, *46*(2), 143–147.

Sodin-Semrl, S., Taddeo, B., Tseng, D., Varga, J., & Fiore, S. (2000). Lipoxin A4 inhibits IL-1β-induced IL-6, IL-8, and matrix metalloproteinase-3 production in human synovial fibroblasts and enhances synthesis of tissue inhibitors of metalloproteinases. *The Journal of Immunology*, *164*(5), 2660–2666.

Soltani, Z., Rasheed, K., Kapusta, D. R., & Reisin, E. (2013). Potential role of uric acid in metabolic syndrome, hypertension, kidney injury, and cardiovascular diseases: Is it time for reappraisal? *Current Hypertension Reports*, *15*(3), 175–181.

Soufli, I., Toumi, R., Rafa, H., & Touil-Boukoffa, C. (2016). Overview of cytokines and nitric oxide involvement in immuno-pathogenesis of inflammatory bowel diseases. *World Journal of Gastrointestinal Pharmacology and Therapeutics*, *7*(3), 353–360.

Tabashsum, Z., Peng, M., Kahan, E., Rahaman, S. O., & Biswas, D. (2019). Effect of conjugated linoleic acid overproducing *Lactobacillus* with berry pomace phenolic extracts on *Campylobacter jejuni* pathogenesis. *Food & Function*, *10*(1), 296–303.

Tiret, L., Ducimetière, P., Bonnardeaux, A., Soubrier, F., Poirier, O., Ricard, S., et al. (1994). Synergistic effects of angiotensin-converting enzyme and angiotensin-II type 1 receptor gene polymorphisms on risk of myocardial infarction. *The Lancet*, *344*(8927), 910–913.

Trivedi, D., Jena, P. K., & Seshadri, S. (2014). Colicin E2 expression in *Lactobacillus brevis* DT24, a vaginal probiotic isolate, against uropathogenic Escherichia coli. *ISRN Urology*, *2014*, 869610. https://doi.org/10.1155/2014/869610.

Vandenbroucke, K., De Haard, H., Beirnaert, E., Dreier, T., Lauwereys, M., Huyck, L., et al. (2010). Orally administered *L. lactis* secreting an anti-TNF Nanobody demonstrate efficacy in chronic colitis. *Mucosal Immunology*, *3*(1), 49–56.

Vandenbroucke, K., Hans, W., Van Huysse, J., Neirynck, S., Demetter, P., Remaut, E., et al. (2004). Active delivery of trefoil factors by genetically modified *Lactococcus lactis* prevents and heals acute colitis in mice. *Gastroenterology, 127*(2), 502–513.

Vésale Pharma, S. A. (2017). *Microencapsulated probiotic substance and process of manufacture.* Patent EP2665377B1.

Wadwa, M., Klopfleisch, R., Adamczyk, A., Frede, A., Pastille, E., Mahnke, K., et al. (2016). IL-10 downregulates CXCR3 expression on Th1 cells and interferes with their migration to intestinal inflammatory sites. *Mucosal Immunology, 9*(5), 1263–1277.

Wang, J., Korber, D. R., Low, N. H., & Nickerson, M. T. (2015). Encapsulation of *Bifidobacterium adolescentis* cells with legume proteins and survival under stimulated gastric conditions and during storage in commercial fruit juices. *Food Science and Biotechnology, 24*(2), 383–391.

Wijeratne, D. T., Lajkosz, K., Brogly, S. B., Lougheed, M. D., Jiang, L., Housin, A., et al. (2018). Increasing incidence and prevalence of World Health Organization groups 1 to 4 pulmonary hypertension: A population-based cohort study in Ontario, Canada. *Circulation Cardiovascular Quality and Outcomes, 11*(2), e003973.

Wu, A. H., Gladden, J. D., Ahmed, M., Ahmed, A., & Filippatos, G. (2016). Relation of serum uric acid to cardiovascular disease. *International Journal of Cardiology, 213*, 4–7.

Xiong, Z. Q., Kong, L. H., Lai, P. F. H., Xia, Y. J., Liu, J. C., Li, Q. Y., et al. (2019). Genomic and phenotypic analyses of exopolysaccharide biosynthesis in *Streptococcus thermophilus* S-3. *Journal of Dairy Science, 102*(6), 4925–4934.

Yadav, R., Kumar, V., Baweja, M., & Shukla, P. (2018). Gene editing and genetic engineering approaches for advanced probiotics: A review. *Critical Reviews in Food Science and Nutrition, 58*(10), 1735–1746.

Yanaba, K., Yoshizaki, A., Asano, Y., Kadono, T., Tedder, T. F., & Sato, S. (2011). IL-10–producing regulatory B10 cells inhibit intestinal injury in a mouse model. *The American Journal of Pathology, 178*(2), 735–743.

Yang, G., Jiang, Y., Yang, W., Du, F., Yao, Y., Shi, C., et al. (2015). Effective treatment of hypertension by recombinant *Lactobacillus plantarum* expressing angiotensin converting enzyme inhibitory peptide. *Microbial Cell Factories, 14*(1), 202. https://doi.org/10.1186/s12934-015-0394-2.

Yang, Y., Liu, Y., Zhou, S., Huang, L., Chen, Y., & Huan, H. (2019). Bile salt hydrolase can improve *Lactobacillus plantarum* survival in gastrointestinal tract by enhancing their adhesion ability. *FEMS Microbiology Letters, 366*(8), fnz100.

Yao, M., Wu, J., Li, B., Xiao, H., McClements, D. J., & Li, L. (2017). Microencapsulation of *Lactobacillus salivarious* Li01 for enhanced storage viability and targeted delivery to gut microbiota. *Food Hydrocolloids, 72*, 228–236.

Yazawa, K., Fujimori, M., Amano, J., Kano, Y., & Taniguchi, S. I. (2000). *Bifidobacterium longum* as a delivery system for cancer gene therapy: Selective localization and growth in hypoxic tumors. *Cancer Gene Therapy, 7*(2), 269–274.

Zhang, H., & Tsao, R. (2016). Dietary polyphenols, oxidative stress and antioxidant and anti-inflammatory effects. *Current Opinion in Food Science, 8*, 33–42.

Zhao, M., & Burisch, J. (2019). Impact of genes and the environment on the pathogenesis and disease course of inflammatory bowel disease. *Digestive Diseases and Sciences, 64*(7), 1759–1769.

Zuo, L., Sypert, D. C., Clark, A. D., Xu, Z., Garrison, D. E., & He, F. (2017). Redox mechanism of reactive oxygen species in gastrointestinal tract diseases. In *Gastrointestinal tissue* (pp. 21–27). Academic Press.

Zurita-Turk, M., Del Carmen, S., Santos, A. C., Pereira, V. B., Cara, D. C., Leclercq, S. Y., et al. (2014). *Lactococcus lactis* carrying the pValac DNA expression vector coding for IL-10 reduces inflammation in a murine model of experimental colitis. *BMC Biotechnology, 14*(1), 73. https://doi.org/10.1186/1472-6750-14-73.

Zwirner, N. W., & Ziblat, A. (2017). Regulation of NK cell activation and effector functions by the IL-12 family of cytokines: The case of IL-27. *Frontiers in Immunology, 8*, 25. https://doi.org/10.3389/fimmu.2017.00025.

Further reading

Dey, G. (2018). Non dairy probiotics foods: Innovations and market trends. In S. K. Panda, & P. K. Shetty Halady (Eds.), *Innovations in Technologies in Fermented Foods and Beverages* (pp. 159–174). Springer International Publishing. ISBN 978-3-319-74820-7.

Dey, G., & Sireswar, S. (2020). Tailoring functional beverages from fruits and vegetables for specific disease conditions – Are we there yet? *Critical Reviews in Food Science and Nutrition*. https://doi.org/10.1080/10408398.2020.1769021.

Sireswar, S., Biswas, S., & Dey, G. (2020). Adhesion and anti-inflammatory potential of *Lactobacillus rhamnosus* GG in a sea buckthorn based beverage matrix. *Food & Function, 11*, 2555–2572. https://doi.org/10.1039/c9fo02249j.

Sireswar, S., & Dey, G. (2019). Matrix-wise evaluation of in vivo and in vitro efficiencies of L. rhamnosus GG-fortified beverages. *Food Research International, 119*, 908–919. https://doi.org/10.1016/j.foodres.2018.10.077.

Sireswar, S., Dey, G., Suondayra, K., & Dipon, S. (2017). Design of probiotic-fortified food matrices influence their antipathogenic potential. *Food Biosciences, 20*, 28–35. https://doi.org/10.1016/j.fbio.2017.08.002.

Sireswar, S., Ghosh, I., & Dey, G. (2019). First and second generation probiotic therapeutics for inflammatory bowel disease. *Pharma Nutrition, 9*, 1–16. https://doi.org/10.1016/j.phanu.2019.100159.

Sireswar, S., Ghosh, I., Dey, K., Behera, L., Rezza, M., Das, S., & Dey, G. (2019). Evaluation of probiotic-food beverage matrix interaction for efficient control of *Enterobacter aerogenes* and *Staphylococcus aureus*. *Journal of Food Protection, 82*(4), 669–676. https://doi.org/10.4315/0362-028X.JFP-18-492.6.

CHAPTER

16

Packaging for probiotic beverages

Natalia Lumby and Jonghun (Jay) Park

School of Graphic Communications Management, Ryerson University, Toronto, ON, Canada

16.1 Introduction

The functional beverage market shows incredible potential for growth (Nazir et al., 2019). What follows is a discussion of the packaging and technology used in probiotic beverages. Before delving into the details of the topic, there are some general packaging truths that apply to this product category. Firstly, while the package has several functions, the most critical is its ability to contain and protect the product. As such, the packaging selected for a product depends on the product itself. Here, we will see that probiotics have their own challenges that require specific packaging solutions. Secondly, it is not uncommon in the consumer goods market that the packaging is the key differentiator on store shelves. As such, many production parameters are protected by brand owners, as they constitute a competitive advantage. This in turn leads to a broad variety of processes and a lack of standardization in the industry overall. Both of these challenges will be discussed as we look more deeply at the packages themselves, the processes used to create them, and finally the future trends for this beverage sector as it pertains to the package.

16.2 The package

The product type often dictates the packaging decisions made. The probiotic beverage market does have a variety of different products that each have their own requirements. Here, we will focus on some of the most popular probiotic beverages such as kefir, kombucha, fresh juice, as well as functional water. There is a broad range of packaging options for probiotics today, which include glass, plastic, aluminum can, and carton options. In addition, there are now less traditional probiotic delivery

Probiotic Beverages
https://doi.org/10.1016/B978-0-12-818588-9.00014-0

methods that result directly from the innovation of the package. When selecting the best option, the brand owner needs to understand, which package will perform best at protecting the product, as well as standing out to the consumer.

16.2.1 Glass packaging

Glass bottles have been used to package and sell beverages for hundreds of years. There are several reasons that glass performs well in the probiotic market. Often the material of choice for pharmaceuticals, glass is both inert and impermeable. Inert packaging is exceptionally safe, with no adverse effects on consumers. Impermeability is especially important for carbonated beverages, such as Kombucha. The acidity level of the beverage also matters, with more acidic drinks faring better in a glass container. Further, glass can withstand high temperatures, which allows for a greater variety of processing options such as pasteurization. In addition to these production advantages, glass is perceived to be premium by consumers (The European Container Glass Federation, n.d.). With the higher price points of probiotic beverages, especially when compared to main-stream soft drinks, the premium look and feel are an important part of the product experience. Lastly, glass is 100% recyclable, which appeals to environmentally friendly consumers. Not only do some packaging value chains, such as beer, allow for the bottle to be reused several times, but glass can also be melted and reused to make a new package. The same cannot be said of paper or plastic, where the materials can be used again, but often not for the same application.

Our ability to recycle glass does not mean that it does not have an environmental impact. More energy is used to produce glass due to the high temperatures required. Further, glass has more complex shipping requirements, with weight and fragility being issues (Soroka, 2014). Lastly, choosing glass can be a financial decision, as glass is more expensive. Thus, the premium look and feel do in fact come at a premium price Fig. 16.1).

16.2.2 Plastic packaging

Plastic bottle packaging dominates the nonalcoholic beverage market, with upwards of 85% of products being packaged in polyethylene terephthalate (PET) bottles (Beverage Packaging, n.d.). Plastic offers unparalleled production flexibility and cost-effectiveness. The functional beverage market has many small craft producers. The small production runs make economies of scale in production difficult and the savings offered by selecting a plastic bottle (especially a standard shape) attractive. However, a package can also be used as a brand differentiator. If the

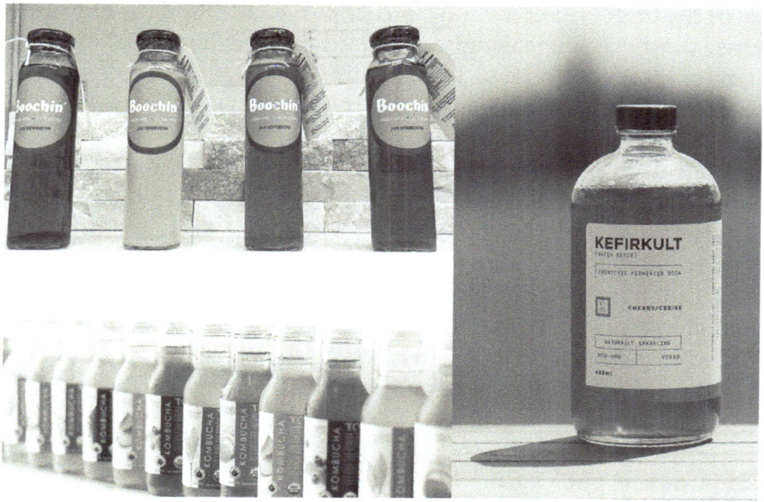

FIG. 16.1 Examples of glass bottle style packaging in probiotic beverages. *Credit: Boochin', Kefirkult, and Tonica Kombucha (left to right).*

package constitutes a competitive advantage, manipulating its shape and look is most easily performed with plastic. An example of this is demonstrated in Fig. 16.2, where the standard yogurt tub has been inverted and transformed as a "beverage shot."

While the look of plastic bottles is more easily changed than glass, single use plastics are increasingly being scrutinized for being heavy pollutants. Sustainability is often a key concern for consumers who are concerned with health and wellness. As such, choosing plastic may not be in line with the

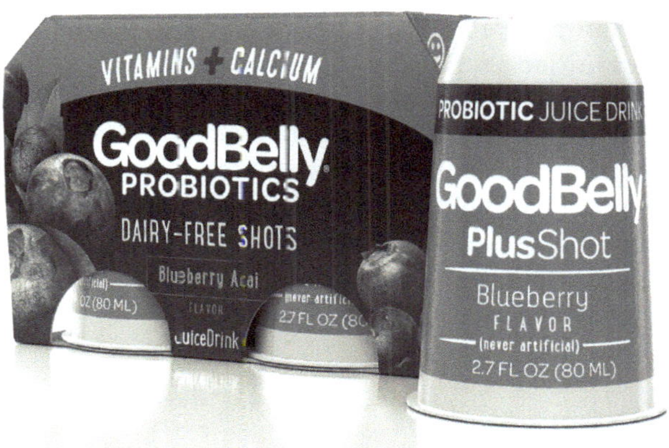

FIG. 16.2 Probiotic shot packaging. *Credit: Good Belly.*

desires of the target market (Crawford, 2019). In addition to environmental concerns, plastic is increasingly criticized from a health perspective for issues of toxicity (such as BPA leaching into food) (Brewer & Prestat, 2002).

The process used to fill the beverage container also dictates the materials that can be used. These processes are evolving. For example, hot filling is one process used for juices, teas, and nectars that are transitioning from glass only, to glass and plastic. This is possible because heavier PET options, with special expandable panels, now exist. These packages are specially designed to allow the container to expand while being heated, without permanently bulging the bottle. High-pressure processing is also dependent on the characteristics of the material used, favoring the flexibility of plastic. Some studies suggest that PET is not suitable for probiotic beverages because of its higher moisture vapor transmission rate (Fenster et al., 2019).

16.2.3 Carton packaging

Cartons are predominantly seen in the dairy and juice categories of functional beverages. Carton packaging consists of a combination of paper and a variety of liners. The layers used in the package will determine what type of product it can be used with, as well as impacting the product's shelf life. Some benefits of cartons include that they are light-weight, often made from sustainable materials, offer a lot of surface area for decoration, as well as being convenient when paired with a plastic closure.

In the carton industry, there are also aseptic packaging lines that result in a shelf-stable package that does not require refrigeration. However, this often means that the product must be heated in order to kill any pathogens, killing along with it any probiotic benefits. Advancements in the preparation of probiotic cultures have had a significant impact in this regard. As an example, probiotic supplier Chr Hansen has developed a strain that can be added aseptically to milk or juice at the last stage of filling, thus avoiding the issue of overheating (Patton, 2005).

Drawbacks of using cartons to package probiotics include a shortened shelf life, the requirement for fairly high volumes, consumer perception of cartons as low quality as well as confusion relating to whether or not they are in fact recyclable (resulting from municipalities not always having access to the appropriate equipment). Fig. 16.3 is an example of a probiotic beverage packaged in a carton.

16.2.4 Aluminum packaging

A rising star in the probiotic container market is the aluminum can traditionally use for beer and soda. Informed by successes in the craft beer market, brands are increasingly turning to canning as an option for Kombucha (Fig. 16.4).

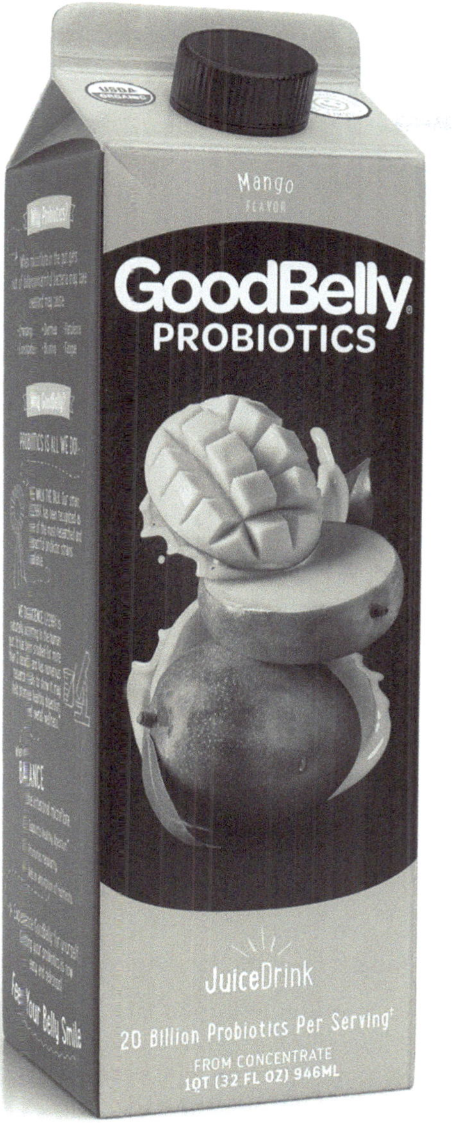

FIG. 16.3 Example of carton packaging in probiotic beverages. *Credit: Good Belly.*

Aluminum offers many advantages including being lightweight, completely blocking light, and maintaining a low cost per container. Cans are also highly recyclable, both from the standpoint of consumer participation rates as well as the material itself. About 70% of a new aluminum

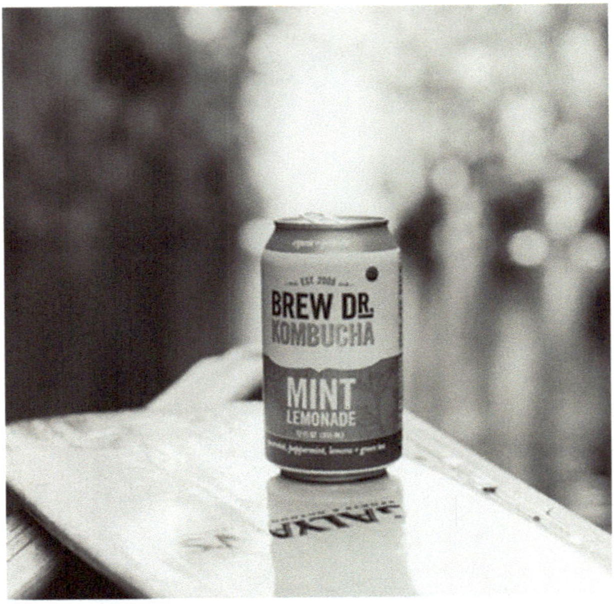

FIG. 16.4 Example of aluminum packaging in probiotic beverages. *Credit: Brew Doctor Kombucha.*

can is made from recycled aluminum. This is much higher than the 20%–30% of recycled glass used to make the average glass bottle (Hines, 2017).

One drawback of this type of process is that it requires higher volumes. Secondly, cans lack the convenience of most bottles as they cannot be resealed once opened.

16.2.5 Closures and other packaging

In addition to the common materials discussed, new innovative solutions are being developed. One can expect that with the growth of the functional beverage market, there will be a corresponding increase in package innovativeness. This is especially true for probiotics because the package can does play an active role in maintaining efficacy. Two such examples are specialty caps and straws.

Caps and closures already play an important role in probiotic beverage packaging. Oxygen scavenging liners placed in a metal crown cap, often used in beer packaging, is one example of how the cap can be used to extend the shelf life of a beverage. Ros-Chumillas, Belissario, Iguaz, and López (2007) found that combining the use of liquid nitrogen and an aluminum foil seal increased the shelf life of a PET bottle to match the capabilities of glass. Cap dispensing technology is another example of innovative packaging in the probiotic market. Here again, a shelf-stable probiotic powder is housed in a cap, separate from the liquid. Unlike the straw, the consumer is purchasing the beverage and not just the probiotic powder. A variety of dispensing caps is being developed. Whether it is a twist or a push, the single unit dose is hermetically sealed and released into the beverage upon opening. An example of a push dispensing cap is the KarmaCap, which is used with both the probiotic and vitamin water products produced by Karma Wellness Water (n.d.) (Fig. 16.5).

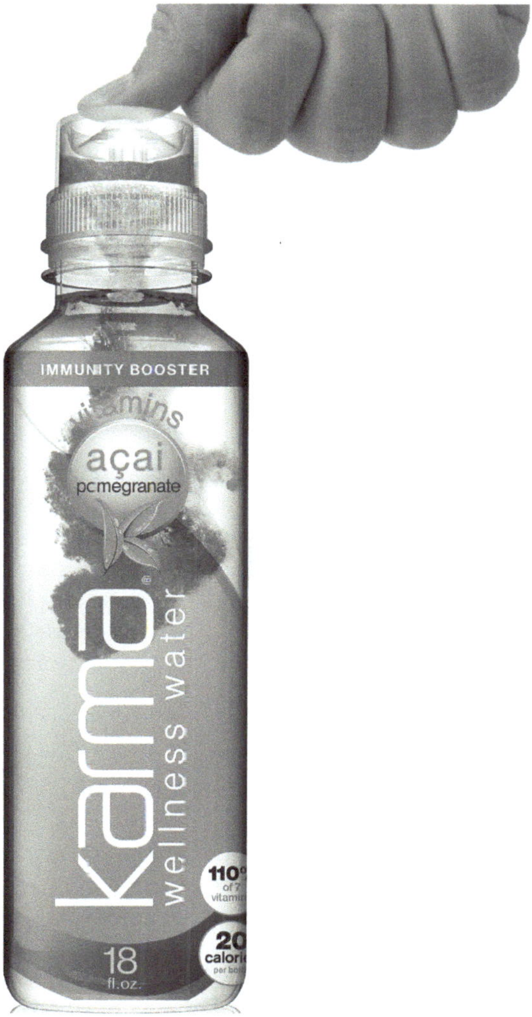

FIG. 16.5 Push dispensing cap. *Credit: KarmaCap.*

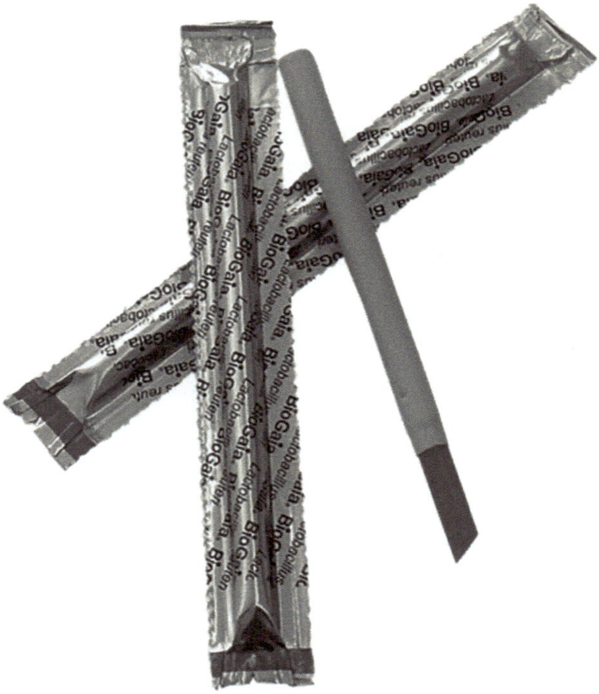

FIG. 16.6 Probiotic straw. *Credit: BioGaia.*

Probiotic straws can be viewed as a separate product, as they are purchased to be used with a beverage. They use a dry probiotic powder housed in an individually wrapped straw. An example of such a straw is the Life Top Straw sold by BioGaia (Fig. 16.6). Here a telescopic straw is extended and the probiotic powder is consumed as a beverage of choice is ingested (BioGaia, n.d.. One advantage of this method of delivery is that the product is shelf-stable and thus has a longer shelf life and does not require complex refrigeration supply chain logistics.

16.3 The packaging process

What makes probiotic beverages unique, from a packaging perspective, is that the package must adequately deliver microorganisms. Where packaging is most often concerned with keeping microbes out to prevent product spoilage, probiotics are microbes that must stay viable in order to deliver on the product promise. Many production conditions such as temperature, water activity, pH level, and moisture vapor transmission rate must all be considered and controlled (Fenster et al., 2019). Optimal production parameters do not apply in the same way with probiotics because we are attempting to maintain some microbes while eliminating others. As such a strict understanding of each process and its impact on the viability of the probiotic is critical.

Unfortunately, there is no one answer formula for what production solution works in the beverage market. This is because the preparation of the probiotic itself, the beverage ingredients, and the package selected will all have an impact. For example, live and active cultures, such as those in Kombucha, will be more sensitive to temperature than spore formers, which are encapsulated and do not become active until ingested. The process starts with the type of probiotic selected and how it is stabilized (whether by freezing, drying, or encapsulation) (Saarela, 2009). Thus a high quality, stabilized probiotic is much more likely to survive and deliver the desirable dosage. All handling and processing will have an impact, as such the product often overdoses in order to end up with approximately the correct live dosage (Fenster et al., 2019). In addition, carefully choosing where the probiotic is added in the production process, and selecting as late in the packaging chain as possible can be helpful.

The scale of a packaging operation will also dictate the type of bottling technology used. In North America, the probiotic beverage market is made up of many craft suppliers, who would not need to invest in high volume bottling lines. This will not remain the case for long, as the probiotic beverage category reached USD 39.56 billion in 2018 and is expected to reach USD 77 billion in 2025 (BusinessWire, 2019). Already, large brands such as Pepsi are launching their own products (Kevita). Often, the probiotic is simply added as just another ingredient. The key is understanding wherein the process it is appropriate to introduce it. For example, if one is working with a pasteurized product, cultures need to be added after pasteurization, otherwise, the microbes would not be viable. Probiotic suppliers can help in this regard. For example, encapsulated probiotics are better able to withstand the temperature and pH levels of processing (Iravani, Korbekandi, & Mirmohammadi, 2014). While many probiotic suppliers provide shelf-stable cultures, once they are combined with other wet ingredients, refrigeration is a must. As such, manufacturing conditions must be controlled and once the product is packaged, refrigerated trucks are needed to deliver the product into stores.

16.3.1 Promising processing technology

What makes packaging probiotics unique is the desire for some microorganisms, namely the probiotic cultures, to survive the packaging process. There are many packages filling processes that fail in this regard unless they are properly sequenced. Traditional approaches such as hot filling, ultra-high temperature (UHT) sterilization, pasteurization, and cold sterilization would kill probiotic microorganisms, thus not delivering on the product promise. This does not mean that they are not used in packaging probiotics, but rather that their sequence is important. If for example, a company is packaging a probiotic juice, it is possible to pasteurize the juice and sterilize the package, then following both processes, to add the probiotic cultures.

There are two methods that are particularly promising for this unique situation: high-pressure processing (HPP) and aseptic packaging.

16.3.2 High-pressure processing

High-pressure processing is a relatively new food processing option that is ideally suited for probiotics. The process uses water pressure to inactivate undesirable microbial content, without compromising the nutrient-rich enzymes of the product. The process can be performed in a bulk format, once the product is packaged. Probiotic juices have seen success in using HPP to extend shelf life. Some of the benefits of using HPP include:

- It is a nonthermal process, with no product heating required
- Shelf life can be extended without chemicals and additives
- The nutrients in the product are preserved (Hiperbanic, n.d.)

One of the disadvantages of HPP processing is that it can dictate the packaging format. Due to the tremendous pressure in the water, the package must be water-resistant and flexible. This means that plastic packaging is most typically used with this processing method.

16.3.3 Aseptic packaging

Aseptic packaging is a food processing technique that allows liquid products to have a nonrefrigerated shelf life of up to approximately 1 year. The advantages of aseptic processing over conventional package processing include longer shelf life, greater variety of packaging sizes and materials, and better nutritional and sensory maintenance functions (Chen & Rosenthal, 2015). Therefore, aseptic packaging is commonly applied to liquid foods and beverages as well as pharmaceutical products. The most well-known aseptic packaging technologies have been introduced by Tetra Pak, which is one of the largest food packaging companies in the world based on sales. The aseptic packages that Tetra Pak developed consist of a multi-layered film, paperboard, and aluminum foil and are hermetically sealed. The aseptic packaging products that Tetra Pak has produced in the past several decades include Tetra Brik Aseptic, with a rectangular shape; Tetra Rex, with a cuboid shape and a gabled top; Tetra Prisma Aseptic, with an octagonal shape; and Tetra Top, with a resealable cuboid package. These packages have been applied to a variety of liquid food products such as milk, soy milk, yogurt, and juice to extend their shelf life even in ambient temperatures and humid conditions (Tetra Pak, 2017). Polyethylene terephthalate (PET) or high-density polyethylene bottles are also commonly used in the aseptic packaging process for dairy and nondairy beverages, as they are easy to handle and reseal, and they have strong shock resistance.

For aseptic processing, food should be sterilized before the filling process and then filled into a sterilized container and sealed under sterile conditions. Thus, the key to aseptic food processing is to sterilize products and packaging containers as well as to keep a commercial sterilization condition throughout the packaging process. The liquid can be thermally sterilized using either high-temperature, short-time (HTST) pasteurization, which sterilizes the food at 72°C for 15s, or ultra-high temperature (UHT) sterilization, which sterilizes the food between 135°C and 150°C for 1–2s (Sanjana, Hemegowda, & Sushma, 2019). Compared to the HTST method, UHT technology provides better preservation in terms of nutritional and sensory quality, as well as a faster processing time. Because of its advantages, UHT sterilization is more commonly used in aseptic processing than in HTST pasteurization. Kept separate from the sterilization of the food products, the packaging materials should be sterilized before being filled. The typical methods used to sterilize the packaging materials are heat, steam, hot water, radiation, and chemical agents such as peracetic acid and peroxide (Hersom, 2009). Peracetic acid is used to sterilize PET bottles. Ansari and Datta (2003) found that the use of hydrogen peroxide, with concentrations of up to 30%, temperatures of up to 80°C, and contact times of up to 15s, was successful for in-line aseptic packaging. All packaging components should be erect, thermoformed, blow-molded, or sealed, and the packages should be filled under commercially sterile conditions (Pillai & Shayanfar, 2015).

There are several heat-transfer methods applied to thermally sterilize and cool food products, including several indirect heat-transfer methods (i.e., tubular, plate, scraped-surface, electrical, and microwave), direct heat transfer methods (i.e., steam injection, steam infusion), and nonheating methods (i.e., high pressure) (Nelson, 2010). A proper heat-transfer method needs to be chosen by considering the food characteristics (i.e., viscosity, particles, and heat sensitivity). For example, the direct heat-transfer method works better for heat-sensitive foods such as milk, while the indirect heat-transfer method, such as the tubular method, works better for viscous food with particulates (Fellows, 2009).

The aseptic packaging process should involve strict cleaning procedures, and those administering the process should have a high level of training and assistance. The equipment, instrumentation, and procedures used in aseptic processing facilities must be maintained and inspected according to government regulatory requirements such as the US Code of Federal Regulations (CFR 21, i.e., CFR 21 Sub-part C [211.42]), the FDA documents for aseptic processing and packaging systems, and the EU GMP's *Rules and Guidance for Pharmaceutical Manufacturers and Distributors* (Sandle, 2013).

There were many challenges to directly inoculating nondairy beverages with probiotics, especially juice products, because of several unfavorable conditions such as juice products' acidity and the thermally sensitive nature of probiotics (Shigematsu et al., 2018). However, technological innovations in this area have led to the possibility of using aseptic processing technology for probiotics. In order to inoculate nondairy beverages, such as juices, with probiotics, special technology using an aseptic dosing system (i.e., Tetra Pak Aseptic Dosing unit F or Tetra Aldose with in-line sterile filtration) is often used to allow bacteria to be added immediately before the filling process (Soccol et al., 2012). This innovative aseptic technology has boosted the development of nondairy probiotic beverages such as juices and fermented beverages.

16.4 Future trends in probiotic beverage packaging

New packaging technologies have emerged in the food and beverage industry to preserve and protect products in more efficient ways, as well as to provide better convenience to the consumers. This is mainly because consumers are constantly changing the way they think and purchase. Therefore, packaging must constantly evolve to meet the changing economic, environmental, and social needs of consumers (Biswas & Roy, 2015). Packaging design change and innovation occur when new technologies emerge.

In this section, future trends in probiotic beverage packaging are discussed based on expected consumers' needs and emerging technologies and that more sustainable, active, and intelligent packaging technologies for diverse supply chains will be applied to probiotic beverage packaging.

16.4.1 Trends towards sustainable packaging design and systems

Consumers are more concerned about environmental sustainability issues and many of them are changing their purchasing behaviors accordingly. In particular, millennials, who are great influencers for the food and beverage industry and have a greater environmental concern than other generations (Tetra Pak, 2017). The environment is becoming a key factor in their purchasing decisions. Other than consumers' needs, increasing public concerns, environmental laws, and environmental campaigns by NGOs also drive environmental concerns about packaging. Therefore, the global food and beverage industry has been under significant pressure to develop and use more environmentally sustainable packaging designs and systems. It appears that sustainable packaging is no longer an optional add-on for brands in the probiotic beverage industry. Like other brand owners in the food and beverage industry, stakeholders in the probiotic beverage industry are continuously looking for more reliable, convenient, and intelligent packaging solutions that have minimal impact on the environment.

Packaging is often targeted as a primary cause of environmental issues in the food and beverage industry due to the large amount of municipal solid waste generated. Some even argue that packaging should not be used at all. This is very difficult to achieve in reality. Distribution of food and beverages without packaging is not feasible and is not the best option to solve the environmental issues existing in the industry from a holistic view. Packaging is an essential component used to preserve and deliver food and beverages to the consumer. It can reduce food waste by expanding the shelf life of food and beverages. In particular, packaging is a critical component needed to maintain the quality of products containing probiotic bacteria (Saarela, Mogensen, Fondén, Mättö, & Mattila-Sandholm, 2000).

Scientific and holistic approaches to analyze the environmental impacts of packaging are becoming more critical, as more consumers become aware of greenwashing strategies often used in the beverage industry. There are several ways to analyze and review the environmental impact of packaging design. Examples include environmental scorecards (e.g., Walmart Scorecard), environmental claims, and life cycle assessments (LCA). Among them, LCA is the most quantitative method used to analyze and compare the environmental impacts of packaging designs and systems, from their raw material extraction to the end-of-life cycle. As the packaging industry is becoming increasingly aware of the importance of data-driven packaging design decisions for environmental sustainability, LCA will be more frequently applied to package design.

Sustainable packaging design ideas are often initiated following the 4Rs guideline of reducing, reuse, recycle, and renew (starting from the highest priority). In this context, it is expected that the probiotic beverage industry will be focusing on using the following packaging materials and systems for probiotic beverages:

16.4.1.1 Reducing packaging materials

Reducing the amount of packaging in weight and volume is known as the best way to eliminate the environmental impacts generated from the packaging. Packaging material reduction also naturally leads to packaging cost reduction. Some studies have found that there was a noticeable reduction in packaging materials in the consumer-packaged-goods (CPG) industry for the last few decades (United Nations Conference on Trade and Development [UNCTAD], 2019; Lipsman, 2019). For example, the weight of a yogurt cup made of polypropylene decreased by approximately 40% from 1990 to 2018. Probiotic beverage brand owners now constantly focus on packaging material reduction in order to obtain economic and environmental benefits.

16.4.1.2 Using reusable (or returnable) packaging systems

A reusable (or returnable) packaging system is another option to reduce the environmental impacts of packaging by extending the life cycle of the package. This system can eliminate the environmental impacts generated from raw material extraction and manufacturing stages of the packaging life cycle. A returnable packaging system that uses reusable containers typically requires durable containers that have more expensive material costs than single-use containers in order to protect products multiple times. This system also requires closed-loop supply chains in order to circulate the reusable containers. Due to these reasons, the returnable packaging system has only been used in limited areas such as the automotive and fresh produce industries, not often for consumer packaged goods (CPG). Although two very successful reusable packaging systems in CPG are seen in the beverage sector (milk and beer).

Recently, some CPG brands have considered using the returnable packaging system by collaborating with a new distribution platform, "Loop," which is a business venture of the waste management company TerraCycle. "Loop" enables the use of durable containers based on returnable supply chains by partnering with brand owners, retailers, couriers, and asset recovery centers. Products in reusable containers are delivered in "Loop's" shipping tote once consumers order them on-line, and the empty containers are collected, cleaned, refilled, and reused by "Loop." The reusable containers used in the "Loop" platform, mostly are made of tin, in order to provide enough durability for containers. Some global food and beverage corporations such as Nestle and large retailers such as Walgreens have joined "Loop's" platform, and they have introduced new reusable containers for existing products such as Häagen-Dazs ice cream. Although there are still many technical and logistical challenges, it is expected that some probiotic beverage brands will participate in the returnable packaging platform in the near future in order to create new and sustainable packaging formats for consumers. At the grass-roots level, small and medium-sized brands have created these closed-loop systems locally. For example, some suppliers reward customers with a free beverage for every 10 glass bottles returned.

16.4.1.3 *Using recyclable materials and increasing recycled content*

Recycling is a typical end-of-life option to reduce the environmental impacts of packaging. Most probiotic beverages use recyclable packaging materials, except for those products using multilayer plastic pouches. For example, most yogurt cups are made of polypropylene with a lid made of either high-density polyethylene (HDPE) or low-density polyethylene (LDPE), all of which are recyclable. Some include a foil lid, which is also recyclable if there is no sticker attached. A glass bottle or container with an aluminum cap, which is the typical packaging format for Kombucha and some yogurt products are also recyclable. Some brands use multilayer packaging materials, such as Tetra Pak's carton, and multilayer pouches for their probiotic beverage packaging. Some of the multilayer packaging materials are technically recyclable, as well, but recycling multilayer packaging is not as simple as recycling packages made of glass and single layer plastics. Therefore, some brands may consider looking for single-layer packaging materials to enhance recyclability.

Many beverage brands are also trying to use more recycled content for packaging made of plastics. In particular, there is an increasing number of beverage brands applying recycled polyethylene terephthalate (rPET) to their probiotic beverages. For instance, the Coca-Cola company, which recently entered the probiotic beverage market (e.g., Kombucha), first introduced rPET into a beverage package in 1991, and it has adapted 100% rPET for some of its beverage products. In 2018, PepsiCo, which produces some probiotic beverages (e.g., probiotics added to juice), also announced a new goal to strive to use 33% recycled content in their PET beverage bottles. As new recycling and polymer technologies are introduced, it is expected that more probiotic beverage brands will apply more recycled content, such as rPET, to their product packaging.

16.4.1.4 *Using renewable packaging materials (e.g., biodegradable plastics)*

Brand owners using plastics for their products often look for alternative packaging materials in order to reduce the use of plastics. Due to the ocean plastic issues recently highlighted by the public, there are many ongoing efforts to eliminate microplastics from the food and beverage industry. In 2019, Yakult, which is a traditional brand in the probiotic beverage industry, announced that it is considering changing its plastic packaging to an alternative form of packaging.

Bioplastics (biodegradable plastics) such as polylactic acid (PLA) are often considered an alternative to other petroleum-based plastic packaging materials in the food and beverage industry. Though it is not common yet, some brands started partially using bioplastics for their probiotic products. Danone has converted some of its yogurt packages from polystyrene to bio-based PLA. Tetra Pak also launched its fully renewable beverage carton, Tetra Rex® Bio-based, which is manufactured solely from paperboard with polymers derived from sugar cane. Even though some challenges still exist for applying bioplastics to probiotic beverage packages (e.g., material costs, safety issues, etc.), bioplastics will be more frequently considered as a sustainable packaging material by food and beverage brands in the future. An example of this market moving forward is Coca Cola's "Plant Bottle," which is made from 30% plant-based materials, and striving towards a 100% plant-based makeup in the future. (Anderson, 2015).

16.4.2 Application of active and intelligent packaging for probiotic beverages

The primary functions of beverage packaging are to perfectly contain the beverage and to help preserve and protect it from environmental hazards that lead to the deterioration of the beverage, such as oxygen, moisture, light, and microbes. Based on these goals, traditional beverage packaging has mostly focused on passive roles, which separate the beverage from the outside environment and prevent the migration of unsafe compounds from entering the beverage. For this reason, inert packaging materials, such as glass, are often considered the best materials for beverage packaging.

Today, however, consumers expect a more active or smarter role when it comes to their beverage packaging. They are not satisfied that the packaging just keeps the beverage up to its natural shelf life or that the packaging just maintains product quality during distribution. The consumers desire packaging that extends the product's shelf life and adds more value to the products after the packaging process. Thus, the importance of active and intelligent packaging technologies has increased in the beverage industry, especially for functional beverages, such as probiotic beverages.

16.4.2.1 Active packaging

Active packaging is defined as "packaging in which subsidiary constituents have been deliberately included in or on either the packaging material or the packaging headspace to enhance the performance of the packaging system" (Robertson, 2005). The goals of active packaging are to primarily gain shelf-life extension for food and beverages and to improve quality. There are three concepts of active packaging for a beverage. First, the active substances can be directly incorporated into the packaging material. Second, the bioactive substances can be coated on the packaging material. Lastly, the active substances can be incorporated into a tablet or sachet (Cooksey, 2001).

Various active packaging techniques have been developed and used for foods and beverages, such as absorbers, releasing systems, self-heating, self-cooling, etc. Among these, the absorbing systems and releasing systems are the two most commonly used active packaging techniques in the beverage sector. Absorbing systems remove or control undesired compounds (e.g., oxygen, water, carbon dioxide, ethylene, etc.) from the packaged food or beverage. The inclusion of oxygen scavengers in packaged food is an example of an absorbing system. Releasing systems emit functional compounds (e.g., preservatives, antioxidants, carbon dioxide, etc.) into the packaged food or beverage or into the head-space of the package (Dobrucka, 2013). Examples of the releasing systems include probiotics that are released into a yogurt drink, nutrients that are released into functional drinks, gases that are released into beer, and flavors that are released into dairy beverages (Ramos, Valdés, Mellinas, & Garrigós, 2015). The absorbers and releasers can also be applied to the packages, such as the film, label, or sachet. In this case, direct contact with the food and beverage is avoided in order to prevent migration issues (Ahvenainen, 2005).

One of the most critical factors affecting the viability of the probiotic bacteria in probiotic beverages is oxygen toxicity (Dave & Shah, 1997; Klaver, Kingma, & Weerkamp, 1993). While bifidobacteria are anaerobes, *Lactobacillus acidophilus* is microaerophilic. The exposure of fermented beverages to oxygen causes the intracellular accumulation of toxic oxygenic metabolites in these bacteria, and this results in a loss in viability in the probiotic beverage (Condon, 1987). The oxygen permeability of the material is the most significant property when considering probiotic beverage packaging. Some commercial barrier packaging has been introduced for probiotic beverages in order to prevent oxygen permeation, such as $ZerO_2$™, which is an active packaging film (OPET/EVOH/OS/CPP) that scavenges oxygen from dairy probiotics (Perkins, Zerdin, Rooney, Darcy, & Deeth, 2007), and Nupak™, which is lined with an oxygen scavenger sheet (EVOH/OS/EVA/$ZerO_2$™) that prevents the diffusion of oxygen into probiotic drinks (Miller, Nguyen, Rooney, & Kailasapathy, 2003). Many probiotic beverage brands are expected to continuously develop and adapt active packaging that is incorporated with oxygen barrier films, which have selective permeability to their products (Cruz, Faria, & Dender, 2007).

16.4.2.2 Intelligent packaging

Consumer needs are becoming more diverse and specific. In particular, they want to use, store, and dispose of packages in more convenient ways. In addition to the primary functions of packaging discussed above, such as containment, preservation, and protection, convenience and communication are becoming critical functions when it comes to beverage packaging.

In order to satisfy the increasing needs of the consumer, the beverage industry has put significant effort into the development of intelligent packaging, which is also called smart packaging.

Often, intelligent packaging is used with the same meaning as active packaging because both pursue the creation of new opportunities for better food safety, food quality, and user convenience. Both also typically require innovative packaging technologies to make them happen. However, the exact definitions and functions of active packaging and intelligence are different. Intelligent packaging is defined as "packaging that contains an external or internal indicator to provide information about aspects of the history of the packaging and/or the quality of the food" (Robertson, 2005). It typically aims to extend the communication functions of packaging using technologies to detect, sense, and record internal or external changes in the packaged products or their supply chains (Dobrucka, 2013). In addition, intelligent packaging also aims to create more convenience, to provide tamper evidence functions, and to improve product quality. Thus, intelligent packaging can lead to value-adding package development.

Smart sensors are the most popular examples of intelligent packaging techniques for beverage products. Various types of smart sensors, such as time–temperature indicators, gas indicators, and shock indicators, are used to monitor the internal and external conditions of products. For probiotic beverages, time–temperature indicators provide information to users via a color change when the beverage is exposed to an undesired temperature, which can lead to faster deterioration of the beverage. These are often used as freshness indicators, which estimate the shelf-life of beverages. The typical ways in which the time–temperature indicators are applied to the packaging are either using adhesive labels or laminating films. While the indicator is actively used for individual pharmaceutical products, it still has some limitations in its application to an individual probiotic beverage package due to the relatively high price. For foods and beverages, these are generally applied to a secondary package or tertiary package. However, some food and beverage brands are expanding the application of these indicators to more food and beverage products. For example, Nestle, one of the leading brand owners in the food and beverage sector, often employs a time–temperature indicator Timestripâ with their product packaging (Huff, 2008; Sharma, Dhiman, Rokana, & Panwar, 2017).

Another common type of smart sensor for beverage products is a gas indicator. The purpose of the gas indicator is to monitor the gas composition (e.g., oxygen, water vapor, ethanol, etc.) inside a beverage package through an enzymatic or chemical reaction (De Jong et al., 2005). It results in a color change if it detects the presence of an unwanted gas, such as oxygen. This sensor is used to verify the efficiency of scavengers, the sealing condition, and provides a tamper evidence function. The application of a gas indicator is expected to increase in the probiotic beverage sector as the presence of the gas, such as oxygen, is the primary cause of oxidative rancidity or allows aerobic microbes to grow inside of the package.

Thermochromic inks are also a form of useful intelligent packaging for probiotic beverages. The temperature-sensitive inks change color as the temperature goes up or down. The color is used to indicate the proper temperature at which consumers can drink the beverage. Thermochromic inks are becoming a much useful technology for functional drinks, such as probiotic beverages.

Often, packaging innovations occur based on a new packaging structure or configuration change. For example, Emerson introduced its "mix-to-drink" probiotic beverages using a new closure in 2017 (Lingle, 2017). A sealed upper closure contains dry probiotics until consumers want to mix them into the drink, and its breakthrough function dispenses the probiotics with the push of a button. This can be a great alternative that avoids the deterioration of probiotics, which typically occurs when probiotics are premixed with water before bottling, due to oxygen, moisture, and UV light exposure.

Other than the active and intelligent packaging technologies discussed above, more innovative technologies are being applied to materials, manufacturing, and the distribution of probiotic beverage packaging, such as biosensors, artificial intelligence, customization through big data analytics, augmented reality, etc.

The primary restriction is that most active and intelligent packaging components add material cost to the package. In order to increase the use of active and intelligent packaging, there needs to be more evidence that proves that the overall benefits of active and intelligent packaging outweigh the additional costs. Also, the active and intelligent packaging often have migration and contamination issues due to the direct contact of the packaging component with the beverage. For example, the direct contact between the packaging material or the sensor and the beverage may cause substances from the sensor to migrate into beverages.

Consumer expectations will continue to increase as society continues to advance. In addition, the technologies and knowledge about active and intelligent packaging systems will constantly improve. Thus, innovations towards active and intelligent packaging and their commercial success are expected to boost the probiotic beverage market by eliminating restrictions, such as concerns about contamination and the sensitive nature of the ingredients.

16.4.3 Packaging for e-commerce

The e-commerce market is booming as the way consumers purchase goods is changing. According to the United Nations Conference on Trade and Development (UNCTAD), global e-commerce sales were estimated at 29 trillion USD in 2018 (2019). One of the most noticeable trends in the current e-commerce market is the growing business-to-consumer (B2C) market. While business-to-business (B2B) still accounts for the majority of the total e-commerce market, the biggest growth segment is the business-to-consumer (B2C) market, increasing by 22% in 2017. The food and beverage industry does not yet represent a large portion of the global e-commerce market, mainly because distributing food and beverages is not as simple as dealing with nonperishable dry goods through online channels. Also, consumers still prefer to buy food and beverages inside retail stores (Ladd, 2019).

However, according to a recent study (Lipsman, 2019), the food and beverage sector, which in 2019 grew 18% to 20 billion USD in the United States, will, in the near future, be ranked as the fastest-growing product category in the e-commerce market. It is anticipated that online sales will make up 15%–20% of the food and beverage industry's overall sales by 2025.

The primary driver leading to the fast growth of the food and beverage segment in e-commerce is giant on-line retailers' recent investments into online grocery distribution channels. Amazon, the industry's leading online retailer, has operated a subplatform to deal with groceries, "Amazon Fresh," since 2007. At first, it did not look like the most optimistic business model, as many complex supply chain puzzles needed to be solved in order to distribute fresh and perishable products that generally require a cold chain environment. However, Amazon is setting up cold chain infrastructures and introducing new supply chain models to solve supply chain issues. Amazon's acquisition of Whole Foods Market in 2017 kickstarted the grocery e-commerce sector once again. Probiotic beverage brands will be actively looking for opportunities to distribute more products through the e-commerce platform.

Probiotic beverage packaging will be evolving for e-commerce grocery supply chains. Packaging materials and packaging structures are designed and selected by considering which distribution channels best prevent product damage and spoilage from various hazards in the distribution environment, such as temperature, humidity, shock, and vibration. Online supply chains typically have a more severe distribution environment than traditional retailers due to more touchpoints and higher handling heights. Therefore, packages distributed through offline channels can have damages if the same packages are distributed through online channels. For example, glass bottles, which are the most common packaging materials for Kombucha, can be broken if they are shipped through online supply chains. If a product is sensitive to temperature and humidity conditions, such as many probiotic beverages, packaging materials need to enable the product to be distributed through cold-chain supply chains. Thus, the different distribution environments between offline and online supply chains often lead to different packaging materials, structures, and configurations for each marketplace.

In this context, many probiotic beverage brands will design or redesign their packages by considering the supply chain environment of omnichannel distribution including both offline and online marketplaces. Not always, but generally, durable packaging such as metal cans and rigid plastic containers and flexible packaging such as multilayer plastic pouches are preferred for online beverage distribution. These materials are relatively light, and they can provide enough protection functions to the beverages when they are exposed to a harsh-handling environment. For the same reason, glass typically is not the best packaging material for probiotic beverages distributed through online channels. For example, various do-it-yourself (DIY) fermented probiotic drink kits, such as yogurt starters and fruit-juice mixes, are actively distributed through e-commerce supply chains. Typical packaging types for dry DIY kits include multiple sticks, sachets, or pouches made of a combination of paper or PET and aluminum contained in a paperboard carton. From the protection and preservation perspectives, these packaging configurations fit into both online and offline channels.

Preshipment testing is a mandatory process to ensure the quality of packaging during distribution The International Safe Transit Association's (ISTA) preshipment packaging test standard is the most frequently used preshipment testing standard. Depending on the packaging type, handling method, and distribution channel, the ISTA preshipment packaging standard is divided into six test series such as ISTA 1 to ISTA 6. Typically, the test standards for parcel types include a drop test, vibration test, compression test, while unit load types include an incline impact test, rotational drop test, vibration test, and compression test. The ISTA 3A test has generally been used for parcel shipment, which is applicable to most probiotic beverage products distributed online. By recently collaborating with Amazon, the ISTA created ISTA 6-Amazon.com, which is a test method for Amazon's supply chain environment. The ISTA also provides testing standards and data for thermal transport packaging used in parcel delivery system shipments such as ISTA 7E, and Thermal Lane Data Package. These preshipment testing standards will greatly help to ensure the packaging quality of some probiotic beverages.

16.5 Conclusion

Packaging plays a critical role in maintaining the efficacy, and by extension, product promise, of probiotic beverages. The packaging system in probiotics is unique because where most food and beverage systems have evolved to eliminate all microbes, this cannot be the approach for this category. A variety of packaging materials exist in the marketplace, each with their own advantages and drawbacks. Further, packaging solutions have been developed to separate probiotics from liquid (for example through the use of a dispensing cap). Most commonly, however, the probiotics are added directly inside the container. Here, the filling/processing technology used can help stabilize the package on-shelf, ensuring that harmful microbes and bacteria are not present, while the beneficial probiotics remain. Examples of innovative processing technologies used today include high-pressure processing and aseptic processing.

Once the product is packaged, it is the role of the particular container to maintain product freshness. This may require producers and retailers to control the environment, such as using a refrigerated supply chain. Innovative components can be added in order to ensure that the product quality has been maintained throughout the system. This can include the use of oxygen scavenging liners and caps, specialty inks that change color as a result of spoilage, and even smart sensors that can indicate when the gas composition of the container has changed. These package innovations continue to evolve, alongside innovations in probiotics themselves, working towards a product that delivers on the promised benefits of probiotics, while simplifying production and storage.

References

Ahvenainen, R. (2005). *Novel food packaging techniques.* Boca Raton: CRC Press.

Anderson, M. (2015). *Great things come in innovative packaging: An introduction to plantbottle packaging.* Retrieved November 13, 2019 from https://www.coca-colacompany.com/stories/great-things-come-in-innovative-packaging-an-introduction-to-plantbottle-packaging.

Ansari, I. A., & Datta, A. K. (2003). An overview of sterilization methods for packaging materials used in aseptic packaging systems. *Food and Bioproducts Processing, 81*(1), 57–65.

Beverage Packaging. (n.d.). Retrieved November, 2020, from https://www.interpack.com/en/TIGHTLY_PACKED/SECTORS/BEVERAGES_PACKAGING/News/Beverage_Packaging?_ga=2.155502267.1686766686.1604511650-1707066182.1604511650.

BioGaia. (n.d.). BioGaia life top straw. Retrieved October 12, 2019 from https://www.biogaia.com/product/biogaia-life-top-straw/.

Biswas, A., & Roy, M. (2015). Green products: An exploratory study on the consumer behaviour in emerging economies of the east. *Journal of Cleaner Production, 87*, 463–468. https://doi.org/10.1016/j.jclepro.2014.09.075.

Brewer, M. S., & Prestat, C. J. (2002). Consumer attitudes toward food safety issues. *Journal of Food Safety, 22*(2), 67–83.

BusinessWire, 2019. Global Probiotics Market To Surpass $77 Billion By 2025—Probiotic Beverages Emerged as the Largest Segment in 2018 with a Revenue of $39.56 Billion—Researchandmarkets.com. Retrieved on November 30, 2019 from https://www.businesswire.com/news/home/20190821005461/en/Global-Probiotics-Market-Surpass-77-Billion-2025.

Chen, J., & Rosenthal, A. (Eds.). (2015). *Modifying food texture: Volume 2: Sensory analysis, consumer requirements and preferences*. Amsterdam: Woodhead Publishing.

Condon, S. (1987). Responses of lactic acid bacteria to oxygen. *FEMS Microbiology Letters, 46* (3), 269–281. https://doi.org/10.1111/j.1574-6968.1987.tb02465.x.

Cooksey, K. (2001). Antimicrobial food packaging materials. *Additives for Polymers, 2001*(8), 6–10. https://doi.org/10.1016/s0306-3747(01)80187-1.

Crawford, E. (2019, January 22). *Consumer push-back against plastic will spur manufacturers to seek new packaging in 2019*. FoodNavigator-USA. Retrieved from https://www.foodnavigator-usa.com/Article/2019/01/22/Consumer-push-back-against-plastic-will-spur-manufacturers-to-seek-new-packaging-in-2019.

Cruz, A. G. D., Faria, J. D. A., & Dender, A. G. V. (2007). Packaging system and probiotic dairy foods. *Food Research International, 40*(8), 951–956. https://doi.org/10.1016/j.foodres.2007.05.003.

Dave, R. I., & Shah, N. P. (1997). Effectiveness of ascorbic acid as an oxygen scavenger in improving viability of probiotic bacteria in yoghurts made with commercial starter cultures. *International Dairy Journal, 7*(6–7), 435–443. https://doi.org/10.1016/s0958-6946(97)00026-5.

De Jong, A., Boumans, H., Slaghek, T., Van Veen, J., Rijk, R., & Van Zandvoort, M. (2005). Active and intelligent packaging for food: Is it the future? *Food Additives and Contaminants: Part A, 22*(10).

Dobrucka, R. (2013). Application of active packaging systems in probiotic foods. *LogForum, 9* (3), 165–167. Retrieved from http://www.logforum.net/vol9/issue3/no5.

Fellows, P. J. (2009). *Food processing technology: Principles and practice*. Amsterdam: Elsevier.

Fenster, K., Freeburg, B., Hollard, C., Wong, C., Laursen, R. R., & Ouwehand, A. (2019). The production and delivery of probiotics: A review of a practical approach. *Microorganisms, 7* (3), 83. https://doi.org/10.3390/microorganisms703008.

Hersom, A. C. (2009). Aseptic processing and packaging of food. *Food Reviews International, 1* (2), 215–270.

Hines, N. (2017, February 12). *Cans or bottles: What's worse for the environment?*. Retrieved from https://vinepair.com/articles/can-versus-bottle-environment/.

Hiperbanic. (n.d.). HPP technology. Retrieved from https://www.hiperbaric.com/en/hpp.

Huff, K. (2008). *Active and intelligent packaging: Innovations for the future*. Blacksburg, VA: Department of Food Science and Technology, Virginia Polytechnic Institute and State University.

Iravani, S., Korbekandi, H., & Mirmohammadi, S. V. (2014). Technology and potential applications of probiotic encapsulation in fermented milk products. *Journal of Food Science and Technology, 52*(8), 4679–4696. https://doi.org/10.1007/s13197-014-1516-2.

Karma Wellness Water. (n.d.). Karma Probiotics. Retrieved from https://drinkkarma.com/productcat/probiotics/.

Klaver, F., Kingma, F., & Weerkamp, A. (1993). Growth and survival of bifidobacteria in milk. *Netherlands Milk and Dairy Journal, 47*, 151–164.

Ladd, B. (2019, January 11). *Amazon to expand whole foods: Is AmazonFresh strategic? Will Amazon acquire a grocery distributor?*. Retrieved from https://www.forbes.com/sites/brittainladd/2018/12/30/amazon-is-expanding-whole-foods-will-amazon-acquire-a-grocery-distributor-as-well/#34a1c6791565.

Lingle, R. (2017, October 11). *Bottled probiotics innovate with push-button cap*. Retrieved from https://www.plasticstoday.com/packaging/bottled-probiotics-innovate-push-button-cap/98470048457637.

Lipsman, A. (2019, April 8). *Grocery ecommerce 2019*. Retrieved from https://www.emarketer.com/content/grocery-ecommerce-2019#page-report.

Miller, C. W., Nguyen, M. H., Rooney, M., & Kailasapathy, K. (2003). The control of dissolved oxygen content in probiotic yoghurts by alternative packaging materials. *Packaging Technology and Science, 16*(2), 61–67. https://doi.org/10.1002/pts.612.

Nazir, M., Arif, S., Khan, R. S., Nazir, W., Khalid, N., & Maqsood, S. (2019). Opportunities and challenges for functional and medicinal beverages: Current and future trends. *Trends in Food Science & Technology, 88*, 513–526. https://doi.org/10.1016/j.tifs.2019.04.011.

Nelson, P. E. (Ed.). (2010). *Principles of aseptic processing and packaging*. West Lafayette: Purdue University Press.

Patton, D. (2005, September 14). *Chr Hansen, Tetra Pak project removes obstacles to probiotic beverages*. DairyReporter. Retrieved from https://www.dairyreporter.com/Article/2005/09/15/Chr-Hansen-Tetra-Pak-project-removes-obstacles-to-probiotic-beverages.

Perkins, M. L., Zerdin, K., Rooney, M. L., Darcy, B. R., & Deeth, H. C. (2007). Active packaging of UHT milk to prevent the development of stale flavour during storage. *Packaging Technology and Science, 20*(2), 137–146. https://doi.org/10.1002/pts.749.

Pillai, S., & Shayanfar, S. (2015). Aseptic packaging of foods and its combination with electron beam processing. *Electron Beam Pasteurization and Complementary Food Processing Technologies*, 83–93. https://doi.org/10.1533/9781782421085.2.83.

Ramos, M., Valdés, A., Mellinas, A., & Garrigós, M. (2015). New trends in beverage packaging systems: A review. *Beverages, 1*(4), 248–272. https://doi.org/10.3390/beverages1040248.

Robertson, G. L. (2005). *Food packaging: Principles and practice*: (pp. 399–425) (2nd ed.). Boca Raton: CRC Press. https://doi.org/10.1201/9781420056150.

Ros-Chumillas, M., Belissario, Y., Iguaz, A., & López, A. (2007). Quality and shelf life of orange juice aseptically packaged in pet bottles. *Journal of Food Engineering, 79*(1), 234–242.

Saarela, M. (2009). Probiotics as ingredients in functional beverages. *Functional and Speciality Beverage Technology*, 55–70. https://doi.org/10.1533/9781845695569.1.55.

Saarela, M., Mogensen, G., Fondén, R., Mättö, J., & Mattila-Sandholm, T. (2000). Probiotic bacteria: Safety, functional and technological properties. *Journal of Biotechnology, 84*(3), 197–215. https://doi.org/10.1016/s0168-1656(00)00375-8.

Sandle, T. (2013). *Sterility, sterilisation and sterility assurance for pharmaceuticals: Technology, validation and current regulations*. Amsterdam: Elsevier.

Sanjana, M. C., Hemegowda, R., & Sushma, R. E. (2019). Aseptic packaging–a novel technology to the food industry. *International Journal of Trend in Scientific Research and Development, 3*(3), 307–310.

Sharma, C., Dhiman, R., Rokana, N., & Panwar, H. (2017). Nanotechnology: An untapped resource for food packaging. *Frontiers in Microbiology, 8*. https://doi.org/10.3389/fmicb.2017.01735.

Shigematsu, E., Dorta, C., Rodrigues, F. J., Cedran, M. F., Giannoni, J. A., Oshiiwa, M., et al. (2018). Edible coating with probiotic as a quality factor for minimally processed carrots. *Journal of Food Science ad Technology, 55*(9), 3712–3720.

Soccol, C. R., Lindner, J. D. D., Yamaguishi, C. T., Spier, M. R., Vandenberghe, L. D. S., & Thomaz-Soccol, V. (2012). Probiotic nondairy beverages. In *Handbook of plant-based fermented food and beverage technology* (pp. 707–728). Boca Raton: CRC Press.

Soroka, W. (2014). *Fundamentals of Packaging Technology* (5th). Herdon, VA: Institute of Packaging Professionals.

Tetra Pak (2017, November 16). Changing world of packaging: Past, present and the future. *The Economic Times*. Retrieved from https://economictimes.indiatimes.com/tetra-pak/tetra-pak-articles/changing-world-of-packaging-past-present-and-the-future/articleshow/61101823.cms?from=mdr.

The European Container Glass Federation. (n.d.). Why choose Glass? Retrieved from https://feve.org/about-glass/.

United Nations Conference on Trade and Development. (2019, March 29). Global e-Commerce sales surged to $29 trillion. Retrieved from https://unctad.org/en/pages/PressRelease.aspx?OriginalVersionID=505.

CHAPTER

17

Microbial safety issues related to probiotic beverages and the organisms used in their manufacture

Md Latiful Bari and Md Arafat Al Mamun

Centre for Advanced Research in Sciences, University of Dhaka, Dhaka, Bangladesh

17.1 Introduction

The term probiotic was derived from the Greek word, meaning "for life" (Reid, Jass, Sebulsky, & McCormick, 2003). Today probiotic bacteria are defined as "live microorganisms," which when administered in adequate amounts confer a health benefit to humans and animals (FAO/WHO, 2006). The Russian born Nobel Prize winner scientist Eli Metchnikoff first postulated that "the dependence of the intestinal microbes on the food makes it possible to adopt measures to modify the flora in our bodies and to replace the harmful microbes by useful microbes" (Metchnikoff, 1908). Similarly, Henry Tissier (a French pediatrician) observed lower counts of "bifid" bacteria (Bifidobacterium) in stool samples of children suffering from diarrhea, in contrast, these bacteria were abundantly present in the stools of healthy children. This finding paved the application for using these bacteria with diarrheal patients for the restoration of gut health (Tissier, 1906).

The fermentation of dairy products is an ancient procedure known to preserve or enhance product shelf life. One of the first fermented products was cheese, known and recommended for consumption by the Greeks and Romans (Fox & Mc Sweeney, 2004). Currently, probiotic microorganisms are gaining special consideration by researchers and the manufacturers of

Probiotic Beverages
https://doi.org/10.1016/B978-0-12-818588-9.00001-2

novel dairy products, as well as the attention of consumers. Today, one-third of the human diet globally consists of fermented foods, and most probiotic foods available are dairy based. Many studies in the past decades have concluded that for the delivery of probiotics, a dairy product is one of the best substrates. Currently, around 78% of sales of probiotics are delivered through yogurt (Rezac, Kok, Heermann, & Hutkins, 2018). The growth of vegetarianism, as well as consumers with lactose intolerance, milk allergies, and high fat and cholesterol levels, has resulted in more research into nondairy probiotic products for consumers.

Fermented beverages (dairy and nondairy) are regarded as alternatives to artificially carbonated drinks in several countries. Fermented dairy beverages such as ayran, kefir, kumis, yakult, villi, etc. contain probiotic microorganisms. These products have long been popular in Europe, North America, and Asia-Pacific countries (Luckow & Delahunty, 2004). Buttermilk and cheese whey are good matrices for the growth and viability of probiotic microorganisms. Also, naturally fermented beverages can be considered as fermented probiotic beverages because they contain some beneficial bacteria and/or yeasts. Currently, consumers throughout the globe are interested in natural food and beverage products and manufacturers often consider limiting sugars and sweeteners from a health perspective. Many traditional fermented beverages use fruits, vegetables, and cereals as these plant products possess vitamins, minerals, antioxidants, and fiber. For example, boza, shalgam, tomato, and pickle juice are rich in phenolics, which impart antioxidative nature and healthful property to human beings. Moreover, these plant products are devoid of cholesterol and lactose, which are usually not preferred by health-conscious consumers.

Hence, by considering the consumer preference for health benefits, the development of advanced technologies and market share for functional foods has paved the formulation of new nondairy probiotic food and beverages products. Moreover, fruit juices, desserts, and cereal-based products featuring nonalcoholic beverages show other suitable media for delivering probiotics (Cargill, 2009). However, product innovation in different food products, such as beverages, bakery products, use of probiotics, is apparent, with trends generally seen in developed countries. On the other hand, Asian diets are traditional in nature and relatively low in non-vegetarian and dairy-based foods, while botanical foods contribute their maximum daily food intake. Besides these dietary habits, lactose intolerance in Asian populations discourages them from consuming milk and allied products. Taking the above-mentioned facts into consideration cereals, fruits, and vegetables–based probiotic beverages can be a positive alternative, where the viable probiotic flora can cover their way. The development of new nondairy probiotic beverages is enormously challenging, as it has to achieve consumer expectations of products that are safe, healthy, as well as tasty (Shah, 2007). Some recently developed nondairy probiotic beverages are listed in Table 17.1. There have been a multitude of nondairy fermented cereal products in the history of human nutrition (Saadiya, Rouf, Jan, & Sharma, 2018). Table 17.2 illustrates the comparative advantages of dairy and nondairy probiotic foods.

TABLE 17.1 List of some nondairy probiotic products developed recently.

Category	Product	Reference
Fruit and vegetable-based	Vegetable-based drinks	Lambo, Oste, and Nyman (2005)
	Beets-based drink	Yoon, Woodamns, and Hang (2005)
	Tomato-based drink	Yoon, Woodamns, and Hang (2004)
	Green coconut water	Prado, Parada, Pandey, and Soccol (2008)
	Peanut milk	Kabeir et al. (2009)
	Cranberry, pineapple, and orange juices	Sheehan, Ross, and Fitzgerald (2007)
	Ginger juice	Chen, Wang, and Chang (2008)
	Grape and passion fruit juices	Saarela, Virkarjarvi, Alakomi, Matilla, and Matto (2006)
	Cabbage juice	Yoon, Woodams, and Hang (2006)
	Carrot juice	Nazzaro, Fratinni, Sada, and Orlando (2008)
	Noni juice	Wang, Ng, Tzeng, and Shyu (2009)
	Onion	Roberts and Kidd (2005)
	Nonfermented fruit juice beverages	Renuka, Kulkarni, Vijayanand, and Prapulla (2009)
	Blackcurrant juice	Luckow and Delahunty (2004)
	Plum juice	Sheela and Suganya (2012)
	Cashew apple juice	Pereira and Gibson (2002)
	Fruit juices (mango, sapota, grape)	Kumar, Sreedharamurthy, and Reddy (2013)
Cereals and pulses based	Fermented soymilk drink	Donkor, Henriksson, Vasiljevic, and Shah (2007)
	Soy-based stirred yogurt-like drinks	Saris, Beasley, and Tourila (2003)
	Soyghurt	Bedani, Vieira, Rossi, and Saad (2014)

Continued

TABLE 17.1 List of some nondairy probiotic products developed recently—cont'd

Category	Product	Reference
	Soy product fermented with Kefir	Baú, Garcia, and Ida (2014)
	Rice-based yogurt	Wongkhalaung and Boonyaratanakornkit (2000).
	Oat-based drink	Angelov, Gotcheva, Kuncheva, and Hristozova (2006)
	Oat milk	Bernat, Cháfer, González-Martínez, Rodríguez-Garcíaez, and Chiralt (2014)
	Mahewu (a sour beverage prepared from corn meal)	McMaste, Kokott, and Abratt (2005)
	Wheat, rye, millet, maize, and other cereals fermented probiotic beverages	Nyanzi and Jooste (2012)
	Malt-based drink	Kedia, Wang, Patel, and Pandiella (2007)
	Boza (a traditional fermented beverage made from cereals)	Moncheva et al. (2003)
	Maize, sorghum, and millet malt fermented probiotic beverages	Nyanzi and Jooste (2012)
	Millet or sorghum flour fermented probiotic beverage	Muyanja, Narvhus, Treimo, and Langsrud (2003)
	Mixed cereal beverage	Rathore, Salmerón, and Pandiella (2012)
	Kombucha probiotic tea drink	Saadiya et al. (2018)
Sorghum based	Sorghum based "Sorghurt"	Sanni et al. (2013)

17.2 Safety of probiotic bacteria

Safety considerations of probiotic bacteria are of high importance, as live microbial products, probiotics are potential sources of risk and there exists a skeptical attitude among medical professionals and consumers who have less than optimal experiences with probiotics (Naidu, Adam, & Govender, 2012). When ingested in sufficient numbers, probiotics are expected to confer one or more proven health benefits on the consumer. Theoretically, the effectiveness of a probiotic food product is the

TABLE 17.2 Comparative advantages of dairy and non-dairy probiotic foods.

Parameter	Dairy probiotic foods	Non-dairy probiotic foods
Lactose intolerance	Negative effect	No issue
Calcium availability	Positive effect	No issue
High fat	Negative effect	No issue
Cholesterol content	Negative effect	No issue
Dietary fiber	No issue	Positive effect
Digestibility	Not easy	Easy to digest
The survival rate of probiotics	High	Low
Flavor (diacetyl/acetaldehyde)	Positive effect	No issue
Phyto-chemicals	No issue	Positive effect
Isoflavones	No issue	Positive effect

sum of its microbial quality and its functional potential. Whereas the latter may vary with the body (target) site, delivery mode, human target population, and health benefit envisaged. Microbial assessment of the probiotic product quality is more straightforward.

Some strains of other LAB groups such as enterococci are agents of opportunistic infections. Rare cases of infection associated with certain Lactobacillus strains have been reported, mostly in immunocompromised patients (Cannon, Lee, Bolanos, & Danziger, 2005). Bifidobacteria are very rarely associated with infections (Hata, Yoshida, Ohkubo, Mochizuki, et al., 1988). Bifidobacterium-associated infections are most likely caused by bifidobacteria from the patients' own microbiota (MacFie, O'Boyle, Mitchell, Buckley, et al., 1999; Wang, Andersson, Soltesz, Leveau, et al., 1996). A recent study reported that the administration of the probiotic *E. coli strain* Nissle 1917 to immunocompromised patients could lead to severe adverse effects (Gronbach, Eberle, Muller, Olschlager, et al., 2010).

The microorganisms used in the production of fermented products have a long history of safe use and are often referred to as "food grade" or GRAS (Generally Recognized as Safe) microorganisms (Holzapfel, Haberer, Snel, Schillinger, et al., 1998). In general, four types of side effects of probiotics can be distinguished: systemic infections, metabolic and enzymatic effects, immunomodulation and adjuvants, and gene transfer. Among these, the most direct safety risk associated with the consumption of microorganisms is infection (e.g., endocarditis), especially in immune-compromised individuals. However, the risk of infection by probiotic *Lactobacillus* or *Bifidobacterium* strains is similar to the risk of infection by commensal strains, and thus products containing such probiotic strains present a negligible risk to consumers (Ouwehand & Vesterlund, 2003).

In recognition of the importance of ensuring their safety for human purposes, even among the LAB that are generally considered to have a very good safety record, new and existing probiotic strains need to be characterized with respect to a number of safety aspects. Important criteria for probiotic bacteria to be used for food are the capacity to survive during passage through the digestive tract (by exhibiting acid and bile tolerance), their ability to withstand digestive enzymes, as well as their ability to proliferate in the gut. In addition, they must be able to exert their benefits on the host through growth and/or activity in the body, and hence, the ability to remain viable at the target site and to be effective should be verified for each strain. In addition to strain identification and characterization, the food matrix is important itself and the applied technology to prepare the food (constituent) and the stability and survival of the strain until the moment of food consumption. This in turn points toward a food matrix dependency (including the amount of food to be consumed for a proven health effect) and the importance of an adequate amount of live active cells (Huys et al., 2013).

There are four main steps in the microbial quality assessment process (FAO/WHO, 2002):

- **(i)** Correct species identification and strain-specific typing of bacterial and yeast strains to be used in probiotic applications
- **(ii)** Probiotic strains must be resistant to factors such as gastric acidity, bile acid, and digestive enzymes, and should possess antimicrobial activity against potentially pathogenic bacteria
- **(iii)** Safety assessment of probiotic strains used for human consumption (proof that a probiotic strain is safe and does not cause any disease to the host)
- **(iv)** Quality of the final probiotic product in terms of its microbial composition, concentration, stability, authenticity, and labeling.

Although still under debate, it is generally agreed that probiotic safety aspects should cover the isolation history and species identity of the probiotic culture and provide phenotypic and/or genotypic evidence showing that the culture does not harbor acquired antibiotic resistance traits, putative virulence factors, or other pathogenic properties (Salminen, Von Wright, Morell, Marteau, et al., 1998; Sanders, Akkermans, Haller, Hammerman, et al., 2010; Vankerckhoven, Huys, Vancanneyt, Vael, et al., 2008). In addition, it has been suggested that translocation, adhesion, and colonization may also contribute to the safety dossier of a probiotic strain. The ideal properties of probiotic bacteria for human consumption are shown in Table 17.3.

TABLE 17.3 Ideal properties of probiotic organisms.

	Ideal properties of a probiotic bacteria
1	Probiotic bacteria should be completely nonpathogenic
2	Probiotic bacteria should be capable of surviving passage through the digestive tract, by exhibiting acid and bile tolerance and withstand digestive enzymes, also they should have the potential to proliferate in the gut
3	Probiotic bacteria should not cause disease in humans
4	Probiotic bacteria should not be able to evolve into pathogenic variants
5	Probiotic bacteria should not have the ability to acquire foreign DNA
6	Probiotic bacteria should not contain transferable resistance to antibiotics [such as glycopeptide (e.g., vancomycin) resistance in enterococci]
7	Probiotic bacteria should not have the capacity to form biogenic amines (such as tyramine, histamine, and phenylethylamine)
8	Probiotic bacteria should not activate procarcinogens (such as activation by azo reductase, nitro reductase, and glucuronidase)
9	Probiotic bacteria should not cause induction and/or destruction of thrombocyte properties (such as specific hydrolases)
10	Probiotic bacteria should not be able to activate platelet aggregation
11	Probiotic bacteria should not be capable of binding to fibrinogen and fibronectin
12	Probiotic bacteria should not be able to reduce mucin (can be regarded as a condition for invasive properties)
13	Probiotic bacteria should not have hemolytic activity
14	Probiotic bacteria should not have the capacity for the deconjugation and dehydroxylation of bile salts

17.2.1 Isolation, identification, characterization, and safety assessment of probiotic strains

Although still a matter of debate, it has been suggested that probiotic strains should originate from the species of intended use. One can argue that a probiotic strain isolated from the gastrointestinal tract of a healthy human can function better in a similar environment. Although this point of view has been supported by the fact that most current successful strains are indeed of human origin, some animal-derived strains have also shown positive effects on humans (Huys et al., 2013). In addition to documenting a strain's history, the first step should be to identify the microorganism (probiotic bacteria) using internationally accepted methodologies, preferably by combining phenotypic and genotypic methods. Correct identification at the species level also implies the use of scientifically recognized names and adequate designations of particular strains. Strain-specific identification and characterization are required to prove the absence of pathogenicity. Furthermore, different strains can possess different features related to different safety risks, implying that it is not possible to identify the specific safety risks associated with a probiotic strain without proper identification. Reliable identification and species-specific or strain-specific safety evaluations must be performed to avoid the inclusion of pathogenic microorganisms in probiotic products (Falkow, 1997).

For characterizing probiotic bacteria, evidence should be provided that particular pathogenic features are absent, notably those involved in invasion and translocation, toxin production, and the ability to survive and multiply in the bloodstream (Bernardeau, Guguen, & Vernoux, 2006). In addition, some bacteria can take up DNA from the environment and incorporate this DNA into their genome. Nonpathogenic bacteria are able to gain virulence genes in this way, especially while inhabiting the human gut (Wassenaar & Klein, 2008). As a consequence of DNA uptake, there is an additional risk that probiotic bacteria could acquire resistance against antimicrobial agents by horizontal gene transfer, which is generally considered undesirable. When residual nonpathogenic bacteria (probiotics or natural microbiota) have gained antimicrobial resistance genes, they could donate such genes to pathogenic or other nonpathogenic bacteria that cause adverse health consequences. Therefore, the safety of probiotic bacteria must be considered in terms of their virulence repertoire, antibiotic resistance, and ability to acquire foreign DNA.

17.2.2 Antimicrobial resistance of probiotic bacteria

Antibiotic resistance in bacteria may be intrinsic or acquired. Intrinsic resistance is a naturally occurring trait that may be characteristic for a given species or genus, whereas acquired resistance derives either from genetic mutations or acquisition of foreign DNA from other bacteria (Verraes, Van Boxstael, Van Meervenne, et al., 2013). Probiotic strains with nontransmissible antibiotic resistances do not usually confer a safety concern. The absence of antibiotic resistance in a given bacterial strain can be proven in a simple manner. Determination of the minimum inhibitory concentration (MICs) for common antibiotics is a routine and highly standardized procedure, and evidence for the absence of resistance genes can be obtained by molecular methods (Huys et al., 2013). In contrast nontransmissible antibiotic resistance might be a useful property, if the probiotic strain is to be used as a prophylactic agent in the treatment of antibiotic-associated diarrhea (Charteris, Kelly, Morelli, & Collins, 1998a; Charteris, Kelly, Morelli, & Collins, 1998b). However, antibiotic resistance linked to transferable plasmids and mobile elements is a different case because of the possibility of resistance plasmid transfer, which could result in potentially harmful bacteria. In the end, such increases in the antibiotic resistance genes can drastically reduce the therapeutic possibilities in infectious diseases. The presence of antibiotic resistance genes in LAB has been reported and the indirect evidence that these genes could be transferred along the food chain (Gevers, Huys, & Swings, 2003; Jacobsen, Wilcks, Hammer, Huys, et al., 2007; Teuber, Meile, & Schwarz, 1999). It is therefore relevant to assess the presence of transferable antibiotic resistances in LAB strains that are or proposed to be used as probiotics for human consumption [EFSA, 2005].

The carriage of plasmids could be considered a potential risk factor because many bacterial virulence genes and antibiotic resistance genes are encoded on plasmids. Nevertheless, assessment of the presence of plasmids can be performed but currently, this is not required for food supplements in Europe (Sanders et al., 2010). When the complete genetic content (chromosomal plus extrachromosomal entities) is included in the analysis for the presence of virulence and resistance genes, the presence of plasmids is not relevant because the genes they carry are already included (Wassenaar & Klein, 2008). An exception could be made for plasmids that enable conjugation because these plasmids would make it easier for the cell to acquire DNA from the environment. The presence of prophages is of less concern, although at some stage prophages may become lytic and may influence the gut microbiota in undesired ways (Salminen, von Wright, Ouwehand, & Holzapfel, 2001; Vankerckhoven et al., 2008). A large proportion of intraspecies bacterial variation appears to be phage related (Brabban, Hite, & Callaway, 2005). Thus, specific risks related to each probiotic strain must be carefully identified.

17.2.3 Virulence and pathogenic properties of probiotic bacteria

Providing evidence of the presence of virulence properties in a given bacterial strain is relatively straightforward. Virulence properties such as hemolytic activity, production of enterotoxins or cytotoxins, or the capacity to invade host epithelial cells can be easily demonstrated, however, the absence of such properties should be equally simple to demonstrate. The genes involved in these activities could be present but not expressed, negative phenotypic results should be confirmed by proving the absence of key genes with PCR techniques and/or DNA hybridization (Peterson, 1996). The PCR primers or oligonucleotide probes used for the detection of genes may be too specific, weak DNA hybridization may occur below detection levels, or chosen cut-offs may result in incorrect interpretations. However, potential probiotic strains should be screened in vitro for their interactions with cell lines to investigate possible cytotoxic or cytopathological effects after being grown in different media, to evaluate for the presence of known virulence genes (e.g., lecithinase activity, toxin genes, etc.) and mobile genetic elements. After these in vitro tests for potentially safe use, in vivo toxicity tests and persistence studies would be required. A study by Hütt et al. (2011) in 2011 evaluated the in vivo safety and persistence of *Lactobacillus* strains in the gastrointestinal tract of healthy adult volunteers after oral consumption of high doses of lactobacilli. The long history of safe use of probiotic LAB (e.g., *Lactococcus* and *Lactobacillus*) is the best evidence for the safety of probiotic products (O'Hara & Shanahan, 2006). Other LAB genera, such as *Streptococcus* and *Enterococcus* and other genera that could be used as probiotics contain opportunistic pathogens (Gueimonde, Ouwehand, & Salminen, 2004). The absence of pathogenicity of any potential probiotic strain must be shown to prove its safety. Furthermore, strains belonging to the *B. cereus* group are known to be able to cause two kinds of foodborne illness. First, there is an emetic (vomiting) illness due to the ingestion of food containing the heat-stable toxin cereulide (Tewari & Abdullah, 2015). The second is a diarrheal infection due to the ingestion of *B. cereus* strains producing heat-labile enterotoxins in the small intestine. Several published PCRs for these virulence genes or toxins could be used to screen *B. cereus* group strains (Wehrle, Moravek, Dietrich, & Burk, 2009). Detection of toxin genes in *B. cereus* allows assessment of the enterotoxic potential of an isolate, but not necessarily of its enteropathogenicity. Cytotoxicity tests can be used as an approximate estimation of the latter in the absence of other valid tests. Nevertheless, the detection of the presence of toxin genes by PCR-based approaches remains important for strain characterization of *B. cereus* (Amor et al., 2019).

17.2.4 Metabolic activities and toxic substance production by probiotic bacteria

Another important requirement of probiotics is that the probiotic bacteria should not produce harmful substances by metabolic activities. One way to test this is to assess whether the strain converts food components or biological secretions into secondary substances harmful to the host. For example, some intestinal bacteria are known to convert proteins and their digested products into ammonia, indole, phenols, and biogenic amines (histamine, tyramine, putrescine, etc.) (Drasar & Hill, 1974). There are no real indications on the production of harmful compounds by *Lactobacillus* and *Bifidobacterium* species. Araya-Kojima, Yaeshima, Ishibashi, Shimamura, et al. (1995, 1996) measured the enzyme activities related to the consumption and generation of ammonia in *Bifidobacterium* species of human origin. Compared with other bacteria of the intestinal microbiota, *Bifidobacterium* species have a lower deaminase activity involved in the production of ammonia from amino acids but a higher ammonia assimilation activity (Ogata et al., 1999). Secondary bile acids are important harmful substances that are produced by intestinal bacterial actions on body secretions. These may exhibit carcinogenicity by acting on the mucous-secreting cells and promoting their proliferation, or they may act as promoters of carcinogenesis (Cheah, 1990). Many intestinal bacteria, including *Bifidobacterium* and *Lactobacillus* species, can deconjugate conjugated bile acids (Midtvedt & Norman, 1967). However, *Bifidobacterium* spp., *Lactobacillus* spp., *Leuconostoc lactis* subsp. lactis and *S. thermophilus* have been reported to lack the 7α-dehydroxylase activity that is related to the production of secondary bile acids (Ferrari, Pacini, & Canzi, 1980; Takahashi & Morotomi, 1994). However, for *Enterococcus*, cytolytic substance and other virulence factors have been reported (Jett, Huycke, & Gilmore, 1994).

17.2.5 Adhesion, translocation, and colonization properties of probiotic Bacteria

In the process of infection and invasion, three aspects are very important: (i) first contact or adhesion between the bacterial strains and the epithelial cells, (ii) further translocation of the strain into or through the intestinal epithelium, and (iii) proliferation in the sterile body site, either at the level of the lamina propria, the mesenteric lymph nodes, or systemically (Berg, 1992; Dietch, Hempa, Specian, & Bery, 1992) leading to sepsis, endocarditis, and bacteremia (Steinberg, 2003). For this reason, it has been suggested that the adhesion and translocation potential of a strain should be considered as part of the safety evaluation of probiotics (Huys et al., 2013). Adhesion has been considered as a possible probiotic characteristic as adhesion can prolong the intestinal colonization of the probiotic strain, improve the beneficial immune interactions, occupy receptors that could otherwise also accommodate pathogens, and fortify the intestinal barrier (Adams & Marteau, 1995). Adhesion may also depend on the local competition with the commensal microbiota and the number of bacteria consumed. Translocation, on the other hand, depends heavily on the immune status of the hosts and thus the effects of translocated bacteria may also be very different, hence, the absence of pathogenicity and infectivity is a prerequisite of probiotic safety (Donohue & Salminen, 1996). As some probiotic bacteria may have the ability to colonize, thus a distinction between colonization properties and virulence properties exists as these activities are related. However, it is not always possible to define the properties that help bacteria colonize and adapt to a niche, i.e., the gut epithelium (an ability that may be pertained in probiotic strains), and the properties that are exclusively or largely responsible for the disease. For this difficulty, identification of virulence factors may be the best solution (Ratna Sudha, Chauhan, Dixit, Babu, et al., 2010). When the integrity of the intestinal barrier is disturbed or when the immune system is not able to confine an infection, pathogenic or commensal bacteria can reach the bloodstream and cause septicemia (Berg, 1999). Antibiotic treatment, administration of immunosuppressive agents, and induction of colitis have been used to measure bacterial translocation (Berg, 1983, 1999; Salminen & Marteau, 1997). While bacterial translocation does not occur easily in healthy specific pathogen-free animals, it is known to occur for a long duration in germ-free mice (Berg & Garlington, 1979; Ishibashi & Yamazaki, 2001; Maejima & Tajima, 1973), linked to the immature intestinal barrier and the underdeveloped immune system of these germ-free animals (Deitch, Xu, Lu, & Berg, 1991; Foo & Lee, 1972). Therefore, the safety assessment of probiotics from various angles is not a simple task (Ishibashi & Yamazaki, 2001). Acute and chronic toxicity tests provide circumstantial evidence. However, observations of the passage of bacteria across the intestinal barrier and invasion of the host body by translocation provide more direct data for determining infectivity.

17.2.6 Genetically modified probiotic microorganisms (GMPM)

Alongside natural bacterial and yeast strains, GMPMs have been designed to treat specific diseases by targeting specific pathogens and/or toxins, or through the delivery of immunosuppressive proteins (Daniel, Roussel, Kleerebezem, & Pot, 2011). The use of these so-called designer probiotics in humans would mean that GMPMs are deliberately released into the environment, which would call for specific measures and monitoring to guarantee their safety. Such measures include well-documented evidence that probiotic GMM (i) do not possess antibiotic selection markers, (ii) cannot accumulate in the environment, and (iii) cannot transfer their genetic modification (s) to other microorganisms (Culligan, Hill, & Sleator, 2009). The most challenging of these is the prevention of environmental accumulation that can be achieved through active and/or passive biological containment. Active containment is achieved by the production of a compound toxic to the GMM under regulation and control of an environmentally responsive element, whereas passive containment relies on complementation of an auxotrophy by supplementation with either an intact gene or an essential metabolite (Kimman, Smit, & Klein, 2008). The latter method was applied in the design of a recombinant interleukin-10-producing *L. lactis* strain for the treatment of Crohn's disease patients (Steidler, Neirynck,

Huyghebaert, & Snoeck, 2003). This recombinant is deficient for the thymidylate synthase gene (thyA), which is essential for the growth of *L. lactis,* and thus holds a negligible risk to accumulate and spread in the environment in the absence of thymine or thymidine.

17.3 Quality control of probiotic beverages

17.3.1 Microbial contamination of the final product

Probiotic foods and beverages have steadily gained popularity over the past decades and a wide variety of foods nowadays contain probiotic cultures. Strains are selected based on their specific health-promoting effects, but it is obvious that the safety aspects are also carefully considered to ensure that they do not pose any health risk for the consumer. The safety evaluation usually includes screening for (transferable) antibiotic resistance genes, virulence or pathogenic properties, undesirable metabolic activities, and collection of evidence to demonstrate a "history of safe use," etc. (Salminen et al., 1998). Once a strain has been approved, it must still be determined whether the analytical methods that are normally used to verify the microbiological safety of the ingredients and the finished products can also be used for the product with the probiotic strains. For microbiological methods, this is not obvious.

Finished products typically contain about 7 to 8 log colony-forming unit (CFU) per gram and the initial starter may contain more than 11 log CFU per gram, so it should be taken into account that the presence of undesirable contaminants is masked by the abundance of the beneficial microorganisms. Theoretically, this problem is most likely to occur with nonselective cultural methods. However, even with selective methods, this possibility should be considered, in particular, because many of these methods include a nonselective pre-enrichment step. This is, for instance, the case for various internationally recognized protocols, for example, for the isolation and detection of *Salmonella* (ISO standard 6579:2002). Joosten, Bidlas, and Garofalo (2006) demonstrated that false-negative results could be obtained for the detection of *Salmonella* in infant powder with probiotics. The high incidence of false-negative results can probably be explained by the metabolic activities, properties of the probiotic bacteria, in particular the production of organic acids, whose accumulation could render the pre-enrichment broth into a hostile environment for *Salmonella*. By using double strength buffered peptone water supplemented with vancomycin (10 μg/mL) and malachite green (100 μg/mL) and non-fat dry milk powder (10 g/L) as a pre-enrichment medium, the recovery of *Salmonella* was much better (Joosten et al., 2006). For the detection of other pathogenic bacteria, especially when a nonselective enrichment is used, a similar problem could be observed. By adding antimicrobial compounds to selectively suppress the growth and/or metabolic activity of the probiotic bacteria, this problem could be resolved, but more research is still needed to optimize such enrichment procedures. For the enumeration of the total microbiota, especially the contaminating microbiota (without the enumeration of the probiotic strain), the addition of 2% sodium phosphate or 5% glycerophosphate could solve the problem (Champagne, Raymond, Gonthier, & Audet, 2009). To study more in detail the problem of detection of contaminants in starter cultures and probiotics, a specific ISO working group was started in 2010 (ISO/TC 34/SC9).

17.3.2 Microbial composition

Several research labs have independently analyzed the microbial composition of probiotic dairy products (Hamilton-Miller, Shah, & Winkler, 1999; Holzapfel et al., 1998; Masco, Huys, De Brandt, Temmerman, et al., 2005; Reuter, 1997; Temmerman, Pot, Huys, & Swings, 2003; Temmerman, Scheirlinck, Huys, & Swings, 2003). Ideally, microbial analysis of probiotic products relies on standardized and accurate procedures for both the isolation and the identification of the implemented strains. In practice, however, microbial quality control of probiotic products is carried out using a culture-dependent or a culture-independent approach, or a combination of both, with each of these approaches having specific drawbacks and limitations. Especially in the case of multispecies products, a reliable taxonomic inventory may be difficult to achieve. In a culture-dependent approach, the most crucial step is the recovery of the probiotic strain(s) from the product matrix, using one or more selective isolation media (Coeuret, Gueguen, & Vernoux, 2004; Schillinger, 1999). Some probiotic strains are the result of isolation campaigns that employed very specific growth conditions that are not always provided by commercial media or by the standard set of incubation parameters used for isolation. In this context, it has been shown that some *Bifidobacterium* strains may be hard to recover from the original products, and that selective isolation of bifidobacteria from products that also contain LAB is not always straightforward (Masco et al., 2005; Temmerman, Scheirlinck, et al., 2003). Although still far from optimal, improved protocols and selective media with higher performance have been proposed for specific enumeration and isolation of bifidobacteria from (probiotic) samples (Masco et al., 2005; Roy, 2001). After isolation, a limited number of colonies are usually subjected to taxonomic characterization for the purpose of species identification as described above. When the most optimal isolation conditions are applied, and culture-dependent analyses are negative, it can be concluded that the targeted bacteria are either absent or are present in numbers beneath 1000 CFU/mL or CFU/g, which is generally considered to be the detection limit of culture-dependent analyses. In order to circumvent the possible pitfalls of conventional culturing, culture-independent methods are increasingly being used for both qualitative and quantitative microbial analysis of probiotic products because it may overcome some of the major disadvantages or limitations of culture-dependent approaches in terms of speed, taxonomic resolution, and reproducibility,

17.3.3 Microbial concentration and stability

The quality of a microbiological product, such as a starter or more generally a powder enriched with microbial cells, is generally quantified by its content of microbial cells, and among these cells two properties being expected: the ability to divide and to display a metabolic activity when introduced into a medium or into a food composition. These properties are generally represented by a term called "viability." However, recent studies have shown that cell division and metabolic activity are not always correlated as microbial cells are able to reach a transient state where no cell division occurs but metabolic activity is maintained (Booth, 2002), leading to a distinction between viability (or ability to divide) and vitality (related to the metabolic activity). These observations have led to the distinction between three classes: viable and cultivable (VC), nonviable (NV), and viable but noncultivable (VBNC). This last class has been the subject of intensive studies followed by the development of a dedicated method in order to make the distinction between the states of VC, NV, and VBNC (Lowder, Unge, Maraha, Jansson, et al., 2000). The correct assignment of a probiotic product to one of these classes is crucial, given the fact that the FAO/WHO definition of probiotics explicitly excludes NV formulations (Sanders, Hamilton, Reid, & Gibson, 2007). According to this definition, dead cells of (beneficial) bacteria that are shown to trigger or modify biological responses such as anti-inflammatory effects (Adams, 2010) should thus not be named probiotics. However, even for quality-checked probiotic products in which the active strains are considered to be in a VC state, it has been shown that a part of the bacterial population may become VBNC during storage (Lahtinen, 2012; Lahtinen, Gueimonde, Ouwehand, Reinikainen, & Salminen, 2005). Although the technological and economical importance of this finding is clear, possible effects of VC-to-VBNC transitions on probiotic efficacy are yet to be studied in more depth.

17.3.4 Strain authenticity and genetic stability

The authenticity of a probiotic culture is an important criterion to ensure the expected quality and thus predicted health-promoting effect of the probiotic product. Linked to strain authenticity is genetic stability, which reflects the susceptibility of the culture concerning genomic rearrangements in the course of its natural evolution. These rearrangements may reflect small variations introduced at specific or random positions of the genome through point mutations, deletions, and insertions, but may also be linked to larger structural variations resulting from homologous recombination (vertical inheritance) and horizontal gene transfer events. Although this is a highly relevant issue in order to ensure that specific health-promoting characteristics and functionalities are not affected during long-term preservation and production, few studies have reported comprehensive data documenting the genetic stability of commonly used probiotic strains. Ideally, a rigorous assessment of a strain's genetic stability requires the availability of its whole-genome sequence. In the absence of this information, however, the use of molecular typing techniques probably provides the best estimate of genetic stability at the individual strain level.

A preliminary verification of bacterial strain authenticity can be obtained by partial 16S rRNA gene sequencing. If this analysis confirms the species identity of the probiotic culture, further characterization at the strain level may be required. Elsewhere in this report, a series of typing methods are discussed that could be used for this purpose. However, as different typing methods offer different levels of genotypic resolution, the choice of the method and the appropriate protocol are crucial. As far as DNA fingerprinting approaches are concerned, amplified-fragment length polymorphism (AFLP) analysis and pulsed-field gel electrophoresis (PFGE) of macro-restriction fragments offer the highest resolution at the strain level. These two methods are excellent tools for genotypic comparisons throughout the production or shelf-life period of a product. Sequence-based approaches such as the multilocus sequence typing (MLST) schemes developed for several *Lactobacillus* and *Bifidobacterium* species are also relevant for typing of probiotic cultures, although their usefulness in strain authenticity matters still needs to be verified. Although not supported by producers and distributors of commercial probiotic products, the deposit of probiotic cultures into an internationally recognized culture collection would provide an enduring source of reference material for confirmation of genetic stability.

17.3.5 Labeling and claims

National food control authorities must ensure verification of compliance with food laws and apart from the risk of using unauthorized strains, product mislabelling is a known problem, partly because of the use of phenotyping or genotyping methods with a lack of discriminative power

(Huys, Vancanneyt, D'Haene, Vankerckhoven, et al., 2006). In addition to official controls, private controls by food-producing companies are important in the frame of protection of patented strains and industrial property rights. In their "Guidelines for the Evaluation of Probiotics in Food" document, the FAO/WHO working group (FAO/WHO, 2002) recommends that the following information should be described on the label of probiotic products:

- Genus, species, and strain designation. Strain designation (definition) should not mislead consumers about the functionality of the strain
- Minimum viable numbers of each probiotic strain at the end of the shelf-life
- The suggested serving size must deliver the effective dose of probiotics related to the health claim
- Health claim(s)
- Proper storage conditions
- Corporate contact details for consumer information.

In most countries, only general health claims are currently allowed on foods containing probiotics. The FAO/WHO working group recommended that specific health claims on foods be allowed relating to the use of probiotics, where sufficient scientific evidence is available. Such specific health claims should be permitted on the label and promotional material (FAO/WHO, 2002). For example, a specific claim that states that a probiotic "reduces the incidence and severity of rotavirus diarrhea in infants" would be more informative to the consumer than a general claim that states "improves gut health." It is recommended that it has to be the responsibility of the product manufacturer that an independent third-party review by scientific experts in the field be conducted to establish that health claims are truthful and not misleading. In line with the suggestions of the FAO/WHO working group, in 2006 the European Parliament and the Council published Regulation (EC) No. 1924/2006 on "Nutrition and Health Claims Made on Foods" (EU, 2006). This regulation applies to all nutritional and health claims relating to all types of food intended for final consumers, thus also including probiotic products brought to the market with a health claim. The regulation aims to harmonize the nutrition and health claims at the European level in order to better protect consumers, including commercial communications (labeling, presentation, and promotional campaigns) and trademarks and other brand names that may be construed as nutrition or health claims. The regulation establishes the authorization procedures required to ensure that claims on food labeling, presentation, and advertising are clear, concise, and based on evidence accepted by the entire scientific community.

17.4 Conclusions

The currently applied systems for safety assessments of bacterial supplements are not standardized. As multiple avenues exist for contamination in such a product, therefore stringent quality control systems and correct product labeling are the key. It is impossible to assess the safety of such a product when the identities of the strains in the product are not known or characterized. In addition to microbiological hazards regarding labels that inaccurately describe contents, excipients used in the formulations of final products can also be problematic. For instance, some children receiving probiotics have developed anaphylactic reactions from cow milk protein allergens present in the probiotic product. There are culture methods to grow lactic acid bacteria that effectively eliminate residual cow milk protein allergens. While it is unclear whether such methods are sufficient to exempt products from food allergen labeling requirements, unless the probiotic product specifically states that it is allergen-free, allergic individuals who wish to use probiotic products should actively seek assurance from manufacturers that a given product does not contain an offending allergen. The concept of Qualified Presumption of Safety (QPS) was developed by the European Commission to facilitate the safety evaluation of microorganisms intentionally introduced into the food chain and the QPS approach is a promising alternative for the safety assessment of bacterial dietary supplements and probiotic food products. Compared with the GRAS system, the QPS system appears more flexible and takes into account additional emerging safety risks, such as the acquisition of antibiotic resistance or virulence determinants. Evaluation of these characteristics is essential, as evidence to prove the absence of virulence genes or traits is by definition never exhaustive. Nevertheless, the risk of adverse effects due to the transfer of virulence genes can be considered low. The QPS system includes additional criteria to evaluate the safety of bacterial additives (such as a history of safe use in the food industry), clearly describes the relationship to a taxonomic unit, and specifies the intended application. Such a system is preferred over a regulatory system that assesses only the presence of certain virulence or resistance factors. However, by choosing the right strains, culture conditions, and product manufacturing process, much can be achieved, and the investigated health benefits can be more safely delivered to the consumer.

References

Adams, C. A. (2010). The probiotic paradox: Live and dead cells are biological response modifiers. *Nutrition Research Reviews*, *23*, 37–46.

Adams, M. R., & Marteau, P. (1995). On the safety of lactic acid bacteria from food. *International Journal of Food Microbiology*, *27*, 263–264.

Amor, M. G. B., Jan, S., Baron, F., Grosset, N., Culot, A., Gdoura, R., et al. (2019). Toxigenic potential and antimicrobial susceptibility of Bacillus cereus group bacteria isolated from Tunisian foodstuffs. *BMC Microbiology, 19*, 196.

Angelov, A., Gotcheva, V., Kuncheva, R., & Hristozova, T. (2006). Development of a new oat-based probiotic drink. *International Journal of Food Microbiology, 112*(1), 75–80. https://doi.org/10.1016/j.ijfoodmicro.2006.05.015.

Araya-Kojima, T., Yaeshima, T., Ishibashi, N., Shimamura, S., et al. (1995). Inhibitory effects of *Bifidobacterium longum* BB536 on harmful intestinal bacteria. *Bifidobacteria Microflora, 14*, 59–66.

Araya-Kojima, T., Yaeshima, T., Ishibashi, N., Shimamura, S., et al. (1996). Inhibitory effects of human-derived *Bifidobacterium* on pathogenic *Escherichia coli* serotype O-111. *Bioscience and Microflora, 15*, 17–22.

Baú, T. R., Garcia, S., & Ida, E. I. (2014). Evaluation of a functional soy product with addition of soy fiber and fermented with probiotic kefir culture. *Brazilian Archives of Biology and Technology, 57*, 402–409.

Bedani, R., Vieira, A. D. S., Rossi, E. A., & Saad, S. M. I. (2014). Tropical fruit pulps decreased probiotic survival to *in vitro* gastrointestinal stress in synbiotic soy yoghurt with okara during storage. *LWT-Food Science and Technology, 55*, 436–443.

Berg, R. D. (1983). Bacterial translocation from the gastrointestinal tracts of mice receiving immune-suppressive chemotherapeutic agents. *Current Microbiology, 8*, 285–292.

Berg, R. D. (1992). In R. Fuller (Ed.), *Probiotics, The scientific basis* (pp. 55–85). London: Chapman & Hall.

Berg, R. D. (1999). Bacterial translocation from the gastrointestinal tract. *Adv Exp Med Biol, 473*, 11–30.

Berg, R. D., & Garlington, A. W. (1979). Translocation of certain indigenous bacteria from the gastrointestinal tract to the mesenteric lymph nodes and other organs in a gnotobiotic mouse model. *Infection and Immunity, 23*, 403–411.

Bernardeau, M., Guguen, M., & Vernoux, J. P. (2006). Beneficial lactobacilli in food and feed: Long-term use, biodiversity and proposals for specific and realistic safety assessments. *FEMS Microbiology Reviews, 30*, 487–513.

Bernat, N., Cháfer, M., González-Martínez, C., Rodríguez-Garcíaez, J., & Chiralt, A. (2014). Optimisation of oat *milk* formulation to obtain fermented derivatives by using probiotic *Lactobacillus reuteri* microorganisms. *Food Science and Technology International, 21*(2), 145–157. https://doi.org/10.1177/1082013213518936.

Booth, I. R. (2002). Stress and the single cell: Intrapopulation diversity is a mechanism to ensure survival upon exposure to stress. *International Journal of Food Microbiology, 78*, 19–30.

Brabban, A. D., Hite, E., & Callaway, T. R. (2005). Evolution of foodborne pathogens via temperate bacteriophages. *Foodborne Pathogens and Disease, 2*, 287–303.

Cannon, J. P., Lee, T. A., Bolanos, J. T., & Danziger, L. H. (2005). Pathogenic relevance of Lactobacillus: A retrospective review of over 200 cases. *European Journal of Clinical Microbiology & Infectious Diseases, 24*, 31–40.

Cargill (2009). *Cargill beverage concepts will address consumer demands. Available from:(2009). https://www.foodingredientsfirst.com/news/cargill-beverage-concepts-will-address-consumer-demands.html. Last accessed June, 2020.*

Champagne, C. P., Raymond, Y., Gonthier, J., & Audet, P. (2009). Enumeration of the contaminating bacterial microbiota in unfermented pasteurized milks enriched with probiotic bacteria. *Canadian Journal of Microbiology, 55*, 410–418.

Charteris, W. P., Kelly, P. M., Morelli, L., & Collins, J. K. (1998a). Antibiotic susceptibility of potentially probiotic *Lactobacillus* species. *Journal of Food Protection, 61*, 1636–1643.

Charteris, W. P., Kelly, P. M., Morelli, L., & Collins, J. K. (1998b). Antibiotic susceptibility of potentially probiotic *Bifidobacterium* isolates from the human gastrointestinal tract. *Letters in Applied Microbiology, 26*, 333–337.

Cheah, P. Y. (1990). Hypotheses for the etiology of colorectal cancer — An overview. *Nutrition and Cancer, 14*, 5–13.

Chen, I. N. C. C., Wang, C. Y., & Chang, T. L. (2008). Lactic fermentation and antioxidant activity of Zingiberaceae plants in Taiwan. *International Journal of Food Sciences and Nutrition, 22*, 1–10.

Coeuret, V., Gueguen, M., & Vernoux, J. P. (2004). Numbers and strains of lactobacilli in some probiotic products. *International Journal of Food Microbiology, 97*, 147–156.

Culligan, E. P., Hill, C., & Sleator, R. D. (2009). Probiotics and gastrointestinal disease: Successes, problems and future prospects. *Gut Pathogens, 1*, 19. https://doi.org/10.1186/1757-4749-1-19.

Daniel, C., Roussel, Y., Kleerebezem, M., & Pot, B. (2011). Recombinant lactic acid bacteria as mucosal biotherapeutic agents. *Trends in Biotechnology, 29*, 499–508.

Deitch, E. A., Xu, D., Lu, Q., & Berg, R. D. (1991). Bacterial translocation from the gut impairs systemic immunity. *Surgery, 109*, 269–276.

Dietch, E. A., Hempa, A. C., Specian, R. D., & Bery, R. D. (1992). A study of the relationships among survival gut origin, sepsis and bacterial translocation in a model of systemic inflammation. *The Journal of Trauma, 32*, 141–147.

Donkor, O. N., Henriksson, A., Vasiljevic, T., & Shah, N. P. (2007). α-Galactosidase and proteolytic activities of selected probiotic and dairy cultures in fermented soymilk. *Food Chemistry, 104*, 10–20.

Donohue, D. C., & Salminen, S. (1996). Safety of probiotic bacteria. *Asia Pacific Journal of Clinical Nutrition, 5*, 25–28.

Drasar, B. S., & Hill, M. J. (1974). *Human intestinal flora*: (pp. 72–102). London: Academic Press.

EU (European Union) (2006). *Regulation (EC) No. 1924/2006 of the European Parliament and of the Council of 20 December 2006 on nutrition and health claims made on foods. OJ L 404, 30.12.2006*: (pp. 9–25). Available from(2006). http://eurlex.europa.eu/LexUriServ/LexUriServ.do?uri=OJ:L:2007:012:0003:0018:EN:PDF.

European Food Safety Authority (EFSA) (2005). Updating of the criteria used in the assessment of bacteria for resistance to antibiotics of human or veterinary importance. Question No. EFSA-Q-2004–079. *EFSA Journal, 223*, 1–12.

Falkow, S. (1997). What is a pathogen? Developing a definition of a pathogen requires looking closely at the many complicated relationships that exist among organisms. *ASM News, 63*, 359–365.

FAO/WHO (2002). *Food and Agriculture Organization – World Health Organization. Report of a Joint FAO/WHO Working Group on Drafting Guidelines for the Evaluation of Probiotics in Food. Available from:(2002). ftp://ftp.fao.org/es/esn/food/wgreport2.pdf.*

FAO/WHO (2006). *Probiotic in foods. Health and nutritional properties and guidelines for evaluation. In FAO food and nutrition* (p. 85). ISBN 92-5-105513-0. Also available at(2006). ftp://ftp.fao.org/docrep/fao/009/a0512e/a0512e00.pdf.

Ferrari, A., Pacini, N., & Canzi, E. (1980). A note on bile acid transformations by strains of Bifidobacterium. *The Journal of Applied Bacteriology, 49*, 193–197.

Foo, M. C., & Lee, A. (1972). Immunological response of mice to members of the autochthonous intestinal microflora. *Infection and Immunity, 6*, 525–532.

Fox, P. F., & Mc Sweeney, P. L. H. (2004). Cheese: An overview. In P. F. Fox, P. L. H. Mc Sweeney, T. M. Cogan, & T. P. Guinee (Eds.), *Cheese: Chemistry, physics and microbiology* (pp. 1–18). Academic Press.

Gevers, D., Huys, G., & Swings, J. (2003). In vitro conjugal transfer of tetracycline resistance from Lactobacillus isolates to other gram-positive bacteria. *FEMS Microbiology Letters, 225*, 125–130.

Gronbach, K., Eberle, U., Muller, M., Olschlager, T. A., et al. (2010). Safety of probiotic *Escherichia coli* strain Nissle 1917 depends on intestinal microbiota and adaptive immunity of the host. *Infection and Immunity, 78*, 3036–3046.

Gueimonde, M., Ouwehand, A. C., & Salminen, S. (2004). Safety of probiotics. *Scandinavian Journal of Nutrition*, *48*, 42–48.

Hamilton-Miller, J. M., Shah, S., & Winkler, J. T. (1999). Public health issues arising from microbiological and labelling quality of foods and supplements containing probiotic microorganisms. *Public Health Nutrition*, *2*, 223–229.

Hata, D., Yoshida, A., Ohkubo, H., Mochizuki, Y., et al. (1988). Meningitis caused by *Bifidobacterium* in an infant. *The Pediatric Infectious Disease Journal*, *7*, 669–671.

Holzapfel, W. H., Haberer, P., Snel, J., Schillinger, U., et al. (1998). Overview of gut flora and probiotics. *International Journal of Food Microbiology*, *41*, 85–101.

Hütt, P., Koll, P., Stsepetova, J., Alvarez, B., Mandar, R., Krogh-Andersen, K., … Mikelsaar, M. (2011). Safety and persistence of orally administered human *Lactobacillus* sp. strains in healthy adults. *Beneficial Microbes*, *2*(1), 79–90. https://doi.org/10.3920/BM2010'0023.

Huys, G., Botteldoorn, N., Delvigne, F., De Vuyst, L., Heyndrickx, M., Pot, B., et al. (2013). Microbial characterization of probiotics–advisory report of the working group "8651 probiotics" of the Belgian superior health council (SHC). *Molecular Nutrition & Food Research*, *57*(8), 1479–1504.

Huys, G., Vancanneyt, M., D'Haene, K., Vankerckhoven, V., et al. (2006). Accuracy of species identity of commercial bacterial cultures intended for probiotic or nutritional use. *Research in Microbiology*, *157*, 803–810.

Ishibashi, N., & Yamazaki, S. (2001). Probiotics and safety. *The American Journal of Clinical Nutrition*, *73*, 465S–470S.

Jacobsen, L., Wilcks, A., Hammer, K., Huys, G., et al. (2007). Horizontal transfer of tet(M) and erm(B) resistance plasmids from food strains of *Lactobacillus plantarum* to *Enterococcus faecalis* JH2–2 in the gastrointestinal tract of gnotobiotic rats. *FEMS Microbiology Ecology*, *59*, 158–166.

Jett, B. D., Huycke, M. M., & Gilmore, M. S. (1994). Virulence of enterococci. *Clinical Microbiology Reviews*, *7*, 462–478.

Joosten, H., Bidlas, E., & Garofalo, N. (2006). Salmonella detection in probiotic products. *International Journal of Food Microbiology*, *110*, 104–107.

Kabeir, B. M., Yazid, A. M., Hakim, M. N., Khahatan, A., Shaborin, A., & Mustafa, S. (2009). Survival of *Bifidobacterium pseudocatenulatum* G4 during the storage of fermented peanut milk (PM) and skim milk (SM) products. *African Journal of Food Science*, *3*(6), 150–155.

Kedia, G., Wang, R., Patel, H., & Pandiella, S. S. (2007). Use of mixed cultures for the fermentation of cereal-based substrates with potential probiotic properties. *Process Biochemistry*, *42*, 65–70.

Kimman, T. G., Smit, E., & Klein, M. R. (2008). Evidence-based biosafety: A review of the principles and effectiveness of microbiological containment measures. *Clinical Microbiology Reviews*, *21*, 403–425.

Kumar, B. V., Sreedharamurthy, M., & Reddy, O. V. S. (2013). Physico-chemical analysis of fresh and fermented fruit juices probioticated with *Lactobacillus casei*. *International Journal of Applied Sciences and Biotechnology*, *1*(3), 127–131. https://doi.org/10.3126/ijasbt.v1i3.8301.

Lahtinen, S. J. (2012). Probiotic viability – Does it matter? *Microbial Ecology in Health and Disease*, *23*, 18567. https://doi.org/10.3402/mehd.v23i0.18567.

Lahtinen, S. J., Gueimonde, M., Ouwehand, A. C., Reinikainen, J. P., & Salminen, J. (2005). Probiotic bacteria may become dormant during storage. *Applied and Environmental Microbiology*, *71*, 1662–1663.

Lambo, A. M., Oste, R., & Nyman, M. G. E L. (2005). Dietary fibre in fermented oat and barley β-glucan rich concentrates. *Food Chemistry*, *85*, 283–293.

Lowder, M., Unge, A., Maraha, N., Jansson, J. K., et al. (2000). Effect of starvation and the viable but nonculturable state on green fluorescent protein (GFP) fluorescence in

GFP-tagged *Pseudomonas fluorescens* A506. *Applied and Environmental Microbiology, 66*, 3160–3165.

Luckow, T., & Delahunty, C. (2004). Which juice is healthier? A consumer study of probiotic non-dairy juice drinks. *Food Quality and Preference, 15*, 751–759.

MacFie, J., O'Boyle, C., Mitchell, C. J., Buckley, P. M., et al. (1999). Gut origin of sepsis, a prospective study investigating associations between bacterial translocation, gastric microflora, and septic morbidity. *Gut, 45*, 223–228.

Maejima, K., & Tajima, Y. (1973). Association of gnotobiotic mice with various organisms isolated from conventional mice. *The Japanese Journal of Experimental Medicine, 43*, 289–296.

Masco, L., Huys, G., De Brandt, E., Temmerman, R., et al. (2005). Culture-dependent and culture-independent qualitative analysis of probiotic products claimed to contain Bifidobacteria. *International Journal of Food Microbiology, 102*, 221–230.

McMaste, L. D., Kokott, S. J., & Abratt, V. R. (2005). Use of traditional African fermented beverages as delivery vehicles for *Bifidobacterium lactis* DSM 10140. *International Journal of Food Microbiology, 102*, 231–237.

Metchnikoff, E. (1908). The prolongation of life. In P. C. Mitchell (Ed.), *Optimistic studies* (pp. 161–183). New York: G P Putnam's Sons.

Midtvedt, T., & Norman, A. (1967). Bile acid transformation by microbial strains belonging to genera found in intestinal contents. *Acta Pathologica et Microbiologica Scandinavica, 7*, 629–638.

Moncheva, P., Chipeva, V., Kujumdzieva, A., Ivanova, I., Dousset, X., & Gocheva, B. (2003). The composition of the microflora of boza, an original Bulgarian beverage. *Biotechnology & Biotechnological Equipment, 17*(1), 164–168. https://doi.org/10.1080/13102818.2003.10819214.

Muyanja, C. M. B. K., Narvhus, J. A., Treimo, J., & Langsrud, T. (2003). Isolation, characterisation and identification of lactic acid bacteria from bushera: A Ugandan traditional fermented beverage. *International Journal of Food Microbiology, 80*, 201–210.

Naidu, K. S., Adam, J. K., & Govender, P. (2012). The use of probiotics and safety concerns: A review. *African Journal of Microbiology Research, 6*(41), 6871–6877.

Nazzaro, F., Fratinni, F., Sada, A., & Orlando, P. (2008). Synbiotic potential of carrot juice supplemented with *Lactobacillus* spp. and inulin or fructo oligosaccharides. *Journal of the Science of Food and Agriculture, 88*, 2271–2276.

Nyanzi, R., & Jooste, P. J. (2012). Cereal-based functional foods. In E. C. Rigobelo (Ed.), *Probiotics*. IntechOpen.

Ogata, T., Kingaku, M., Yaeshima, T., Teraguchi, S., Fukuwatari, Y., Ishibashi, N., et al. (1999). Effect of *Bifidobacterium longum* BB536 yogurt administration on the intestinal environment of healthy adults. *Microbial Ecology in Health and Disease, 11*(1), 41–46. https://doi.org/10.1080/089106099435916.

O'Hara, A. M., & Shanahan, F. (2006). The gut flora as a forgotten organ. *EMBO Reports, 7*, 688–693.

Ouwehand, A. C., & Vesterlund, S. (2003). Health aspects of probiotics. *I Drugs, 6*, 573–580.

Pereira, D. I. A., & Gibson, G. R. (2002). Cholesterol assimilation by lactic acid bacteria and Bifidobacteria isolated from the human gut. *Applied and Environmental Microbiology, 68*(9), 4689–4693. https://doi.org/10.1128/AEM.68.9.4689-4693.2002.

Peterson, J. W. (1996). *Bacterial pathogenesis. In S. Baron (Ed.), Medical Microbiology*. (4th ed.). Galveston, TX: University of Texas Medical Branch at Galveston (Chapter 7). Available from:(1996). *https://www.ncbi.nlm.nih.gov/books/NBK8526/*.

Prado, F. C., Parada, J. L., Pandey, A., & Soccol, C. R. (2008). Trends in non-dairy probiotic beverages. *Food Research International, 41*, 111–123.

Rathore, S., Salmerón, I., & Pandiella, S. S. (2012). Production of potentially probiotic beverages using single and mixed cereal substrates fermented with LAB cultures. *Food Microbiology, 30*, 239–244.

Ratna Sudha, M., Chauhan, P., Dixit, K., Babu, S., et al. (2010). Molecular typing and probiotic attributes of a new strain of *Bacillus coagulans* – Unique IS-2: A potential biotherapeutic agent. *Genetic Engineering and Biotechnology Journal, GEBJ-7*.

Reid, G., Jass, J., Sebulsky, M. T., & McCormick, J. K. (2003). Potential use of probiotics in clinical practice. *Clinical Microbiology Reviews, 16*, 658–672.

Renuka, B., Kulkarni, S. G., Vijayanand, P., & Prapulla, S. G. (2009). Fructo oligosaccharide fortification of selected fruit juice beverages: Effect on the quality characteristics. *LWT-Food Science and Technology, 43*, 1031–1033.

Reuter, G. (1997). Present and future of probiotics in Germany and in Central Europe. *Bioscience and Microflora, 16*, 43–51.

Rezac, S., Kok, C. R., Heermann, M., & Hutkins, R. (2018). Fermented foods as a dietary source of live organisms. *Frontiers in Microbiology, 9*, 1785. https://doi.org/10.3389/fmicb.2018.01785.

Roberts, J. S., & Kidd, D. R. (2005). Lactic acid fermentation of onions. *Food Science and Technology, 38*, 2185–2190.

Roy, D. (2001). Media for the isolation and enumeration of bifidobacterial in dairy products. *International Journal of Food Microbiology, 69*, 167–182.

Saadiya, Rouf, A., Jan, T., & Sharma, P. (2018). Non-dairy probiotics – An emerging trend in health care products. *International Journal of Current Microbiology and Applied Sciences, 7*(10), 131–145. https://doi.org/10.20546/ijcmas.2018.710.015.

Saarela, M., Virkarjarvi, I., Alakomi, H. L., Matilla, P. S., & Matto, J. (2006). Stability and functionality of freeze-dried probiotic *Bifidobacterium* cells during storage in juice and milk. *International Dairy Journal, 16*, 1477–1482.

Salminen, S., & Marteau, P. (1997). Safety of probiotic lactic acid bacteria and other probiotics. In: *Lactic 97 (Proceedings). Adria Normandie Caen*, pp. 71–72.

Salminen, S., Von Wright, A., Morell, L., Marteau, P., et al. (1998). Demonstration of safety of probiotics–a review. *International Journal of Food Microbiology, 44*, 93–106.

Salminen, S., von Wright, A. J., Ouwehand, A. C., & Holzapfel, W. H. (2001). In M. R. Adams, & M. J. R. Nout (Eds.), *Fermentation and food safety* (pp. 239–251). (1st ed.). Gaithersburg, MD: Aspen.

Sanders, M. E., Akkermans, L. M. A., Haller, D., Hammerman, C., et al. (2010). Safety assessment of probiotics for human use. *Gut Microbes, 1*, 164–185.

Sanders, M. E., Hamilton, J., Reid, G., & Gibson, G. (2007). A nonviable preparation of *Lactobacillus acidophilus* is not a probiotic. *Clinical Infectious Diseases, 44*, 886.

Sanni, A., Franz, C., Schillinger, U., Huch, M., Guigas, C., & Holzapfel, W. (2013). Characterization and technological properties of lactic acid bacteria in the production of "Sorghurt," a cereal-based product. *Food Biotechnology, 27*(2), 178–918.

Saris, P. E. J., Beasley, S., & Tourila, H. (2003). Fermented soymilk with a monoculture of *Lactococcus lactis*. *International Journal of Food Microbiology, 81*, 159–162.

Schillinger, U. (1999). Isolation and identification of lactobacilli from novel-type probiotic and mild yoghurts and their stability during refrigerated storage. *International Journal of Food Microbiology, 47*, 79–87.

Shah, N. P. (2007). Functional cultures and health benefits. *International Dairy Journal, 17*, 1262–1277.

Sheehan, V. M., Ross, P., & Fitzgerald, G. F. (2007). Assessing the acid tolerance and the technological robustness of probiotic cultures for fortification in fruit juices. *Innovative Food Science and Emerging Technologies, 8*(2), 279–284. https://doi.org/10.1016/j.ifset.2007.01.007.

Sheela, T., & Suganya, R. S. (2012). Studies on anti-diarrhoeal activity of synbiotic plums juice. *International Journal of Scientific and Research Publications, 2*, 1–5.

Steidler, L., Neirynck, S., Huyghebaert, N., & Snoeck, V. (2003). Biological containment of genetically modified Lactococcus lactis for intestinal delivery of human interleukin 10. *Nature Biotechnology, 21*, 785–789.

Steinberg, S. M. (2003). Bacterial translocation: What it is and what it is not. *American Journal of Surgery, 186*, 301–305.

Takahashi, T., & Morotomi, M. (1994). Absence of cholic acid 7-dehydroxylase activity in the strains of Lactobacillus and Bifidobacterium. *Journal of Dairy Science, 77*, 3275–3286.

Temmerman, R., Pot, B., Huys, G., & Swings, J. (2003). Identification and antibiotic susceptibility of bacterial isolates from probiotic products. *International Journal of Food Microbiology, 81*, 1–10.

Temmerman, R., Scheirlinck, I., Huys, G., & Swings, J. (2003). Culture-independent analysis of probiotic products by denaturing gradient gel electrophoresis. *Applied and Environmental Microbiology, 69*, 220–226.

Teuber, M., Meile, L., & Schwarz, F. (1999). Acquired antibiotic resistance in lactic acid bacteria from food. *Antonie Van Leeuwenhoek, 76*, 115–137.

Tewari, A., & Abdullah, S. (2015). *Bacillus cereus* food poisoning: International and Indian perspective. *Journal of Food Science and Technology, 52*(5), 2500–2511.

Tissier, H. (1906). Intestinal infections treatment. *Comptes Rendus de la Societe de Biologie Paris, 60*, 359–361.

Vankerckhoven, V., Huys, G., Vancanneyt, M., Vael, C., et al. (2008). Biosafety assessment of probiotics used for human consumption: Recommendations from the EU-PROSAFE project. *Trends in Food Science and Technology, 19*, 102–114.

Verraes, C., Van Boxstael, S., Van Meervenne, E., et al. (2013). Antimicrobial resistance in the food chain: A review. *International Journal of Environmental Research and Public Health, 10* (7), 2643–2669.

Wang, X., Andersson, R., Soltesz, V., Leveau, P., et al. (1996). Gut origin sepsis, macrophage function, and oxygen extraction associated with acute pancreatitis in the rat. *World Journal of Surgery, 20*, 299–307.

Wang, C., Ng, C. C., Tzeng, W., & Shyu, Y. T. (2009). Probiotic potential of noni juice fermented with lactic acid bacteria and bifidobacteria. *International Journal of Food Sciences and Nutrition, 1*, 1–9.

Wassenaar, T. M., & Klein, G. (2008). Safety aspects and implications of regulation of probiotic bacteria in food and food supplements. *Journal of Food Protection, 71*(8), 1734–1741.

Wehrle, E., Moravek, M., Dietrich, R., & Burk, C. (2009). Comparison of multiplex PCR, enzyme immunoassay and cell culture methods for the detection of enterotoxinogenic *Bacillus cereus*. *Journal of Microbiological Methods, 78*, 265–270.

Wongkhalaung, C., & Boonyaratanakornkit, M. (2000). Development of a yogurt-type product from saccharified rice. *Kasetsart Journal (Natural Science), 34*, 107–116.

Yoon, K. Y., Woodamns, E. E., & Hang, Y. D. (2004). Probiotication of tomato juice by LAB. *Journal of Microbiology, 42*, 315–318.

Yoon, K. Y., Woodamns, E. E., & Hang, Y. D. (2005). Fermentation of beet juice by beneficial LAB. *LWT- Food Science and Technology, 38*, 73–75.

Yoon, K. Y., Woodams, E. E., & Hang, Y. D. (2006). Production of probiotic cabbage juice by lactic acid bacteria. *Bioresource Technology, 97*(12), 1427–1430.

CHAPTER

18

Quality control of probiotic beverages and organisms

Martins Ajibade Adefisoye, Ezekiel Green, Patrick Berka Njobeh, Ajibola Bamikole Oyedeji, and Oluwafemi Ayodeji Adebo

Department of Biotechnology and Food Technology, Faculty of Science, University of Johannesburg, Gauteng, South Africa

18.1 Introduction

Thousands of probiotic mixtures, drinks, or collectively "probiotic products" exist, contributing to the health of numerous consumers spread over the globe. Sequel to the different desirable and appreciable qualities of probiotics, the numbers are ever-growing with every year, new products, additives, or ingredients containing probiotic microorganisms being developed and subsequently made available in the market. With such growth and availability of this vital product arises the daunting task of effectively classifying and grouping these beneficial food groups. Not only might some claims be "untrue" but also, they might not necessarily confer the acclaimed functional properties of probiotics. Table 18.1 lists some commercially available beverages and their claimed probiotic content.

The majority of the available studies have looked at probiotics from other perspectives but a question that remains unanswered is "how well are these products truly conferring the claimed benefits?" Does the number indicated on the label accurately correspond to the microbial levels present in the product? A number of studies conducted independently have shown that the majority of probiotic products do not contain the specified strains, rather they contain mostly other bacteria, and/or they do not contain the acclaimed number of probiotic bacteria (Hamilton-Miller & Shah, 2002; Majeed et al., 2016; Weese, 2002). Therefore, the

Probiotic Beverages
https://doi.org/10.1016/B978-0-12-818588-9.00006-1

TABLE 18.1 Some commercially available beverage probiotic products and manufacturers' claims of their contents.

Beverage product	Country and manufacturer	Claim of probiotics content by manufacturers
AB Jogurtti yoghurt drink	Finland, Juustoportti	*Lactobacillus acidophilus, Bifidobacterium* spp. https://www.juustoportti.fi/ab-jogurtti_1_kg_maustamaton
Actimel	France, Danone	*Lactobacillus casei* Immunitas https://www.danone.com/brands/dairy-plant-based-products/actimel.html
Activia shot probiotic drinks	France, Danone	*Bifidobacterium lactis* https://www.activia.ca/en/activia-probiotic-drinks/
Benecol Jogurtti yoghurt drinks	Finland, Benecol	*Bifidobacterium* spp. https://www.benecol.fi/tuotteet/jogurtit
Biola mild yoghurt	Norway, Tine	*Lactobacillus rhamnosus* GG, *Lactobacillus acidophilus, Bifidobacterium* spp. https://www.tine.no/merkevarer/biola/produkter/biola-pluss-mild-yoghurt
Fjall yoghurt	Sweden, Milko	*Lactobacillus acidophilus, Bifidobacterium bifidum* https://www.norrmejerier.se/produkter/fjallfil-och-fjallyoghurt/fjallyoghurt-hjortron/397
Gefilus, Valio Probiotic juices	Finland, Valio	*Lactobacillus rhamnosus* GG https://www.valio.com/news/valio-gefilus-for-building-the-inner-strength/
Kombucha green tea	South Africa, Nature's Choice	Symbiotic culture of bacteria and yeast https://www.natureschoice.co.za/products/kombucha-green-tea/
L. Casei - Piima	Finland, SataMaito	*Lactobacillus casei* https://satamaito.fi/tuotteet/piimat/laktoositon-l-casei-piima/
Lc1 Nestlé yoghurt	Switzerland (CH) Nestlé	*Lactobacillus johnsonii* https://world.openfoodfacts.org/product/7613196007574/lc1-nestle
Rawbiotics	South Africa, Faithful to Nature	*Bifidobacterium animalis, Bi. bifidum, Bi. longum, Lactobacillus acidophilus, L. buchneri, L. bulgaricus, L. casei, L. delbrueckii, L. fermentum, L. plantarum, Lactococcus diacetylactis, L. lactis, Bacillus subtilis, Saccharomyces cerevisiae, Streptococcus thermophilus* https://www.faithful-to-nature.co.za/

majority of the claims should be reassessed, especially the quantity of "live" microorganisms (probiotic) present in a product.

From a broader perspective and across industries, quality control (QC) is a critical activity needed to ensure the reliability of products. For the food industry, QC covers raw materials, the different unit operations involved in the manufacturing process, finished products, as well as packaging. With probiotics, it is equally similar and vital as probiotics are considered beneficial microorganisms that influence the gut of the host and thus are expected to possess some specific characteristics for them to be called "a probiotic" or being "probiotic." Some of these benefits have already been discussed in this book, but summarily it involves conferring a beneficial influence on the health of the host, especially in the gut (digestive system).

The general misnomer is usually assuming that one can evaluate probiotic efficacy by using cell viability and that cell counts would also suffice. While this is vital, it should not be the only case for a QC test of a probiotic product, as other aspects such as the ability to metabolize certain substrates, ability to tolerate acidic conditions, survival of these probiotic strains in the bile, as well as adhesion properties are equally important (Tuomola, Crittenden, Playne, Isolauri, & Slaminen, 2001). QC of probiotics should involve all of these aforementioned areas and numerous others that are discussed in the ensuing sections of this chapter.

18.2 Criteria for quality control of probiotics

Different studies have been presented in literature regarding the need for continuous monitoring of the important QC criteria for the selection of probiotics in order to ensure their effectiveness for human use, as well as the need to ensure the selection of more stable strains of probiotics for commercial purposes. For instance, the Food and Agriculture Organization of the United Nations (FAO) and the World Health Organization (WHO) highlighted important in vitro tests to be used in the study of probiotics strains, most importantly for safety purposes (FAO/WHO, 2002). These tests are vital in probiotic strain selection in order to ensure the functionality of probiotic microorganisms, as well as ensure the acclaimed properties of probiotics for quality assurance reasons. It should be noted however that the use of in vitro testing to ascertain the quality or stability of probiotic strains is often not sufficient and requires substantiation of efficacy with in vivo or human trials. The major quality assurance/control characteristics or criteria summarized in Fig. 18.1, are discussed below.

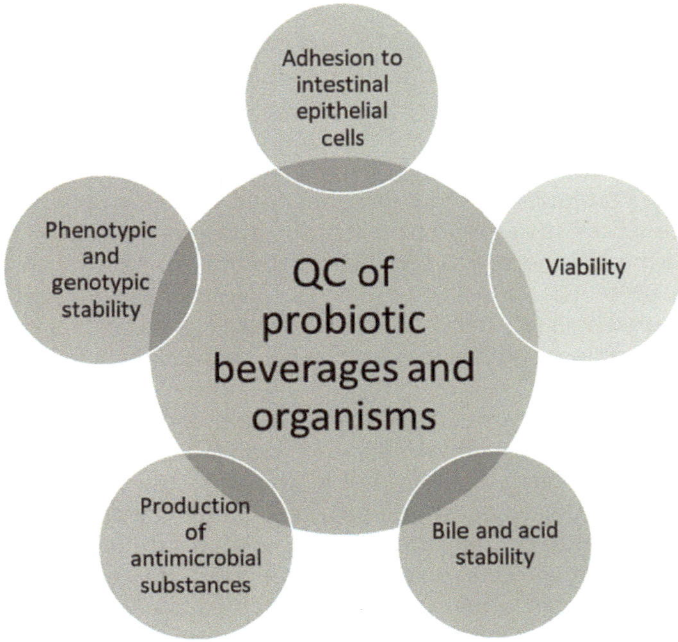

FIG. 18.1 QC criteria of probiotic beverages/organisms.

18.2.1 Adhesion to intestinal epithelial cells

The outermost intestinal layer, which acts mainly as a protective barrier and filter, is a secreted and hydrated mucus gel, consisting mainly of a diverse mixture of highly glycosylated membrane-associated glycoproteins known as mucins. The preferential adherence of probiotic microorganisms to the intestinal mucosa is a necessary precondition for the eventual colonization of the human GI. This phenomenon generally prolongs and stabilizes the intestinal habitat and possibly elicits diverse defensive host cell immune responses, thus eliminating pathogenic microorganisms via competitive inhibition or steric hindrance. This ability also extends to the promotion of immunomodulatory effects as well as the stimulation of gut barrier and metabolic functions (Monteagudo-Mera, Rastall, Gibson, Charalmpopoulos, & Chatzifragkou, 2019). Even though some studies have shown that probiotic bacteria adhere initially to the mucus gel layer, relatively little knowledge is available about the entire molecular mechanism of adhesion. However, different studies have noted that a probiotic's adherence to the mucosal layer is often due to a surface protein-mediated interaction (do Carmo et al., 2018; Hickey, 2012; von Ossowski et al., 2010; Wang, Zhang, Xia, Lai, & Ai, 2018). This adhesion ability could also increase the opportunity of the probiotic bacteria to interact with the host leading to a temporary colonization, thereby increasing their transit time in the gut (Monteagudo-Mera et al., 2019). Such temporary colonization favors the production of short chain fatty acids and immunomodulatory effects. Since adhesion of pathogens to specific mucosal receptors is vital for the initiation of infection, a competitive adhesion by an adhesive probiotic with specific adhesion analogues may hinder the subsequent adhesion of pathogenic organisms, a process referred to as competitive exclusion. For instance, Spencer and Chesson (1994) documented the inhibition of *Escherichia coli* to porcine enterocytes. Chan, Reid, Irvin, Bruce, and Costerton (1985) reported the inhibition of adhesion of human uropathogens to uroepithelial cells in vitro by some strains of *lactobacillus*. As reported in the literature, the presence of fibronectin-binding and surface-layer proteins could further increase this adhesion ability (Hymes, Johnson, Barrangou, & Klaenhammer, 2016; Lehri, Seddon, & Karlyshev, 2015). An in vitro assay, which involves the co-culturing of probiotic bacteria and enterocyte-like Caco-2 tissue culture cells, has been used to test the effective adherence of probiotic strains. The assay involves the preparation of 17-day-old, well-differentiated Caco-2 cells, which are then incubated with standardized probiotic strains for 90 min, under standard conditions. The number of the adhering probiotic bacteria is then calculated based on the number of the bacteria used for the inoculum (%) and the number of adhering bacteria per one Caco-2 epithelial cell (Piatek et al., 2012). Additionally, since the adhesion of probiotic microbes is important in stimulating the immune system, Tuomola et al. (2001) suggested the inclusion of intestinal biopsy samples as a final in vitro test of adhesion or colonization, which is most similar to in vivo conditions.

18.2.2 Viability

Probiotics need to either adapt to the dynamic gut environment and/or be protected in order to survive and become available in adequate quantities to deliver their health benefits. Viability is generally considered a prerequisite for the functionality of probiotics. Each probiotic strain may differ in response to various stress factors. Such factors include, but are not limited to, the digestive enzymes, certain ions, bile and bile salts, gastric acid, temperature digestive enzymes, the highly proteolytic gastric juice environment, the food matrix, as well as the manufacturing processes, all of which tend to reduce the viability and functionality of probiotic bacteria. A number of reports have shown that the survival and viability of probiotic strains in a gastric juice environment is very poor, with only a small number exhibiting stability and resistance to adverse environmental conditions (Corcoran, Stanton, Fitzgerald, &

Ross, 2005; Park, Lee, Jun, Son, & Kang, 2016). The loss of viability by the strains constitutes a significant economic burden for manufacturers due to the compromise of product efficacy, thus hindering the inclusion of probiotics in several product categories (Gueimonde & Sánchez, 2012). Therefore, in order to improve the survival and stability of probiotics during processes and the gastro-juice environment, new technological approaches have been developed, such as the alteration of production parameters or the reformulation of products, microencapsulation, as well as microbiological strategies focusing on the intrinsic resistance of probiotic strains. The various approaches at enhancing the viability and stability of bacterial cells can be grouped into three broad categories, which include the selection of naturally occurring probiotic strains, stress adaptation of naturally occurring bacterial strains, and genetic modification of strains.

18.2.3 Bile and acid stability

The potential of microorganisms to exhibit acid tolerance is one of the important desirable characteristics for the selection of probiotic strains. Probiotics need to be able to survive in the bile and acidic gastric environment of the host GI before they can reach and colonize the small intestine and impart their health benefits. Though different strains behave differently in an acid environment, microorganisms generally show higher sensitivity at pH levels below 3.0 (Rönkä et al., 2003). For instance, *Lactobacillus rhamnosus* GG reportedly survives gastric transit and is able to resist acidity as low as 2.5 for about 4h (Jacobsen et al., 1999). The increased acid tolerance of lactic acid bacteria has been attributed to the existence of a constant gradient between the extracellular and cytoplasmic pH.

Even though bile tolerance is generally strain-dependent, some probiotic bacteria, such as bifidobacteria and lactobacilli, can adapt progressively when exposed to bile salts. Sensitive wild type strains of these bacteria can be become resistant derivatives by subculturing them in gradually increasing bile concentrations. Cross-resistance due to strain exposure to other stressful conditions, such as low or acidic pH, can also lead to the development of bile resistance. This phenomenon is a reflection of the occurrence of common strains' response mechanisms to different stress conditions, suggesting that, the enhancement of bile tolerance in probiotic organisms could assist in developing more robust strains, which may show improved resistance to other GI factors that could compromise the survival of the probiotics (Ruiz, Margolles, & Sánchez, 2013).

Human and animal gastric juices, as well as simulated gastric juices, have been used for gastric transit studies of probiotics. These two approaches, however, have different limitations. The use of simulated gastric juice does not consider the effects of nonacid and other dietary constituents of the gastric secretions on the survival of the probiotics; human and animal gastric juices, on the contrary, are limited by the non-availability of fresh materials. Reformulation of foods and ingredients have been used extensively to enhance the survival of probiotic strains during the gastric transit phase; however, little information is available on the influence of individual food constituents and their underlying mechanisms of action at enhancing probiotic survival (Corcoran et al., 2005).

Bile is a yellowish-green aqueous fluid, functioning mainly as a biological detergent, which emulsifies and solubilizes lipids. The detergent property of bile also makes it a potent antimicrobial, mostly through the dissolution of bacterial membranes. Hydrolysis of bile salts by probiotic strains is an important property that has been used for probiotic selection. Common probiotic strains (lactobacillus and bifidobacteria) and other commensal GI bacteria, such as *Bacteriodes*, *Enterococcus* and *Clostridium* species, have been reported with bile salt hydrolase (BSH) activities (Kawamoto, Horibe, & Uchida, 1989; Kim, Brochet, & Lee, 2005; McAuliffe, Cano, & Klaenhammer, 2005; Pereira, McCartney, & Gibson, 2003; Wijaya et al., 2004). However, BSH activity has generally not been reported in bacteria from environments lacking bile salts. Despite the inclusion of BSH activity in the selection of probiotics, this property has been argued to be potentially harmful to human hosts; therefore, it is not clear whether this trait should be a desirable quality for probiotic selection (Begley, Hill, & Gahan, 2006).

18.2.4 Production of antimicrobial substances

The ability of bacteria to produce antimicrobial substance with antagonistic potentials against enteric pathogens is often considered an important criterion for the selection of probiotic strains. The production of compounds with broad spectrum antimicrobial potential, as well as antagonism against pathogens with strong antimicrobial activity, is a functional desirable property of a probiotic bacterium. Probiotic strains may produce antimicrobial compounds that have bacteriostatic or bactericidal effects against potential pathogens by maintaining the homeostasis of the gastrointestinal flora. The antagonistic activity of probiotics against other microorganisms can be through the stimulation of host defense systems, exclusion by competition, production of hydrogen peroxides or organic acids that lower pH, immune system modulation, production of signaling substances that trigger changes in gene expression, and production antimicrobials, such as short chain fatty acids, antioxidants, nitric oxide, bacteriocins, and bacteriocin-like inhibitory substances (Fijan, 2016). The production of bacteriocins, which are ribosomally-synthesized bacterial antimicrobial peptides with antagonistic activity against other bacterial strains, is traditionally considered an important criterion for the selection of probiotics. Even though the precise ecological function of bacteriocins as antimicrobials is still very much in debate, the noticeable ubiquitous nature of this characteristic indicates that bacteriocins play a vital role in spite of the energy cost associated with their production. Common examples of bacteriocins include colicin, enterolysin, plantaricin, pediocin, lactocin, pisciolin, lacticin, reuterin, enterocin, and nisin among others (Arqués, Rodríguez, Langa, Landete, & Medina, 2015; Šušković et al., 2010). Bacteriocins have been broadly classified into four groups designated Class I to IV (Kumariya et al., 2019); however, in terms of their antagonist actions, they function as colonizing peptides that promote the introduction and/or dominance of a bacteriocin producer into an already occupied habitat. Second, they may act as signaling peptides that either signal to the immune system of the host or signal to other bacterial cells via quorum sensing. Last, bacterial-produced bacteriocins may function as killing or antimicrobial peptides, directly suppressing competing microbes (Dobson, Cotter, Ross, & Hill, 2012). In vitro tests for probiotics' antagonistic effects against other strains include the agar well diffusion test, agar spot or spot-on lawn antimicrobial test, and a co-culturing test to determine antagonistic potential. For in vivo antimicrobial testing, animal models, placebo-controlled human trials, and randomized double blind studies have been used. However, it should be noted that due to obvious reasons, such as species-specific variation in physiology, anatomy, toxic responses, and pharmacokinetics, animal model results might not necessarily give a scientifically appropriate and applicable human outcome.

18.2.5 Phenotypic and genotypic stability

Safety concerns of probiotics requires validation of their phenotypic and genotypic stability over time. Probiotics have mainly been characterized over the years using phenotypic approaches, which always leave some uncertainties. Traditionally, probiotics strains, such as lactobacilli and bifidobacteria, have been characterized based on their cell morphology, ability to metabolize different carbohydrate substrates, as well as the analysis of their products of fermentation and related enzymatic activities. A number of studies have reviewed the limitations and narrow reproducibility of these phenotypic approaches (Sgorbati, Biavati, & Palenzona, 1995; Tannock, 1999). The classical phenotypic typing methods (morphological, physiological, and biochemical) often provide important data for the preliminary characterization of microbes for the description of their taxa from species up to genus and family levels. Nevertheless, the phenotypic characterization must be complemented by genotyping (Donelli, Vuotto, & Mastromarino, 2013).

The bacterial genome generally contains a very large number of insertion sequence (IS) elements that can cause major problems in sequence assembly and which may lead to genome "reshuffling" during growth and stressful conditions. This may potentially trigger variability between batches of production over a period, hence the need to assess the phenotypic and genotypic consistency of probiotics regularly (Majeed et al., 2016). A recent study into genetic drift within bacterial strains, including probiotics, suggests the need for probiotic manufacturers to address the risks associated with genetic drift in the probiotic industry. To this end, genetic drift can be described as a divergence in genetic components through DNA mutation of a microbial strain over time. However, mutation in DNA is generally believed to occur at a constant low rate unless there is an application of selective pressure. The genetic stability assurance of a probiotic strains will boost consumer confidence and preserve the efficacy of the product. To reduce the risk of genetic drift and phenotypic variations within a probiotic population, process control must be strictly controlled during growth and scale up in order to ensure the fewest number of generations as possible from the mother seed culture (Sanders et al., 2019).

The integrity of manufacturer's claims of the microbiological quality of probiotics has been tested by many researchers (Aureli, Fiore, Scalfaro, Casale, & Franciosa, 2010; Chen et al., 2014; Marinova, Rasheva, Kizheva, Dermenzhieva, & Hristova, 2019; Patro et al., 2016). Commercial probiotic foods and beverages, with different claims of microbial contents by manufacturers as stipulated on the labels of these products, were purchased from shelves and subjected to microbial analysis. These researchers carried out their studies in different countries of different continents and used different microbial evaluation methods, from plate count to high-throughput next-generation sequencing in the analysis of the microbiological quality of manufacturers' claims of probiotics. Table 18.2 provides information on the microbiological quality of some commercially available probiotic products as elucidated by different researchers.

18.3 Conclusion and future perspectives

Probiotic product regulations are generally not established on an international basis and there is often a lack of label control, as well as the absence of time-to-time screening of products for quality and safety purposes. Quality assurance checks are vital steps to ensure the efficacy of probiotic products and to ascertain the conferment of acclaimed health benefits. Even though general opinions tend to emphasize the major health benefits of probiotics, by and large, it should be noted that the majority of the recognized functionality of probiotic foods are often strain

TABLE 18.2 Assessment of microbiological quality of some commercially available probiotic products (supplements, foods, and beverages) by different researchers from different locations.

Number of products	Country/ location	Method of evaluation	Major findings	Reference
Ten (two are in powder form)	Online products (study carried out in the United States)	Whole genome sequencing	Products generally adhered to manufacturers' ingredient claim with minimal differences. Discrepancies in naming closely related *Lactobacillus* and *Bifidobacterium* species were observed and one product contained *Enterococcus* contamination	Patro et al. (2016)
Twenty-eight (eight yoghurt products)	China	Culture dependent and culture-independent methods	Inconsistencies with the bacterial counts of some species with the labelling information was observed. *Bifidobacteria* were not detected in any product that claimed to contain them, degradation of probiotic prowess of species and contamination by *Enterobacter* sp., *Klebsiella* sp., and *Serratia* spp. Was detected	Chen et al. (2014)
Seventy-two (some bottled as probiotic supplements)	Italy	Culture dependent isolation and enumeration of viable cells and PCR identification	*Bifidobacteria* were sporadically detected. In some samples as dead cells despite the claim of their presence by most labeled samples. Spore forming and toxin producing	Aureli et al. (2010)

TABLE 18.2 Assessment of microbiological quality of some commercially available probiotic products (supplements, foods, and beverages) by different researchers from different locations—cont'd

Number of products	Country/ location	Method of evaluation	Major findings	Reference
			Bacillus cereus was detected in some samples. Eighty-seven percent of samples did not conform with Italian guidelines	
Twenty-six (ten powdered products)	Bulgaria	Isolation using culture-dependent methods and molecular identification using PCR based methods and DNA sequencing	None of the commercial products tested contained all of the LAB as claimed on their labels, and there was a presence of contaminants. Only ten of the isolates exhibited slight antimicrobial activities against *Escherichia coli*, *Salmonella enterica* and *Bacillus subtilis*	Marinova et al. (2019)
Sixteen (some are powdered products)	United States (online and local stores)	Genomic DNA extraction coupled with different PCR assays. Also, isolation of Bifidobacterial strains coupled with identification by MALDI-TOF mass spectrometry and genome sequencing	Contents of most samples differed from the claims on the labels. Only one of the sixteen samples perfectly matched its Bifidobacterial claims	Lewis et al. (2016)

dependent. Notwithstanding, it is essential that the specific characteristics of a probiotic product originally used in the strain selection process should also be targeted for quality assurance purposes. Therefore, one should take into account, the specific characteristics of probiotic strains as well as their stability during processing and usage. Accurate methods of identification and documentation are mandatory during each manufacturing step, from strain identification to functionality testing such as viability during industrial processing, stability in acid and bile environment, adhesion to the mucosal epithelial cells, and viability by the end of shelf life. An important emerging issue related to probiotic quality is the problem of contamination by "foreign" strains. Contaminating strains can invalidate and skew study results making them irreproducible in the QC of the same probiotic product with undesirable clinical outcomes. With the current advances in omics technologies, a range of high-throughput applications of omics in the study of functionality of probiotics will revolutionize and further enhance the understanding of the specific interactions between the human host and probiotics strains. The prospect to study completely sequenced and annotated bacterial genomes will greatly help in understanding the important genetics and functional aspects of probiotic foods.

Acknowledgment

This work was partly supported by the University of Johannesburg Global Excellence and Stature (GES) Post Doctoral Research Fellowship, GES 4.0 Catalytic Initiative Grant and the National Research Foundation (NRF) of South Africa Thuthuka Grant (grant number: 121826).

References

Arqués, J. L., Rodríguez, E., Langa, S., Landete, J. M., & Medina, M. (2015). Antimicrobial activity of lactic acid bacteria in dairy products and gut: Effect on pathogens. *BioMed Research International, 2015*, 9. https://doi.org/10.1155/2015/584183.

Aureli, P., Fiore, A., Scalfaro, C., Casale, M., & Franciosa, G. (2010). National survey outcomes on commercial probiotic food supplements in Italy. *International Journal of Food Microbiology, 137*(2–3), 265–273.

Begley, M., Hill, C., & Gahan, C. G. (2006). Bile salt hydrolase activity in probiotics. *Applied and Environmental Microbiology, 72*(3), 1729–1738.

Chan, R. C. Y., Reid, G., Irvin, R. T., Bruce, A. W., & Costerton, J. W. (1985). Competitive exclusion of uropathogens from human uroepithelial cells by Lactobacillus whole cells and cell wall fragments. *Infection and Immunity, 47*, 84–89.

Chen, T., Wu, Q., Li, S., Xiong, S., Jiang, S., Tan, Q., et al. (2014). Microbiological quality and characteristics of probiotic products in China. *Journal of the Science of Food and Agriculture, 94*(1), 131–138.

Corcoran, B. M., Stanton, C., Fitzgerald, G. F., & Ross, R. P. (2005). Survival of probiotic lactobacilli in acidic environments is enhanced in the presence of metabolizable sugars. *Applied and Environmental Microbiology, 71*(6), 3060–3067.

do Carmo, F. L., Rabah, H., de Oliveira Carvalho, R. D., Gaucher, F., Cordeiro, B. F., da Silva, S. H., et al. (2018). Extractable bacterial surface proteins in probiotics in probiotic-host interaction. *Frontiers in Microbiology, 9*, 645.

Dobson, A., Cotter, P. D., Ross, R. P., & Hill, C. (2012). Bacteriocin production: A probiotic trait? *Applied and Environmental Microbiology, 78*(1), 1–6.

Donelli, G., Vuotto, C., & Mastromarino, P. (2013). Phenotyping and genotyping are both essential to identify and classify a probiotic microorganism. *Microbial Ecology in Health and Disease, 24*(1)20105.

FAO/WHO (2002). *Report of a joint FAO/WHO working group on drafting guidelines for the evaluation of probiotics in food London, Ontario, Canada April 30 and May 1, 2002.* .

Fijan, S. (2016). Antimicrobial effect of probiotics against common pathogens. *Probiotics and Prebiotics in Human Nutrition and Health*. https://doi.org/10.5772/63141.

Gueimonde, M. & Sánchez, B. (2012). Enhancing probiotic stability in industrial processes. Microbial Ecology in Health and Disease, 23, https://doi.org/10.3402/mehd.v23i0.18562. doi:https://doi.org/10.3402/mehd.v23i0.18562.

Hamilton-Miller, J. M. T., & Shah, S. (2002). Deficiencies in microbiological quality and labelling of probiotic supplements. *International Journal of Food Microbiology*, *72*, 175–176.

Hickey, R. M. (2012). The role of oligosaccharides from human milk and other sources in prevention of pathogen adhesion. *International Dairy Journal*, *22*(2), 141–146.

Hymes, J. P., Johnson, B. R., Barrangou, R., & Klaenhammer, T. R. (2016). Functional analysis of an S-layer-associated fibronectin-binding protein in *Lactobacillus acidophilus* NCFM. *Applied and Environmental Microbiology*, *82*, 2676–2685.

Jacobsen, C. N., Nielsen, V. R., Hayford, A. E., Møller, P. L., Michaelsen, K. F., Paerregaard, A., et al. (1999). Screening of probiotic activities of forty-seven strains of *Lactobacillus* spp. by in vitro techniques and evaluation of the colonization ability of five selected strains in humans. *Applied and Environmental Microbiology*, *65*(11), 4949–4956.

Kawamoto, K., Horibe, I., & Uchida, K. (1989). Purification and characterization of a new hydrolase for conjugated bile acids, chenodeoxycholyltaurine hydrolase, from *Bacteroides vulgatus*. *The Journal of Biochemistry*, *106*(6), 1049–1053.

Kim, G. B., Brochet, M., & Lee, B. H. (2005). Cloning and characterization of a bile salt hydrolase (bsh) from *Bifidobacterium adolescentis*. *Biotechnology Letters*, *27*(12), 817–822.

Kumariya, R., Garsa, A. K., Rajput, Y. S., Sood, S. K., Akhtar, N., & Patel, S. (2019). Bacteriocins: Classification, synthesis, mechanism of action and resistance development in food spoilage causing bacteria. *Microbial Pathogenesis*, *128*, 171–177.

Lehri, B., Seddon, A. M., & Karlyshev, A. V. (2015). *Lactobacillus fermentum* 3872 genome sequencing reveals plasmid and chromosomal genes potentially involved in a probiotic activity. *FEMS Microbiology Letters*, *362*(11), fnv068.

Lewis, Z. T., Shani, G., Masarweh, C. F., Popovic, M., Frese, S. A., Sela, D. A., et al. (2016). Validating bifidobacterial species and subspecies identity in commercial probiotic products. *Pediatric Research*, *79*(3), 445.

Majeed, M., Nagabhushanam, K., Natarajan, S., Sivakumar, A., Eshuis-de Ruiter, T., Booij Veurink, J., et al. (2016). Evaluation of genetic and phenotypic consistency of *Bacillus coagulans* MTCC 5856: A commercial probiotic strain. *World Journal of Microbiology and Biotechnology*, *32*(4), 60.

Marinova, V. Y., Rasheva, I. K., Kizheva, Y. K., Dermenzhieva, Y. D., & Hristova, P. K. (2019). Microbiological quality of probiotic dietary supplements. *Biotechnology & Biotechnological Equipment*, *33*(1), 834–841.

McAuliffe, O., Cano, R. J., & Klaenhammer, T. R. (2005). Genetic analysis of two bile salt hydrolase activities in *Lactobacillus acidophilus* NCFM. *Applied and Environmental Microbiology*, *71*(8), 4925–4929.

Monteagudo-Mera, A., Rastall, R. A., Gibson, G. R., Charalmpopoulos, D., & Chatzifragkou, A. (2019). Adhesion mechanisms mediated by probiotics and prebiotics and their potential impact on human health. *Applied Microbiology and Biotechnology*, *103*, 6463–6472.

Park, H. J., Lee, G. H., Jun, J., Son, M., & Kang, M. J. (2016). Multiple-unit tablet of probiotic bacteria for improved storage stability, acid tolerability, and in vivo intestinal protective effect. *Drug Design, Development and Therapy*, *10*, 1355.

Patro, J. N., Ramachandran, P., Barnaba, T., Mammel, M. K., Lewis, J. L., & Elkins, C. A. (2016). Culture-independent metagenomic surveillance of commercially available probiotics with high-throughput next-generation sequencing. *MSphere*, *1*(2). e00057-16.

Pereira, D. I., McCartney, A. L., & Gibson, G. R. (2003). An in vitro study of the probiotic potential of a bile-salt-hydrolyzing *Lactobacillus fermentum* strain, and determination of its cholesterol-lowering properties. *Applied and Environmental Microbiology, 69*(8), 4743–4752.

Piatek, J., Gibas-Dorna, M., Olejnik, A., Krauss, H., Wierzbicki, K., Zukiewicz-Sobczak, W., et al. (2012). The viability and intestinal epithelial cell adhesion of probiotic strain combination-in vitro study. *Annals of Agricultural and Environmental Medicine, 19*(1).

Rönkä, E., Malinen, E., Saarela, M., Rinta-Koski, M., Aarnikunnas, J., & Palva, A. (2003). Probiotic and milk technological properties of *Lactobacillus brevis*. *International Journal of Food Microbiology, 83*(1), 63–74.

Ruiz, L., Margolles, A., & Sánchez, B. (2013). Bile resistance mechanisms in Lactobacillus and Bifidobacterium. *Frontiers in Microbiology, 4*, 396.

Sanders, M. E., Jackson, S., Schoeni, J. L., Vegge, C., Pane, M., Stahl, B., et al. (2019). Improving end-user trust in the quality of commercial probiotic products. *Frontiers in Microbiology, 10*, 739.

Sgorbati, B., Biavati, B., & Palenzona, D. (1995). The genus *Bifidobacterium*. In B. J. B. Wood, & W. H. Holzapfel (Eds.), *The lactic acid bacteria. Volume 2. The genera of lactic acid bacteria* (pp. 279–306). London: Blackie Academic and Professional.

Spencer, R. J., & Chesson, A. (1994). The effect of *Lactobacillus* spp. on the attachment of enterotoxigenic *Escherichia coli* to isolated porcine enterocytes. *Journal of Applied Bacteriology, 77*, 215–220.

Šušković, J., Kos, B., Beganovič, J., Leboš Pavunc, A., Habjanič, K., & Matošić, S. (2010). Antimicrobial activity—The most important property of probiotic and starter lactic acid bacteria. *Food Technology and Biotechnology, 48*(3), 296–307.

Tannock, G. W. (1999). *Probiotics: A critical review*. Wymondham, UK: Horizon Scientific Press.

Tuomola, E., Crittenden, R., Playne, M., Isolauri, E., & Slaminen, S. (2001). Quality assurance criteria for probiotic bacteria. *American Journal of Clinical Nutrition, 73*, 393S–398S.

von Ossowski, I., Reunanen, J., Satokari, R., Vesterlund, S., Kankainen, M., Huhtinen, H., et al. (2010). Mucosal adhesion properties of the probiotic *Lactobacillus rhamnosus* GG SpaCBA and SpaFED pilin subunits. *Applied and Environmental Microbiology, 76*(7), 2049–2057.

Wang, G., Zhang, M., Xia, Y., Lai, P. F. H., & Ai, L. (2018). A surface protein from *Lactobacillus plantarum* increases the adhesion of Lactobacillus strains to human epithelial cells. *Frontiers in Microbiology, 9*, 2858.

Weese, J. S. (2002). Microbiologic evaluation of commercial probiotics. *Journal of the American Veterinary Medical Association, 220*, 794–797.

Wijaya, A., Hermann, A., Abriouel, H., Specht, I., Yousif, N. M., Holzapfel, W. H., et al. (2004). Cloning of the bile salt hydrolase (bsh) gene from *Enterococcus faecium* FAIR-E 345 and chromosomal location of bsh genes in food enterococci. *Journal of Food Protection, 67* (12), 2772–2778.

Further reading

Tamime, A. Y., Saarela, M., Wszolek, M., Ghoddousi, H., Linares, D. M., & Shah, N. P. (2018). Production and maintaining viability of probiotic microorganisms in dairy products. In A. Y. Tamime, & L. V. Thomas (Eds.), *Probiotic dairy products* (pp. 67–164). Hoboken, NJ: Wiley Blackwell.

Vecchione, A., Celandroni, F., Mazzantini, D., Senesi, S., Lupetti, A., & Ghelardi, E. (2018). Compositional quality and potential gastrointestinal behavior of probiotic products commercialized in Italy. *Frontiers in Medicine, 5*, 59.

CHAPTER

19

Legalities, intellectual property, ethical concerns and regulatory aspects in probiotics

Sripathi Rao Kulkarni

Business Development-Intellectual Property Unit, CSIR-Central Drug Research Institute, Lucknow, Uttar Pradesh, India

19.1 Introduction

Humans can thrive on this planet because of what they consume, digest, and assimilate, deriving energy from metabolic activities. Human pursuits towards understanding on what to eat and what not to, have been based on observational patterns since the advent of the species. In the olden days, most of the food and food-based cottage industries were more local than global, as the food was more region-specific. The taste and preference of food changes from state to state, country to country, and region to region, and the availability of food in diverse forms led to mankind exploring food's nutritional and medicinal benefits. It has been thought that roughly 100 trillion bacteria that symbiotically inhabit the body of a human and which were earlier considered to be parasites, significantly contribute to maintaining and managing human health. Speculation is that perhaps the human role is to host bacteria and not the other way around, as they are known to show an impact on our growth, metabolism, digestion, immunity, longevity, and even brain health. Thus, comes the importance of "Probiotics" in the lives of humans and animals. Although the knowledge of probiotics is known from the Neolithic age, nearly 10,000 years ago (Ozen & Dinleyici, 2015; Santacroce, Charitos, & Bottalico, 2019), the significant documented evidence comes from the beginning of the 20th century.

Probiotic Beverages
https://doi.org/10.1016/B978-0-12-818588-9.00012-7

A Russian scientist, Elie Metchnikoff, observed the extraordinary health of Bulgarians who inhabited the mountains, and who were reported to be among the longest-lived people on the Earth. He speculated that this affinity towards live bacterial cultured yogurts was the main reason behind their longevity. His studies proclaimed that taking fermented milk along with lactic acid bacteria (LAB) resulted in the presence of abundant good bacteria in the human intestine, these were later identified as the "Bulgarian bacillus." Metchnikoff further suggested that the harmful microbes found in the gut flora could be replaced with useful microbes, and in 1905, he started a consumer rush to consume yogurt in France when he hypothesized that the toxic substances that are produced because of putrefaction by microbes in the gut flora affect the aging process (Fig. 19.1).

Werner Kollath in 1953, described the first use of additives in probiotics, specifically relating to the significance of organic and inorganic supplements, in the restoration of health of malnourished patients. Today, researchers are moving towards microbiome-focused approaches in enhancing gut health ecosystems (WGO, 2017).

In 2001, a panel of experts, at the behest of the Food and Agriculture Organization (FAO) and World Health Organization (WHO) was convened and they defined probiotics as follows: "Live microorganisms *which* when administered in adequate amounts confer a health benefit on the host." Later, in 2014, another panel reiterated the definition part, with

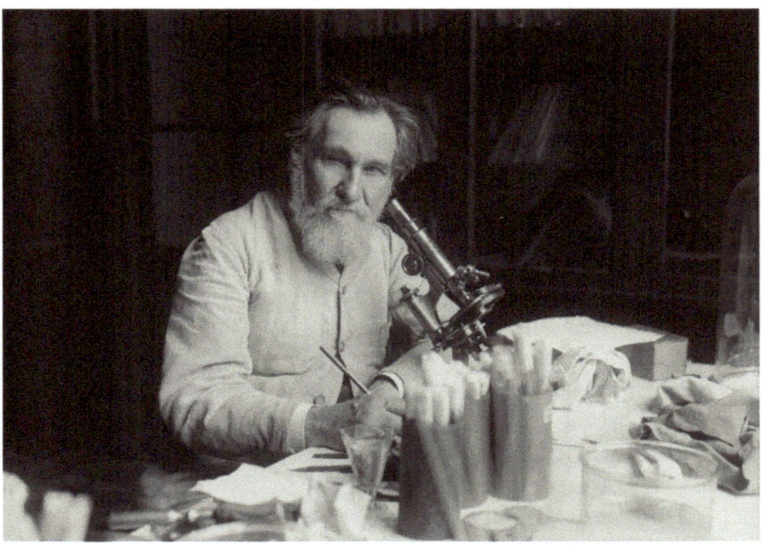

FIG. 19.1 Russian Scientist and Nobel prize winner, Elie Metchnikoff of the Pasteur Institute.

one minor change replacing "*which*" with "*that*" (Hill et al., 2014). Traditionally, for humans, the use of probiotics in the food industry has been deemed safe with no risk upon consumption. Theoretically, some probiotics could pose certain side-effects (such as infections, disturbing metabolic activities, immunity related issues, and gene transfer) in susceptible individuals. The scientific understanding and application of probiotics is known to be an eco-friendly alternative. Probiotics can be bundled with several types of products, which can include dietary supplements, foods, and drugs. *Lactobacilli* and *Bifidobacteria* are commonly known probiotics; however, some strains of yeasts such as *Saccharomyces cerevisiae* and bacteria such as certain serovars of *Escherichia coli* and other *Bacilli* are also employed as probiotics. Food and pharmaceutical industries have obtained patents on the use and application of certain strains and combinations of novel probiotic strains. Humans have used lactic acid bacteria (LAB) for several thousands of years for food-preservation and fermentation techniques and they serve dual functions, acting as fermentation agents of foods and giving benefits relating to health (WGO, 2017).

This chapter offers the reader a glimpse into the complexities of legality and regulations when the market for probiotic products is now more global than local and yet regulations tend to be very much still local, with very little consensus between government policies in different parts of the globe. In addition, the rapid growth of newer genetic technologies, which were not even on the horizon just 10 years ago, further makes it difficult to interpret what is covered by older definitions.

19.2 Probiotic markets

Several market reports at different time points reveal a steady growth in the overall probiotic market. In 2016, the global probiotic ingredient market was $1.5 billion USD and was expected to increase by another $1 billion USD by the year 2021. The estimates from a discussion group held in 2017, by the International Scientific Association for Probiotics and Prebiotics, suggested that the manufacture and sales of all probiotic product ingredients could reach $50 billion USD by the year 2024, while Grand View Research (2019) estimated it could reach $77 billion USD by 2025. In 2018, probiotic beverages emerged as the largest market segment, with a revenue of USD $39.6 billion USD, with consumption of probiotic cereal-based beverages on the rise (Grand View Research, 2019). Several commercial probiotic preparations, with more than one live microorganism in combination, have been introduced to enhance the quality and to further the overall global market for foods, their supplements, and probiotic ingredients.

According to the International Probiotics Association (IPA) (http://internationalprobiotics.org/), the ingredient markets can be divided as follows.

(a) Fermentation and bacteria production:

Major economies including Australia, Brazil, Canada, China, India, Japan, South Korea, UK, and the USA have fermentation capabilities and facilities. The fermentation capacity of these facilities ranges from 20 metric tons to 500 metric tons.

(b) Ingredient market revenue:

The food and beverage segment is the biggest revenue-earning market in all regions. Probiotic ingredients are generally marketed as capsules, tablets, powders, and gels, based on ingredients, form, end-user, and application.

Significant players in the probiotics market include companies such as Biena, Dow, DuPont, Lallemand, and UAS Labs from North America; Bifodan, Biogaia, Probi, CHR Hansen, and Kerry from Europe; Glac Biotech from Asia.

19.2.1 Nomenclature

There has been a consensus towards nomenclature of probiotic strains and these are identified by genus, species, and an alphanumeric strain designation (Table 19.1).

The best documented probiotic, at the global level is *Lactobacillus rhamnosus* GG, which has been in use in food and dietary supplements markets since 1990. It has proven beneficial effects on overall immunity enhancement and gut-health. It has been one of the most extensively studied strains over the past 30 years, with a plethora of clinical studies and scientific publications (Capurso, 2019).

TABLE 19.1 Examples of nomenclature of probiotic species.

Genus	Species	Alphanumeric or strain designation
Bacillus	*coagulans*	GBI-30
Bifidobacterium	*animalis*	DN 173010
Bifidobacterium	*longum*	MM-2
Lactobacillus	*rhamnosus*	GG
Lactobacillus	*casei*	DN-114001
Lactococcus	*lactis*	L1A

19.3 Health claims

19.3.1 Probiotics in human health

For centuries, the use of probiotics has been known for fermented food products and to impart important health benefits, in turn providing nutritional support. Such health benefits by the probiotic bacteria can be attributed to strain specificity. There is no known single universal strain that provides all health benefits as each bacterial strain has its individual effect. Even though we have pieces of evidence for the role of probiotics in other areas such as cardio-metabolic diseases, the strongest clinical evidence comes from their use in gut-health and immunity enhancement.

19.4 Intellectual property and probiotics—Some examples of products

USPTO Patent Classification (CPC) specifically deals with "A23V 2200/3204: Probiotics, living bacteria to be ingested for action in the digestive tract."

Many strains of bacteria have been patented and used for commercial products. In 1899, Henry Tissier, from the Pasteur Institute, first reported on the isolation of *Bifidobacterium* from a breast-fed baby and named it "*Bacillus bifidus* communis" and further proclaimed that it would displace the proteolytic bacteria causing diarrhea. He recommended that it be given to babies suffering from diarrhea. Further, in 1900, Moro described *Lactobacillus acidophilus* focusing on intestinal problems and solutions for children's health. A patent on "a method of culturing" indicating the use of *Lactobacillus acidophilus* LA-5, was issued to TransAgra Corporation with patent number 4349569 in 1982. Similarly, in 1983, a U.S. Patent 4,689,226 was issued claiming a preparation with bacteria towards prophylactic intestinal disturbances, especially *Salmonella* infections in poultry, containing several strains including *Lactobacillus acidophilus*. A patent on *Lactobacillus rhamnosus* was issued in 1988 and subsequently published in 1989 by Gorbach and Goldin, relating to a preparation addressing gastric disorder–related issues. In 1987, the company Valio came into a license agreement with Gorbach and Goldin to use the strain under trade name *Lactobacillus rhamnosus* LGG. The GG derives from the first letters of their surnames. The patents about the use of probiotics with *Lactobacillus acidophilus*, as studied in North Carolina State University for human applications by Gorbach and Goldin, relate to US4839281 and US5032399, which disclose that when ingested by humans or animals, the strain exhibits beneficial effects on several GI tract–related functions.

In 1930, Minoru Shirota isolated and cultivated a *Lactobacillus* strain, later called *Lactobacillus casei* Shirota, which had been proven to have the potential to survive the journey through harsh conditions in the stomach and travel safely to the large intestine. The first patent, coming from Yakult, dates back to 1973. The Patent Cooperation (PCT) publication WO 96/020607 applied by Compagnie Gervais Danone, describes the strain *Lactobacillus casei* DN-114001 and was deposited with the National Collection of Cultures of Microorganisms (CNCM) relates to the Pasteur Institute, Paris, claiming beneficial properties in treating diarrhea (Boschloo, 2011).

19.4.1 Innovation examples

The Naked Juice Co. from Azusa, CA (USA) filed a patent application at USPTO in 2008 (application no. 12/110,746) entitled "juice beverages with probiotic bacteria" with bacteria selected from the group consisting of *Bifidobacterium animalis* (lactis), *Lactobacillus rhamnosus*, and mixtures thereof.

The University of Saskatchewan filed a PCT application (6th August 2014) entitled "Microcapsules containing probiotics and methods of making same" describing a microcapsule for protecting a probiotic and/or delivering a probiotic to an intestine.

Danone and Yakult are well-known probiotic yogurt drink brands globally and they both incorporate *L. casei and L. acidophilus* strains in their probiotic products.

Nestle launched its first US baby formula named "Good Start Natural Cultures," containing probiotics. It also launched probiotic drops for infant colic relief under the name "BioGaia."

An Irish company called "Alimentary Health" secured a patent on "Zenflore" involving a bacterial strain *B. Longum 1714* that claims to address stress-related issues.

FitBiomics is a company that specializes in sequencing the microbiome and identifying and isolating novel bacteria towards the improvement of sports-related performances. On similar lines, Sun Genomics focuses on the concept of personalized "precision" probiotics by analyzing the gut flora signatures.

An Australian company, Prota Therapeutics is developing a unique oral immunotherapy technology to use probiotic foods in addressing allergy-related issues, specifically to peanuts.

Unibiome, a company that specializes in products relating to yeasts, created a baker's yeast variety that is known to enhance iron absorption from bread and further enhances the bioavailability of nutrients, vitamins, and trace elements that are commonly found in fermented foods.

Novalact, a Chilean-based start-up company, focuses on the development of products for lactose intolerants using probiotic engineering for the alleviation of the symptoms relating to gastrointestinal complications.

19.5 Summary of patents and patent applications for probiotics

In the following section, there are a number of tables that list patent record searches for the various probiotic beverages to illustrate the activity in this area in terms of legal submissions.

19.5.1 Kefir

To date, there were around 1245 patent records when searched with the keyword "Kefir" in title, abstract, and claims, with the following assignees in their order of filing patents (Table 19.2).

19.5.2 Koumiss

About 109 patents pertaining to Koumiss have been issued to date and the first known patent was issued in the year 1954, wherein the applicant was Fedorov. It was entitled "Method of the preparation of the koumiss" (Table 19.3).

TABLE 19.2 Major assignees of Kefir related patents.

	Assignee	Number of patents
1	Konkuk University Industrial Cooperation	13
2	Yakult Honsha	13
3	Sudzucker	11
4	Yingshang Haoyuan Food	11
5	Chr Hansen	11
6	Jilin University	10
7	Gorsky State Agrarian University	10
8	Nutrinova Nutrition Specialties & Food Ingredients	9
9	Pepsico	9
10	Tianjin University of Science & Technology	9

TABLE 19.3 Major assignees of Koumiss related patents.

	Assignee	Number of patents
1	Chelyabinsk State Agroengineering Academy	5
2	Inner Mongolia Agricultural University	5
3	Bashkir State Medical University	2
4	Abaga Zhaofu Economic & Trade	2
5	Bashkirskij Institute Patentovedeni	2
6	Beijing Scientific Plus Biotech	2
7	Chr Hansen	2
8	Inner Mongolia Zhongyun Horse Industry Development	2
9	Jiangnan University	2
10	Kubansk University	2

19.5.3 Kombucha

The first known patent pertaining to "Kombucha" dates back to the year 1998, wherein the applicant was Mao Wengzu. It was entitled "Black tea fungus-mineral water beverage." To date, there are over 589 patent records when one searches with the keyword "Kombucha" in title, abstract, and claims.

19.5.4 Probiotic water

The first known patent application pertaining to "Probiotic Water" was submitted in 2010, wherein the applicant was PROBIOTIKI. It was entitled "Probiotic water: water with microorganisms added." To date, there are ~28 patent records when one searches with the keyword "Probiotic water" in title, abstract, and claims (Table 19.4).

TABLE 19.4 Major assignees of probiotic water-related patents.

	Assignee
1	Hangzhou Yiru Information Technology
2	Hunan Institute of Microbiology
3	Binzhou Ocean & Fisheries Research Institute
4	Dalian University of Technology
5	Daren Environment Protection Science & Technology Co. Ltd., Shanghai

19.5.5 Lactic acid fermented (probiotic) fruit and vegetable juice

To date, there were ~3272 patent records when searched with the keyword ((probiotic AND fruit) OR (Probiotic AND vegetable)) in the title, abstract, and claims. However, when restricted to ((probiotic AND fruit) OR (probiotic AND vegetable)) AND (juice)) the records reduced to 830. The first known patent application in this domain was made in 2003 entitled "Sobering and liver-protecting liquid product and its production method" by L. Fangbin and Yonglongshan Biotechnology Engineering, China (Table 19.5).

19.5.6 Probiotic yogurts

To date, there are ~566 patent records when searched with the keyword (probiotic AND yogurt) in the title, abstract and claims, and the first known patent application in this domain was made in 1987 entitled "Biophysically derived Ascomycetes, Schizomycetes and yeast preparation contained in the food and growth material of plants, and their use in treating the skin and in probiotic activation" by A. Wank with Socop Nahrungsmittel (Radolf Nahrungsmittel) (Table 19.6).

TABLE 19.5 Major assignees of lactic acid fermented (probiotic) fruit and vegetable juice related patents.

	Assignee	Number of patents
1	Jinshanmei Biotechnology	26
2	Bright Dairy & Food	20
3	Shandong Bohua Highly Efficient Ecological Agriculture Science & Technology	12
4	Genmont Biotech	8
5	Gervais Danone	8
6	Anhui Sun Pharmaceutical	7
7	Chr Hansen	7
8	Tianjin Zhongtian Jingke Science & Technology	7
9	Food Industry Research & Development Institute	6
10	Sudzucker	6

TABLE 19.6 Major assignees of probiotic yogurt related patents.

	Assignee	Number of patents
1	Alimentary Health	21
2	Nestec	14
3	Nestle	14
4	Bright Dairy & Food	12
5	Dupont Nutrition Biosciences	12
6	Tianjin Zhongtian Jingke Science & Technology	10
7	Chr Hansen	9
8	Fonterra	7
9	Junlebao Dairy	6
10	Procter & Gamble	6

19.5.7 Sour beer

The activity around IP protection pertaining to "Sour Beer" is still in the early stages. The first known patent application was made in the year 2011, with the applicant S—H Park. It was entitled "Method of preparing sour beer using Korean traditional microorganism." To date, there are around 14 patent records when searched with the keyword "Sour Beer"in title, abstract, and claims from groups such as Dalian Polytechnic University, Danstar Ferment, Joseph Allen Pickard, Metafiltration, and Sapporo Breweries.

19.5.8 Plant-based probiotic beverages

These are currently commercialized in the EU markets.

To date, there were around 769 patent records when searched with the string ((plant) AND (based) AND (probiotic)) in the title, abstract, and claims (Table 19.7).

19.6 Intellectual property related disputes

The next section relates some examples of intellectual property disputes to illustrate what a difficult area this is for companies to navigate and what organisms/products were in dispute (Table 19.8).

TABLE 19.7 Major assignees of plant-based probiotic beverages related patents.

	Assignee	Number of patents
1	Jinshanmei Biotechnology	36
2	Nestec	18
3	Tianjin Zhongtian Jingke Science & Technology	18
4	Nestle	14
5	Beijing Kehuitong Wisdom Technology	10
6	Gervais Danone	8
7	Ubiome	8
8	Evonik Degussa	7
9	Tianjin Zhongtian Jingke Science & Technology	7
10	Advanced Bionutrition	6

19.7 Regulations: The need for probiotic guidelines

A "Joint FAO/WHO Expert Consultation on Evaluation of Health and Nutritional Properties of Probiotics in Food" was held in 2001 to examine several aspects of the usage of probiotic foods and they came up with a definition of probiotics, which was later revised in 2014, stating that probiotics are "Live microorganisms that, when administered in adequate amounts, confer a health benefit on the host." However, there is a global presence of products that are sold as "probiotics" which do not meet this definition. Because of the increasing popularity of probiotic foods, and the lack of international consensus on assessment methodologies as to their efficacy and safety, FAO/WHO then initiated examining the safety aspects of probiotics in foods. Establishing the eligibility criteria is the ultimate goal towards acceptable implementation at national and international levels by Codex member countries for the promotion of human health and well-being (FAO/WHO, 2019).

Included in the food and dietary supplements category, currently, probiotics are not established on an international basis as they are consumed orally, as foods. These products are different from drugs in several ways, especially with respect to claims. In order to understand where probiotic products currently fall in terms of regulatory agencies, their health claims along with their use, have to be understood more clearly:

- A "health claim" characterizes the relationship between a substance and a disease or condition and these should be based upon scientific evidence and broad-based social acceptance and/or recommendations from national or international public health bodies.

TABLE 19.8 Some examples of legal difficulties over claims of probiotic products, labels, and intellectual property.

Parties	Organism	Product
Ganeden Biotech, Inc., Plaintiff, v. American Brewing Company, Inc. and B&R Liquid Adventure, LLC, Defendants	*Bacillus coagulans* GBI-30 strain of *Bacillus coagulans*	Brewer's Kombucha teas infringed its intellectual property
Simone v. VSL Pharmaceuticals, Inc. et al.	Lactic acid bacteria	Combination of eight LAB strains used as a treatment for gastrointestinal disorders and hypercholesteremia The basis for the probiotic called VSL# 3
Brew dr. Kombucha	Probiotic bacteria	The claim of falsely advertised and labeled as containing significantly higher quantities of probiotic bacteria than the US products actually contained
US Class action suit against Procter & Gamble	Bifantis (*Bifidobacterium infantis* 35,624)	"Align" product for abdominal discomfort and to balance the digestive system
US Class action suit and Bayer	*Lactobacillus gasseri KS-13, Bifidobacterium bifidum G9-1,* and *Bifidobacterium longum MM-2*	Phillips' Colon Health Probiotic Capsules - Defense against four occasional digestive issues: gas, bloating, constipation, and diarrhea
US Class action against Dannon in 2008	Probiotic bacteria	Yogurt regulating digestion and boosting the immune system
US Class action against Yoplait in 2009	Probiotic bacteria	Yoplait's Yo-Plus probiotic yogurt Digestion claims

- Further, a "structure/function" claim characterizes the mechanism with which a nutrient or dietary ingredient act to maintain such structure or function.

Science-based risk assessment and risk analysis are important in the regulatory food safety domain with an emphasis on more transparency in decision making for food safety (FAO/WHO, 2001, 2002). The development of Codex guidelines for probiotics guides for global regulatory agencies to build probiotic-focused regulations. The establishment of global requirements is needed to satisfy authorities, consumers, and industry, and further would certainly lead to better consumer satisfaction, health, and well-being.

Wherever claimed, the health claims must be truthful, not misleading, and substantiated by scientific evidence. Normally, probiotics are considered safe by the European Food Safety Authority (EFSA) for human consumption, however, there is no guidance on their relationship with their increasing use for medical conditions. The U.S. Food and Drug Administration (FDA) considers probiotics generally as safe for use in foods. Though there is a similarity in the regulation of probiotics in the US & European Union, there is no agreed framework. In the European Union, the probiotics come under the Food Products Directive and Regulation and all the health-related claims for probiotics have to be authorized by the EFSA. The European Union does not allow structure/function claims relating to dietary supplements. Whereas, in the USA, most of the probiotic products are categorized as foods or dietary supplements and comply with Good Manufacturing Practice guidelines, however, these do not extend to the quality or efficacy testing. In the US, dietary supplements are allowed based on structure/function claims provided they are accompanied by a disclaimer, as mandated by the FDA.

Foods with medicinal values are not normally considered as drugs; therefore, they are not subject to any regulatory demands applying to drugs. However, foods with medicinal values that bear a false or misleading claim would be considered misbranded. Both in the EU and USA, in view of the complexity pertaining to probiotic products, wherein live microorganisms are dealt with, the present situation has created a regulatory void. This is further applicable to the dynamic nature of the probiotics and their species and strain specificity. The current approach towards the regulation of probiotics is inadequate and can lead to quality, safety, and claim validity issues in commercial probiotic products that are used in a medical context. The manufacturing process hugely affects the quality of probiotic products and it is imperative that the manufacturing process and packaging procedures are meticulously controlled to prevent contamination impacting efficacy. Any change or variation in the manufacturing parameters could have a serious effect on the life of the bacterial cultures and the presence of dead bacteria would have direct say on the quality of the probiotic product.

Dead bacteria can originate from any part of the manufacturing process including harvesting, lyophilization, etc., and they accompany the live bacteria. They cannot easily be separated or eliminated from the finished product. To address the issue of the presence of the dead bacteria in the finished product, most manufactures routinely adopt an "over-filling" process to maintain the advertised numbers, as it was mandated that industry should advertise the proportionate numbers of live bacteria present as colony-forming units (CFU) per dose.

Biochemical and immunological profiles of the probiotic strains are also affected by variations in the manufacturing process. The safety and efficacy of the finished product will depend on the manufacturing conditions and facilities. Even with the same number of live and dead bacteria present per dose; there might still not be the same degree of safety and efficacy. For example, a recent study showed that a probiotic formulation from the USA differed significantly from one manufactured in Italy (Trinchieri et al., 2017). Further, efforts are being made to establish meaningful standards or guidelines for probiotic products worldwide.

19.7.1 Brazil

In American countries, Brazil was one of the first countries to issue legislation regarding functional foods. In Brazil, probiotics are considered to be different from food and are regarded as functional foods. Regulations governing probiotics as functional foods/supplements have undergone modernization for several years (Agencia Nacional de Vigilancia Sanitaria [ANVISA], 2019). Regulations require a demonstration of the safety and efficacy of the food products and hence all these products must be registered and further approved by the Brazilian Health Regulatory Agency (ANVISA).

19.7.2 Canada

In 2016, Canada announced amendments to nutrition labeling, a list of ingredients and food color requirements of their Food and Drug Regulations. Requirements for probiotic claims were clearly elucidated and listed under the food labeling requirements (CFIA, 2019; Powers, Farrell, McMullin, Retik, & White, 2019; CFD, 2009). In Canada, specific guidelines on regulations of probiotics in foods have to be worked out however, general provisions of the "Food and Drugs Act and Regulations" apply to foods containing microorganisms including those microorganisms represented as probiotics. Canada recognizes strain-specific and/or nonstrain specific health claims over probiotic beverages. The statements on validation of health claims are to be supported by strain-specific evidence including the functionality aspects of products such as safety, stability, viability, etc.

19.7.3 China

Presently, China has a well-developed market for functional foods (CIRS, 2018), which is based on traditional dietary cultures and there are strict standards of performance along with rapid growth. Recently, China adopted the State Food and Drug Administration's (SFDA) guidelines regulating all health foods, which includes all kinds of functional foods and nutraceuticals. It defines functional foods as foods that have special health functions or can supply vitamins or minerals and possess the function of regulating human body functions. Health foods are different from drugs, and health foods give health benefits but cannot be claimed to cure a disease. As per the Probiotics Health Food Review Regulations, probiotics refer to "a micro-ecological preparation that can promote the ecological balance of intestinal flora and has a beneficial effect on the human body," which is slightly different from the FAO/WHO definition. A probiotic must be a member of the normal human flora, either in its live/dead form or its metabolite. Recently, China's State Administration for Market Regulation (SAMR) has started permitting the individual firms to provide their proof of evidence on health claims and after assessment, the authorities shall determine the validity of health claims (Chinese Approach to Regulating Health Foods, Chenlei He, Master Food Safety (https://edepot.wur.nl/310333)).

19.7.4 Europe

Europe was the second entity to establish a definition of functional foods and to bring a regulatory commission on functional food science in Europe (FUFOSE) into practice in 1995. Even in absence of an EU-wide harmonized legal framework, the EU can be considered as one of the most strict implementers of regulations relating to probiotics. Europe already has a developed market for probiotics with the rapid growth of functional foods, whose largest segment is composed of probiotic food products, especially dairy products such as yogurts and fermented milks. As per European laws, even microbial cultures present in food need to comply with the regulatory requirements (Bröring, Khedkar, & Ciliberti, 2017). The European food safety authority introduced Qualified Presumption of Safety (QPS), to ensure a premarket safety assessment in foods and food supplements. European guidelines conclude that probiotics do not have any legal definition or specific legislation, rather they belong to the category of functional foods. The European regulatory framework is still not harmonized for probiotics because these are regulated by the Food Products Directive and Regulation, whether they are to be marketed as food supplements under Herbal Medicinal Products Directive, or marketed as traditional herbal products. For the use of probiotic products as an herbal medicinal product, they must apply and obtain a drug registration, otherwise, they are transferred to the category of food supplements.

19.7.5 India

In India, probiotics are consumed as foods and pharmaceuticals, but because of varying categories, probiotics are regulated differently as per their intended use (Bhupathiraju et al., 2019). Currently, food and drugs are regulated by the Prevention of Food Adulteration Act (PFA) and the Food and Drug Administration (FDA), respectively. The Food Safety and Standards Act (FSSA) came into force in 2006 and defines the foods for special dietary uses or functional foods, nutraceuticals, or health supplements. Presently, probiotics are characterized as functional foods rather than as pharmaceutical drugs and therefore are regulated by food laws. FSSA was passed by the Indian government to regulate different varieties of eatables with regulations covering nutraceuticals, foods, and dietary supplements. According to the FSSA, functional foods are defined legally, however, the bundling of food categories, including nutraceuticals and biotherapeutics, is still unclear. Existing PFA rules set down minimum standards relating to the quality and content of food products. The PFA also mandates that the labeling and packaging information of food products should be disclosed to the consumer. In India, in the absence of any specific regulatory guidelines, there was a need for guidelines and regulations towards the evaluation of safety and efficacy of probiotics and also towards the prevention of marketing products with false claims. Keeping in view the above, a Task Force was constituted in association with the Indian Council of Medical Research (ICMR) and the Department of Biotechnology (DBT) to frame regulatory guidelines for the evaluation of probiotics in food in India. These guidelines have a set of parameters to define a product/strain as an actual "probiotic."

19.7.6 Japan

In Japan, probiotics are recognized as both foods and drugs. Japan was the very first global jurisdiction to implement a robust regulatory system for functional foods and nutraceuticals (Farid et al., 2019). Foods with health claims are categorized into two groups, namely "Food with Nutrient Function Claims" and "Food for Specified Health Uses (FOSHU)," with probiotics included under FOSHU. For a product to be considered FOSHU, and making any claim on safety and efficacy, one must obtain special permission from the Ministry of Health and Welfare (MHLW).

Depending on the degree of the claim and substantiated scientific evidence, FOSHU categorizes applications based on food claims, as follows:

Grade "A": both medically and nutritionally established evidence.
Grade "B": evidence confirmed at the level previously required for the approval of existing FOSHU.
Grade "C": evidence not established, but efficacy is suggested.

Further, the FOSHU health claims are subcategorized based on GI-health, lipid, salt, sugar moderation, and bone health–related claims. Regular FOSHU registration is based on information relating to safety, efficacy, processing, formulation data, analytical methods, chemical and physical analysis, as well as other specific information along with product samples, and proposed labels and claims. All of this information must be published in a Japanese scientific journal. The information should also speak about beneficial effects on dietary ingredients that have physiological functions in the human body, maintain and promote health, and improve health-related conditions.

19.7.7 Malaysia

Currently, functional food products do not have an official definition in Malaysia. In Malaysia, all foods and drugs are regulated by a well-established legal system. Functional foods are classified as foods and must, therefore, comply with food regulations. The Food Safety and Quality Division (FSQD), the Drug Control Authority, the National Pharmaceutical Control Bureau (NPCB), and the Committee for the Classification of Food-Drug Interface Products are the regulatory agencies that are responsible for the implementation and enforcement of regulations on food and drugs. Malaysian regulations are developed locally with reference to CODEX, and for functional foods, there are complex regulatory guidelines, however, there are no separate guidelines for the probiotic category (Nor, 2016).

19.7.8 New Zealand and Australia

New Zealand and Australia have a joint framework agency, the Food Standards Australia and New Zealand (FSANZ) (https://www.foodstandards.gov.au/Pages/default.aspx). Earlier, functional foods were defined as foods that are similar in appearance to conventional foods and are intended to be consumed as part of a normal diet; but as per recent rules, these are now supposed to serve physiological roles beyond the provision of simple nutrient requirements.

19.7.9 USA

Probiotic products in the United States are generally sold to a healthy population as foods/beverages or as dietary supplements. In the case of dietary supplements, demonstration of safety and efficacy before marketing and approval by the Food and Drug Administration is not required. The regulations, in addition to nutrient content claims, allows the manufacturers of dietary supplements to make structure/function or health claims for their products. The "health claims" must go through a regulatory examination process. The guidelines that were developed by the Joint FAO/WHO Expert Consultation on Evaluation of Health and Nutritional Properties of Probiotics, could be used as the global standard for evaluation of probiotics in foods that could lead to the substantiation of health claims (Song, Ibrahim, & Hayek, 2012). Currently, in the USA regulation of probiotics is carried out by the Dietary Supplement Health and Education Act (DSHEA) and Food and Drug Administration (FDA) through the Center for Food Safety and Applied Nutrition.

As per existing guidelines in the USA:

a. A probiotic, which is used as a dietary supplement, is recognized as "food," and is regulated by the DSHEA
b. In the case of a dietary supplement having any new dietary ingredient, without prior market presence, it then becomes the responsibility of the manufacturer to notify the FDA
c. If the probiotics are considered to be probiotic drugs for therapeutic purposes, then there must be proof of safety and efficacy, before being marketed, and then it will be regulated by the FDA
d. In the case of a biological product, one needs to have approval via the Biologic License Application (BLA). The FDA applies the current good manufacturing practices (cGMP) and investigational new drug (IND) approval process.

19.8 Genetically modified microorganisms

The use of recombinant DNA technology to come up with genetically modified microorganisms (GMMs) is a significant milestone in scientific developments and includes simultaneous advancements in sensitive analytical methods. With the help of recombinant DNA technologies, the very basic properties of microorganisms can now be changed with the utmost precision and subsequent selection procedures. Production process optimization, product quality enhancement, and safety establishment, as well as enlargement of product diversity, play a major role in such technological advancements. This enormous potential of genetic engineering has aided in the application of microorganisms in functional foods, such as probiotics, demonstrating enhanced use of microorganisms in the food industry.

Even though several strains of bacteria have been employed for improved performance by genetic engineering, GMO strains have been applied to a limited extent as there is a lack of risk assessment procedures, knowledge on gene transfer, understanding of adverse effects of genetic modifications, and unpredictability on the effect of spreading of the genetically modified bacteria when they come into interaction with human systems. Efforts are being in the development of tools for GMOs in their applications to food fermentations or as probiotics. By using site-specific recombination methods, the development of food-grade genetically modified bacteria is possible. The use of sophisticated analytical genomic tools, such as DNA microarrays contributes immensely towards the development of robust risk assessment procedures by the stakeholders such as manufacturers and consumers. Such developments facilitate applications of GMOs in foods with enhanced consumer benefits.

The Cartagena Protocol on Biosafety (https://bch.cbd.int/protocol/text/), an international treaty, recognizes standards in a process that aims at regulating and monitoring of the movement of GM crops/seeds/foods. In all countries, but especially within the EU, the use of GMOs in the food industry invites strong debate, as there is still a very low level of acceptance from the consumers. On the other hand, in the United States, the regulations on genetically modified foods are based on end products, rather than the process of preparation (https://www.fda.gov/food/agricultural-biotechnology/how-gmos-are-regulated-food-and-plant-safety-united-states). In Canada, the regulations are based on end products, however, they treat all GM foods as "novel" (https://www.canada.ca/en/health-canada/services/food-nutrition/genetically-modified-foods-other-novel-foods/safety.html). The genetically modified foods are passed through premarketing safety assessment, however, when approved they are considered as conventional and are subjected to the same regulations as those for traditional foods.

The Canadian and the United States regulatory framework recognizes that the foods that are produced with interventions relating to biotechnology, and which do not necessarily present any greater risk in comparison to traditional foods regarding the safety of these GM foods, for this risk assessment is termed as equivalent to that of traditional foods. The EU, however, considers that the development of GM foods comes with unprecedented risks for mankind and must be dealt in a different manner. The regulators in the EU recognize and approve these GM foods with caution, considering that GM foods might pose specific risks and ought to be treated separately and differently from conventional foods (http://www.efsa.europa.eu/en/topics/topic/gmo). Most of the countries have regulations based on the process of production and further require a specific set of approval and labeling regulations when it comes to considering GM foods as "novel" (Alexandraki, Tsakalidou, Papadimitriou, & Holzapfel, 2013).

19.9 Gaps in policies

At the global level, as far as implementation of regulations and policies relating to probiotics is concerned, for products such as GM foods and beverages, there are several gaps. It is more or less established that health claims on foods should show scientific validation, however, it should not jeopardize the pace of innovations in the areas of probiotics and functional foods. A European Union project entitled, "Process for the Assessment of Scientific Support for Claims on Foods (PASSCLAIM)" (https://ilsi.eu/passclaim/), engaged scientists, academicians, experts from industry, research institutes, public interest groups, and the regulatory set-up, to produce a set of criteria for the validation of health claims on foods, emphasizing the need for direct evidence on benefits of scientific approaches to humans.

In the EU, any such application through the national food authority is forwarded to the EFSA, which in turn provides opinion on the validity of the health claim, and further sends it to the European Commission. The Commission then decides whether to authorize the application for a health claim or not as per the regulatory guidelines. Health claims thus approved, in compliance with the requirements, can subsequently be used by producers.

In the USA, claims pertaining to food and dietary supplements related labels can be broadly categorized into:

a. nutrient content related.
b. structure/function related.
c. health-related.

These are slightly different from the European equivalent regulatory procedures and approval processes. In the USA, a qualifying statement of disclaimer on the level of scientific evidence is required for "qualified health claims (QHC)."

In Japan, FOSHU foods typically contain dietary ingredients having beneficial effects on the physiological functions in humans, and maintain and improve health-related conditions in humans. Any application that is submitted for approval for a product must mention both published information, internal reports proving the efficacy (including in-vitro and in-vivo studies), and results of trials on Japanese consumers.

Japan and the USA have relatively liberal regulatory provisions for health claims, whereas Europe displays requirements for a high level of scientific substantiation.

19.10 Summary

In view of the fast-changing lifestyles and environments, the need for probiotics in foods and beverages has been positively accepted by society. However, their use has to comply with the regulatory guidelines, across the globe, under specified health claims.

Acknowledgment

The author sincerely thanks CSIR-CDRI, Lucknow, India.

References

Alexandraki, V., Tsakalidou, E., Papadimitriou, K., & Holzapfel, W. (2013). *Commission on genetic resources for food and agriculture. Background study paper no. 65. (2013). http://www.fao.org/3/mg309e/mg309e.pdf.*

ANVISA (2019). *Guide for procedural instruction for probiotic assessment request for food use (2019). (2019). http://portal.anvisa.gov.br/documents/10181/5280930/21.pdf/1c99eeb1-7143-469a-93ff-7b2b0f9187c0.*

Bhupathiraju, K., Krishnaraju, A. V., Sengupta, K., Golakoti, T., Akolkar, S. K., & Datla, P. (2019). Regulations on nutraceuticals, functional foods, and dietary supplements in India. In *Nutraceutical and functional food regulations in the United States and around the world* (pp. 445–464). Academic Press.

Boschloo, H. (2011). *Probiotics: From patent to consumer product–a dairy case.* Wageningen, the Netherlands: Wageningen University.(2011). *https://edepot.wur.nl/176628.*

Bröring, S., Khedkar, S., & Ciliberti, S. (2017). Reviewing the nutrition and health claims regulation (EC) No. 1924/2006: What do we know about its challenges and potential impact on innovation? *International Journal of Food Sciences and Nutrition, 68*(1), 1–9.

Capurso, L. (2019). Thirty years of *Lactobacillus rhamnosus* GG: A review. *Journal of Clinical Gastroenterology, 53*, S1–S41.

CFD (Canada Food Directorate, Health Products and Food Branch) (2009). *Guidance document—The use of probiotic microorganisms in food. (2009). https://www.canada.ca/en/health-canada/services/food-nutrition/legislation-guidelines/guidance-documents/guidance-document-use-probiotic-microorganisms-food-2009.html.*

CFIA (2019). *Probiotic claims. (2019). https://www.inspection.gc.ca/food-label-requirements/labelling/industry/health-claims-on-food-labels/eng/1392834838383/1392834887794?chap=10.*

CIRS (2018). *China health food regulations in present and future. 20 June (2018). http://www.cirs-reach.com/news-and-articles/China-Health-Food-Regulations-in-Present-and-Future.html.*

FAO/WHO (2001). *Joint FAO/WHO expert consultation on evaluation of health and nutritional properties of probiotics in food including powder milk with live lactic acid bacteria, 1–4 October 2001 Cordoba, Argentina. (2001). http://pc.ilele.hk/public/pdf/20190225/bd3689dfc2fd663bb36def1b672ce0a4.pdf.*

FAO/WHO (2002). *Joint FAO/WHO working group report on drafting guidelines for the evaluation of probiotics in food, London, Ontario, Canada, April 30 and May 1, 2002. (2002). https://www.who.int/foodsafety/fs_management/en/probiotic_guidelines.pdf.*

FAO/WHO (2019). *Report of the Joint FAO/WHO food standards programme codex committee on nutrition and foods for special dietary uses, 41st Session, 24–29 November 2019 in Dusseldorf, Germany. (2019). http://www.fao.org/fao-who-codexalimentarius/sh-proxy/en/?lnk=1&url=https%253A%252F%252Fworkspace.fao.org%252Fsites%252Fcodex%252FMeetings%252FCX-720-41%252FReport%252FAdoption%252FREP20_NFSDUe.pdf.*

Farid, M., Kodama, K., Arato, T., Okazaki, T., Oda, T., Ikeda, H., et al. (2019). *Comparative study of functional food regulations in Japan and globally. (2019). https://pdfs.semanticscholar.org/1510/77184b769d57d695cf2e01d1d445a470d616.pdf.*

Grand View Research (June 2019). *Press release—Probiotic market worth $77.09 billion by 2025. (June 2019). https://www.grandviewresearch.com/press-release/global-probiotics-market.*

Hill, C., Guarner, F., Reid, G., Gibson, G. R., Merenstein, D. J., Pot, B., et al. (2014). Expert consensus document: The International Scientific Association for Probiotics and Prebiotics consensus statement on the scope and appropriate use of the term probiotic. *Nature Reviews Gastroenterology & Hepatology, 11*(8), 506–514.

Nor, N. (2016). *The functional food industry in Malaysia. FFTC agricultural policy articles. (2016). http://ap.fftc.agnet.org/ap_db.php?id=607&print=1.*

Ozen, M., & Dinleyici, E. C. (2015). The history of probiotics: the untold story. *Beneficial Microbes, 6*(2), 159–165.

Powers, J. P., Farrell, M., McMullin, C., Retik, L., & White, J. (2019). Regulation of dietary supplements and functional foods in Canada. In *Nutraceutical and functional food regulations in the United States and around the world* (pp. 235–252). Academic Press.

Santacroce, L., Charitos, I. A., & Bottalico, L. (2019). A successful history: probiotics and their potential as antimicrobials. *Expert Review of Anti-Infective Therapy, 17*(8), 635–645.

Song, D., Ibrahim, S., & Hayek, S. (2012). Recent application of probiotics in food and agricultural science. *Probiotics, 10*, 1–34.

Trinchieri, V., Laghi, L., Vitali, B., Parolin, C., Giusti, I., Capobianco, D., et al. (2017). Efficacy and safety of a multistrain probiotic formulation depends from manufacturing. *Frontiers in Immunology, 8*, 1474. https://doi.org/10.3389/fimmu.2017.01474.

WGO (2017). *World gastroenterology organisation global guidelines on probiotics and prebiotics. (2017). https://www.worldgastroenterology.org/UserFiles/file/guidelines/probiotics-and-prebiotics-english-2017.pdf.*

PART VI

Marketing probiotic beverages

CHAPTER

20

Marketing probiotic beverages

Julie Kellershohn

Ted Rogers School of Hospitality and Tourism Management, Ryerson University, Toronto, ON, Canada

20.1 Introduction

In this chapter, the goal is to provide an overview of the marketing of probiotic beverages. Areas examined include the market size, the probiotic consumer target, wants and needs of probiotic consumers, and how to use marketing to connect with probiotic consumers. Examples of new products on the market are used to illustrate the latest trends, how these products are currently being marketed, and what opportunities exist but are still in their infancy. Mainstream products such as kombucha and yogurt drinks are well-covered elsewhere in this book; therefore, the main focus in this chapter is on trending and novel probiotic beverages.

20.2 Global market size

By 2022, the overall global beverage category is expected to grow to a value of $1 trillion USD (Euromonitor, 2018). Within global beverages, the functional beverage category is one of the fastest-growing segments, growing from $55 billion USD in 2010 to over $94 billion USD in 2019 (Grand View Research, 2020). This growth is a reflection of the rising consumer interest in functional beverages and the market opportunity that this is creating.

There are two key drivers growing the global probiotic beverage market: a rise in disposable personal income and an increasing geriatric population. The total global population in 2020 is 7.8 billion, of which ~780 million are geriatric. The UN estimates that by the year 2050, there will be 1.5 billion people over the age of 65, and the global life expectancy beyond 65 is projected to increase by 19 years (UN-DESA, 2020). This will

Probiotic Beverages
https://doi.org/10.1016/B978-0-12-818588-9.00019-X

result in a shift from 1 in 11 people over the age of 65 in 2019 to 1 in 6 people over the age of 65 by 2050. This change in demographic composition creates a new market opportunity, especially for products such as probiotic beverages. When surveyed by age group, the current consumer age bracket with the highest interest in probiotic beverages are those aged 18–34 (32%) (FoodNavigator, 2017). While the current geriatric consumers are underserved in terms of marketing efforts on probiotic beverages, as today's younger high-interest group ages over the next several years, more targeted marketing and product positioning will be required to appeal to this rapidly expanding age group's needs.

While the North American probiotic market is still in the early growth stage, an already well-established market exists in Asia where consumers buy probiotics for their health benefits. Over 42% of Chinese consumers purchase beverages marketed as having digestive benefits (Mintel, 2017). The market growth opportunity in Asia is expected to come not only from products targeting the growing geriatric market but also from consumer demand for products offering health benefits to young children. Europe, the second biggest market for probiotic beverages after Asia, is expected to have consistent but moderate growth over the next few years as probiotics move out of specialty retailers into mainstream supermarkets and convenience stores. In Latin America, the expanding middle-class is driving growth in the probiotic market, with Brazil representing both the highest market share in Latin America as well as the fastest-growing market.

20.3 Consumer needs and wants

In April of 2020, the International Food Information Council Foundation carried out a food and health survey in which American consumers ranked in terms of importance what they were seeking from food and beverages. The highest consumer priorities were as follows: weight loss management (>60%), feeling better with more energy (>55%), and products that offered digestive health benefits, and these were third in importance (45%). Standing out as distinctive in their consumer benefits, probiotics were perceived as healthy (65%), as were prebiotics (~45%) (IFIC, 2020). The FMCG Gurus, a UK market research company, in April of 2020, surveyed 23,000 respondents across 18 countries providing a broader, international perspective on consumer preferences (FMCG Gurus, 2020). Consumers reported having become more conscious about their overall health (59%) and more concerned about their health immunity status due to COVID-19. As this study was conducted during the early months of the COVID-19 global pandemic, the increased interest in overall health and immunity could have been heightened by the global health environment at the time of the survey. Globally, 57% of the consumers reported their health concern level was growing, with rising concerns in South America (61%), North America (59%), Europe (58%), Asia Pacific (55%), and Africa and the Middle East (51%). Boosting immunity to reduce vulnerability to disease is a topic that is more important to consumers in 2020 than it ever was in the previous years.

Consumers are no longer thinking just about digestive health. They are seeking both physical and mental health benefits and regard them as having equal importance. The 2018 Innova Market Insights Survey reported that eight out of ten consumers agreed that mental health was as important as physical health to them, with an even higher agreement in China and Brazil (nine out of ten respondents) (Innova, 2018). This consumer interest in mental health creates a growing market opportunity for products that address brain health in addition to physical health in both their components and in their marketing material.

Consumers are looking for more than hydration from beverages. Time-crunched and convenience-driven consumers are seeking beverages that offer additional benefits, such as energy, nutrients, health, and wellness. This desire for *hydration + benefits* is especially true for the millennial cohort. In a survey by the Hartman Group (2019), 65% of millennial respondents agreed to the statement "beverages play a very important role in my health and wellness." While the *+benefits* element of beverage preferences vary by consumer, top consumer benefit preferences include the following: a source of calcium (63%), fiber (61%), reduced sugar (61%), source of antioxidants (60%), increased protein (57%), source of omega 3 (55%), and a beverage that contains probiotics (46%) (Winsight, 2018).

20.4 The market for probiotic beverages spans dayparts, occasions, and consumer preferences

Kerry research surveys in 2019 noted that the majority (68%) of the consumers surveyed said that they would prefer to consume foods with immunity-boosting benefits at breakfast. The potential for probiotic beverages to span dayparts and occasions is vast. Already, probiotic beverages are often consumed as a part of breakfast, or a mid-morning or mid-afternoon snack (Kerry, 2020). Beverages are consumed seated, on-the-go as snacks, and as meal replacements. The drinking of beverages is becoming increasingly acceptable in most spaces be that at work, in cars, on public transit, in public places, and walking. Cultural norms about drinking behavior have changed over the past years. Consumers no longer drink beverages during fixed time points during the day and instead, they have evolved into "constant sippers," with 65% of the consumers saying that they always have a beverage on hand (Hartman Group, 2019).

When considering consumers of different ages, incomes, life stages, and geographies, there will be differences based on multiple factors, but a number of common themes still emerge. The importance of convenience cannot be overstated. When consumers are seeking convenience, a probiotic beverage can be an easy option to add to their daily routine.

Consumers want products that are safe, trustworthy, and efficacious. They want to be able to trust that the product will deliver upon the marketing promises. Probiotic drink consumers are looking not only for information on product ingredients and benefits, but they are also expecting that the information will be communicated in an accessible way and offer full transparency. They want the information to be available on the product packaging and access to information about the manufacturer as well.

Consumers are seeking products that are sustainable for the planet and offer an assurance that the company producing the product demonstrates corporate social responsibility. In 2018, 65% of global consumers said they expect companies to invest in sustainability and by 2019 this had increased to 87% of consumers (Innova, 2020). How consumers interpret corporate social responsibility is evolving over time. What was once a heavy focus on environmental impacts and sustainable business practices in 2020 has expanded in the mind of the consumers to include a focus on how corporations are protecting and supporting their employees, as well as consumers and first responders, especially in the time of COVID-19 (Mintel, 2020).

With the growing variety of options available in the global beverage market, in parallel, a consumer interest in novelty and taste exploration has developed. Often referred to as "food explorers" or "flavor explorers," many consumers seek novelty or unique experiences in their beverage choices. The potential to customize a drink to one's own specific needs, ranks high as a future market opportunity (Innova Market Insights Trends for 2020).

Finally, and arguably most important, great taste remains the strongest driver of consumer purchase intent and satisfaction. Offering *Hydration + Benefits* without great taste is a hard sell to any consumer, and with the wide range of available products, to be competitive in the global marketplace, ensuring that the product tastes great to the target consumer cannot be ignored. Great taste, followed by the product specialization that best addresses the consumer's specific priorities/beliefs, has led to an abundance of new products on the market (e.g., vegan, gluten-free, dairy-free, certified organic). *Taste + Hydration + Benefits* has led to the development of hybrid beverage products, such as drinks containing a blend of dairy milk and almond milk as well as the introduction of cosmeceutical drink products promising muscle health, hair health, and skin health all in the market space of traditional probiotic drinks (Innova, 2020).

20.5 Beyond probiotics

While this book focuses largely on probiotic beverages, the range of beverages associated with some form of "biotics" is vast. Beyond probiotics, the beverage market has expanded to include products with added prebiotics, postbiotics, psychobiotics, paraprobiotics, adaptogens, and nootropics. All of these are offered in various symbiotic combinations, which are proposed to make them more effective.

Prebiotics encourage the growth of probiotic bacteria in the digestive tract. In beverages, prebiotics are typically soluble fibers (e.g., inulin) or oligosaccharides (e.g., fructooligosaccharides (FOS)). Prebiotics can aid with beverage stability, and some prebiotics add a sweetness level that allows for a reduction in the need for added sugars. Some products now feature a suite of prebiotics from "different families," which lend themselves to "clean-label, food-based" functional benefits, making resistant starch and polyphenols (which have an antioxidant function) consumer-valued additions to traditional prebiotics.

There is no overall consensus on the term "postbiotic." Postbiotics are most often described as metabolites of probiotics although what falls into this classification is not well defined. Postbiotics are bioactive compounds produced by food-grade microorganisms during a fermentation process and can include microbial cells, cell constituents, and metabolites (Wegh, Geerlings, Knol, Roeselers, Belzer, 2019). Interest in the role of postbiotics is expected to grow as early research shows that postbiotics appear to have a direct positive effect in healthy individuals to improve their overall health and they may increase the potency of the probiotics.

The terms "psychobiotics," "paraprobiotics," "adaptogens," and "nootropics" are new additions to the terms making their way into consumer marketing language. Psychobiotics are probiotics that offer benefits to mental health. Parabiotics are nonviable microorganisms or metabolites able to provide physiological health benefits to consumers, or the term "parabiotic" may refer to the therapeutic action related to probiotics. Adaptogens are promoted as supporting the body in handling mental and physical stress. Adaptogens are often herbs or roots. Nootropics are compounds for improving cognitive function (brain health and performance), such as enhancing memory and facilitating learning. As an example, caffeine is a compound that has been shown to improve both mental function and physical performance.

New-to-market probiotic beverages increasingly consist of blends of probiotics with psychobiotics, paraprobiotics, adaptogens, or nootropics. These product-line expansions are growing in popularity as they offer convenience and a fast and easy route to a cognitive boost or stress-ameliorating effect.

Probiotic drinks can be categorized into a number of groupings, which include (but are not limited to): alcohol/fermented, dairy, nondairy, high pressure-processed (HPP) juices, vegan, and sport (protein). Within these groups, taste and convenience remain the top consumer priority, but the secondary claims also have enough consumer importance to warrant unique probiotic drink subcategories.

20.6 "Clean label" and "absence of"

Consumers will often speak of a desire for a product with a *clean label,* but the idea of a *clean label* has no regulatory definition for a marketer or a manufacturer. Consumers generally think of a *clean label* product as having ingredients that are recognizable, generally considered to be wholesome in nature, and contain as few ingredients as possible. It involves moving away from highly processed ingredients and moving towards ingredients from natural sources.

Marketers have embraced the *clean label* product positioning by focusing on the "absence of" ingredients. Depending on the consumer group's specific concerns, common examples of "absence of" communications include the absence of added sugar, lactose, gluten, genetically modified organisms (GMO), etc. The rise in plant-based probiotic beverages ties in with the "cleaner living" movement as plant-based products continue to move into the realm of mainstream consumer products. Consumers look to manufacturers expecting transparency of ingredients as well as ingredient education where appropriate. Consumers expect transparency of ingredient information on both the product website as well as on the product packaging, with an understanding that consumers will use this information to make their purchase decisions.

"Better-for-you" renditions of familiar products are also a growing category (e.g., probiotic sodas and waters). These beverages have a marketing focus not on the "absence of" things such as sugars or fats, but rather on the benefits of additions such as live probiotics. As the consumer is already familiar with the traditional product, this has the potential to be an opportunity for consumer upsell in terms of appeal.

20.7 Benefit stacking and health halos in new product development

Benefit stacking for probiotic beverages refers to the marketing practice of expanding a product's promoted features by adding other desirable features to the probiotic bacteria in the drink. This can expand the product's appeal, and the additions can take many forms, including prebiotics, postbiotics, and psychobiotics.

While a single product may offer multiple benefits to the consumer, often one benefit is perceived as having more importance than the others. A "health halo" is the term for a single health benefit that causes a consumer to have a favorable impression of the overall product. The presence of a "health halo" distinguishes a product from its competitors and may result in the consumer perceiving the product as being virtuous in all respects.

The Irish food company ***Kerry*** approaches new product development marketing as a three-part process using something familiar to the customer and combining it with "benefit stacking" and a "health halo." New products developed by Kerry have the following: (1) the welcome mat (an ingredient familiar to the consumer such as strawberry), (2) the "health halo" (a trending ingredient associated with benefits to the immune system such as ginger) and (3) "the hero" (a scientifically proven ingredient supporting immunity or gut health, such as a live probiotic bacteria) (Kerry, 2020). The inclusion of the scientifically proven ingredient, or as Kerry calls it the "hero," also addresses the consumers' desire for a transparent and trustworthy ingredient that offers benefits and convenience.

20.8 New technologies

Globally, over 2.25 billion cups of coffee and over 3 billion cups of tea are consumed daily, creating a robust hot beverage market filled with product variations and where new innovative products are brought to market every year. Coffee and tea infused with probiotics offer a benefit-driven familiar product that is easy for consumers to incorporate into their daily routines. For example, US consumers, who currently average three cups of coffee per day can substitute a current coffee product for a probiotic-enhanced coffee without substantially impacting their daily habits while easily incorporating additional health benefits into their lives. The technology that has allowed for the production of probiotic hot drinks is the use of spore-forming strains of probiotic bacteria. The spores are more resistant to the extremes of heat, cold, pH, and pressure than vegetative cells. Even in the highly acidic and high-temperature environment of coffee or tea, these hardier bacteria now offer the opportunity for live probiotics to find their way into the consumer's gut.

The addition of a probiotic to a hot drink can be introduced at various stages in the beverage making process. The US company ***JÙS by Julie*** launched a probiotic cold brew coffee product, and US ***Tipton Mills*** launched a probiotic instant coffee. Both incorporate a probiotic branded *Bacillus coagulans* strain (Ganeden BC30) from Ganeden Biotech (Cleveland).

Offering a probiotic beverage in a nontraditional format, ***Vitacup*** created a probiotic-infused coffee k-cup pod. These pods quickly produce a probiotic hot coffee product using the already popular standard coffee pod equipment. Incorporated into the coffee pods are probiotic strains with spores that can survive the high brewing temperature. The marketing material claims that there are 1 billion colony-forming units (CFUs) of heat-stable probiotic bacteria present in each pod (heat-resistant *Bacillus coagulans*), and the pods also include aloe vera and B vitamins (an example of benefit stacking).

Vitacup also markets probiotic tea bags with aloe vera and B vitamins. There is a wide variety of probiotic teas on the marketplace, especially herbal and organic options, using heat-tolerant spores with probiotic strains. It is easy to benefit stack tea by incorporating high nutrient ingredients, such as vitamin C and ginger, further adding to their consumer appeal.

Targeting the consumer's desire for convenience, in 2020, Nestlé embarked on a group of innovative drinks called "***nesQino***," drink sachets that can be used with Q-cup machines to quickly make hot or cold drinks. The base sachets can be dairy milk, cereals, or plant-based materials along with sachets that contain probiotics. Consumers choose one "superfood sachet" and "one base sachet" to make a drink, allowing for a wide range of customization (21 options) and a drink ready in under 2 minutes. Initially launched in China, ***nesQino*** was aimed at Millennials and Gen-Z consumers, known for their high interest in personalized nutrition products. The product claims on the packaging include highlighting the absence of additives, preservatives, artificial colors, and artificial flavors. Further personalization of the beverages is supported through a ***nesQino*** smartphone app for the Q-cup machine, which allows for the personalization of drink temperature, recipe combinations, and nutritional information.

AliveBiome, a UK start-up, launched a probiotic water drink with an innovative cap, which contains a blend of probiotics, vitamins, and minerals in an airtight container to maintain viability. With a twist of the cap, the seal breaks, the probiotics are released into the water, and the drink is ready for consumption. As the probiotic market continues to expand, technological innovations will continue to create new delivery methods to add probiotics into previously microbe unfriendly environments.

20.9 Developing market opportunities—The young, the old, and the athlete

While there is an emphasis on the role that probiotic beverages can play in helping consumers age well, they also appeal to a younger demographic focused on preventative care at an earlier life stage. There is a lack of probiotic beverages designed specifically for the senior consumers despite the growing geriatric population.

Child-focused probiotic beverages are also an area of opportunity for future market growth. There appears to be a gap in functional beverages that target this young group, but that is slowly starting to change. The Californian company ***Once upon a Farm*** is marketing dairy-free smoothies designed for babies, toddlers, and young children. The refrigerated smoothie is made with organic fruits and vegetables, cold-pressed, and with probiotics added for gut and immune health. The packaging for this group is in bisphenol A (BPA)-free and recyclable pouches, but also with some smoothies offered in child-friendly bottles for older children.

The sports drink market is well-developed and continues to expand in its product offerings. Sports nutrition has often focused on antioxidants and energy claims in their marketing material. However, probiotics as a part of a sports nutrition drink is an area of new product innovation, usually through the combination of probiotics with protein drinks for workout recovery. Probiotics in protein drinks can increase the absorption of critical nutrients, such as amino acids from proteins, decrease the incidence of upper respiratory infections, and improve recovery from muscle-damaging exercise; all sought after health benefits for the sports drink consumer (Jäger et al., 2019; Jäger, Mohr, & Pugh, 2020).

20.10 The market message in 2020

Successful marketing plans adjust to the needs of the times to stay relevant to the consumers. Social media and social media influencers have changed how probiotic beverages are being marketed, especially in the time of COVID-19.

Social media—Marketing to Millennials and Gen Z—One of the most effective ways to reach Millennials when considering marketing options is social media. Millennials are a large consumer target market, with strong purchasing power. With Millennials being the largest purchasers of probiotics, this demographic sector is a key market focus.

Globally, over 4.5 billion people use the internet, and active social media users number over 3.8 billion. In 2020, Instagram is one of the most popular social media platforms with over 1 billion monthly active users. Millennials reinforce new trends on their social media platforms where they like to document their healthy lifestyle. They like third party recommendations, dislike traditional advertising, and value brand authenticity. As they check their smartphones on an average over 43 times a day, social media marketing is a key pathway to reach Millennials through advertising, peer reviews, and social media influencer recommendations (Social Toaster, 2020). Gen Z (52%) and Millennials (62%) often turn to social media health influencers when looking for health information and new wellness trends, such as probiotic beverages (Specialty Enzymes and Probiotics, 2020).

Millennials have shown a high interest in purchasing probiotic beverages due to the tie in with their social media accounts and other internet platform links. Influencer marketing (ranging from celebrities to health specialists) is an area that continues to grow. Influencers are shaping trends, and online health advice and social media generate awareness in this consumer group.

Storytelling—One of the most effective and popular marketing techniques is selling with "storytelling," and 56% of global consumers say the stories around a brand influence their purchase decisions (Innova, 2020). "Storytelling" is a way to connect to the consumer, build trust in a product, and create top of mind awareness. A well-crafted story can teach the consumer about the product's origin, history, and ingredient provenance, and it can be tied into a company's work around sustainability and corporate social responsibility.

A successful use of storytelling and capturing current trends is illustrated by ***Skyr***, a company that produces traditional Icelandic dairy products. With their drinkable yogurt-like smoothies, they communicate an exciting story about Viking history and about their production process. They teach the consumer how the beverage is traditionally made in Iceland using a low-temperature fermentation, live and active probiotics, and they connect the beverage to the unique local history associated with their microbial cultures. Consumers are educated about how the product is low-fat as it is made from skim milk as well as the fact that it has more protein and less sugar than similar traditional products. Nordic fruits such as lingonberry and bilberry are used, enabling the marketers to advertise the product as low-lactose, gluten-free, and free of artificial ingredients such as sweeteners, vegan friendly, and non-GMO. Although the product sold in the United States is not produced in Iceland, there is transparency about this fact on the US website. This product is also an excellent example of benefit stacking and "absence of" and "better-for-you" claims. It contains "halo" ingredients, as well as adventuresome and health trending fruits (lingonberry and bilberry), and of course, probiotic bacteria with a special story, and the presence of yeast. This high protein source of fermented dairy makes it appealing to the sports consumer segment as well. One can see how this product hits many of the key touchstones identified as important to consumers.

Convenient shots—Convenience is a key priority to consumers. Many prefer not to take supplements in the form of pills or powders but still seek convenient ways to get the benefit of live probiotic organisms into their daily diet. The class of probiotic drinks called "shots" addresses this consumer need. A popular example is Activia's probiotic yogurt drink, marketed as "***Activia Shots***," which emphasizes that it has "the least sugar on the market" and that the probiotic organisms contribute to healthy gut flora. Under the Actimel brand, there are 100% dairy-free ***Actimel Shots*** containing roasted almonds, oats, and two probiotic live cultures (incl. *Lactobacillus casei*) along with vitamins D and B6. The shots are advertised as low in sugar, no additives, and suitable for vegans.

An example of both sustainability and social responsibility can be seen in the actions of the Minneapolis-based company "***So Good So You***." The company uses botanical ingredients for their organic, plant-based, probiotic, cold-pressed juice shots—marketed as vegan and non-GMO, with names such as "immunity," "longevity," and "sleep," and with key ingredients of ginger, turmeric, and California poppy, respectively. What makes this company stand out from competitive companies with similar products is how much their communications focus on the importance of sustainability as shown with their drink shots. They were the first to use a biodegradable polyethylene terephthalate (PET) product for their packaging. During the time of COVID-19, they have been actively donating care packages containing their immune-boosting juice shots to the local medical workers and others in hard-hit areas. In addition, they use Instagram as a way for consumers to nominate frontline workers to receive care packages of probiotic shot drinks. In a recent interview, the company cofounders said that it was about more than just helping the frontline workers stay healthy, that it was about making certain they felt supported and remembered.

Waters and sodas—In the development of new probiotic beverages, it is important to consider the consumer's desire for a multisensory experience that includes not only taste, appearance, and aroma, but also mouthfeel and even sound.

Sparkling waters and soda pops are now available as probiotic beverages. For mouthfeel, seltzer, and sparkling waters tingle on the taste buds and offer the sound of small bubbles popping, adding to the drinking experience. An example of a probiotic soda that falls into the "better-for-you" marketing category is ***Culture Pop***. Launched in the summer of 2020, with its brightly decorated aluminum can, it has the look of regular soda pop, with a tag line of "*it's a soda that is actually good for you.*" On the can, it calls itself "*a fizzy and gutzy probiotic soda.*" It targets many current consumer desires such as: live probiotic organisms, low in calories (40 calories), gluten-free, vegan, plant-based, non-GMO, and offers a mix of fruit flavors. "Better-for-you" renditions of familiar products that mimic iconic sodas include the brand ***Live Soda***, which offers typical soda pop flavors such as cola and root beer and promotes the products as zero sugar by using monk fruit as the sweetener. This particular drink contains live probiotics, and it uses the familiarity of well-loved flavors combined with a new added benefit.

Prebiotic sodas—A "better-for-you" US prebiotic soda is ***Poppi,*** which has a loyal following of Generation X and Millennial consumers after it was made famous on the television (TV) show "Shark Tank." Currently, on track to become the show's first billion-dollar company, ***Poppi*** is marketed as a prebiotic soda. It is a fruit-juice product combined with apple cider vinegar. Apple cider vinegar is very popular in the "alternative" and "natural health" community, with the prebiotic factor ascribed to the fermented apples and pectin. The resulting product is a very drinkable beverage with an array of famous social media influencers touting its tastes and benefits on Instagram.

Another example of a prebiotic beverage is ***Clue*** prebiotic water, where the prebiotic is not apple cider vinegar but rather an added fructooligosaccharide. Most prebiotics included in beverages are oligosaccharides and ***Clue*** prebiotic water contains 4 g of fructooligosaccharides (also called FOS) in each 16 oz bottle. Fructooligosaccharides are believed to aid in digestive functions, immune health, calcium absorption, and are a good source of fiber that is then available as food for the beneficial bacteria already present in the gut microbiome, thus, stimulating an increase in these beneficial bacteria.

Probiotic juice drinks—Popular new products in this area are the high pressure-processed (HPP) juice drinks (i.e., the juice has been cold pasteurized). The process kills 99.9% of the microorganisms present. It is a nonthermal process that helps the product retain a fresh-squeezed taste while giving it a longer shelf life than one would get with a cold-pressed juice. Certain strains of sporulated commercially available probiotic organisms (such as *Bacillus coagulans* from GanedenBC30) can survive high pressure while problem organisms that cause spoilage, such as molds, are inactivated. The HPP processing of fruit and vegetable juices for probiotic drinks has gained additional momentum during the COVID-19 pandemic. Consumers are looking for products to boost their immune system, support a clean eating lifestyle, and that have a longer shelf life, which means fewer trips to the grocery store.

In 2014, ***Garden of Flavor*** was one of the first probiotic juices on the US market using HPP technology and the GanedenBC30 probiotic strain. Their first three flavors at that time were marketed as Green Harmony, Appleade, and Turmeric Tonic. Their product line has expanded, with a profusion of organic ingredients. As an example, their cold-pressed energy wheatgrass pineapple juice is described as containing all organic ingredients (guayusa, pineapple juice, wheatgrass juice, kale juice, spinach juice, romaine juice, lemon juice, and mint-leaf juice) and water and a probiotic organism content of *Bacillus coagulans* GBI-30 at a level of 500 million per serving.

Advertising and social media—The power of social media to connect with key target consumers should not be underestimated. Of the paid ads in Q4 2019, 96.1% of ads were seen on mobile devices and 3.9% on desktop access. Facebook received 58% of the relative ad spend in Q1 of 2019, followed by Instagram feed and Instagram stories, which combined received 28.4% of relative ad spend. For brands mentioned by influencers, data shows that in Q4 2019, there was considerable growth in influencer marketing (using #AD or local language version). In the last quarter of 2019, Instagram's total audience surpassed Facebook with the higher engagement of posts on Instagram. Women aged 25–34 were the largest group engaging with brands on Facebook in terms of interacting with brand pages.

Instagram stories and tap backs—Instagram stories are an important format for brand communications. The tap back rate is the number of times a viewer taps on the left side of a screen to rewatch a previous story. Socialbakers reports that the industries that got the most viewers to tap back to rewatch their Instagram stories were e-Commerce and beverages (both with a median rate of 2.72%), followed by alcohol (2.66%) (SocialBakers, 2020). Storytelling, combined with social media marketing, when performed well can be so engaging that consumers choose to rewatch the advertising more than once.

20.11 Concluding thoughts

With COVID-19, there has never been a better time for brands to promote immune-supporting drinks, especially in the underdeveloped senior market. COVID-19 immunity support is on the consumer's mind. While the effects of COVID-19 in the coming year on consumer preferences and purchases are yet to be determined, early indications are that there will be even more interest in well-produced and well-marketed probiotic beverages if the consumer is confident that their consumption will lead to a tasty and convenient way to reach better health outcomes in daily life.

References

Jäger, R., Mohr, A. E., Carpenter, K. C., Kerksick, C. M., Purpura, M., Moussa, A., et al. (2019). International society of sports nutrition position stand: Probiotics. *Journal of the International Society of Sports Nutrition, 16*(1), 62.

Jäger, R., Mohr, A. E., & Pugh, J. N. (2020). Recent advances in clinical probiotic research for sport. *Current Opinion in Clinical Nutrition & Metabolic Care, 23*(6), 428–436.

Wegh, C. A., Geerlings, S. Y., Knol, J., Roeselers, G., & Belzer, C. (2019). Postbiotics and their potential applications in early life nutrition and beyond. *International Journal of Molecular Sciences, 20*(19), 4673.

Organization links

Euromonitor (2018). *Passport analysis. August 2018(2018).* https://www.euromonitor.com/

FMCG Gurus (2020). (2020). https://fmcggurus.com/top-trends-2020/

FoodNavigator (2017). *Market research group packaged facts 2017 survey. (2017).* https://www.foodnavigator-usa.com
Grand View Research (2020). (2020). https://www.grandviewresearch.com/
Hartman Group (2019). (2019). https://www.hartman-group.com/blogs/44453216/beverages-as-snacks-you-are-what-you-drink
IFIC (2020). (2020). https://ific.org/
Innova (2018). *Innova market insights survey. (2018).* https://www.innovamarketinsights.com/
Innova (2020). *Innova market insights top trends for 2020. (2020).* https://www.innovamarketinsights.com/
Kerry (2020). (2020). https://www.kerry.com/
Mintel (2017). (2017). https://www.mintel.com/the-chinese-consumer-2017
Mintel (2020). (2020). https://www.mintel.com/global-food-and-drink-trends
Social Toaster (2020). (2020). https://www.socialtoaster.com/tips-marketing-to-millennials/
SocialBakers (2020). *Social media trends report. (2020).* www.socialbakers.com
Specialty Enzymes and Probiotics (2020). (2020). http://www.specialtyenzymes.com/blog/millennials-probiotics
UN-DESA (2020). (2020). https://www.un.org/en/desa
Winsight (2018). *Winsight grocery business magazine—February*: (p. 70).. (2018). https://www.winsightgrocerybusiness.com/magazine

Product website links

Actimel Shots. https://www.actimel.co.uk/yogurt-drink/100-dairy-free
Activia Shots. https://www.activia.ca/en/products/shot/yogurt-drink/
AliveBiome. https://alivebiome.com
Clue. https://drinkclue.com/
Culture Pop. https://drinkculturepop.com/
Garden of Flavor. https://gardenofflavor.com/
JÙS by Julie. https://www.jusbyjulie.com/
Live Soda. https://livesoda.com/products/live-probiotic-soda
nesQino. https://www.nestle.com/media/news/nestle-launches-nesqino-healthy-customizable-drinks
Once upon a Farm. https://onceuponafarmorganics.com/
Poppi. https://www.drinkpoppi.com
Skyr. https://www.icelandicprovisions.com/what-is-skyr/
So Good So You. https://sogoodsoyou.com/probiotic-shots/
Tipton Mills. https://www.tiptonmills.com/products
Vitacup. https://www.vitacup.com

CHAPTER

21

Thoughts on the future of probiotic beverages

Spiros Paramithiotis, Maria K. Syrokou, and Eleftherios H. Drosinos

Laboratory of Food Quality Control and Hygiene, Department of Food Science and Human Nutrition, Agricultural University of Athens, Athens, Greece

21.1 Introduction

Consumer awareness regarding food safety and quality is constantly increasing. In addition, nutritional trends, such as vegetarianism, veganism, refrain from certain nutrients such as gluten, lactose etc., without these being directed by an underlying medical condition, are also gaining ground. However, there is a concept that is widely accepted and stands above this splintering of the food preferences sphere. This concept includes the consumption of food that according to Roberfroid (1999) "has been modified to sub-serve physiological roles beyond the provision of simple nutrient requirements", i.e., functional food. Within this frame, the use of microorganisms in order to increase the nutritional content and functionality of food has been widely exercised. The probiotic concept was conceived long before those nutritional movements appeared; the term was first used in 1953 by Werner Kollath to describe substances that could ameliorate the symptoms of malnutrition. Since then, various modifications of the term were proposed, until in 2001 FAO/WHO provided the definition currently in use (Gogineni, Morrow, Gregory, & Malesker, 2013). This concept is undeniably one of the favorites among researchers worldwide because of the high importance and the constant need and capacity for improvement. The latter has been greatly favored by the technical and conceptual advances in the field of molecular biology that allowed massive data generation and the ability to assess them by alternative points of view.

Probiotic Beverages
https://doi.org/10.1016/B978-0-12-818588-9.00022-X

Probiotic products have met commercial acceptance and success; it is most likely that the market will continue to grow, at least in the near future. This growth will be based on four cornerstones:

1. Further development of probiotic beverages. Although yogurt is considered as the traditional probiotic delivery vehicle, beverages fit better for the "on the go" generation with their elevated daily working rhythms, which demand nutrition-dense but effortless foods.
2. Expansion of probiotic delivery matrices beyond dairy products. Dairy products with their long history of use, have familiarized the public with the probiotic drink concept. Although there is still room for improvement, fruit and vegetable juices are currently serving better the demand for multifunctional products.
3. Improved culture selection. The criteria for the selection of potentially probiotic cultures involve (a) technological properties that are associated with the delivery matrix and the production procedure of the microorganism itself, (b) properties associated with the capacity of a microbial strain to reach the target colonization site, (c) safety aspects, and (d) functional properties. The latter two are in the epicenter of intensive study. The safety of commercially available probiotic cultures is being reconsidered as in some cases such products may not be suitable for the general population, and certain categories may be excluded from their consumption.
4. Similarly, functional properties include a wide variety of health-promoting attributes that are constantly updated.
5. Next-generation probiotics. This is a concept developed to distinguish between "traditional" probiotics, i.e., those cultures that confer a health benefit upon consumption from those that may restore a health phenotype. Although this concept is still far from being effectively implemented, the idea alone is capable of further boosting product development and acceptability.

The aim of the present chapter is to present thoughts regarding the future of probiotic beverages and the data on which these are based.

21.2 Isolation of strains and the in vitro characterization of probiotic potential

There are hundreds of publications assessing the probiotic potential of isolates through *in vitro* experimentation. The criteria used for the characterization of probiotic potential are being constantly updated; an update on the selection criteria and the methods employed was recently offered by De Melo Pereira, de Oliveira Coelho, Júnior, Thomaz-Soccol, and Soccol (2018). In general, these criteria may be distinguished into three categories: safety aspects, efficiency to reach colonization site and colonization capacity, as well as functional properties.

Regarding the first category, the properties most frequently assessed are antibiotic resistance, hemolytic activity, production of biogenic amines, toxins (e.g., cytolysin), or enzymes (e.g., hyaluronidase, gelatinase). Despite the extensive scrutiny that strains bearing the "probiotic" label have been through, a reappraisal of their safety is currently ongoing. The reason for this is the accumulation of data regarding some adverse effects that have been associated with their consumption. The majority of the cases refer to immunocompromised individuals, infants, and elderly people and involve a wide range of conditions including gastrointestinal disorders, systemic infections, skin irritation, etc. Available data on the adverse effects of probiotics were recently collected and comprehensively reviewed by Sotoudegan, Daniali, Hassani, Nikfar, and Abdollahi (2019). This issue is of utmost importance and careful safety evaluation of the microorganisms intended for use as probiotics is suggested.

The efficiency to reach the colonization site is predicted through an assessment of the strain's ability to withstand the hurdles encountered during digestion; while at the same time maintenance of high populations is desired. These hurdles include the enzymes present in the saliva (mostly focused on lysozyme), the low pH, and pepsin of the gastric juice in the stomach, as well as pancreatin and the bile salts of the intestine. Adhesion to epithelial cells is predicted through an assessment of the ability to form biofilms on various surfaces, adherence to intestinal mucin and various cell lines, cell surface hydrophobicity, and cellular autoaggregation.

The functional properties is a constantly expanding list. It includes antagonistic ability against pathogens, as well as a series of properties and functions that are beneficial to the host. The latter may possess either a prophylactic or a therapeutic character (Varankovich, Nickerson, & Korber, 2015).

In Table 21.1, the properties assessed in recent representative studies are summarized.

Even though the majority of these studies did not reach experimentation in animal models or clinical trials, and thus they do not address the aim of providing new probiotic cultures, such studies are very important for the following reasons:

a. They contribute to our knowledge on ordinary properties of food-related microbial species and the development of respective databases,

b. They show that some strains are capable of extraordinary activities; the underlying molecular mechanisms of which may improve our understanding regarding microbial physiology and responses under optimal and stressful conditions

TABLE 21.1 Recent representative studies on the in vitro evaluation of probiotic potential.

Microorganisms assessed	Isolation matrix	Properties studied	Reference
F. pseudoficulneus, *F. fructosus*, *F. durionis*, *Lb. kunkeei*	Fruits and flowers	Auto-aggregation, antibiotic resistance, production of antimicrobial compounds, low pH tolerance, cell surface hydrophobicity, bile salts tolerance, cholesterol assimilation	Sakandar, Kubow, and Sadiq (2019)
Lb. pentosus, *Lb. plantarum*, *Lb. fermentum*, *Lb. rhamnosus*	Fruits, fermented food, human	pH, bile, NaCl, phenol tolerance, mucin adhesion, biofilm formation, antibacterial and antifungal activity, hydrolysis of bile salts, production of GABA, β-galactosidase and DNAse activity, antibiotic resistance, haemolysis, biogenic amine production, mucin degradation	Boricha, Shekh, Pithva, Ambalam, and Vyas (2019)
B. longum, *B. breve*, *B. bifidum*	New-born infant feces	pH, bile tolerance, biogenic amine production, haemolysis, antibiotic resistance, adhesion to Caco-2 cell lines (and presence of associated genes), antibacterial activity	Achi and Halami (2019)
Lb. plantarum, *Lb. brevis*, *Pd. acidilactici*	Aguamiel and pulque	Antibiotic resistance, bile, pH tolerance, antibacterial activity	Cervantes-Elizarraras et al. (2019)
Lb. plantarum, *M. luteus*	fermented milled-mixed corn-soybean wastes-meal	Bile, pH tolerance, antibacterial activity, hydrolysis of bile salts, haemolysis	Nwachukwu, George-Okafor, Ozoani, and Ojiagu (2019)
Lb. plantarum	Infant feces	Bile, pH tolerance, antibacterial activity, antibiotic resistance, biofilm formation on glass and plastic surfaces, adhesion to intestinal mucin and Caco-2 lines, stimulation of THP-1 macrophages	Gheziel et al. (2019)

TABLE 21.1 Recent representative studies on the in vitro evaluation of probiotic potential—cont'd

Microorganisms assessed	Isolation matrix	Properties studied	Reference
E. faecalis, Lb. fermentum, Lb. plantarum, Lb. paracasei, Str. thermophilus	Infant feces	Bile and low pH tolerance, adhesion to Caco-2 lines, antibiotic resistance, stimulation of murine macrophage cells	Kook, Chung, Lee, Lee, and Kim (2019)
Lc. lactis, Lc. garvieae	Goat cheese	Bile and low pH tolerance, resistance to pepsin and pancreatin, antibiotic resistance, auto- and co-aggregation	Kazancıgil, Demirci, Öztürk-Negiş, and Akin (2019)
S. cerevisiae	Suan-yu (fermented fish)	Survival in pH 2.5 medium with 0.3% bile salts, antimicrobial activity, hydrophobicity, biofilm formation	Zeng, Fan, He, Duan, and Xia (2019)
Lb. curvatus	Sliced cooked ham	Bile and low pH tolerance, resistance to pepsin and pancreatin, antibiotic resistance, auto- and co-aggregation, hydrophobicity, antimicrobial activity, haemolytic and DNAse activity	Funck et al. (2019)
Lb. casei, Lb. paracasei, Lb. plantarum. Lb. pentosus, Lb. brevis	Jeot-gal (high-salt fermented seafood)	Cinnamoyl esterase production, antimicrobial activity, auto-aggregation, hydrophobicity, adhesion to Caco-2 cells	Kim and Baik (2019)
P. guilliermondii, P. membranifaciens, P. kluyveri, H. opuntiae, H. uvarum, K. marxianus, C. orphopsilosis, C. quercitrusa, S. cerevisiae	Fermented foods	Bile and low pH tolerance, hydrophobicity, auto- and co-aggregation, haemolytic and antioxidant activity, adhesion to Caco-2 cells	Menezes et al. (2019)

Continued

TABLE 21.1 Recent representative studies on the in vitro evaluation of probiotic potential—cont'd

Microorganisms assessed	Isolation matrix	Properties studied	Reference
Lb. plantarum, Lb. pentosus, Lb. rhamnosus, Lb. paracasei, Pd. pentosaceus, Ln. lactis	Piacentinu Ennese cheese	DNAse, gelatinase, hemolytic and mucin degradation activities, biogenic amine production, antibiotic susceptibility, lysozyme, acidic and bile salts tolerances, antimicrobial activity, hydrophobicity, auto- and co-aggregation abilities, adhesion to Caco-2 cells, antioxidant activity, anti-inflammatory activity	Pino et al. (2019)

B.: Bifidobacterium; C.: Candida; En.: Enterococcus; F.: Fructobacillus; H.: Hanseniaspora; K.: Kluyveromyces; Lb.: Lactobacillus; Lc.: Lactococcus; Ln.: Leuconostoc; M.: Micrococcus; P.: Pichia; Pd.: Pediococcus; S.: Saccharomyces; Str.: Streptococcus.

c. Addressed through a time point of view, they depict the research trends that concomitantly reflect, at least to some extent, societal needs.

Another issue of interest is the methodology applied to assess probiotic potential. Identification of the genes responsible for some actions has led to the belief that phenotypic experimentation could be replaced by the detection of the respective encoding genes. However, such an approach must be exercised with extreme caution, as the presence or absence of a gene, or group of genes, may not predict whether or not that phenotype is active; it has become common knowledge that the cell may find alternative ways to perform an action that may offer a competitive advantage. However, in some cases, a good indication may be offered, and thus the detection of specific enzymes such as *gelE* encoding gelatinase, *hyl* encoding hyaluronidase, *cylA*/B encoding cytolysins, *tetM*, *tetK*, and *tetW* responsible for tetracycline resistance, as well as virulence-associated genes, such as *ace* (collagen protein adhesin), *agg* (aggregation protein), *asa1* (aggregation substance), *efaAfs* (cell wall adhesin), and *esp* (enterococcal surface protein) are now commonly reported in the literature (Guo et al., 2017; Hwanhlem, Ivanova, Biscola, Choiset, & Haertle, 2017; Motahari, Mirdamadi, & Kianirad, 2017; Ojekunle, Banwo, & Sanni, 2017; Perumal & Venkatesan, 2017; Rzepkowska, Zielińska, Ołdak, & Kolozyn-Krajewska, 2017).

Selection criteria very often include a set of technological properties that assess the ability of the microbial strains to reach high numbers during industrial-scale production and to withstand freezing or drying, which are the most commonly applied preservation practices. Retaining viability during storage and a high resuscitation capacity, as well as a high population and functionality during food processing and storage are also important. As mentioned previously, a wealth of literature is available on this topic. Regarding heat and osmotic stresses, which are very often encountered during the industrial production and preservation of both starter and adjunct cultures, as well as fermented products, it has been reported that *Streptococcus* spp. are often more resistant than *Lactobacillus* spp. (Bielecka & Majkowska, 2000; Kumar & Mishra, 2004; Wang, Yu, & Chou, 2004), *Propionibacterium* spp. than *Bifidobacterium* spp., *Lactobacillus* spp. and *Lactococcus* spp. (Huang et al., 2016; Schuck, Dolivet, Mejean, Herve, & Jeantet, 2013), and *Bifidobacterium longum* than *Bf. infantis* (Lian, Hsiao, & Chou, 2002). Enhancement of this ability, through the addition of several additives, mostly proteins and polysaccharides, has been examined, leading to the conclusion that this property is rather a strain- than species-dependent (Bedani, Vieira, Rossi, & Saad, 2014; Blaiotta et al., 2017; Buriti, Okazaki, Alegro, & Saad, 2007; Coda, Laner, Trani, Gobbetti, & Di Cagno, 2012; Donkor, Tsangalis, & Shah, 2007; El-Nagga, & Abd El-Tawab, 2012; Kailasapathy, Harmstorf, & Phillips, 2008; Liu et al., 2017; Marafon, Sumi, Alcantara, Tamime, & Oliveira, 2011; Mazinani, Fadaei, & Khosravi-Darani, 2016; Oliveira, Florence, Perego, De Oliveira, & Converti, 2011; Phillips, Kailasapathy, & Tran, 2006; Pino et al., 2017; Radulovic et al., 2017; Ranadheera, Evans, Adams, & Baines, 2012; Zare, Champagne, Simpson, Orsat, & Boye, 2012). Although the prediction of such behavior through the application of "omic" approaches is considered, it is a difficult task mainly due to the complexity of the physiological responses involved.

21.3 Advances in dairy probiotic beverages

Dairy beverages in general, and probiotic-containing beverages in particular, have been extensively studied. As a result, several classification schemes are currently available; among the most recent is the one proposed by Turkmen, Akal, and Ozer (2019), in which dairy beverages can be distinguished into traditional (including kefir, koumiss, buttermilk, etc.), value-added (including high protein, carbonated, energy, etc.), and functional (enriched or supplemented with functional ingredients). Probiotic-containing beverages can be found in all groups, and they hold an important position from a commercial perspective. Currently, the probiotic products that are commercially available are mostly based on very well-characterized strains of the species *Lb. acidophilus, Lb. casei, Lb. plantarum, Lb. rhamnosus, Bf. animalis, Bf. bifidum, Bf. longum* and their combinations (Turkmen et al., 2019).

Research is very active within this topic, spanning from the isolation and evaluation of novel cultures to the development of novel products. The latter, along with a reassessment of the criteria employed for safety characterization of a culture, as already mentioned in the previous paragraph, has drawn specific attention. In Table 21.2, recent representative studies that depict current trends are shown.

Fruit pulps and juices, as well as cereals, are added to milk to improve organoleptic properties, increase the functional ingredient content, and in some cases protect the starter, or the adjunct cultures possessing the probiotic properties, during storage.

TABLE 21.2 Recent representative studies on the development of novel dairy-based products.

Potential probiotic beverage	Comment	Reference
Milk whey with orange juice	A functional beverage combining orange juice and milk whey was fermented by the potential probiotic strain *Lb. fermentum* pH 5. After a cold storage period for approximately one month, the bacterium retained its viability (above 6 log CFU mL^{-1}). The 40 (whey):60 (orange juice) proportion, displayed higher sensory quality properties, compared to the rest	Thakkar, Vaghela, Patel, Modi, and Prajapati (2018)
Whole cow's milk with mango juice	A *Lb. acidophilus* dairy fermented beverage supplemented with increasing levels of mango juice was developed. Its fortification with 10% mango juice improved the probiotic strain's viable population during a 5-week cold storage period and enhanced *Lb. acidophilus* gastrointestinal tolerance. However, higher concentrations of juice led to better organoleptic characteristics	Ryan et al. (2020)
Semi-skimmed sheep milk with strawberry puree	Semi-skimmed sheep milk was combined with strawberry puree at a ratio of ca. 5:4 and fermented by the potential probiotic strain *Lb.*	Balthazar et al. (2019)

TABLE 21.2 Recent representative studies on the development of novel dairy-based products—cont'd

Potential probiotic beverage	Comment	Reference
	plantarum CECT8328. In addition, the beverage was fortified with the prebiotics, inulin, and potato starch. *Lb. plantarum* kept its viability after cold storage for 30 days and after simulated digestion. The blend of prebiotics with *Lb. plantarum*, CECT8328 enhanced the beverage's health promoting attributes	
Skimmed milk supplemented with pomegranate peel extract	A *Lb. acidophilus* dairy fermented beverage supplemented with pomegranate peel extracts (PPE), was developed. PPE addition at 2 % (w/v) did not adversely influence bacterial strain viability. In addition, antioxidant activity and phenolic concentration exhibited elevated rates, during fermentation, thus promoting a symbiotic relationship in the food matrix	Chan, Gan, Shah, and Corke (2018)
Dairy beverage supplemented with oat	A dairy beverage supplemented with oat, fermented by the potential probiotic *Lb. curvatus* P99 was developed. The bacterial strain, inoculated in the dairy substrate supplemented with oat extract, kept its viability after 35 days storage at 4°C	Funck et al. (2019)

Lb.: *Lactobacillus.*

21.4 Development of nondairy probiotic beverages

Probiotic delivery through nondairy beverages has been extensively considered. Fruit and vegetable pulps and juices, cereal extracts, soybean products, and some of their combinations have been used for this purpose. In the majority of the cases, procedures derived from tradition are followed with only slight modifications. In Table 21.3, recent representative studies on the development of such products are summarized.

Probiotic or potential probiotic strains belonging to the species *Lb. casei*, *Lb. paracasei*, *Lb. acidophilus*, *Lb. delbrueckii*, *Lb. plantarum*, *Bf. animalis*, *Bf. lactis*, and *Bf. longum* are more often included in these studies. These may be accompanied by technologically important species, such as

TABLE 21.3 Recent representative studies on the development of non-dairy probiotic beverages.

Potential probiotic beverage	Comment	Reference
Sugary kefir	Spontaneously formed milk kefir grains were gradually acclimatized from a milk to sucrose fermentation and used to ferment apple juice (NAJ), cherry juice (SCN), and a solution of sugary water enriched with plums (BSS). Yeasts dominated fermentation and enumerated at 6.28-6.58 log CFU g^{-1}, while bacteria were enumerated at 4.32-4.85 log CFU g^{-1}. *S. cerevisiae* dominated all three sugary kefir grains with *K. marxianus* forming a secondary microbiota in BSS and NAJ. *Lb. rhamnosus* dominated BSS and *Bacillus amyloliquefaciens* NAJ and SCN. Several yeast and bacteria strains exhibited proteolytic and lipolytic activities	Syrokou, Papadelli, Ntaikou, Paramithiotis, and Drosinos (2019)
Pomegranate juice	*Lb. paracasei* K5, bound to delignified wheat bran, was tested for its ability to ferment pomegranate juice at escalating pH levels. After a one-month cold storage the strain presented a viable population above 10^6 CFU mL^{-1}. The moderately alcoholic fermented beverage (EtOH levels less than 1%) presented increased phenol content and antifungal capacity, during its shelf life	Mantzourani et al. (2020)
Apricot juice	An apricot juice-based beverage was developed through fermentation by strains of *Bf. longum*, *Bf. lactis*, *Lb. acidophilus*, and *Lb. casei* used as single or combined cultures. Bacterial strains presented higher cell yields in mixed fermentations. Lactic acid levels were similar between fermentations by single and combined cultures, but acetic acid was double in the latter	Bujna, Farkas, Tran, Dam, and Nguyen (2018)

TABLE 21.3 Recent representative studies on the development of non-dairy probiotic beverages—cont'd

Potential probiotic beverage	Comment	Reference
Sea buckthorn berries juice	Sea buckthorn berries juice was supplemented with wheat protein concentrate, soy protein isolate, and skim milk, inoculated with 8.5 log CFU mL^{-1} *Lb. rhamnosus* GG and stored at 4°C for two weeks. The probiotic strain retained a population above 8 log CFU mL^{-1} throughout the storage period and at the same time diminished the *E. coli* population when co-inoculated at 6 log CFU mL^{-1}	Sireswar, Dey, Dey, and Kundu (2017)
Lemon juice	Lemon juice was fermented by *Lb. casei*, *Lb. delbrueckii*, *Lb. plantarum*, and *Lb. helveticus* as single cultures or in combinations, as free cells or microencapsulated. The beverage was then stored at 4°C for up to six weeks. The beverage was then administered to wild type C57BL/6 (B6) mice that were infected by *Sh. flexneri* and *Sh. dysenteriae*. The combination of all four lactic acid bacteria prolonged the shelf life of lemon juice by two weeks. In addition, the inflammatory haematological profiles of the mice were improved	Islam, Hasan, Al Mamun, Kudrat-E-Zahan, and Al-Bari (2015)
Coconut water	The development of a functional beverage based on the synergistic action of the liquid coconut water and *Lb. plantarum* AC-1 was described. After cold storage for approximately one month, *Lb. plantarum* AC-1 maintained its cellular viability (8 log CFU mL^{-1}). In addition, the antimicrobial effect against *E. coli*, *Sa.* Typhi and *St. aureus*, combined with the high organoleptic acceptability, resulted in the proposal of a potential probiotic product	Prado et al. (2015)
Litchi juice	A high hydrostatic pressure (HHP) approach was investigated in litchi juice, for the development of a potential probiotic beverage fermented by *Lb. casei*. The	Zheng et al. (2014)

Continued

TABLE 21.3 Recent representative studies on the development of non-dairy probiotic beverages—cont'd

Potential probiotic beverage	Comment	Reference
	appropriateness of this method was evidenced by high viability rates of *Lb. casei* (more than 8.0 log CFU mL^{-1}) after storage at 4°C for 4 weeks. In addition, the HPP-employed litchi beverage maintained its antioxidant activity and phenolic content and good sensory properties	
Orange juice	The effect of different probiotic addition methodologies (lyophilized commercial culture, culture activated through propagation, alginate encapsulated) on the quality parameters of orange juice, was studied. It was reported that direct addition of the commercial culture resulted in improved organoleptic acceptance as well as physicochemical characteristics	Miranda et al. (2019)
Maoluang juice	The protective action of *T. triandra* gum, maltodextrin, and inulin on *Lb. casei* 01 and *Lb. acidophilus* LA5 viability after their addition to pasteurized Maoluang juice at 10^{10} CFU mL^{-1}, spray drying and subjected to simulated stomach and small intestinal fluids was studied. Efficacy of this treatment to protect the cells during simulated GIT passage, compared to free cells, was exhibited. In addition, evidence suggesting prebiotic action of *T. triandra* gum was presented	Chaikham, Kemsawasd, and Seesuriyachan (2017)
Maize-based	The development of a beverage based on the Brazilian indigenous "calugi" prepared with *Lb. paracasei* LBC-81 alone or in combination with the yeasts *S. cerevisiae* CCMA 0731 and CCMA 0732 and *P. kluyveri* CCMA 0615 was reported. After fermentation at 37°C for 24 h, storage at 4°C for 28 d took place. With the exception of the *P. kluyveri* strain, all strains retained populations above 6 log CFU mL^{-1}	Menezes, Ramos, Dias, and Schwan (2018)

TABLE 21.3 Recent representative studies on the development of non-dairy probiotic beverages—cont'd

Potential probiotic beverage	Comment	Reference
	throughout storage. In addition, sensory evaluation raised an encouraging outcome, given the fact that no flavouring agents were added	
Rice-based	The development of a cassava-rice beverage based on the Brazilian indigenous "cauim" prepared with *Lb. plantarum* CCMA0743, *Lb. acidophilus* LAC-04 and *To. delbrueckii* CCMA0235, alone or in combination, was reported. After fermentation at 37°C for 48 h, the populations of bacteria were at 8 log CFU mL^{-1}. The combination with *To. delbrueckii* exhibited enhanced functional properties	Freire, Ramos, Souza, Cardoso, and Schwan (2017)
Oat, barley, malt-based	Fermentation of oat, barley and malt–water suspensions inoculated with *Lb. acidophilus*, *Lb. plantarum*, and *Lb. reuteri* human isolates at 37°C for 10 h, was reported. LAB reached populations of approx. 10^8 CFU mL^{-1}. The physicochemical characteristics of the products were encouraging for further development of the products	Salmeron, Thomas, and Pandiella (2015)
Drumstick, beetroot-based	A blend of drumstick leaves and beetroot was fermented by *Lb. plantarum* and *En. hirae* at 37°C for 48 h. The resulting beverage was reported to be rich in minerals and to exhibit good antimicrobial properties and radical scavenging capacity	Vanajakshi, Vijayendra, Varadaraj, Venkateswaran, and Agrawal (2015)
Carrot juice	Carrot juice was fermented overnight at 37°C by commercially available probiotic strains of *Lb. plantarum*, *Lb. paracasei*, *Bf. lactis*, and *Lb. rhamnosus*. After fermentation, lactobacilli reached a population of 10^9–10^{10} CFU mL^{-1}; after a 12-week storage *Lactobacillus* strains displayed viability populations at 10^7–10^9 CFU mL^{-1}. In contrast, bifidobacteria failed to grow and were undetectable after storage	Tamminen, Salminen, and Ouwehand (2013)

Continued

TABLE 21.3 Recent representative studies on the development of non-dairy probiotic beverages—cont'd

Potential probiotic beverage	Comment	Reference
Soybean waste-based	A promising approach for valorization of soybean waste was reported. It was initially treated with a carbohydrase to reduce insoluble fibre and then fermented by *Lb. paracasei* and *Li. saturnus* at 30°C for 48 h. The final product had increased concentrations of free amino acids, isoflavone aglycones, and significant probiotic populations, even after a 6-week storage at 5°C	Vong and Liu (2019)
Soymilk	Soymilk was fermented by the probiotic strains *Lb. acidophilus* La-5, *Bf. animalis* Bb-12 in the presence of *Str. thermophilus*. After a 28-day storage at 5°C, the *Bf. animalis* Bb 12 population remained above 10^8 CFU mL^{-1}, whereas *Lb. acidophilus* La 5 presented a decrease by one log. Use of inulin and fructooligosaccharides (FOS) did not impair the viability of probiotic bacteria	Battistini et al. (2018)
Soymilk-apple juice	Soymilk supplemented or not with apple juice was fermented by *Lb. acidophilus*. After a 21-day storage at 4°C, the strain retained its population in both cases above 8 log CFU mL^{-1}. The soymilk beverage, fortified with apple juice, gained the approval of panellists in sensory evaluation	Icier, Gündüz, Yılmaz, and Memeli (2015)
Green tea	The survival of *Lb. paracasei* LAFTI-L26, *Lb. acidophilus* LAFTI-L10, and *Bf. animalis* LAFTI-B94 during fermentation at 37°C for 72 h of extracts of six green tea varieties was assessed. In general, strain viability was affected by green tea variety with the highest survival presented by the *Lb. paracasei* strain after fermentation of the Gyokuro Asahi variety. Green tea substrates fermented with the potential probiotic bacteria did not improve either their angiotensin converting enzyme (ACE) inhibitory activity, or their antioxidant attributes	Lopez de Lacey, Pérez-Santín, López-Caballero, and Montero (2014)

TABLE 21.3 Recent representative studies on the development of non-dairy probiotic beverages—cont'd

Potential probiotic beverage	Comment	Reference
Tofu whey	The ability of *Lb. paracasei*, *Ln. mesenteroides*, *Lb. rhamnosus* GG, and *Lb. plantarum* strains to ferment tofu whey at 37°C for 24 h on the basis of their isoflavone bioconversion was examined. The *Lb. rhamnosus GG* and *Lb. paracasei* mixture exhibited great potential, increasing bioactive isoflavone aglycones from 4.6 to 93.8%. The bacteria population increased to 9.13 log CFU mL^{-1} with a significant improvement in tofu whey odor	Zhu, Wang, and Zhang (2019)

Bf.: Bifidobacterium; E.: Escherichia; En.: Enterococcus; K.: Kluyveromyces; Lb.: Lactobacillus; Li.: Lindnera; Ln.: Leuconostoc; P.: Pichia; S.: Saccharomyces; Sa.: Salmonella; Sh.: Shigella; St.: Staphylococcus; Str.: Streptococcus; T.: Tiliacora; To.: Torulaspora.

Streptococcus thermophilus, or yeast strains with specific attributes such as *Saccharomyces cerevisiae*, *Torulaspora delbrueckii*, and *Lindnera saturnus*. In most of the cases, strains indigenous to the matrix under consideration are utilized; incorporation of commercially available ones has also been applied. An interesting approach was described by Syrokou et al. (2019) regarding the gradual acclimatization of kefir grains formed during spontaneous kefir fermentation, from milk to sucrose fermentation. These grains were then used to ferment apple juice, cherry juice, and a sugary solution enriched with plums. This acclimatization affected the microbial composition of the kefir grains and facilitated yeast dominance over lactic acid bacteria due to the elevated carbohydrate concentration. Similarly, Tu et al. (2019) reported on the fermentation of a soy whey-based beverage by water kefir grains. Improvement of the nutritional, functional, and organoleptic characteristics of the product, after 2 days of fermentation at 25°C, compared to the unfermented control, was reported.

Lactic acid fermentation has been reported as an ideal approach to enhance the functional potential of plant matrices by using lactic acid bacteria metabolism (Gobbetti, Di Cagno, & De Angelis, 2010). Indeed, metabolites such as lactate, short chain fatty acids, and mannitol have been reported to exert specific health-promoting actions (Peters et al., 2019; Ruiz Rodríguez et al., 2019). In addition, the production of γ-aminobutyric acid, vitamin K, and vitamins of the B complex (Dhakal, Bajpai, & Baek, 2012; Leblanc et al., 2011; Morishita, Tamura, Makino, & Kudo, 1999), as well as a series of metabolic pathways that may convert compounds of the food matrix into their functional derivatives (Filannino, Di Cagno, & Gobbetti, 2018), make LAB very attractive. Such actions have been reported to nutritionally and functionally enhance matrices containing the necessary precursors for the production of these bioactive compounds. Indeed, improvement of the functional potential of fruit and vegetable juices through lactic acid fermentation has been reported for the following: apple, cactus pear, cantaloupe, cashew apple, cherry, cranberry, feijoa, grape, jujube, litchi, mulberry, orange, papaya, pear, pomegranate, beetroot, broccoli, carrot, echinacea, tomato, as well as some of their mixtures (Ankolekar, Pinto, Greene, & Shetty, 2012; Chen, Chen, Chen, Chen, & Zhang, 2018; Cui et al., 2019; de Godoy Alves Filho et al., 2017; Espirito-Santo, Carlin, & Renard, 2015; Filannino et al., 2013; Filannino, Bai, Di Cagno, Gobbetti, & Gänzle, 2015; Klewicka & Czyzowska, 2011; Kwaw et al., 2018; Li et al., 2014; Liu et al., 2018; Mantzourani et al., 2019; Rizzello et al., 2013; Valero-Cases, Roy, Frutos, & Anderson, 2017; Vergara, Honorato, Maia, & Rodrigues, 2010; Veron et al., 2019; Xu et al., 2019; Zhao, Zhang, Zhang, Liu, & Meng, 2019; Zheng et al., 2014). In the majority of these cases, fermentation took place by *Lb. plantarum*, a species of great adaptability and metabolic capacity.

Similarly, several literature reports are currently available on the development of a variety of cereal- and soy-based beverages with functional properties. The development process is relatively simple; a liquid substrate is formed and allowed to be fermented by lactic acid bacteria.

21.5 Next-generation probiotics

"Next-Generation Probiotics" (NGPs) is a term that has emerged to distinguish between those cultures that may result in amelioration of a specific disease from those that belong to the traditional probiotic selection process and where in statistical and biological terms, disease amelioration is merely marginal (Chang et al., 2019; Lin et al., 2019). The term "live biotherapeutic products" (LBPs) has been suggested as a synonym for NGPs as the latter fits very well into the definition of the former by the US FDA (O'Toole, Marchesi, & Hill, 2017). To achieve the aim of the NGPs concept, a causal relationship between a bacterial population (at a strain level) and a health phenotype has to be established. Such a relationship should be carefully examined and clear of any possible irrelevant correlations that misuse of a statistical analysis may lead to. Given that our knowledge on the human gastrointestinal tract (GIT) microbiome is largely a result from next-generation sequencing studies and that the underlying molecular mechanisms of disease phenotypes are not yet completely understood, a lot of research is still required before such a causal relationship can be established and the NGPs concept is actually effective.

Probiotic research is dominated by three genera, *Lactobacillus* and *Bifidobacterium* regarding bacteria and *Saccharomyces* regarding yeasts. This is understandable as the selection criteria involve technological criteria that need to be fulfilled by the incorporation of a culture either as a starter or as an adjunct culture. However, from the NGP point of view, only microorganisms that already consist as a part of the human GIT microbiome would be regarded as candidates for use for that purpose. As a result, a significant amount of data has been accumulated regarding the role of bacteria such as *Bacteroides* spp., *Faecalibacterium prausnitzii*, and *Akkermansia muciniphila* that constitute a significant part of the GIT microbiota and appear to possess a role in GIT health as reduction of their population has been associated with specific syndromes. Although a causal relationship has not been yet indisputably established, these bacteria have drawn attention and data are accumulating regarding their capacity to restore the healthy phenotype. Thus, these bacteria are considered as emerging novel cultures, mainly adjunct, despite the fact that some safety concerns have been raised (Brodmann et al., 2017; El Hage, Hernandez-Sanabria, & Van de Wiele, 2017).

Faecalibacterium prausnitzii has been suggested to possess an important role in GIT homeostasis, mostly due to the correlation that has been reported between its reduction or depletion and occurrence of syndromes such as celiac disease, inflammatory bowel diseases, irritable bowel syndrome, etc. (De Palma et al., 2010; Rajilic-Stojanovic et al., 2011; Sokol et al., 2008). Studies in model systems have reported anti-inflammatory effects and improved intestinal permeability upon administration of this bacterium (Carlsson et al., 2013; Laval et al., 2015; Martin et al., 2014, 2015; Miquel et al., 2016; Rossi et al., 2015, 2016; Sokol et al., 2008). These beneficial effects have been attributed to the production of metabolites such as butyrate, salicylic acid, shikimik acid, raffinose, a series of peptides derived from a protein named "microbial anti-inflammatory molecule," as well as an extracellular polymeric matrix that is formed (Martin, Bermúdez-Humarán, & Langella, 2018). These properties appear to be very promising within the concept of Next-Generation Probiotics; however, this species is also characterized as extremely oxygen-sensitive, as well as difficult to grow (Duncan, Hold, Harmsen, Stewart, & Flint, 2002). Thus, these difficulties need to be addressed before incorporation as an adjunct culture is assessed.

Akkermansia muciniphila is a mucin degrading microorganism that also possesses an important role in GIT health. The reduction of its population has been correlated with type-2 diabetes, obesity, and inflammatory bowel disease (Cani & Everard, 2014; Png et al., 2010; Schneeberger et al., 2015). Moreover, administration in mice has resulted in the prevention of metabolic disorders resulting from a high fat diet (Everard et al., 2013). In addition, tolerance to oxygen as well as stability to stressful conditions simulating passage through the GIT (Machado et al., 2020; Marcial-Coba et al., 2018) makes this microorganism a good candidate for the NGP concept. Indeed, Marcial-Coba, Saaby, Knochel, and Nielsen (2019) reported that *A. muciniphila* presented with population reduction of less than 1 log CFU g^{-1} after 60-day storage in chocolate at 4°C, after microencapsulation in a xanthan/gellan gum matrix. In addition, the population remained high after a simulated gastric transit, providing promising results.

Bacteroides xylanisolvens, B. acidifaciens, and *B. uniformis* have been reported to exhibit health-promoting properties. More accurately, heat-treated preparation of *B. xylanisolvens* has been reported to increase the levels of Tfα-specific immunoglobulin M serum antibodies in healthy humans after oral administration (Ulsemer et al., 2016), *B. acidifaciens* has been reported to promote IgA production in the large intestine (Yanagibashi et al., 2013) and *B. uniformis* has been reported to ameliorate metabolic and immunological dysfunction in mice fed a high fat diet. The latter took place after oral administration of the bacterium, which resulted in a reduction of body weight gain, liver cholesterol, and triglyceride concentration, liver steatosis, as well as an increase in the number of small adipocytes (Gauffin Cano, Santacruz, Moya, & Sanz, 2012).

21.6 Conclusions

Probiotic beverages are expected to become a leading vehicle for probiotic delivery. Among them, strong development is expected for non-dairy beverages. Our knowledge of ordinary and extraordinary properties, mainly of lactic acid bacteria, is also expected to improve in the future. However, only a few, if any, of the newly characterized strains may reach commercial application and availability. Nonconventional species will continue to be examined for their probiotic potential; among them research on NGPs is expected to further reveal their physiological attributes.

References

Achi, S. C., & Halami, P. M. (2019). In vitro comparative analysis of probiotic and functional attributes of indigenous isolates of *Bifidobacteria*. *Current Microbiology*, *76*, 304–311.

Ankolekar, C., Pinto, M., Greene, D., & Shetty, K. (2012). In vitro bioassay based screening of antihyperglycemia and antihypertensive activities of *Lactobacillus acidophilus* fermented pear juice. *Innovative Food Science and Emerging Technologies*, *13*, 221–230.

Balthazar, C. F., Santillo, A., Guimarães, J. T., Capozzi, V., Russo, P., Caroprese, M., et al. (2019). Novel milk–juice beverage with fermented sheep milk and strawberry (*Fragaria × ananassa*): Nutritional and functional characterization. *Journal of Dairy Science, 102*, 10724–10736.

Battistini, C., Gullón, B., Ichimura, E. S., Gomes, A. M. P., Ribeiro, E. P., Kunigk, L., et al. (2018). Development and characterization of an innovative synbiotic fermented beverage based on vegetable soybean. *Brazilian Journal of Microbiology, 49*, 303–309.

Bedani, R., Vieira, A. D. S., Rossi, E. A., & Saad, S. M. I. (2014). Tropical fruit pulps decreased probiotic survival to in vitro gastrointestinal stress in symbiotic soy yoghurt with okara during storage. *LWT-Food Science and Technology, 55*, 436–443.

Bielecka, M., & Majkowska, A. (2000). Effect of spray drying temperature of yoghurt on the survival of starter cultures, moisture content and sensoric properties of yoghurt powder. *Nahrung – Food, 44*, 257–260.

Blaiotta, G., Murru, N., Di Cerbo, A., Succi, M., Coppola, R., & Aponte, M. (2017). Commercially standardized process for probiotic "Italico" cheese production. *LWT-Food Science and Technology, 79*, 601–608.

Boricha, A. A., Shekh, S. L., Pithva, S. P., Ambalam, P. S., & Vyas, B. R. M. (2019). In vitro evaluation of probiotic properties of *Lactobacillus* species of food and human origin. *LWT-Food Science and Technology, 106*, 201–208.

Brodmann, T., Endo, A., Gueimonde, M., Vinderola, G., Kneifel, W., de Vos, W. M., et al. (2017). Safety of novel microbes for human consumption: practical examples of assessment in the European Union. *Frontiers in Microbiology, 8*, 1725. https://doi.org/10.3389/fmicb.2017.01725.

Bujna, E., Farkas, N. A., Tran, A. M., Dam, M. S., & Nguyen, Q. D. (2018). Lactic acid fermentation of apricot juice by mono- and mixed cultures of probiotic *Lactobacillus* and *Bifidobacterium* strains. *Food Science and Biotechnology, 27*, 547–554.

Buriti, F. C., Okazaki, T. Y., Alegro, J. H., & Saad, S. M. (2007). Effect of a probiotic mixed culture on texture profile and sensory performance of Minas fresh-cheeses in comparison with the traditional products. *Archivos Latinoamericanos de Nutrición, 57*, 179–185.

Cani, P. D., & Everard, A. (2014). *Akkermansia muciniphila*: a novel target controlling obesity, type 2 diabetes and inflammation? *Medical Science, 30*, 125–127.

Carlsson, A. H., Yakymenko, O., Olivier, I., Hakansson, F., Postma, E., Keita, A. V., et al. (2013). *Faecalibacterium prausnitzii* supernatant improves intestinal barrier function in mice DSS colitis. *Scandinavian Journal of Gastroenterology, 48*, 1136–1144.

Cervantes-Elizarraras, A., Cruz-Cansino, N. S., Ramírez-Moreno, E., Vega-Sanchez, V., Velazquez-Guadarrama, N., Zafra-Rojas, Q. Y., et al. (2019). In vitro probiotic potential of lactic acid bacteria isolated from Aguamiel and Pulque and antibacterial activity against pathogens. *Applied Sciences, 9*, 601. https://doi.org/10.3390/app9030601.

Chaikham, P., Kemsawasd, V., & Seesuriyachan, P. (2017). Spray drying probiotics along with maoluang juice plus *Tiliacora triandra* gum for exposure to the in vitro gastrointestinal environments. *LWT-Food Science and Technology, 78*, 31–40.

Chan, C.-L., Gan, R.-Y., Shah, N. P., & Corke, H. (2018). Enhancing antioxidant capacity of *Lactobacillus acidophilus*-fermented milk fortified with pomegranate peel extracts. *Food Bioscience, 26*, 185–192.

Chang, C.-J., Lin, T.-L., Tsai, Y.-L., Wu, T.-R., Lai, W.-F., Lu, C.-C., et al. (2019). Next generation probiotics in disease amelioration. *Journal of Food and Drug Analysis, 27*, 615–622.

Chen, W., Chen, R., Chen, W., Chen, H., & Zhang, G. (2018). Comparative evaluation of the antioxidant capacities, organic acids, and volatiles of papaya juices fermented by *Lactobacillus acidophilus* and *Lactobacillus plantarum*. *Journal of Food Quality, 2018*, 1–12.

Coda, R., Laner, A., Trani, A., Gobbetti, M., & Di Cagno, R. (2012). Yogurt-like beverages made of a mixture of cereals, soy and grape must: Microbiology, texture, nutritional and sensory properties. *International Journal of Food Microbiology, 155*, 120–127.

Cui, S., Zhao, N., Lu, W., Zhao, F., Zheng, S., Wang, W., et al. (2019). Effect of different *Lactobacillus* species on volatile and nonvolatile flavor compounds in juices fermentation. *Food Science & Nutrition*, 2214–2223.

de Godoy Alves Filho, E., Rodrigues, T. H. S., Fernandes, F. A. N., Pereira, A. L. F., Narain, N., de Brito, E. S., et al. (2017). Chemometric evaluation of the volatile profile of probiotic melon and probiotic cashew juice. *Food Research International, 99*, 461–468.

De Melo Pereira, G. V., de Oliveira Coelho, B., Júnior, A. I. M., Thomaz-Soccol, V., & Soccol, C. R. (2018). How to select a probiotic? A review and update of methods and criteria. *Biotechnology Advances, 36*, 2060–2076.

De Palma, G., Nadal, I., Medina, M., Donat, E., Ribes-Koninckx, C., Calabuig, M., et al. (2010). Intestinal dysbiosis and reduced immunoglobulin-coated bacteria associated with coeliac disease in children. *BMC Microbiology, 10*, 63. https://doi.org/10.1186/1471-2180-10-63.

Dhakal, R., Bajpai, V. K., & Baek, K.-H. (2012). Production of GABA (γ-aminobutyric acid) by microorganisms: a review. *Brazilian Journal of Microbiology, 43*, 1230–1241.

Donkor, O. N., Tsangalis, D., & Shah, N. P. (2007). Viability of probiotic bacteria and concentrations of organic acids in commercial yoghurts during refrigerated storage. *Food Australia, 59*, 121–126.

Duncan, S. H., Hold, G. L., Harmsen, H. J., Stewart, C. S., & Flint, H. J. (2002). Growth requirements and fermentation products of *Fusobacterium prausnitzii*, and a proposal to reclassify it as *Faecalibacterium prausnitzii* gen. nov., comb. nov. *International Journal of Systematic and Evolutionary Microbiology, 52*, 2141–2146.

El Hage, R., Hernandez-Sanabria, E., & Van de Wiele, T. (2017). Emerging trends in "Smart Probiotics": functional consideration for the development of novel health and industrial applications. *Frontiers in Microbiology, 8*, 1889. https://doi.org/10.3389/fmicb.2017.01889.

El-Nagga, E. A., & Abd El-Tawab, Y. A. (2012). Compositional characteristics of date syrup extracted by different methods in some fermented dairy products. *Annals of Agricultural Science, 57*, 29–36.

Espirito-Santo, A. P., Carlin, F., & Renard, C. M. G. C. (2015). Apple, grape or orange juice: Which one offers the best substrate for lactobacilli growth? A screening study on bacteria viability, superoxide dismutase activity, folates production and hedonic characteristics. *Food Research International, 78*, 352–360.

Everard, A., Belzer, C., Geurts, L., Ouwerkerk, J. P., Druart, C., Bindels, L. B., et al. (2013). Cross-talk between *Akkermansia muciniphila* and intestinal epithelium controls diet-induced obesity. *Proceedings of the National Academy of Sciences of the United States of America, 110*, 9066–9071.

Filannino, P., Azzi, L., Cavoski, I., Vincentini, O., Rizzello, C. G., Gobbetti, M., et al. (2013). Exploitation of the health-promoting and sensory properties of organic pomegranate (*Punica granatum* L) juice through lactic acid fermentation. *International Journal of Food Microbiology, 163*, 184–192.

Filannino, P., Bai, Y., Di Cagno, R., Gobbetti, M., & Gänzle, M. G. (2015). Metabolism of phenolic compounds by *Lactobacillus* spp during fermentation of cherry juice and broccoli puree. *Food Microbiology, 46*, 272–279.

Filannino, P., Di Cagno, R., & Gobbetti, M. (2018). Metabolic and functional paths of lactic acid bacteria in plant foods: get out of the labyrinth. *Current Opinion in Biotechnology, 49*, 64–72.

Freire, A. L., Ramos, C. L., Souza, P. N. C., Cardoso, M. G. B., & Schwan, R. F. (2017). Nondairy beverage produced by controlled fermentation with potential probiotic starter cultures of lactic acid bacteria and yeast. *International Journal of Food Microbiology, 248*, 39–46.

Funck, G. D., Marques, J. D. L., Cruxen, C. E. D. S., Sehn, C. P., Haubert, L., Dannenberg, G. D. S., et al. (2019). Probiotic potential of *Lactobacillus curvatus* P99 and viability in fermented oat dairy beverage. *Journal of Food Processing & Preservation, 43*, e14286.

Gauffin Cano, P., Santacruz, A., Moya, Á., & Sanz, Y. (2012). *Bacteroides uniformis* CECT 7771 ameliorates metabolic and immunological dysfunction in mice with high-fat-diet induced obesity. *PLoS One, 7*, e41079.

Gheziel, C., Russo, P., Arena, M. P., Spano, G., Ouzari, H.-I., Kheroua, O., et al. (2019). Evaluating the probiotic potential of *Lactobacillus plantarum* strains from Algerian infant feces: towards the design of probiotic starter cultures tailored for developing countries. *Probiotics and Antimicrobial Proteins, 11*, 113–123.

Gobbetti, M., Di Cagno, R., & De Angelis, M. (2010). Functional microorganisms for functional food quality. *Critical Reviews in Food Science and Nutrition, 508*, 716–727.

Gogineni, V. K., Morrow, L. E., Gregory, P. J., & Malesker, M. A. (2013). Probiotics: History and evolution. *Journal of Infectious Diseases & Preventive Medicine, 1*, 107. https://doi.org/10.4172/2329-8731.1000107.

Guo, H., Pan, L., Li, L., Lu, J., Kwok, L., Menghe, B., et al. (2017). Characterization of antibiotic resistance genes from *Lactobacillus* isolated from traditional dairy products. *Journal of Food Science, 82*, 724–730.

Huang, S., Cauty, C., Dolivet, A., Le Loir, Y., Chen, X. D., Schuck, P., et al. (2016). Double use of highly concentrated sweet whey to improve the biomass production and viability of spray-dried probiotic bacteria. *Journal of Functional Foods, 23*, 453–463.

Hwanhlem, N., Ivanova, T., Biscola, V., Choiset, Y., & Haertle, T. (2017). Bacteriocin producing *Enterococcus faecalis* isolated from chicken gastrointestinal tract originating from Phitsanulok, Thailand: Isolation, screening, safety evaluation and probiotic properties. *Food Control, 78*, 187–195.

Icier, F., Gündüz, G. T., Yılmaz, B., & Memeli, Z. (2015). Changes on some quality characteristics of fermented soy milk beverage with added apple juice. *LWT-Food Science and Technology, 63*, 57–64.

Islam, M. K., Hasan, M. S., Al Mamun, A., Kudrat-E-Zahan, M., & Al-Bari, M. A. A. (2015). Lemon juice synergistically preserved with lactobacilli ameliorates inflammation in shigellosis mice. *Advances in Pharmacology and Pharmacy, 3*, 11–21.

Kailasapathy, K., Harmstorf, I., & Phillips, M. (2008). Survival of *Lactobacillus acidophilus* and *Bifidobacterium animalis* ssp. *lactis* in stirred fruit yogurts. *LWT-Food Science and Technology, 41*, 1317–1322.

Kazancıgil, E., Demirci, T., Öztürk-Negiş, H. İ., & Akin, N. (2019). Isolation, technological characterization and in vitro probiotic evaluation of *Lactococcus* strains from traditional Turkish skin bag Tulum cheeses. *Annales de Microbiologie, 69*, 1275–1287.

Kim, J.-H., & Baik, S.-H. (2019). Probiotic properties of *Lactobacillus* strains with high cinnamoyl esterase activity isolated from jeot-gal, a high-salt fermented seafood. *Annales de Microbiologie, 69*, 407–417.

Klewicka, E., & Czyzowska, A. (2011) Biological stability of lactofermented beetroot juice during refrigerated storage. *Polish Journal of Food and Nutrition Sciences, 61*, 251–256.

Kook, S.-Y., Chung, E.-C., Lee, Y., Lee, D. W., & Kim, S. (2019). Isolation and characterization of five novel probiotic strains from Korean infant and children faeces. *PLoS One, 14*, e0223913.

Kumar, P., & Mishra, H. N. (2004). Yoghurt powder-a review of process technology, storage and utilization. *Food and Bioproducts Processing, 82*, 133–142.

Kwaw, E., Ma, Y., Tchabo, W., Apaliya, M. T., Wu, M., Sackey, A. S., et al. (2018). Effect of lactobacillus strains on phenolic profile, color attributes and antioxidant activities of lactic-acid fermented mulberry juice. *Food Chemistry, 250*, 148–154.

Laval, L., Martin, R., Natividad, J. N., Chain, F., Miquel, S., Desclee de Maredsous, C., et al. (2015). *Lactobacillus rhamnosus* CNCM I-3690 and the commensal bacterium *Faecalibacterium prausnitzii* A2-165 exhibit similar protective effects to induced barrier hyperpermeability in mice. *Gut Microbes, 6*, 1–9.

Leblanc, J. G., Laiño, J. E., del Valle, M. J., Vannini, V., van Sinderen, D., Taranto, M. P., et al. (2011). B-Group vitamin production by lactic acid bacteria—current knowledge and potential applications. *Journal of Applied Microbiology*, *111*, 1297–1309.

Li, C., Ding, Q., Nie, S. P., Zhang, Y. S., Xiong, T., & Xie, M. Y. (2014). Carrot juice fermented with *Lactobacillus plantarum* NCU116 ameliorates type 2 diabetes in rats. *Journal of Agricultural and Food Chemistry*, *62*, 11884–11891.

Lian, W. C., Hsiao, H. C., & Chou, C. C. (2002). Survival of bifidobacteria after spray-drying. *International Journal of Food Microbiology*, *74*, 79–86.

Lin, T.-L., Shu, C.-C., Lai, W.-F., Tzeng, C.-M., Lai, H.-C., & Lu, C.-C. (2019). Investiture on next generation probiotics on amelioration of diseases-strains do matter. *Medicine in Microecology*, *1-2*, 100002. https://doi.org/10.1016/j.medmic.2019.100002.

Liu, Y., Chen, H., Chen, W., Zhong, Q., Zhang, G., & Chen, W. (2018). Beneficial effects of tomato juice fermented by *Lactobacillus plantarum* and *Lactobacillus casei*: antioxidation, antimicrobial effect, and volatile profiles. *Molecules*, *23*, 1–18.

Liu, L., Chen, P., Zhao, W., Li, X., Wang, H., & Qu, X. (2017). Effect of microencapsulation with the Maillard reaction products of whey proteins and isomaltooligosaccharide on the survival rate of *Lactobacillus rhamnosus* in white brined cheese. *Food Control*, *79*, 44–49.

Lopez de Lacey, A. M., Pérez-Santín, E., López-Caballero, M. E., & Montero, P. (2014). Survival and metabolic activity of probiotic bacteria in green tea. *LWT-Food Science and Technology*, *55*, 314–322.

Machado, D., Almeida, D., Seabra, C. L., Andrade, J. C., Gomes, A. M., & Freitas, A. C. (2020). Uncovering *Akkermansia muciniphila* resilience or susceptibility to different temperatures, atmospheres and gastrointestinal conditions. *Anaerobe*, *61*, 102135. https://doi.org/10.1016/j.anaerobe.2019.102135.

Mantzourani, I., Bontsidis, C. A., Plessas, S., Alexopoulos, A., Theodoridou, E., Tsigalou, C., et al. (2019). Comparative susceptibility study against pathogens using fermented cranberry juice and antibiotics. *Frontiers in Microbiology*, *10*, 1294. https://doi.org/10.3389/fmicb.2019.01294.

Mantzourani, I., Terpou, A., Bekatorou, A., Mallouchos, A., Alexopoulos, A., Kimbaris, A., et al. (2020). Functional pomegranate beverage production by fermentation with a novel synbiotic *L. paracasei* biocatalyst. *Food Chemistry*, *308*, 125658. https://doi.org/10.1016/j.foodchem.2019.125658.

Marafon, A. P., Sumi, A., Alcantara, M. R., Tamime, A. Y., & Oliveira, M. N. (2011). Optimization of the rheological properties of probiotic yoghurts supplemented with milk proteins. *LWT-Food Science and Technology*, *44*, 511–519.

Marcial-Coba, M. S., Cieplak, T., Cahu, T. B., Blennow, A., Knochel, S., & Nielsen, D. S. (2018). Viability of microencapsulated *Akkermansia muciniphila* and *Lactobacillus plantarum* during freeze-drying, storage and in vitro simulated upper gastrointestinal tract passage. *Food & Function*, *9*, 5868–5879.

Marcial-Coba, M. S., Saaby, L., Knochel, S., & Nielsen, D. S. (2019). Dark chocolate as a stable carrier of microencapsulated *Akkermansia muciniphila* and *Lactobacillus casei*. *FEMS Microbiology Letters*, *366*, fny290.

Martin, R., Bermúdez-Humarán, L. G., & Langella, P. (2018). Searching for the bacterial effector: the example of the multi-skilled commensal bacterium *Faecalibacterium prausnitzii*. *Frontiers in Microbiology*, *9*, 346. https://doi.org/10.3389/fmicb.2018.00346.

Martin, R., Chain, F., Miquel, S., Lu, J., Gratadoux, J. J., Sokol, H., et al. (2014). The commensal bacterium *Faecalibacterium prausnitzii* is protective in DNBS induced chronic moderate and severe colitis models. *Inflammatory Bowel Diseases*, *20*, 417–430.

Martin, R., Miquel, S., Chain, F., Natividad, J. M., Jury, J., Lu, J., et al. (2015). *Faecalibacterium prausnitzii* prevents physiological damages in a chronic low grade inflammation murine model. *BMC Microbiology*, *15*, 67. https://doi.org/10.1186/s12866-015-0400-1.

Mazinani, S., Fadaei, V., & Khosravi-Darani, K. (2016). Impact of *Spirulina platensis* on physicochemical properties and viability of *Lactobacillus acidophilus* of probiotic of feta cheese. *Journal of Food Processing & Preservation, 40*, 1318–1324.

Menezes, A. G. T., Ramos, C. L., Cenzi, G., Melo, D. S., Dias, D. R., & Schwan, R. F. (2019). Probiotic potential, antioxidant activity, and phytase production of indigenous yeasts isolated from indigenous fermented foods. *Probiotics and Antimicrobial Proteins*. https://doi.org/10.1007/s12602-019-9518-z.

Menezes, A. G. T., Ramos, C. L., Dias, D. R., & Schwan, R. F. (2018). Combination of probiotic yeast and lactic acid bacteria as starter culture to produce maize-based beverages. *Food Research International, 111*, 187–197.

Miquel, S., Martin, R., Lashermes, A., Gillet, M., Meleine, M., Gelot, A., et al. (2016). Antinociceptive effect of *Faecalibacterium prausnitzii* in non-inflammatory IBS-like models. *Scientific Reports, 6*, 19399. https://doi.org/10.1038/srep19399.

Miranda, R. F., de Paula, M. M., da Costa, G. M., Barão, C. E., da Silva, A. C. R., Raices, R. S. L., et al. (2019). Orange juice added with *L. casei*: is there an impact of the probiotic addition methodology on the quality parameters? *LWT-Food Science and Technology, 106*, 186–193.

Morishita, T., Tamura, N., Makino, T., & Kudo, S. (1999). Production of menaquinones by lactic acid bacteria. *Journal of Dairy Science, 82*, 1897–1903.

Motahari, P., Mirdamadi, S., & Kianirad, M. (2017). Safety evaluation and antimicrobial properties of *Lactobacillus pentosus* 22C isolated from traditional yogurt. *Food Measure, 11*, 972–978.

Nwachukwu, U., George-Okafor, U., Ozoani, U., & Ojiagu, N. (2019). Assessment of probiotic potentials of *Lactobacillus plantarum* CS and *Micrococcus luteus* CS from fermented milled corn-soybean waste-meal. *Scientific African, 6*, e00183.

O'Toole, P. W., Marchesi, J. R., & Hill, C. (2017). Next-generation probiotics: the spectrum from probiotics to live biotherapeutics. *Nature Microbiology, 2*, 17057. https://doi.org/10.1038/nmicrobiol.2017.57.

Ojekunle, O., Banwo, K., & Sanni, A. I. (2017). In vitro and in vivo evaluation of *Weissella cibaria* and *Lactobacillus plantarum* for their protective effect against cadmium and lead toxicities Lett. *Applied Microbiology, 64*, 379–385.

Oliveira, R. P. S., Florence, A. C. R., Perego, P., De Oliveira, M. N., & Converti, A. (2011). Use of lactulose as prebiotic and its influence on the growth, acidification profile and viable counts of different probiotics in fermented skim milk. *International Journal of Food Microbiology, 145*, 22–27.

Perumal, V., & Venkatesan, A. (2017). Antimicrobial, cytotoxic effect and purification of bacteriocin from vancomycin susceptible *Enterococcus faecalis* and its safety evaluation for probiotization. *LWT-Food Science and Technology, 78*, 303–310.

Peters, A., Krumbholz, P., Jaeger, E., Heintz-Buschart, A., Cakir, M. V., Rothemund, S., et al. (2019). Metabolites of lactic acid bacteria present in fermented foods are highly potent agonists of human hydroxycarboxylic acid receptor 3. *PLoS Genetics, 15*, e1008145.

Phillips, M., Kailasapathy, K., & Tran, L. (2006). Viability of commercial probiotic cultures (*L. acidophilus, Bifidobacterium* sp., *L. casei, L. paracasei* and *L. rhamnosus*) in Cheddar cheese. *International Journal of Food Microbiology, 108*, 276–280.

Pino, A., Russo, N., Van Hoorde, K., De Angelis, M., Sferrazzo, G., Randazzo, C. L., et al. (2019). Piacentinu Ennese PDO cheese as reservoir of promising probiotic bacteria. *Microorganisms, 7*, 254. https://doi.org/10.3390/microorganisms7080254.

Pino, A., Van Hoorde, K., Pitino, I., Russo, N., Carpino, S., Caggia, C., et al. (2017). Survival of potential probiotic lactobacilli used as adjunct cultures on Pecorino Siciliano cheese ripening and passage through the gastrointestinal tract of healthy volunteers. *International Journal of Food Microbiology, 252*, 42–52.

Png, C. W., Lindén, S. K., Gilshenan, K. S., Zoetendal, E. G., McSweeney, C. S., Sly, L., et al. (2010). Mucolytic bacteria with increased prevalence in IBD mucosa augment in vitro utilization of mucin by other bacteria. *The American Journal of Gastroenterology, 105*, 2420–2428.

Prado, F. C., Lindner, J. D. D., Inaba, J., Thomaz-Soccol, V., Brar, S. K., & Soccol, C. R. (2015). Development and evaluation of a fermented coconut water beverage with potential health benefits. *Journal of Functional Foods, 12*, 489–497.

Radulovic, Z., Miocinovic, J., Mirkovic, N., Mirković, M., Paunović, D., Ivanović, M., et al. (2017). Survival of spray-dried and free-cells of potential probiotic *Lactobacillus plantarum* 564 in soft goat cheese. *Animal Science Journal, 88*, 1849–1854.

Rajilic-Stojanovic, M., Biagi, E., Heilig, H. G., Kajander, K., Kekkonen, R. A., Tims, S., et al. (2011). Global and deep molecular analysis of microbiota signatures in fecal samples from patients with irritable bowel syndrome. *Gastroenterology, 141*, 1792–1801.

Ranadheera, C. S., Evans, C. A., Adams, M. C., & Baines, S. K. (2012). In vitro analysis of gastrointestinal tolerance and intestinal cell adhesion of probiotics in goat's milk ice cream and yogurt. *Food Research International, 49*, 619–625.

Rizzello, C. G., Coda, R., Macías, D. S., Pinto, D., Marzani, B., Filannino, P., et al. (2013). Lactic acid fermentation as a tool to enhance the functional features of *Echinacea* spp. *Microbial Cell Factories, 12*, 44.

Roberfroid, M. B. (1999). What is beneficial for health? The concept of functional food. *Food and Chemical Toxicology, 37*, 1039–1041.

Rossi, O., Khan, M. T., Schwarzer, M., Hudcovic, T., Srutkova, D., Duncan, S. H., et al. (2015). *Faecalibacterium prausnitzii* strain HTF-F and its extracellular polymeric matrix attenuate clinical parameters in DSS-induced colitis. *PLoS One, 10*, e0123013.

Rossi, O., van Berkel, L. A., Chain, F., Tanweer Khan, M., Taverne, N., Sokol, H., et al. (2016). *Faecalibacterium prausnitzii* A2-165 has a high capacity to induce IL-10 in human and murine dendritic cells and modulates T cell responses. *Scientific Reports, 6*, 18507. https://doi.org/10.1038/srep18507.

Ruiz Rodríguez, L. G., Mohamed, F., Bleckwedel, J., Medina, R., De Vuyst, L., Hebert, E. M., et al. (2019). Diversity and functional properties of lactic acid bacteria isolated from wild fruits and flowers present in Northern Argentina. *Frontiers in Microbiology, 10*, 1091. https://doi.org/10.3389/fmicb.2019.01091.

Ryan, J., Hutchings, S. C., Fang, Z., Bandara, N., Gamlath, S., Ajlouni, S., et al. (2020). Microbial, physico-chemical and sensory characteristics of mango juice-enriched probiotic dairy drinks. *International Journal of Dairy Technology, 73*, 182–190.

Rzepkowska, A., Zielińska, D., Ołdak, A., & Kolozyn-Krajewska, D. (2017). Safety assessment and antimicrobial properties of the lactic acid bacteria strains isolated from polish raw fermented meat products. *International Journal of Food Properties, 20*, 2736–2747.

Sakandar, H. A., Kubow, S., & Sadiq, F. A. (2019). Isolation and in-vitro probiotic characterization of fructophilic lactic acid bacteria from Chinese fruits and flowers. *LWT-Food Science and Technology, 104*, 70–75.

Salmeron, I., Thomas, K., & Pandiella, S. S. (2015). Effect of potentially probiotic lactic acid bacteria on the physicochemical composition and acceptance of fermented cereal beverages. *Journal of Functional Foods, 15*, 106–111.

Schneeberger, M., Everard, A., Gomez-Valades, A. G., Matamoros, S., Ramirez, S., Delzenne, N. M., et al. (2015). *Akkermansia muciniphila* inversely correlates with the onset of inflammation, altered adipose tissue metabolism and metabolic disorders during obesity in mice. *Scientific Reports, 5*, 16643. https://doi.org/10.1038/srep16643.

Schuck, P., Dolivet, A., Mejean, S., Herve, H., & Jeantet, R. (2013). Spray drying of dairy bacteria: new opportunities to improve the viability of bacteria powders. *International Dairy Journal, 31*, 12–17.

Sireswar, S., Dey, G., Dey, K., & Kundu, A. (2017). Evaluation of probiotic *L. rhamnosus* GG as a protective culture in sea buckthorn-based beverage. *Beverages, 3*, 48. https://doi.org/10.3390/beverages3040048.

Sokol, H., Pigneur, B., Watterlot, L., Lakhdari, O., Bermudez-Humaran, L. G., Gratadoux, J. J., et al. (2008). *Faecalibacterium prausnitzii* is an antiinflammatory commensal bacterium identified by gut microbiota analysis of Crohn disease patients. *Proceedings of the National Academy of Sciences of the United States of America, 105*, 16731–16736.

Sotoudegan, F., Daniali, M., Hassani, S., Nikfar, S., & Abdollahi, M. (2019). Reappraisal of probiotics' safety in human. *Food and Chemical Toxicology, 129*, 22–29.

Syrokou, M. K., Papadelli, M., Ntaikou, I., Paramithiotis, S., & Drosinos, E. H. (2019). Sugary kefir: Microbial identification and technological properties. *Beverages, 5*, 61.

Tamminen, M., Salminen, S., & Ouwehand, A. C. (2013). Fermentation of carrot juice by probiotics: viability and preservation of adhesion. *International Journal of Biotechnology for Wellness Industries, 2*, 10–15.

Thakkar, P., Vaghela, B., Patel, A., Modi, H. A., & Prajapati, J. B. (2018). Formulation and shelf life study of a whey-based functional beverage containing orange juice and probiotic organisms. *International Food Research Journal, 25*, 1675–1681.

Tu, C., Azi, F., Huang, J., Xu, X., Xing, G., & Dong, M. (2019). Quality and metagenomic evaluation of a novel functional beverage produced from soy whey using water kefir grains. *LWT-Food Science and Technology, 113*, 108258. https://doi.org/10.1016/j.lwt.2019.108258.

Turkmen, N., Akal, C., & Ozer, B. (2019). Probiotic dairy-based beverages: A review. *Journal of Functional Foods, 53*, 62–75.

Ulsemer, P., Toutounian, K., Kressel, G., Goletz, C., Schmidt, J., Karsten, U., et al. (2016). Impact of oral consumption of heat-treated *Bacteroides xylanisolvens* DSM 23964 on the level of natural TFα-specific antibodies in human adults. *Beneficial Microbes, 7*, 485–500.

Valero-Cases, E., Roy, N. C., Frutos, M. J., & Anderson, R. C. (2017). Influence of the fruit juice carriers on the ability of *Lactobacillus plantarum* DSM20205 to improve in vitro intestinal barrier integrity and its probiotic properties. *Journal of Agricultural and Food Chemistry, 65*, 5632–5638.

Vanajakshi, V., Vijayendra, S. V. N., Varadaraj, M. C., Venkateswaran, G., & Agrawal, R. (2015). Optimization of a probiotic beverage based on Moringa leaves and beetroot. *LWT-Food Science and Technology, 63*, 1268–1273.

Varankovich, N. V., Nickerson, M. T., & Korber, D. R. (2015). Probiotic-based strategies for therapeutic and prophylactic use against multiple gastrointestinal diseases. *Frontiers in Microbiology, 6*, 685. https://doi.org/10.3389/fmicb.2015.00685.

Vergara, C. M. D. A. C., Honorato, T. L. Maia, G. A., & Rodrigues, S. (2010). Prebiotic effect of fermented cashew apple (*Anacardium occidentale* L) juice. *LWT - Food Science and Technology, 43*, 141–145.

Veron, H. E., Gauffin, C. P., Fabersani, E., Sanz, Y., Isla, M. I., Fernández Espinar, M. T., et al. (2019). Cactus pear (*Opuntia ficus-indica*) juice fermented with autochthonous *Lactobacillus plantarum* S-811. *Food & Function, 10*, 1085–1097.

Vong, W. C., & Liu, S.-Q. (2019). The effects of carbohydrase, probiotic *Lactobacillus paracasei* and yeast *Lindnera saturnus* on the composition of a novel okara (soybean residue) functional beverage. *LWT-Food Science and Technology, 100*, 196–204.

Wang, Y. C., Yu, R. C., & Chou, C. C. (2004). Viability of lactic acid bacteria and bifidobacteria in fermented soymilk after drying, subsequent rehydration and storage. *International Journal of Food Microbiology, 93*, 209–217.

Xu, X., Bao, Y., Wu, B., Lao, F., Hu, X., & Wu, J. (2019). Chemical analysis and flavor properties of blended orange, carrot, apple and Chinese jujube juice fermented by selenium-enriched probiotics. *Food Chemistry, 289*, 250–258.

Yanagibashi, T., Hosono, A., Oyama, A., Tsuda, M., Suzuki, A., Hachimura, S., et al. (2013). IgA production in the large intestine is modulated by a different mechanism than in the small intestine: *Bacteroides acidifaciens* promotes IgA production in the large intestine by inducing germinal center formation and increasing the number of IgA+ B cells. *Immunobiology, 218*, 645–651.

Zare, F., Champagne, C. P., Simpson, B. K., Orsat, V., & Boye, J. I. (2012). Effect of the addition of pulse ingredients to milk on acid production by probiotic and yoghurt starter cultures. *LWT-Food Science and Technology*, *45*, 155–160.

Zeng, X., Fan, J., He, L., Duan, Z., & Xia, W. (2019). Technological properties and probiotic potential of yeasts isolated from traditional low-salt fermented Chinese fish Suan yu. *Journal of Food Biochemistry*, *43*, e12865.

Zhao, M. N., Zhang, F., Zhang, L., Liu, B. J., & Meng, X. H. (2019). Mixed fermentation of jujube juice (*Ziziphus jujuba* Mill.) with *L. rhamnosus* GG and *L. plantarum*-1: effects on the quality and stability. *International Journal of Food Science and Technology*, 2624–2631.

Zheng, X., Yu, Y., Xiao, G., Xu, Y., Wu, J., Tang, D., et al. (2014). Comparing product stability of probiotic beverages using litchi juice treated by high hydrostatic pressure and heat as substrates. *Innovative Food Science and Emerging Technologies*, *23*, 61–67.

Zhu, Y., Wang, Z., & Zhang, L. (2019). Optimization of lactic acid fermentation conditions for fermented tofu whey beverage with high-isoflavone aglycones. *LWT-Food Science and Technology*, *111*, 211–217.

Index

Note: Page numbers followed by *f* indicate figures and *t* indicate tables.

A

Absorbers, 355
ACE inhibitory peptides (ACEIPs), 193–194, 273–274, 322–323
Acetaldehyde, 134, 149, 270
Acetic acid bacteria (AAB), 12, 136, 295–296
Active packaging, 354–356
Adaptogens, 431
Additives, 18, 84, 161, 404, 447
Adenosine monophosphate-activated protein kinase (AMPK), 176, 179–183
Adhesion
  to intestinal epithelial cells, 392–393
  probiotic bacteria, 375–376
Africa, plant-based non-alcoholic beverages in, 139–149, 144–145*t*
  cereal-based beverages, 143–146
  fruit-based beverages, 148–149
  vegetable and legume-based beverages, 146–148
Agência Nacional de VigilânciaSanitária (ANVISA), 168–169, 416
Age-related diseases, probiotics for
  cardiovascular disease (CVD), 194–199, 196–198*t*
  diabetes mellitus, 199–202
  macular degeneration, 187–188
  osteoporosis, 188–194, 190–192*t*
Age-related macular degeneration (AMD), 187–188
Aging, 176
  brain, 184–187
  healthy, 179–187
  longevity extension, 179–183
  muscle, 183
Akkermansiamuciniphila, 201, 457–458
Alcoholic fermentation, 23, 103–107, 108*f*, 111
Allyl isothiocyanate (AITC), 224, 228
Aluminum packaging, 342–344, 344*f*
α-Amino-3-hydroxy-5-methyl-4-isoxazolepropionic acid (AMPA), 186
Amplified-fragment length polymorphism (AFLP), 380
Amylase, 85–86, 270
Angiotensin-converting enzymes (ACEs), 273–274, 322–323
Anti-cytotoxic T-lymphocyte associated protein-4 (CTLA-4), 325
Anti-inflammatory compounds, production of, 318–321
Anti-inflammatory cytokine IL-10, 321–322
Anti-inflammatory markers, 315–316
Antimicrobial resistance, of probiotic bacteria, 372–373
Aopopitha, 22–23
Apong (rice beer), 22–23
Apple juice, 14–16*t*, 19, 25–26, 105–107*t*, 132–133*t*, 138–139
Apricot juice, 271–272*t*, 450–455*t*
N-Arachidonoylethanolamine (AEAs), 217–220
Argentina
  Biosec, 169
  Chocolet, 169
  Social Development Ministry, 169
  Yogurito, 169
  Yogurito Social Program, 169
Artificial intelligence (AI), 302, 357
Aseptic packaging, 348–350
Atherosclerosis, 196–198*t*
Atoleagrio, 165
Australia, probiotic guidelines, 419
Ayran, 105–107*t*, 109–110

B

Bacteria
  genomes, 312–314
  as starter cultures, 263–269
Bacterial lipopolysaccharides, 221–223
Bacterial toxins, 221–223
Bacteriocins, 262–263, 395–396
Bacteroides, 178, 189
Barley-based beverages, 450–455*t*

Barnesiella, 183
Bastanga, 23
Beer, 105–107*t*, 114–116
Beetroot-based beverages, 450–455*t*
Benefit stacking, 432–433, 436
β-glucosidase, 270
Beverage shot, 340–341, 341*f*
Bhaatijaanr, 18
Bifidobacterium, 241, 287, 369, 394, 396
Bile, 395
Bioactive compounds
  isoflavones, 147–148
  postbiotics, 431
  produced by starter cultures, 272–274
Bioactive peptides, 268–270, 273–274, 298
Biodegradable plastics, 353–354
Bioextract juice, 84
Bioinformatics
  databases, 247
  tools, 246
Biologic License Application (BLA), 420
Bioplastics, 353–354
Biopolymers, 276
Blending, of beverages, 300–301
Botulinum toxin, 222–223
Boza, 105–107*t*, 116, 131
Brain-derived neurotropic factors (BDNF), 185
Brazil
  Agência Nacional de VigilânciaSanitária (ANVISA), 168–169
  probiotic market, 168
  regulations, 416
Business-to-business (B2B) market, 358
Business-to-consumer (B2C) market, 358

C

Caenorhabditis elegans, 176
Canada
  Food and Drugs Act and Regulations, 416
  probiotic market, value of, 162
  regulations, 163–164, 416
  sour milk drinks, 162
  yogurt, 162
Canadian Food Inspection Agency, 163
Cancer
  checkpoint inhibitors, 325
  kefir for, 288–289
  makgeolli for, 65
Cannabinoid (CB) receptors, 217–218
Cap dispensing technology, 344–345
Capsaicin, 214, 224, 226–227
Cardiovascular disease (CVD), 194–199, 196–198*t*
Carrot juice, 20, 85, 105–107*t*, 132–133*t*, 450–455*t*
Cartagena Protocol on Biosafety, 421
Carton packaging, 342, 343*f*
Cas9 endonuclease, 312–314
Catalase (CAT), 317–318
CD4+ T-cells, 218–219
Cell immobilization, 275–276
Cereal-based beverages, 17–18
  in Africa, 143–146
  in China, 55–57
  in Europe, 128–139
  in Thailand, 89–91
Chhang, 14–16*t*, 17
Chhu, 12
Chhurpi, 12, 13*t*
China
  cereal beverages, 55–57
    development, 55–56
    industrial progress, 57
    research advances, 56–57
  dietary guidelines, 55
  fruit and vegetable beverages, 51–55
  milk beverages, 49–51
    history, 49–50
    market overview, 50–51
  regulations, 417
Chobani probiotic, 161
Cholesterol 7α-hydroxylase (CYP7A1), 200–201
Cinnamaldehyde, 224, 228
Clean label, 432
Clostridia, 189
Clue prebiotic water, 438
Clustered Regularly Interspaced Short Palindromic Repeats (CRISPR), 312
Coconut water, 264–268*t*, 273, 450–455*t*
Coculture, 270–271
Coffee, 300–301, 433–434
Cognitive decline, 184–185
Collagen-binding proteins (Cbp), 315
Colonization, of probiotic bacteria, 375–376
Colony-forming units (CFUs), 377–378, 415–416, 434
Committee for the Classification of Food-Drug Interface Products, 419
Conjugated linoleic acid (CLA), 273, 324
Consumer packaged goods (CPG), 351–352
Consumers, 5–6, 428–430
  millennial, 4
Convenient shots, 436–437

Corn milk, fermented, 88–89
COVID-19, 5–6, 168, 428–429
CRISPR-Cas systems, 312–314
Culture selection, 442
Current good manufacturing practices (cGMP), 420
Cyclic AMP response element-binding protein (CREB), 185
Cytotoxicity tests, 373–374

D

Dahi, 12, 13*t*
Dairy-based beverages, 12–13, 13*t*, 103–113, 104*f*
  advances in, 447–448, 448–449*t*
  Ayran, 105–107*t*, 109–110
  Doogh, 105–107*t*, 108–109
  fermented, 103
  in India, 12–13, 13*t*
  Kefir, 105–107*t*, 112
  Koumiss, 105–107*t*, 111
  Leben, 110–111
  Matzun, 113
  non-fermented, 103
  Qatiq, 111
  Sameel milk, 113
  Shubat, 112
  in Thailand, 83
Dairy fermented milk products, 65–66, 66*t*
Dairy Home Synbiotic Drinking Yoghurt, 92–93, 93*f*
Danger-associated molecular patterns (DAMPs), 223
Defined strain starters (DSS), 261
Diabetes mellitus, probiotics for, 199–202
Dietary pattern, 176–177
Dietary Supplement Health and Education Act (DSHEA), 420
Direct heat-transfer method, 349
Disc diffusion assay, 85–86
DNA fingerprinting, 380
DNA hybridization, 373–374
DNA microarrays, 421
Do-it-yourself (DIY) kits, 359
Doogh, 105–107*t*, 108–109
Drinkable yogurts, 37
  in Japan, 39–40
  Joie, 40
  Mil-Mil, 40
  with probiotic strains, 38–40, 71–72
Drumstick-based beverages, 450–455*t*
Dutch Mill Delight, 91–92, 92*f*

E

E-commerce, packaging for, 358–359
Elafin, 319–320
Encapsulation, 86–87, 89–90, 276
Enterococcus, 69*t*, 373–374
Environmental claims, 351
Environmental scorecards, 351
Epigallocatechin gallate, 228
Estrogen deficiency, 188–189
Europe
  plant-based non-alcoholic beverages in, 128–139, 132–135*t*
    cereal-based beverages, 128–139
    fruit-based beverages, 137–139
    vegetable based beverages, 136–137
  regulations, 417–418
European Food Safety Authority (EFSA), 27, 129, 262, 415
Exopolysaccharides (EPS), 272–273, 312–314

F

Facebook, 438–439
Faecalibacteriumprausnitzii, in GIT homeostasis, 457
Fecal microbiota, 189
Fermentation, 101, 103, 138, 142, 259–261, 287
  kefir, 294–295
  kombucha, 292–293, 295–296
  lactic acid, 103–107, 108*f*
  lambic beer, 296–297
  malolactic, 119
  sour beer, 293–294, 296–297
Fermented beverages
  bioactive compounds, 273–274, 274–275*t*
  mixed cultures, 271, 271–272*t*
  starter cultures
    enzymes in LAB and yeast species used as, 268–269, 269*t*
    functionality of, 263, 263*f*
Fermented red ginseng, 75–76
Fermented yak milk, 50
Fibronectin-binding proteins (Fbp), 315
Flavor explorers, 430
Floradapt, 164
Food and Agriculture Organization (FAO), 159, 391, 404–405
Food and Drug Administration (FDA), 139–140, 262, 415, 420
Food and Drugs Act and Regulations, 416
Food and health supplements, 26–27
Food-borne pathogens, 309–310

Food, Drug, and Cosmetic Act, 27
Food explorers, 430
Food for Specified Health Uses (FOSHU), 36–37, 44–45, 128–129, 418–419, 422
Food grade, 369–370
Food Safety and Quality Division (FSQD), 419
Food Safety and Standards Act (FSSA), 418
Food Standards Australia and New Zealand (FSANZ), 419
Food supplements, and effects on TRPs, 226–227
Food with Nutrient Function Claims, 418–419
FOSHU. *See* Food for Specified Health Uses (FOSHU)
Fructooligosaccharides (FOS), 26, 241, 431, 438
Fruit-based beverages
  in Africa, 148–149
  in China, 51–55
  in Europe, 137–139
  in India, 18–19
  in Thailand, 83–89
Functional foods, 99–100, 441
Functional Food Science in Europe (FuFoSE), 128–129, 417–418

G

Gallic acid equivalents (GAEs), 85–86
γ-Aminobutyric acid (GABA), 18, 88–89, 273
Garlic, 147
Gas indicator, 356–357
Gastric juices, 394–395
Gefilus fruit beverages, 139
Generally Recognized as Safe (GRAS), 10–11, 129, 139–140, 262, 369–370
Genetically modified microorganisms (GMMs), 420–422
Genetically modified organisms (GMO), 432
Genetically modified probiotic microorganisms (GMPM), 376–377
Genetically modified probiotic strains
  anti-tumor activity, 325
  for bacterial and viral infections, 323–325
  for diagnostics as biosensor, 325–326
  for hypertension, 322–323
  for inflammatory bowel disease (IBD), 315–322
  for irritable bowel syndrome (IBS), 315–322
  for phenylketonuria, 323
Genome reshuffling, 397
Genome-sequencing, 226
Genomics, 5, 236*f*, 237–244, 242–243*t*, 301–302
Gen Z, 435–436
Ghrelin, 224
Gilaburu, 137–138
Ginger, 20, 62, 144–145*t*, 147
Glass packaging, 340, 341*f*
Global probiotics market, 70–71
Glucose transporter-4 (GLUT-4), 200–201
Glucosinolates (GSLs), 228
Glutathione peroxidase (GPx), 185, 317–318
Glutathione reductase (GR), 317–318
Glutathione-s-transferase (GST), 317–318
Granulocyte macrophage-colony stimulating factor (GM-CSF), 316–317
Green tea, 292, 390*t*, 450–455*t*
groESL, 312–314
Gut
  function and transient receptor potential (TRP), 225
  transient receptor potential (TRP) in, 215
Gut-brain axis, 223–224
Gut epithelial cells, 215–216
Gut-immune system, TRP as regulators of, 217–219
Gut inflammation, 219–221
Gut microbiota
  age-related macular degeneration (AMD), 187–188
  aging, 177–178
  metagenomic analysis, 178
Gut-neuronal system, TRP as regulators of, 216–217
Gut-retina axis, 187–188

H

Hardaliye, 117–119, 137–138
Haria, 22*t*, 24
Health benefits, 101–102, 102*f*
Health Canada, 163–164
Health claims, 381, 407
Health functional foods (HFF), 66–69, 72–73
Health halo, 433
Healthy aging, probiotics for, 179–187
Heat-transfer methods, 349
α-Hemolysin (Hla), 222
Hi-C sequencing, 297
High-density polyethylene (HDPE), 348–349, 353

High-pressure processing (HPP), 342, 348, 438
High-resolution throughput screening (HTS) analysis, 295–296
High-temperature, short-time (HTST) pasteurization, 349
Host gut-proteome, 246
Hot filling, 342
Human gut microbiota, 312–314
Human health, probiotics in, 407
Human milk oligosaccharides (HMO), 241
Hydration, 429
Hypertension
  angiotensin-converting enzymes (ACEs) inhibitors, 322–323
  genetically modified probiotic strains for, 322–323

I

IL-27, in immune suppression, 319
Immobilization technology, 275–276
Immunoglobulins A (IgA), 321
Immunosenescence, 179
Immunotherapy, 325
India
  dairy-based beverages, 12–13, 13*t*
  ethnic beverages in, 21–25, 22*t*
    bastanga, 23
    haria, 24
    kanji, 23–24
    raabadi, 24–25
    rice beer, 22–23
    rice wine, 23
  food and health supplements, 26–27
  fruit-based beverages in, 18–19
  in modern India, 25–26
    application of modern techniques, 25
    nanotechnology application, 26
    prebiotics effect, 25–26
  non-dairy probiotic beverages, 13–21
    cereal and legume-based probiotic beverages, 17–18
    fruit-based probiotic beverages, 18–19
    mixed probiotic juices, 21
    vegetable-based probiotic beverages, 20–21
  probiotic market, 27
  regulations, 27–28, 418
Indian Council of Medical Research (ICMR), 28, 418
Indirect heat-transfer method, 349
Individual Certification Approval Procedures, 69
Inert packaging, 340
Infections, bacterial and viral, 323–325
Inflammatory bowel disease (IBD), genetically modified probiotic strains for, 315–322
Ingredient markets
  fermentation and bacteria production, 406
  revenue, 406
Insertion sequence (IS), 397
In-silico analysis, 246
Instagram, 435–436, 439
Intellectual property, 407–409
  disputes, 412, 414*t*
  innovation, 408–409
Intelligent packaging, 355–357
International Classification of Disease (ICD) codes, 247
International Diabetes Federation (IDF), 199–200
International Food Information Council Foundation, 428–429
International Probiotics Association (IPA), 129, 406
International Safe Transit Association (ISTA), 359
International Scientific Association for Probiotics and Prebiotics, 405
Intestinal epithelial cells, 392–393
Inulin, 86–87, 431
Investigational new drug (IND), 420
In vitro evaluation, of probiotics, 442–447, 444–446*t*
Irritable bowel syndrome (IBS)
  genetically modified probiotic strains for, 315–322
  transient receptor potential (TRP) in, 219–221
Isoflavones, 193–194
Isoleucyl-prolyl-proline (IPP), 193–194

J

Japan
  beverages with paraprobiotic strains, 42–43, 43–44*t*
  lactic acid drink, 35–36, 36*f*
  market trends, 37–38
  overview, 35–37
  probiotic strains
    drinkable yogurts with, 38–40

Japan *(Continued)*
drinks based on fermented milk with, 40–41
regulations, 418–419
Joint FAO/WHO Expert Consultation on Evaluation of Health and Nutritional Properties of Probiotics, 413, 420

K

Kaentawan juice, 85
Kanji, 23–24
Kefir, 112, 288–290
consumers' preference, 299–300
current market status, 299–300
flavored, 301
future of, 299–300
grains, 288, 288*f*
health claims, 290–291*t*
health-promoting potentials of, 298–299
microbial dynamics during fermentation, 294–295
organic, 299
patents, 409, 409*t*
processing of, 291–292
regular, 301
KetoA, 228
Khalpi, 14–16*t*, 20
Kimchi, 62–63
Kombucha, 4–5, 120, 136, 288–290
consumers' preference, 299–300
current market status, 299–300
future of, 299–300
health claims, 290–291*t*
health-promoting potentials of, 298–299
manufacturing, 292–293, 292*f*
microbial dynamics during fermentation, 295–296
patents, 410
pellicle, 292, 292*f*
Korea
dairy fermented milk products, 65–66, 66*t*
fermented herbal and plant-based products, 75–76
plant-based products, 76
red ginseng, 75–76
fermented soybean paste, 63–64
health functional foods (HFFs), 66–69, 72–73, 74*t*
definition and regulations, 66–67
probiotics as, 67–69, 68–70*t*
kimchi, 62–63
makgeolli, 64–65
market perspectives, 77
milk and vegetable beverages, 74–75, 75*t*
opportunities and restraints of global probiotics market, 70–71
overview, 61–62
probiotic drinkable yogurts, 71–72, 73*t*
Korea Food and Drug Administration, 66–67
Koumiss, 111
patents, 409, 410*t*
Kvass, 131

L

LAB. *See* Lactic acid bacteria (LAB)
Lactate, 220
Lactic acid, 103–107
Lactic acid bacteria (LAB), 12, 18–19, 261, 287, 370, 404–405
B-group vitamins, 272–273
CRISPR-Cas system in, 312–314
fermented beverages, 52
hetero-fermentative, 268
homo-fermentative, 268
with proteolytic activity, 268–269
sequencing of, 237–238
as starter cultures, 263–264
in wine-making process, 119
Lactic acid (LA) fermentation, 18, 20, 103–107, 108*f*
Lactobacillus, 237–238, 287, 394, 396
Lactobacillus strains
cellfree supernatant (CFS) of, 179–183
non-dairy probiotic products based on, 310, 311*t*
Lambic beer fermentation, 296–297
Lassi, 12–13
Latin America
per capita consumption of probiotics, 167
probiotic market, value of, 168
regulations, 167
Leben, 110–111
Legume-based probiotic beverages, 17–18, 146–148
Lemon juice, 438, 450–455*t*
Life cycle assessments (LCA), 351
Lipopolysaccharides (LPS), 195–199, 214–215
Lipoxin A_4 (LXA_4), 320–321
15-Lipoxygenase-1 (15-LOX-1), 320–321
Litchi juice, 264–268*t*, 450–455*t*
Live biotherapeutic products (LBPs), 456–457

Long-term potentiation (LTP) deficits, 185–186
"Loop" platform, 352
Low-density lipoprotein (LDL) receptors, 200–201
Low-density polyethylene (LDPE), 353
Lysozyme (LYS), 119, 134

M

Macrophages, 219–220, 226–227
Maize-based beverages, 450–455*t*
Makgeolli, 64–65
Malaysia, probiotic guidelines, 419
Malee brand fruit juice, 94, 94*f*
Malolactic fermentation (MLF), 119, 258
Malt-based beverages, 450–455*t*
Malting processes, 11
Manganese superoxide dismutase (MnSOD), 318
Maoluang juice, 86–87, 450–455*t*
Marketing
- benefit stacking, 432–433
- clean label product, 432
- consumer preferences, 428–430
- developing opportunity, 434–435
- global market size, 427–428
- health halos, 432–433
- influencer, 436
- social media, 435–439

Matrix-assisted laser desorption ionization-time-of-fiight (MALDI-TOF), 298
Mature coconut water (MCW), 89
Matzun, 113
Melatonin, 317–318
Menthol, 214
Metformin, 176
Methyl-β-cyclodextrin, 222–223
Mexico
- Atoleagrio, 165
- Pozol, 165–166, 166*f*
- Pulque, 166–167, 167*f*
- Tejuino, 166
- Tepache, 166

Microbial cells, 379
Microbial contamination, 377–378
Microbial Genome Database (MGD), 247
Microencapsulation, 69, 117, 326–329
Microglia, activation of, 184–185
Middle East
- dairy beverages, 103–113, 104*f*
  - *Ayran*, 109–110
  - *doogh*, 108–109
  - *Kefir*, 112
  - *Koumiss*, 111
  - *Leben*, 110–111
  - *Matzun*, 113
  - *Qatiq*, 111
  - *Sameel milk*, 113
  - *Shubat*, 112
- non-dairy beverages, 104*f*, 113–120
  - cereal-based, 114–117, 115*f*
  - fruit/vegetable-based, 117–120, 118*f*
- regulatory and application of probiotic microorganisms in, 120–121

Milk-based beverages
- in China, 49–51
- in Thailand, 91–93

Minimum inhibitory concentration (MICs), 372–373
Ministry of Food and Drug Safety, 66–67
Ministry of Health and Welfare (MHLW), 418–419
Mitochondria, 183
Mixed culture, 270–271
- defined, 270–271
- in fermented beverages, 271, 271–272*t*

Mixed probiotic juices, 21
Mixed strain starters (MSS), 261
Mohi, 13
Monocyte chemoattractant protein-1 (MCP-1), 185
Monosodium glutamate (MSG), 89
mTOR inhibitor, 176
Mucins, 392–393
Mulberry leaf extract (MLE), 90–91
Multilocus sequence typing (MLST) scheme, 380
Multi-omics approaches, 247–248
Myocardial infarction, 195–199

N

Nanotechnology, application of, 26
N-arachidonoyl-dopamine (NADA), 217–218
National Bureau of Statistics, 54
National Center for Biotechnology Information (NCBI), 247
National Pharmaceutical Control Bureau (NPCB), 419
Naturally fermented milk (NFM) products, 12
Natural Product Number (NPN), 164
"*NesQino*,", 434
New Zealand, probiotic guidelines, 419

Next-generation probiotics (NGPs), 442, 456–458
Next-generation sequencing (NGS), 177, 295–296
Nisin (NIS), 134
Nitric oxide (NO), 316–317
Nitrofurantoin, 84
N-methyl-D-aspartate receptor (NMDA), 186
Non-dairy beverages, 13–21, 14–16*t*, 104*f*, 113–120, 449–456, 450–455*t*
  cereal-based, 114–117, 115*f*
  fruit/vegetable-based, 117–120, 118*f*
Nonviable (NV), 379
Nootropics, 431
Nordic fruits, 436
Nuclear hormone receptor (NHR), 179–183
Nuruk, 64–65
Nutrition and Health Claims Made on Foods, 381
Nutrition claims, 129

O
Oat-based beverages, 450–455*t*
Olfactory neurons, transient receptor potential (TRP) as regulators of, 216–217
Oligosaccharides, 431
Olvanil, 224
"Omics" approaches, 236–246, 236*f*, 248*f*
  genomics, 236*f*, 237–244, 242–243*t*
  proteomics, 236*f*, 245–246
  transcriptomics, 236*f*, 244–245
Orange juice, 448–455*t*
Osteoclastogenesis, 189–193
Osteoporosis
  estrogen deficiency, 188–189
  probiotics for, 188–194, 190–192*t*
Oxacillin, 84
Oxidative stress, 317–318
10-Oxo-12(Z)-octadecenoic acid, 228
Oxygen scavengers, 355

P
Packaging
  active, 354–355
  aluminum, 342–344, 344*f*
  aseptic, 348–350
  cap dispensing technology, 344–345
  carton, 342, 343*f*
  closures, 344–346
  for e-commerce, 358–359
  environmental issues, 351
  future trends in, 350–359
  glass, 340, 341*f*
  high-pressure processing (HPP), 348
  inert, 340
  intelligent, 355–357
  material reduction, 351–352
  plastic, 340–342
  process, 346–350
  push dispensing cap, 344–345, 345*f*
  returnable, 352
  reusable, 352
  sustainable packaging design and systems, 350–354
  traditional approaches, 347–348
  using recyclable materials, 353
  using renewable materials, 353–354
Paraprobiotics, 431
Paraprobiotic strains, beverages with, 42–43, 43–44*t*
Parathyroid hormone (PTH), 193–194
Pathogen-associated molecular patterns (PAMPs), 223
Pattern-recognition receptors (PRR), 223
Peracetic acid, 349
Peripheral neurons, 223–224
Peroxisome proliferator-activated receptor-α (PPAR-α), 200–201
Phenylalanine hydroxylase (PAH), 323
Phenylketonuria
  genetically modified probiotic strains for, 323
  phenylalanine hydroxylase (PAH), 323
Photoreceptor cell death, 187–188
Plant-based beverages
  patents, 412, 413*t*
  in Thailand, 93–94
Plant-based non-alcoholic beverages
  in Africa, 139–149, 140–141*t*, 144–145*t*
  in Europe, 128–139, 132–135*t*
Plasmids, 312–314, 373
Plastic packaging, 340–342
Policy, gaps in, 422–423
Polyethylene terephthalate (PET) bottles, 340–341, 348–349
Polylactic acid (PLA), 353–354
Pomegranate juice, 450–455*t*
Pore-forming toxins (PFT), 222
Postbiotics, 431
Pozol, 165–166, 166*f*
Prebiotics, 25–26, 431
Prebiotic sodas, 438

Prevention of Food Adulteration Act (PFA), 418
PROBIO, 247
Probiogenomics, 237
Probiotic bacteria, 178
  adhesion, 375–376
  antimicrobial resistance of, 372–373
  in beer, 299
  colonization, 375–376
  defined, 365
  DNA uptake, 372
  metabolicactivitiy, 374–375
  properties of, 370, 371*t*
  safety of, 368–377
  toxic substance production, 374–375
  translocation, 375–376
  virulence and pathogenic properties of, 373–374
Probiotic drinkable yogurts, 71–72, 73*t*
Probiotic markets, 405–406
Probiotic products
  commercial
    claim of probiotics content by manufacturers, 390*t*
    microbiological quality of, 397, 398–399*t*
  dairy *vs.* non-dairy, 369*t*
  global, 310, 311*t*
  label of, 380–381
  microbial quality control of, 378–379
Probiotics, 61, 129, 365
  for age-related diseases, 187–202
  antagonistic activity of, 395–396
  bioinformatics databases, 247
  Codex guidelines for, 414–415
  defined, 127
  emerging techniques for, 310–329
  encapsulation, challenges of, 328–329
  as health functional food, 67–69, 68–70*t*
  for healthy aging, 179–187
  in human health, 407
  intellectual property, 407–409
  patents and patent applications for, 409–412
  side-effects, 369–370, 404–405
  species in food market, 100
Probiotics Database (PBDB), 247
Probiotics Health Food Review Regulations, 417
Probiotic strains
  antimicrobial compounds, production of, 395–396
  bifidobacteria, 394, 396
  characterization, 371–372
  in cognitive decline, 185
  drinkable yogurts with, 38–40
  drinks based on fermented milk, 40–41
  in Europe, 130*t*
  genetic engineering techniques for, 312–315
  healthy aging, promotion of, 180–182*t*
  hydrolysis of bile salts, 395
  identification, 371–372
  isolation, 371–372
  lactobacilli, 394, 396
  nomenclature, 406, 406*t*
  safety assessment, 371–372
Probiotic straws, 346, 346*f*
Probiotic water, patents, 410, 410*t*
Probiotic yogurts, patents, 411, 412*t*
Probyo, 148–149
Programmed cell death protein-ligand 1 (PD-L1), 325
Pro-inflammatory markers, 315–316
Proteome, 245–246
Proteomics, 236*f*, 245–246, 301–302
Prunusnepalensis, 19
Psychobiotics, 431
Pulque, 166–167, 167*f*
Pulsed-field gel electrophoresis (PFGE), 380
Pure-fermentation inoculation techniques, 52
Push dispensing cap, 344–345, 345*f*

Q

Qatiq, 111
Qualified health claims (QHC), 422
Qualified Presumption of Safety (QPS), 129, 382, 417–418
Quality control (QC)
  criteria for, 391–397, 392*f*
    adhesion to intestinal epithelial cells, 392–393
    antimicrobial substance production, 395–396
    bile and acid stability, 394–395
    phenotypic and genotypic stability, 396–397
    viability, 393–394
  genetic stability, 379–380
  labeling and claims, 380–381
  microbial composition, 378–379
  microbial concentration and stability, 379
  microbial contamination of final product, 377–378

Quality control (QC) *(Continued)*
reliability, 391
strain authenticity, 379–380
Quinoa-based beverage, 133

R

Raabadi, 24–25
Recombinant DNA technology, 420–421
Recycling, 353
Red clover extract (RCE), 193–194
Regulations, 4, 413–420
Releasing systems, 355
Retinal pigment epithelium (RPE), 187–188
Returnable packaging system, 352
Reusable packaging system, 352
Riboflavin, 240–241
Rice-based beverages, 450–455*t*
Rice beer, 22–23
Riceberry malt extract (RME), 89–90
Rice wine, 23

S

Saccharomyces cerevisiae, 270, 302
Safety, of probiotic bacteria, 368–377
Salgam, 119–120
Salmonella, 377–378
Sameel milk, 113
Sea buckthorn berries juice, 450–455*t*
Secretory leukocyte protease inhibitor (SLPI), 319–320
Semi-skimmed sheep milk, 448–449*t*
Shalgam, 136
Short-chain fatty acid (SCFA), 86–87, 178
Shotgun Proteomics, 298
Shubat, 112
SignalP, 246
Simulated gastrointestinal (SGI) model, 86–87
Simulator of Human Intestinal Microbial Ecosystem (SHIME), 86–87
Skeletal muscle, 183
Skimmed milk, 36, 448–449*t*
Smart sensors, 356
Sobia, 116–117
Social media, 435–439
Sodas, prebiotic, 438
Sohiong fruit, 19
Sonication, 25
Sorghum, 114, 143–146
Sour bamboo, 23
Sour beer, 288–290
consumers' preference, 299–300
current market status, 299–300
fermentation, 293–294
brewing, 293
malting, 293
microbial dynamics during, 296–297
future of, 299–300
health claims, 290–291*t*
health-promoting potentials of, 298–299
patents, 412
Soybean paste, 63–64
Soybean waste-based beverages, 450–455*t*
Soymilk, 450–455*t*
Soymilk-apple juice, 450–455*t*
Soyoghurt, 90–91
Soy-whey, 302
SpaA protein, 240
SpaC protein, 240
Spray drying process, 327
Stability
bile and acid, 394–395
genetic, 379–380
phenotypic and genotypic, 396–397
Starter cultures, 260–263
bacteria as, 263–269
bioactive compounds produced by, 272–274
enzymes in LAB and yeast species, 268–269, 269*t*
in fermented food production, 261
functionality of, 263, 263*f*
immobilization technology for, 275–276
mesophilic, 261
organic substrates, 262–263
selection criteria for, 262–263
thermophilic, 261
traditional, 261
types and characteristics, 261, 262*f*
yeasts as, 270
State Administration for Market Regulation (SAMR), 417
State Food and Drug Administration (SFDA), 417
Strain authenticity, 379–380
Strains, isolation of, 442–447
Streptococcus, 373–374, 447
Structural Classification of Proteins (SCOP), 246
Sugar cane juice, 87–88
Sugary kefir, 450–455*t*
Superoxide dismutase (SOD), 185, 317–318

Sustainable Development Goals (SDGs), 127–128
Sutterella, 183

T

Tea, 433
Tejuino, 166
Tepache, 166
Terminal restriction fragment length polymorphism (T-RFLP) analysis, 295–296
Thailand
  cereal-based beverages, 89–91
  commercial market in, 91–94
  current and future trends in research development, 82–91
  dairy-based beverages, 83
  fruit- and vegetable-based beverages, 83–89
  milk-based beverages, 91–93
  plant-based beverage products, 93–94
Thermochromic inks, 357
Time-temperature indicators, 356
Tofu whey, 450–455*t*
Tomato juice, 137
Transcriptome, 244
Transcriptomics, 236*f*, 244–245
Transient receptor potential (TRP) channels, 213–215
  ankyrin, 213–214
  bacterial lipopolysaccharides on, 221–223
  bacterial toxins on, 221–223
  canonical, 213–214
  classification, 213–214
  fermented metabolite products, 229*t*
  food/beverage selections, 225–226
  food supplements on, 226–227
  in gut, 215
    epithelia, 215–216
    function, evolution of, 225
    inflammation, 219–221
    related disorders, 219–221
  in human population, 225–226
  in irritable bowel syndrome, 219–221
  melastatin, 213–214
  mucolipins, 213–214
  parasitic, 214
  polycystins, 213–214
  probiotic factors target in gut, 227–229
  as regulators
    of gut-brain axis, 223–224
    of gut-immune system, 217–219
    of gut-neuronal system, 216–217
  vanilloid, 213–214
Translocation, probiotic bacteria, 375–376
Transmembrane Helices Hidden Markov Models (TMHMM), 246
Trefoil peptides, 320
Trimethylamine oxide (TMAO), 199
Trinitrobenzene-sulfonic acid (TNBS), 317
TRP. *See* Transient receptor potential (TRP) channels
Tumor necrosis factor-alpha (TNF-α), 185
Tuna frame protein (TFP), 322–323
Two-dimensional gel electrophoresis (2-DE), 245–246
Type 2 diabetes (T2D), 199–202

U

Ultra-high temperature (UHT) sterilization, 349
Uncoupling protein 1 (UCP1), 228
United Nations Conference on Trade and Development (UNCTAD), 351–352, 358
United States of America (USA)
  health claims, 422
  probiotic market, value of, 160
  regulations, 160–161, 420

V

Valyl-propyl-proline (VPP), 193–194
Vegetable based beverages
  in Africa, 146–148
  in Europe, 136–137
  in India, 20–21
  in Thailand, 83–89
Vegetable juices, 20–21
Viability, 379, 393–394
Viable and cultivable (VC), 379
Viable but noncultivable (VBNC), 379
Virulence, of probiotic bacteria, 373–374
Vitality, 379
Vitamin C, 317–318
Vitamin C equivalent antioxidant capacity (VCEAC), 85–86
Vitamin E, 317–318

W

Waters, 437
  sparkling, 437
Whole cow's milk, 448–449*t*
Wine, 119
Wine fermentation, 11
World Health Organization (WHO), 159, 180, 391, 404–405

X

Xylose-inducible expression system (XIES), 322

Y

Yakult bottled product, 162–163
Yanang gum, 86–87
Yeasts, 261
  β-Glucosidase, 270
  as starter cultures, 263–264, 270
Yellowfin sole frame protein (YFP), 322–323
Yogurito, 169
Yogurt, 12, 37–38, 40, 66, 70–71, 76, 411, 442

FSC
www.fsc.org
MIX
Papier | Fördert
gute Waldnutzung
FSC® C083411

Kolibri 360 GmbH
Ferdinand-Jühlke-Straße 7
99095 Erfurt, Deutschland
produktsicherheit@kolibri360.de